KT-165-548

General Anatomy
and Musculoskeletal System

THIEME
Atlas of Anatomy

Consulting Editors

Lawrence M. Ross, M.D., Ph.D.,
The University of Texas Medical School at Houston

Edward D. Lamperti, Ph.D.,
Boston University School of Medicine

Authors

Michael Schuenke, M.D., Ph.D.,
University of Kiel Medical School

Erik Schulte, M.D.,
University of Mainz Medical School

Udo Schumacher, M.D.,
FRCPath, CBiol, FIBiol, DSc,
Hamburg University Medical Center

In collaboration with Jürgen Rude

Illustrations by

Markus Voll

Karl Wesker

1694 Illustrations
100 Tables

YORK ST. JOHN
COLLEGE LIBRARY

Thieme
Stuttgart · New York

Library of Congress Cataloging-in-Publication Data is available from the publisher.

This book is an authorized and revised translation of the German edition published and copyrighted 2005 by Georg Thieme Verlag, Stuttgart, Germany. Title of the German edition: Schuenke et al.: Allgemeine Anatomie und Bewegungssystem: Prometheus Lernatlas der Anatomie.

Illustrators
Markus Voll, Fürstenfeldbruck, Germany;
Karl Wesker, Berlin, Germany (homepage: www.karlwesker.de)

Translator
Terry Telger, Fort Worth, Texas, USA

© 2006 Georg Thieme Verlag
Rüdigerstraße 14
D-70469 Stuttgart
Germany
http://www.thieme.de
Thieme New York, 333 Seventh Avenue,
New York, NY 10001 USA
http://www.thieme.com

Typesetting by weyhing digital, Ostfildern-Kemnat
Printed in Germany by Appl, Wemding

Softcover
ISBN 1-58890-387-7 (The Americas)
ISBN 3-13-142081-2 (Rest of World)

Hardcover
ISBN 1-58890-358-3 (The Americas)
ISBN 3-13-142071-5 (Rest of World)

Important note: Medicine is an ever-changing science undergoing continual development. Research and clinical experience are continually expanding our knowledge, in particular our knowledge of proper treatment and drug therapy. Insofar as this book mentions any dosage or application, readers may rest assured that the authors, editors, and publishers have made every effort to ensure that such references are in accordance with **the state of knowledge at the time of production of the book**.

Nevertheless, this does not involve, imply, or express any guarantee or responsibility on the part of the publishers in respect to any dosage instructions and forms of applications stated in the book. **Every user is requested to examine carefully** the manufacturers' leaflets accompanying each drug and to check, if necessary in consultation with a physician or specialist, whether the dosage schedules mentioned therein or the contraindications stated by the manufacturers differ from the statements made in the present book. Such examination is particularly important with drugs that are either rarely used or have been newly released on the market. Every dosage schedule or every form of application used is entirely at the user's own risk and responsibility. The authors and publishers request every user to report to the publishers any discrepancies or inaccuracies noticed. If errors in this work are found after publication, errata will be posted at www.thieme.com on the product description page.

Some of the product names, patents, and registered designs referred to in this book are in fact registered trademarks or proprietary names even though specific reference to this fact is not always made in the text. Therefore, the appearance of a name without designation as proprietary is not to be construed as a representation by the publisher that it is in the public domain.

This book, including all parts thereof, is legally protected by copyright. Any use, exploitation, or commercialization outside the narrow limits set by copyright legislation, without the publisher's consent, is illegal and liable to prosecution. This applies in particular to photostat reproduction, copying, mimeographing, preparation of microfilms, and electronic data processing and storage.

Foreword

Our enthusiasm for the THIEME Atlas of Anatomy began when each of us, independently, saw preliminary material from this Atlas. Both of us were immediately captivated by the new approach, the conceptual organization, and by the stunning quality and detail of the images of the Atlas. We were delighted when the editors at Thieme offered us the opportunity to cooperate with them in making this outstanding resource available to our students and colleagues in North America.

As consulting editors we were asked to review, for accuracy, the English edition of the THIEME Atlas of Anatomy. Our work involved a conversion of nomenclature to terms in common usage and some organizational changes to reflect pedagogical approaches in anatomy programs in North America. This task was eased greatly by the clear organization of the original text. In all of this, we have tried diligently to remain faithful to the intentions and insights of the original authors.

We would like to thank the team at Thieme Medical Publishers who worked with us. Heartfelt thanks go first to Cathrin E. Schulz, M.D., Senior Editor, for her assistance and constant encouragement and availability.

We would also like to extend our thanks to Stefanie Langner, Production Manager, and Annie Hollins, Assistant Editor, for checking and correcting our work and preparing this volume with care and speed.

Lawrence M. Ross,
Edward D. Lamperti

Preface

As it started planning this Atlas, the publisher sought out the opinions and needs of students and lecturers in both the United States and Europe. The goal was to find out what the "ideal" atlas of anatomy should be—ideal for students wanting to learn from the atlas, master the extensive amounts of information while on a busy class schedule, and, in the process, acquire sound, up-to-date knowledge. The result of this work is this Atlas. The THIEME Atlas of Anatomy, unlike most other atlases, is a comprehensive educational tool that combines illustrations with explanatory text and summarizing tables, introducing clinical applications throughout, and presenting anatomical concepts in a step-by-step sequence that allows for the integration of both system-by-system and topographical views.

Since the THIEME Atlas of Anatomy is based on a fresh approach to the underlying subject matter itself, it was necessary to create for it an entirely new set of illustrations—a task that took eight years. Our goal was to provide illustrations that would compellingly demonstrate anatomical relations and concepts, revealing the underlying simplicity of the logic and order of human anatomy without sacrificing detail or aesthetics.

With the THIEME Atlas of Anatomy, it was our intention create an atlas that would guide students in their initial study of anatomy, stimulate their enthusiasm for this intriguing and vitally important subject, and provide a reliable reference for experienced students and professionals alike.

"If you want to attain the possible, you must attempt the impossible"
(Rabindranath Tagore).

Michael Schünke, Erik Schulte, Udo Schumacher,
Markus Voll, and Karl Wesker

Acknowledgments

First we wish to thank our families. This atlas is dedicated to them.

We also thank Prof. Reinhard Gossrau, M.D., for his critical comments and suggestions. We are grateful to several colleagues who rendered valuable help in proofreading: Mrs. Gabriele Schünke, Jakob Fay, M.D., Ms. Claudia Dücker, Ms. Simin Rassouli, Ms. Heinke Teichmann, and Ms. Sylvia Zilles. We are also grateful to Dr. Julia Jürns-Kuhnke for helping with the figure labels.

We extend special thanks to Stephanie Gay and Bert Sender, who composed the layouts. Their ability to arrange the text and illustrations on facing pages for maximum clarity has contributed greatly to the quality of the Atlas.

We particularly acknowledge the efforts of those who handled this project on the publishing side:

Jürgen Lüthje, M.D., Ph.D., executive editor at Thieme Medical Publishers, has "made the impossible possible." He not only reconciled the wishes of the authors and artists with the demands of reality but also managed to keep a team of five people working together for years on a project whose goal was known to us from the beginning but whose full dimensions we came to appreciate only over time. He is deserving of our most sincere and heartfelt thanks.

Sabine Bartl, developmental editor, became a touchstone for the authors in the best sense of the word. She was able to determine whether a beginning student, and thus one who is not (yet) a professional, could clearly appreciate the logic of the presentation. The authors are indebted to her.

We are grateful to Antje Bühl, who was there from the beginning as project assistant, working "behind the scenes" on numerous tasks such as repeated proofreading and helping to arrange the figure labels.

We owe a great dept of thanks to Martin Spencker, Managing Director of Educational Publications at Thieme, especially to his ability to make quick and unconventional decisions when dealing with problems and uncertainties. His openness to all the concerns of the authors and artists established conditions for a cooperative partnership.

Without exception, our collaboration with the entire staff at Thieme Medical Publishers was consistently pleasant and cordial. Unfortunately we do not have room to list everyone who helped in the publication of this atlas, and we must limit our acknowledgments to a few colleagues who made a particularly notable contribution: Rainer Zepf and Martin Waletzko for support in all technical matters; Susanne Tochtermann-Wenzel and Manfred Lehnert, representing all those who were involved in the production of the book; Almut Leopold for the Index; Marie-Luise Kürschner and her team for creating the cover design; to Birgit Carlsen and Anne Döbler, representing all those who handled marketing, sales, and promotion.

The Authors

Table of Contents

General Anatomy

Trunk Wall

Upper Limb

Lower Limb

Appendix

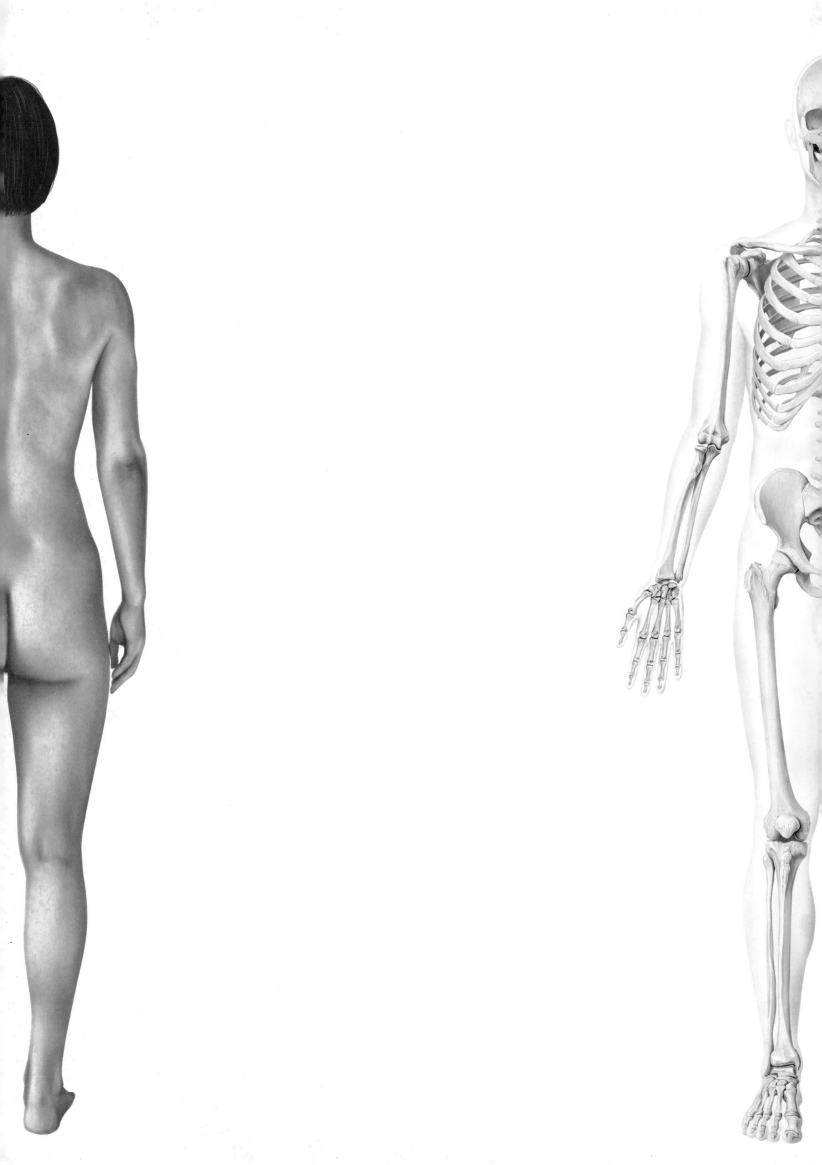

General Anatomy

1.1 Human Phylogeny

A Brief overview of human phylogenetic development
To better understand the evolution of the human body, it is helpful to trace its phylogenetic development. Humans and their closest relatives belong to the **phylum Chordata**, which includes approximately 50,000 species. It consists of two subphyla:

- Invertebrata: the tunicates (Tunicata) and chordates without a true skull (Acraniata or Cephalochordata)
- Vertebrata: the vertebrates (animals that have a vertebral column)

Although some members of the chordate phylum differ markedly from one another in appearance, they are distinguished from all other animals by characteristic morphological structures that are present at some time during the life of the animal, if only during embryonic development (see **G**). Invertebrate chordates, such as the cephalochordates and their best-known species, the lancelet (*Branchiostoma lanceolatum*) are considered the *model of a primitive vertebrate* by virtue of their organization. They provide clues to the basic structure of the vertebrate body and thus are important in understanding the general organization of vertebrate organisms (see **D**).

All the **members of present-day vertebrate classes** (jawless fish, cartilaginous fish, bony fish, amphibians, reptiles, birds, and mammals) have a number of characteristic features in common (see **H**), including a row of vertebrae arranged in a *vertebral column*, which gives the subphylum its name (*Vertebrata*). The evolution of an *amniotic egg*, i. e., the development of the embryo within a fixed shell inside a fluid-filled amniotic cavity, was a critical evolutionary breakthrough that helped the vertebrates to survive on land. This reproductive adaptation enabled the terrestrial vertebrates (reptiles, birds, and mammals) to live out their life cycles entirely on land and sever the final ties with their marine origin. When we compare the embryos of different vertebrate classes, we observe a number of morphological and functional similarities, including the formation of branchial arches (see **B**).

Mammals comprise **three major groups**: monotremes (egg-laying mammals), marsupials (mammals with pouches), and placentals (mammals with a placenta). The placental mammals, which include humans, have a number of characteristic features (see **I**), including a tendency to invest much greater energy in the care and rearing of their young. Placental mammals complete their embryonic development inside the uterus and are connected to the mother by a placenta. Humans belong to the mammalian order of **primates**, whose earliest members were presumably small tree-dwelling mammals. Together with lemurs, monkeys, and the higher apes, human beings have features that originate from the early adaptation to an arboreal way of life. For example, primates have movable shoulder joints that enable them to climb in a hanging position while swinging from branch to branch. They have dexterous hands for grasping branches and manipulating food, and they have binocular, broadly overlapping visual fields for excellent depth perception.

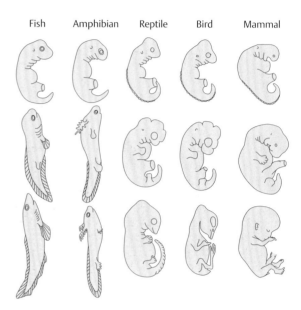

Fish   Amphibian   Reptile   Bird   Mammal

B Different stages in the early embryonic development of vertebrates
The early developmental stages (top row) of fish, amphibians, reptiles, birds, and mammals (as represented by humans) present a series of striking similarities that suggest a common evolutionary origin. One particularly noteworthy common feature is the set of branchial or pharyngeal arches in the embryonic regions that will develop into head and neck. Although it was once thought that the developing embryo of a specific vertebrate would sequentially display features from organisms representing every previous step in its evolution ("ontogeny recapitulates phylogeny", the "biogenetic law" of Ernst Haeckel (1834–1919)), subsequent work has shown that the vertebrates share common embryonic components that have been adapted to produce sometimes similar (fins and limbs) and sometimes radically different (gills vs. neck cartilages) adult structures.

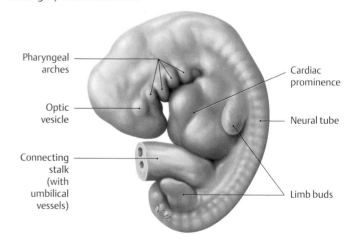

C Formation of the branchial or pharyngeal arches in a five-week-old human embryo
Left lateral view. The branchial or pharyngeal arches of the vertebrate embryo have a *metameric* arrangement (similar to the somites, the primitive segments of the embryonic mesoderm); this means that they are organized into a series of segments that have the same basic structure. Among their other functions, they provide the raw material for the species-specific development of the visceral skeleton (maxilla and mandible, middle ear, hyoid bone, larynx), the associated facial muscles, and the pharyngeal gut (see p. 11).

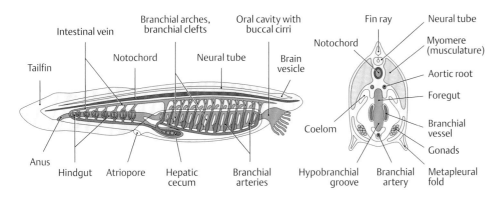

G Characteristic features of chordates

- Development of an axial skeleton (notochord)
- Dorsal neural tube
- Segmental arrangement of the body, particularly the muscles
- Foregut pierced by slits (branchial gut)
- Closed circulatory system
- Postanal tail

D Basic chordate anatomy, illustrated for the lancelet *(Branchiostoma lanceolatum)*

The vertebrates (including humans) are a subphylum of the chordates (Chordata), of which the lancelet is a typical representative. Its anatomy displays relatively simple terms of structures common to all vertebrates. The characteristic features of chordates include the development of an axial skeleton called the *notochord*. The human body still has remnants of the notochord, such as the nucleus pulposus of the intervertebral disks. The notochord is present in humans only during embryonic life, however, and is not a fully developed structure. Its remnants may give rise to developmental tumors called *chordomas*. Chordates have a *tubular nervous system* lying dorsal to the notochord. The body and particularly the muscles are composed of multiple segments called *myomeres*. In humans, this myomeric pattern of organization is most clearly apparent in the trunk. Another distinguishing feature of chordates is the presence of a closed circulatory system.

H Characteristic features of vertebrates

- Nerve cells, sensory organs, and oral apparatus concentrated in the head (cephalization)
- Multipart brain with a pituitary gland
- Replacement of the notochord by the vertebral column
- Generally, two pairs of limbs
- Development of branchial arches
- Presence of neural crest cells
- Closed circulatory system with a ventral, chambered heart
- Labyrinthine organ with semicircular canals
- Stratified epidermis
- Liver and pancreas always present
- Complex endocrine organs such as the thyroid and pituitary
- Complex immune system
- Sexes almost always separate

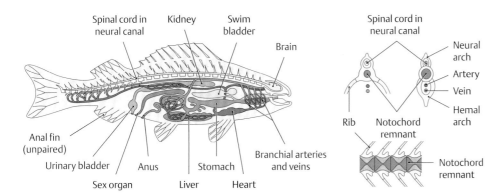

E Basic vertebrate anatomy, exemplified by the bony fish

The vertebrates are the *subphylum of chordates* from which humans evolved. With the evolution of fish, the notochord was transformed into a vertebral column (spinal column). The segmentally arranged bony vertebrae of the spinal column encircle remnants of the notochord and have largely taken its place. Dorsal and ventral arches arise from the vertebral bodies. The dorsal arches (vertebral or neural arches) in their entirety make up the neural canal, while the ventral arches (hemal arches) form a caudal "hemal canal" that transmits the major blood vessels. The ventral arches in the trunk region are the origins of the ribs.

I Characteristic features of mammals

- Highly glandular skin covered with true hair (terminal hair)
- Females always have mammary glands for nursing offspring, which are usually born live (viviparous)
- Well-developed cerebrum
- Well-developed cutaneous muscles
- Diaphragm is the major respiratory muscle and separates the thoracic and abdominal cavities
- Heterogenous and specialized teeth
- Four-chambered heart with a (left-sided) aortic arch
- Constant body temperature (homeothermy)

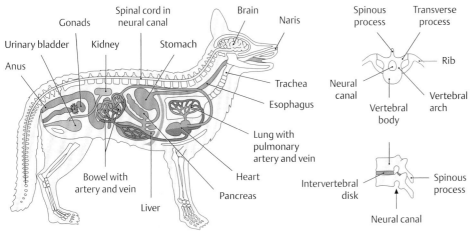

F Basic vertebrate anatomy, the dog

1.2 Human Ontogeny: Overview, Fertilization, and Earliest Developmental Stages

Besides gross and microscopic anatomy, the developmental history of the individual organism (ontogeny) is of key importance in understanding the human body. Ontogeny is concerned with the formation of tissues (*histogenesis*), organs (*organogenesis*), and the shape of the body (*morphogenesis*).

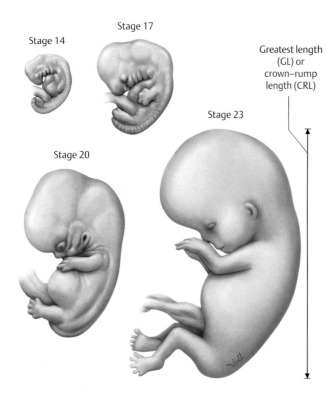

A Five- to eight-week-old human embryos
Streeter (1942) and O'Rahilly (1987) classified early human development and the embryonic period into 23 stages based on specimens from the Carnegie Collection. The Carnegie stages are defined by morphological characteristics that can be closely correlated with specific age (postovulatory days or weeks) and size (measured as the greatest length, excluding lower limb (GL), or crown-rump length (CRL) (see **C**).

Stage 14: Fifth week, GL 5–7 mm, future cerebral hemispheres become identifiable

Stage 17: Sixth week, GL 11–14 mm, digital rays become visible.

Stage 20: Seventh week, GL 18–22 mm, upper arms bent at the elbow, hands in a pronated position.

Stage 23: Eighth week, GL 27–31 mm, eyelids fuse, external genitalia begin differentiation.

B Longitudinal growth and weight gain during the fetal period

Age (weeks)	Crown–rump length, CRL (cm)	Weight (g)
9–12	5–8	10–45
13–16	9–14	60–200
17–20	15–19	250–450
21–24	20–23	500–820
25–28	24–27	900–1300
29–32	28–30	1400–2100
33–36	31–34	2200–2900
37–38	35–36	3000–3400

C Timetable of antenatal human development
(The Carnegie stages are shown in parentheses.)

Weeks 1–3:	Early development
Week 1:	Tubal migration, segmentation, and blastocyst formation (stages 1–3)
Week 2:	Implantation and bilaminar embryonic disk, yolk sac (stages 4–5)
Week 3:	Trilaminar embryonic disk, start of neurulation (stages 6–9)
Weeks 4–8:	**Embryonic period**
Week 4:	Folding of the embryo, neurulation concluded, axial organs, basic body shape (stages 10–13)
Weeks 5–8:	Organogenesis (formation of all essential external and internal organs, elongated limb buds) (stages 14–23)
Weeks 9–38:	**Fetal period**
Weeks 9–38:	Organ growth and functional maturation (sex-specific differentiation of the external genitalia)

Length of gestation

- p.o. = postovulatory age — 266 days = 38 weeks
- p.m. = postmenstrual age — 280 days = 40 weeks

Size

- GL = greatest length, excluding lower limb — simplest, most consistent ultrasound measure
- CRL = crown-rump length — similar to GL in embryonic period, used in most descriptions of the fetal period

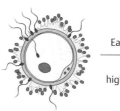

Fertilization — Early development (weeks 1–3) — Low rate of malformations, high rate of spontaneous abortion — Embryonic disc

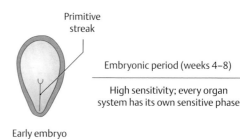
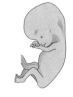
Primitive streak — Embryonic period (weeks 4–8) — High sensitivity; every organ system has its own sensitive phase — Early embryo — Embryo

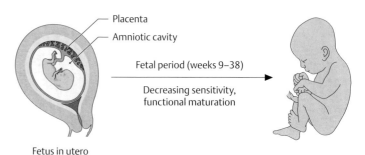
Placenta — Amniotic cavity — Fetal period (weeks 9–38) — Decreasing sensitivity, functional maturation — Fetus in utero

D Stages sensitive to teratogenic influences (after Sadler)

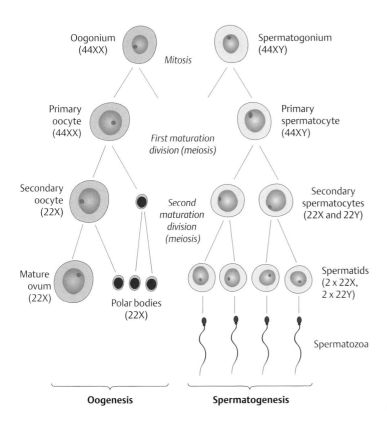

Oogenesis **Spermatogenesis**

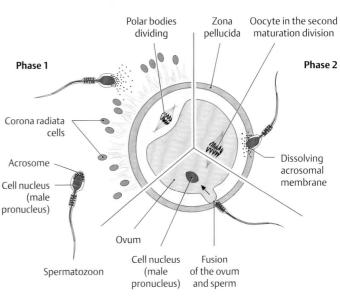

Polar bodies dividing   Zona pellucida   Oocyte in the second maturation division

Phase 1   **Phase 2**

Corona radiata cells

Acrosome

Cell nucleus (male pronucleus)

Ovum

Spermatozoon   Cell nucleus (male pronucleus)   Fusion of the ovum and sperm

Dissolving acrosomal membrane

Phase 3

F Schematic representation of the fertilization process
(after Sadler)

In *phase 1*, the spermatozoon penetrates the corona radiata cells. In *phase 2*, the acrosome dissolves, releasing enzymes that digest the zona pellucida. In *phase 3*, the cell membranes of the ovum and sperm fuse, and the spermatozoon enters the egg.

E Formation of the ovum and sperm (after Sadler)

During the formation of the gametes (sex cells), two successive cell divisions occur (the first and second meiotic maturation divisions). This results in cells having a chromosome set that is reduced by one-half (haploid). When fertilization occurs, a diploid (full) chromosome set is restored. During meiosis, extensive chromosal rearrangement occurs, thus recombining the internal genetic information into new and different subsets.

Oogenesis: The initial oogonia first undergo a mitotic division to form primary oocytes, which still have a diploid chromosome number (44 XX). Later the primary oocytes undergo a first and second maturation division by meiosis, resulting in four haploid cells (22 X): one mature ovum and three polar bodies.

Spermatogenesis: Diploid spermatogonia undergo mitosis to form primary spermatocytes (44 XY). These cells then divide meiotically to form four haploid spermatids, two of which have an X chromosome (22 X) and two a Y chromosome (22 Y). The spermatids develop into motile spermatozoa (spermatohistogenesis).

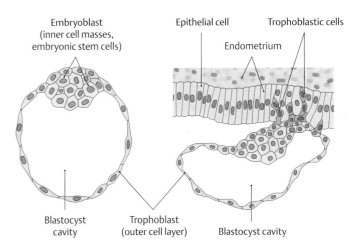

Embryoblast (inner cell masses, embryonic stem cells)   Epithelial cell   Trophoblastic cells

Endometrium

Blastocyst cavity   Trophoblast (outer cell layer)   Blastocyst cavity

G Implantation of the blastocyst in the uterine mucosa on postovulatory day 5–6 (after Sadler)

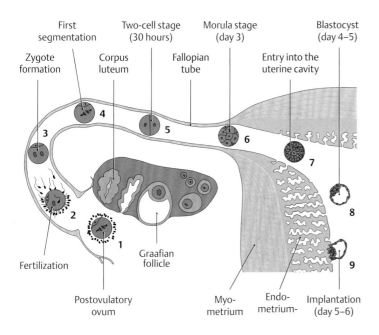

First segmentation   Two-cell stage (30 hours)   Morula stage (day 3)   Blastocyst (day 4–5)

Zygote formation   Corpus luteum   Fallopian tube   Entry into the uterine cavity

Fertilization

Graafian follicle

Postovulatory ovum   Myo-metrium   Endo-metrium   Implantation (day 5–6)

H Developmental processes during the first week of development (after Sadler)

1. Ovum immediately after ovulation
2. Fertilized within approximately 12 hours
3. Male and female pronucleus with subsequent zygote formation
4. First segmentation
5. Two-cell stage
6. Morula stage
7. Entry into the uterine cavity
8. Blastocyst
9. Early implantation

1.3 Human Ontogeny: Gastrulation, Neurulation, and Somite Formation

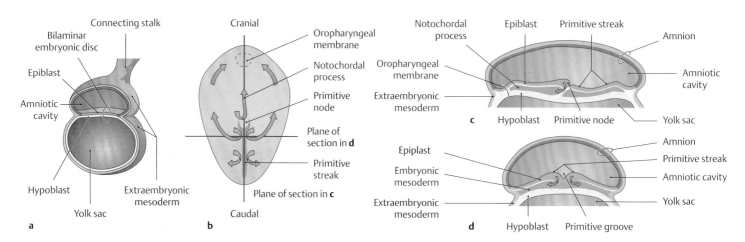

A Formation of the trilaminar human embryonic disk (gastrulation) at the start of the third postovulatory week (after Sadler)
As a result of gastrulation, the cell layers become differentiated into an *ectoderm*, *endoderm*, and *mesoderm*, from which all structures of the human body are derived (e.g., the endoderm gives rise to the central nervous system and the sensory organs). Gastrulation also establishes the primary axes of the body (ventral–dorsal, cranial–caudal, and left–right).

a Sagittal section through a conceptus at 2 postovulatory weeks. The embryonic disk is *still bilaminar* and is stretched between the amniotic cavity and yolk sac. The extraembryonic mesoderm, whose formation commences at the posterior pole of the embryonic disk, already covers the entire conceptus, which is attached to the chorionic cavity by a connecting stalk.

b Dorsal view of a human embryonic disk at the start of gastrulation. The amnion has been removed. The cell layer facing the amniotic cavity, the *epiblast*, will form the embryo itself; the other layer, the *hypoblast*, will generate extra-embryonic structures. In the third week, the epiblast sequentially develops a *primitive streak* and a *primitive node*; some epiblast cells dive into the streak, detach, and migrate as indicated by the arrows to generate the embryonic endoderm and mesoderm; a mass of cells expands cranially from the node to the *oropharyngeal membrane* to form the *notochordal process*. The remaining epiblast cells become the ectoderm, part of which will give rise to the *neuroectoderm* in the next development phase, *neurulation*.

c Sagittal section: embryonic disk along the notochordal process.

d Cross section: embryonic disk at the level of the primitive groove (arrows in **c** and **d**: direction of gastrulation movements by the mesoderm).

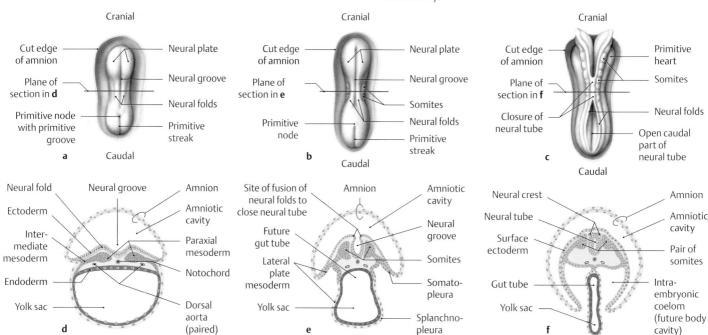

B Neurulation during early human development (after Sadler)
a–c Dorsal view after removal of the amnion.
d–f Schematic cross sections of the corresponding stages at the planes of section marked in **a–c**. Age in postovulatory days. During neurulation, the neuroectoderm differentiates from the surface ectoderm due to inductive influences from the notochord.
a, d Embryonic disk at 19 days. The neural tube is developing in the area of the neural plate.

b, e Embryonic disk at 20 days. The first somites have formed, and the neural groove is beginning to close to form the neural tube, with initial folding of the embryo.
c, f Embryo at 22 days. Eight pairs of somites are seen flanking the partially closed neural tube, which has sunk below the ectoderm. At the sites where the neural folds fuse to close the neural tube, cells form a bilateral neural crest which detaches from the surface and migrates into the mesoderm.

C Somite derivatives and spinal nerve formation during the embryonic period (weeks 4–8), shown in schematic cross sections (after Drews)

D Differentiation of the germ layers (after Christ and Wachtler)

Ectoderm	Neural tube		Brain, retina, spinal cord
	Neural crest	Neural crest of the head	Sensory and parasympathetic ganglia, intramural nervous system of the bowel, parafollicular cells, smooth muscle, pigment cells, carotid body, bone, cartilage, connective tissue, dentin and cementum of the teeth, dermis and subcutaneous tissue of the head
		Neural crest of the trunk	Sensory and autonomic ganglia, peripheral glia, adrenal medulla, pigment cells, intramural plexuses
		Ectodermal placodes	Anterior pituitary, cranial sensory ganglia, olfactory epithelium, inner ear, lens
	Surface ectoderm		Enamel organ of the teeth, epithelium of the oral cavity, salivary glands, nasal cavities, paranasal sinuses, lacrimal passages, external auditory canal, epidermis, hair, nails, cutaneous glands
Mesoderm	Axial	Notochord, prechordal mesoderm	Extraocular muscles
	Paraxial		Spinal column, ribs, skeletal muscle, connective tissue, dermis and subcutis of the back and part of the head, smooth muscle, blood vessels
	Intermediate		Kidneys, gonads, renal and genital excretory ducts
	Lateral plate mesoderm	Visceral (splanchopleura)	Heart, blood vessels, smooth muscle, bowel wall, blood, adrenal cortex, visceral serosa
		Parietal (somatopleura)	Sternum, limbs without muscles, dermis and subcutaneous tissue of the anterolateral body wall, smooth muscle, connective tissue, parietal serosa
Endoderm			Epithelium of the bowel, respiratory tract, digestive glands, pharyngeal glands, eustachian tube, tympanic cavity, urinary bladder, thymus, parathyroid glands, thyroid gland

(For clarity, the surrounding amnion is not shown.) The first pairs of somites appear at approximately 20 postovulatory days. All 34 or 35 of the somites ("primitive segments") have formed by day 30.

a When differentiation begins, each of these somites subdivides into a dermatome, myotome, and sclerotome (i.e., a cutaneous, muscular, and vertebral segment).

b At the end of 4 weeks, the sclerotome cells migrate toward the notochord and form the anlage of the spinal column.

c The neural tube—the precursor of the spinal cord and brain—differentiates to form a rudimentary spinal cord with dorsal and ventral horns. Cells within the ventral horn differentiate into motor neurons that sprout axons which form the *ventral root*. The neural crest has multiple derivatives, including sensory neurons which form dorsal root (spinal) ganglia, which send central processes into the spinal cord via the *dorsal root*. The myotomes become segregated into a dorsal part (epimere = epaxial muscles) and a ventral part (hypomere = hypaxial muscles).

d Each pair of dorsal and ventral roots unites to form a spinal nerve, which then divides into two main branches (a dorsal ramus and a ventral ramus). The epaxial muscles are supplied by the dorsal ramus, the hypaxial muscles by the ventral ramus.

e Cross section at the level of the future abdominal muscles. The epaxial muscles become the intrinsic back muscles, while the hypaxial muscles develop into structures that include the lateral abdominal muscles (external and internal oblique, transversus abdominis) and the anterior abdominal muscles (rectus abdominis).

7

1.4 Human Ontogeny: Development of the Fetal Membranes and Placenta

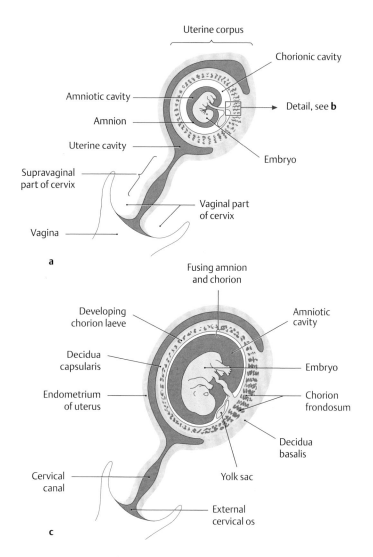

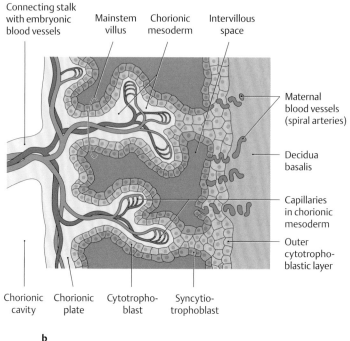

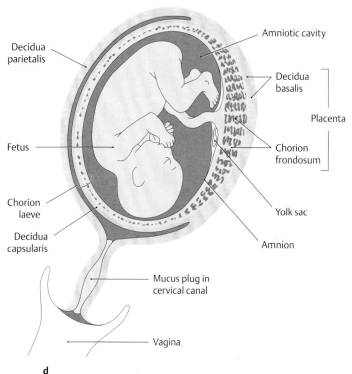

A Development of the fetal membranes and placenta (after Sadler and Drews)

a, c, and **d** Schematic sections through a pregnant uterus at different points in gestation.
b Detail from **a**.

a Embryo at 5 weeks: After the blastocyst has implanted in the uterine mucosa, the embryo initially derives its nutrition through the developing trophoblast and chorionic mesoderm. Chorionic villi are formed which surround the entire chorionic sac and embryo. They develop from primary to secondary villi and finally to tertiary villi (see close-up in **b**).

b Detail from a: The mainstem villi of the chorionic plate are attached on the maternal side to the basal plate of the decidua basalis by compact columns of trophoblastic cells. Like the small villous trees that sprout and branch from them, these mainstem villi have a syncytial covering (syncytial trophoblast), which in turn rests on a continuous layer of trophoblastic cells. Inside the villi, capillaries develop in the chorionic mesoderm and communicate with the vessels in the connecting stalk. Maternal blood flows through spiral arteries into the intervillous spaces.

c Embryo at 8 weeks: While the chorionic villi continue to grow and arborize at the embryonic pole, forming the chorion frondosum, the villi outside of this zone begin to regress, forming the nonvillous chorion laeve directly below the decidua capsularis. The amniotic cavity has enlarged at the expense of the chorionic cavity, and the amnion fuses with the chorion.

d Fetus at 20 weeks: The placenta is fully formed and consists of two parts: a fetal part formed by the chorion frondosum and a maternal part, the decidua basalis.

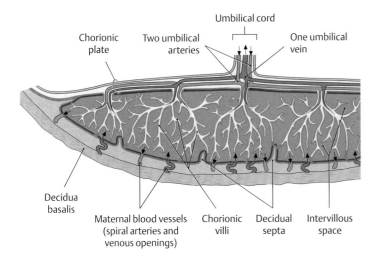

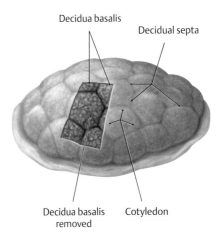

B Schematic cross section of a mature human placenta

The mature placenta is shaped like a frying pan, the maternal decidua basalis (basal plate) forming the base of the pan and the fetal chorionic plate forming the "lid." Some 40 arborizing villous trees containing fetal vessels project from the chorionic plate into the portions of the placenta that are filled with maternal blood (intervillous spaces). The maternal blood flows through approximately 80–100 spiral arteries into the intervillous spaces, which are divided into cotyledons by incomplete decidual septa. After the blood has bathed the villi, it is collected by irregularly distributed venous openings in the basal plate and returned to the material circulation.

C The postpartum placenta (after Sadler)

View of the maternal side of the delivered placenta (with a piece of the decidua basalis removed). The bulging cotyledons on the maternal surface are separated from one another by decidual septa.

E Characteristics of a mature human placenta

Size:	18–23 cm in diameter
	2–3 cm in thickness
Weight:	450–500 g
Total placental volume:	approximately 500 mL
Volume of the intervillous spaces:	approximately 150 mL
Villous surface area:	approximately 11–13 m²
Blood circulation on the maternal side:	500–600 mL/min

Structure of the placental barrier

- Endothelium of the fetal capillaries and basal lamina
- Fibrous villous stroma
- Syncytiotrophoblast and basal lamina
- Continuous trophoblast cell layer (becomes discontinuous after 20 weeks of gestation)

Diffusion distance approx. 5 μm (initially approx. 50 μm)

Primary functions of the mature placenta

1. Transport of substances and exchange of metabolic products

Mother-to-fetus	**Fetus-to-mother**
O_2, water, electrolytes, carbohydrates, amino acids and lipids, hormones, antibodies, vitamins and trace elements, but also drugs, toxins, and certain viruses	CO_2, water, electrolytes, urea, uric acid, bilirubin, creatinine, hormones

2. Hormone production (syncytiotrophoblast)

- Human chorionic gonadotropin (HCG)
  → maintenance of the corpus luteum
- Estrogens
  → growth of the uterus and breasts
- Progesterone
  → inhibits uterine muscle contractions

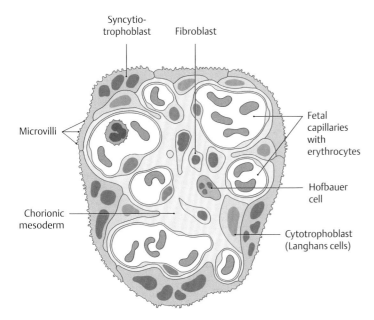

D Cross section through a terminal villus from a mature human placenta (after Kaufmann)

Clinical note: The HCG formed in the syncytiotrophoblast prevents premature breakdown of the corpus luteum and sustains the pregnancy. HCG can be detected in the maternal urine at an early stage, providing the basis for early pregnancy testing.

1.5 Development of the Pharyngeal (Branchial) Arches in Humans

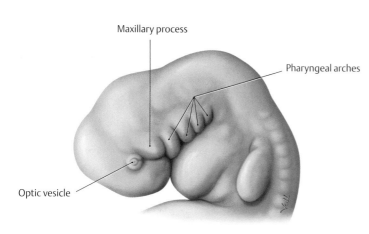

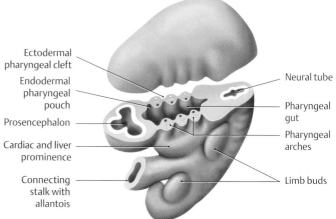

A Head and neck region of a five-week-old human embryo, demonstrating the pharyngeal arches and clefts

Left lateral view. The pharyngeal arches are instrumental in the development of the neck and face. In *fish* and *amphibians*, the branchial arches develop into a respiratory organ (gills) for exchanging oxygen and carbon dioxide between the blood and water. *Land-dwelling vertebrates* (including humans) have *pharyngeal arches* rather than true branchial arches. Development of the pharyngeal arches begins in the fourth week of embryonic life as cells migrate from the neural crest to the future head and neck region. Within one week, a series of four oblique ridges (first through fourth pharyngeal arches) form that are located at the level of the cranial segment of the foregut and are separated externally by four deep grooves (pharyngeal clefts). The pharyngeal arches and grooves are prominent features of the embyro at this stage. Although the human embryo has no equivalent to the fifth and sixth branchial arches of other vertebrates, some of their components are incorporated into the human fourth pharyngeal arch.

B Cross section through a human embryo at the level of the pharyngeal gut (after Drews)

Left superior oblique view. Due to the craniocaudal curvature of the embryo, the cross section passes through the pharyngeal arches and pharyngeal gut as well as the prosencephalon and spinal cord.
The pharyngeal gut is bounded on both sides by the pharyngeal arches (see also **A**), which contain a mesodermal core. They are covered externally by ectoderm and internally by endoderm. Ectodermal pharyngeal *clefts* and endodermal pharyngeal *pouches* lie directly opposite one another. Because the embryo is curved craniocaudally, the pharyngeal gut and pharyngeal arches overlie the prominence of the rudimentary heart and liver.

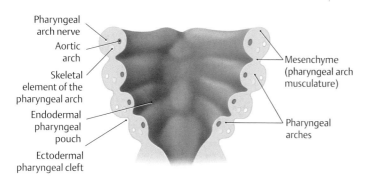

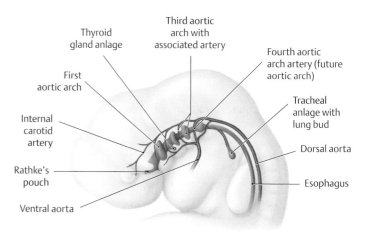

C Structure of the pharyngeal arches (after Drews)

View of the floor of the pharyngeal gut and the transversely sectioned pharyngeal arches. The typical components of a pharyngeal arch are easily identified: the aortic arch, musculature and associated nerves, and a cartilaginous skeletal element of each pharyngeal arch. The derivatives of these structures are of key importance in the formation of the face, neck, larynx, and pharynx. Because the developmental transformation of pharyngeal arch structures is complex, it is readily disrupted, causing malformations that may involve a cluster of related derivatives. Defects in pharyngeal arch development result in branchial and lateral cervical cysts and fistulas and in a group of "first arch syndromes" involving mandibulofacial deformities.

D Location of the aortic arch and pharyngeal pouches (after Sadler)

The aortic arches (branchial arch arteries) *arise* from the paired embryonic *ventral aorta* and run between the pharyngeal pouches. They *open* dorsally into the *dorsal aorta*, which is also paired. The definitive aortic arch develops from the fourth aortic arch on the left side (the development of the aortic arch is described on p. 12). The pharyngeal pouches are paired, diverticula-like outpouchings of the endodermal pharyngeal gut. A total of four distinct pharyngeal pouches develop on each side; the fifth is often absent or rudimentary.
Note: the pouch protruding from the roof of the oral cavity is called *Rathke's pouch* (precursor of the anterior pituitary). Note also the *lung bud* extending ventrally from the pharyngeal gut, and the anlage of the *thyroid gland*.

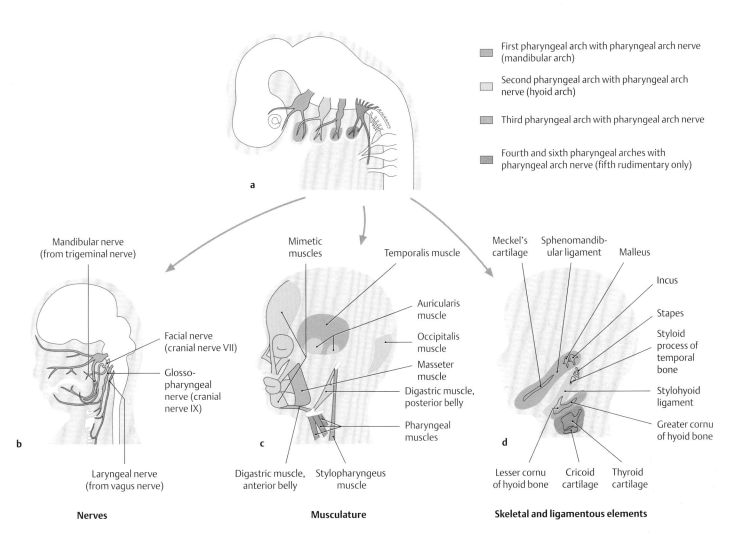

First pharyngeal arch with pharyngeal arch nerve (mandibular arch)

Second pharyngeal arch with pharyngeal arch nerve (hyoid arch)

Third pharyngeal arch with pharyngeal arch nerve

Fourth and sixth pharyngeal arches with pharyngeal arch nerve (fifth rudimentary only)

Mandibular nerve (from trigeminal nerve)

Facial nerve (cranial nerve VII)

Glosso-pharyngeal nerve (cranial nerve IX)

Laryngeal nerve (from vagus nerve)

Nerves

Mimetic muscles

Temporalis muscle

Auricularis muscle

Occipitalis muscle

Masseter muscle

Digastric muscle, posterior belly

Pharyngeal muscles

Digastric muscle, anterior belly

Stylopharyngeus muscle

Musculature

Meckel's cartilage

Sphenomandibular ligament

Malleus

Incus

Stapes

Styloid process of temporal bone

Stylohyoid ligament

Greater cornu of hyoid bone

Lesser cornu of hyoid bone

Cricoid cartilage

Thyroid cartilage

Skeletal and ligamentous elements

E The system of pharyngeal or branchial arches (after Sadler and Drews)

a Anlage of the embryonic pharyngeal arches with the associated pharyngeal arch nerves.

b Definitive arrangement of the future cranial nerves V, VII, IX, and X.

c Muscular derivatives of the pharyngeal arches.

d Skeletal derivatives of the pharyngeal arches.

F Derivatives of the pharyngeal (branchial) arches in humans

Pharyngeal arch	Nerve	Muscles	Skeletal and ligamentous elements
First (mandibular arch)	Cranial nerve V (mandibular nerve from the trigeminal)	Masticatory muscles – Temporalis – Masseter – Lateral pterygoid – Medial pterygoid Mylohyoid Digastric (anterior belly) Tensor tympani Tensor veli palatini	Malleus and incus Portions of the mandible Meckel's cartilage Sphenomandibular ligament Anterior ligament of malleus
Second (hyoid arch)	Cranial nerve VII (facial nerve)	Mimetic facial muscles Stylohyoid muscle Digastric muscle (posterior belly)	Stapes Styloid process of the temporal bone Lesser cornu of hyoid bone Upper part of hyoid body
Third	Cranial nerve IX (glossopharyngeal nerve)	Stylopharyngeus muscle	Greater cornu of hyoid bone Lower part of hyoid body
Fourth and sixth	Cranial nerve X (superior and recurrent laryngeal nerve)	Pharyngeal and laryngeal muscles	Laryngeal skeleton (thyroid cartilage, cricoid cartilage, arytenoid cartilage, corniculate and cuneiform cartilages)

1.6 Early Embryonic Circulation and the Development of Major Blood Vessels

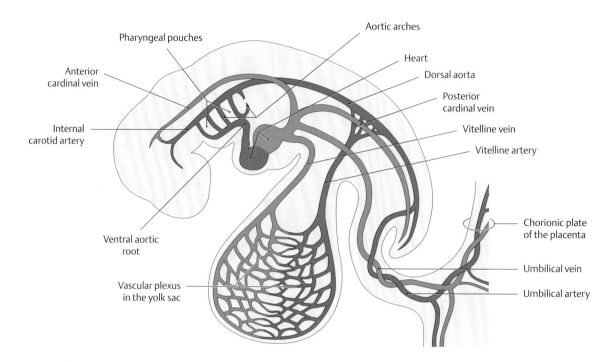

A Circulatory system of a 3- to 4-week-old human embryo
(after Drews)

Lateral view. The cardiovascular system of a 3- to 4-week-old human embryo consists of a well-functioning two-chambered heart and three distinct circulatory systems:

1. An **intraembryonic systemic circulation** (ventral and dorsal aorta, branchial arch and aortic arches, anterior and posterior cardinal veins)
2. An **extraembryonic vitelline circulation** (omphalomesenteric arteries and veins)
3. A **placental circulation** (umbilical arteries and veins)

The vascular pathways still show a largely symmetrical arrangement at this stage.

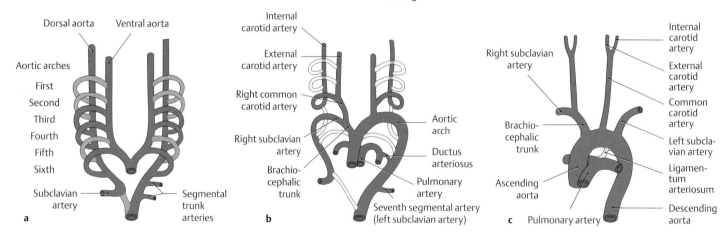

B Development of the arteries derived from the aortic arch
(after Lippert and Pabst)

a **Initial stage** (4-week-old embryo, ventral view). An artery develops in each of the pharyngeal arches, proceeding in the craniocaudal direction. These arteries arise from the paired ventral aortic roots, course through the mesenchyme of the pharyngeal arches, and open into an initially paired dorsal aorta. These vessels give rise to segmental trunk arteries. The six aortic arches are not all present at any one time, however. For example, while the fourth arch is forming, the first two arches are already beginning to regress. The development proceeds in such a way that the original symmetry is lost in favor of a preponderance on the left side.

b **Structures that regress or persist:** The first, second, and fifth aortic arches on both sides regress with continued development. The third

aortic arch gives rise to a common carotid artery on each side and the proximal portion of the internal carotid artery. The left fourth aortic arch later becomes the definitive *aortic arch*, while the artery on the right side becomes the brachiocephalic trunk and the right subclavian artery. The left subclavian artery is derived from the seventh segmental artery. The trunk of the pulmonary arteries and the ductus arteriosus are derived from the sixth aortic arch.

c **Variants in the adult:** Besides the typical case pictured here (77%), there are numerous variants of the brachiocephalic trunk that occur with different frequencies. In the second most common pattern (13%), the left common carotid artery also arises from the brachiocephalic trunk. A right-sided aortic arch and a duplicated aortic arch each occur with a frequency of about 0.1%.

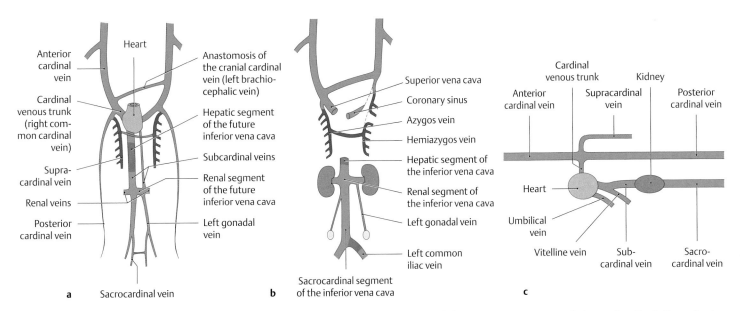

C Development of the cardinal venous system from weeks 5–7 to birth (after Sadler)

a At 5–7 weeks (ventral view), **b** at term (ventral view), **c** lateral view at 5–7 weeks.

Up until the fourth week of development, three paired venous trunks return the blood to the heart: the vitelline, umbilical, and cardinal veins. The cardinal venous system at this stage consists of the anterior, posterior, and common cardinal veins. The following additional cardinal venous systems are formed between weeks 5 and 7:

- **Supracardinal veins:** These vessels replace the posterior cardinal veins and receive blood from the intercostal veins (future azygos system: azygos and hemiazygos veins).
- **Subcardinal veins:** These vessels develop to drain the kidneys—the right subcardinal vein becoming the middle part of the inferior vena

cava, and the transverse anastomosis becoming the left renal vein. The distal segment of the left subcardinal vein persists as a gonadal vein (testicular vein or left ovarian vein).

- **Sacrocardinal veins:** These vessels develop during the formation of the lower limbs, their transverse anastomosis becoming the left common iliac vein.

Characteristic transverse anastomoses are formed between the individual cardinal venous systems. These connections transfer blood from the right to the left side, channeling it to the inflow tract of the heart. The transverse anastomosis between the anterior cardinal veins, for example, forms the future left brachiocephalic vein. The future superior vena cava develops from the right anterior and common cardinal veins, while the left common cardinal vein contributes to the venous drainage of the heart (coronary sinus).

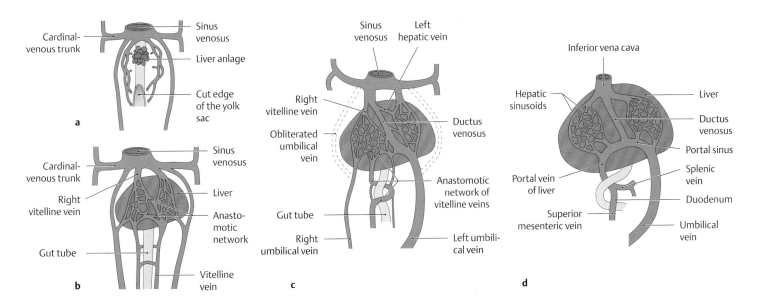

D Development of the vitelline and umbilical veins (after Sadler)
a Fourth week, **b** fifth week, **c** second month, **d** third month (ventral view).

Before the vitelline veins (omphalomesenteric veins) open into the venous sinus, they form a venous plexus around the duodenum, perfuse the embryonic liver anlage, and form the first hepatic sinusoids. At this stage the two umbilical veins still course on both sides of the liver anlage. With further development, however, they establish a connection with the hepatic sinusoids. While the right umbilical vein regresses

completely during the second month, the left umbilical vein assumes the function of transporting all blood back from the placenta to the fetus. The blood flows through a shunt (ductus venosus) into the *proximal* trunk of the right vitelline vein (the future post–hepatic part of the inferior vena cava) and back to the sinus venosus. The *distal* portion of the right vitelline vein develops into the future portal vein, by which blood is conveyed from the unpaired abdominal organs to the liver (superior and inferior mesenteric veins, splenic vein).

13

1.7 Bone Development and Remodeling

Bone development and bone remodeling are closely interrelated. During growth, for instance, bone undergoes a constant remodeling process in which immature woven bone tissue is replaced by "mature" lamellar bone. Continual remodeling also occurs in the mature skeleton, particularly in cancellous bone (called also trabecular or spongy bone, see **F**). In this way, on average, approximately 10% of the entire adult skeleton is remodeled each year, meaning that the skeleton is completely renewed over about a 10-year period. This process is basically a functional adaptation of the bones to the dominant stress patterns to which they are exposed (and which vary over time). It also serves to prevent material fatigue, repair microinjuries to bone, and provide a rapidly available source of calcium.

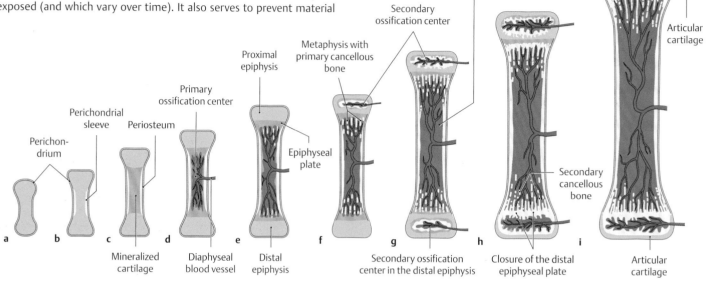

A Development of a long bone

The long bones (humerus, tibia, etc.) are mainly a product of *indirect* bone formation, i.e., they form by replacing a preexisting cartilaginous model of the bone (*endochondral osteogenesis*). But portions of the long bones (the perichondrial bone collar, which allows the bone to grow in thickness) are a product of *direct* bone formation, i.e., they form from the direct transformation of condensed mesenchyme (*membranous osteogenesis*, see **E**).

a Cartilaginous model of a bone in the embryonic skeleton. **b** Formation of a perichondrial bone collar (directly from mesenchyme). **c** Differentiation to hypertrophic chondrocytes and mineralization of the cartilaginous extracellular matrix. **d** Ingrowth of a diaphyseal vessel and formation of a primary ossification center. **e** Development of the proximal and distal growth centers (epiphyseal plates). **f** Appearance of the proximal epiphyseal ossification center (secondary ossification center). **g** Formation of the distal epiphyseal ossification center. **h** Closure of the distal epiphyseal plate. **i** Closure of the proximal epiphyseal plate (occurs at the end of skeletal growth, between about 18 and 23 years of age for most tubular bones).

Note: Osteogenesis = the formation of an individual bone; ossification = the formation of bone tissue.

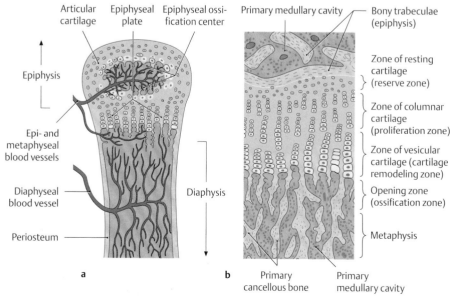

B Structure of the epiphyseal plate
a Blood supply, **b** detail from **a**: zones of the epiphyseal plate.

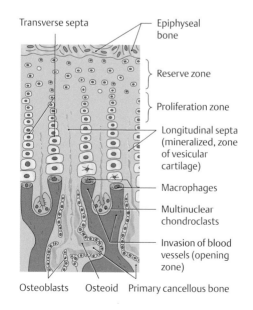

C Schematic representation of cellular processes within the epiphyseal plate

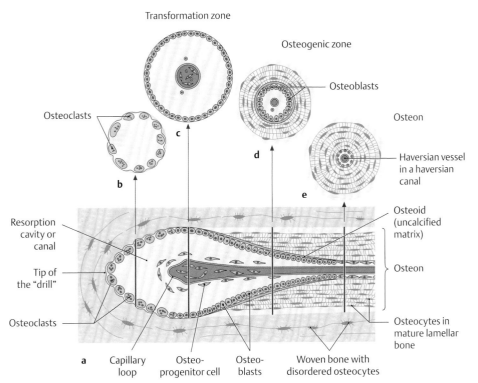

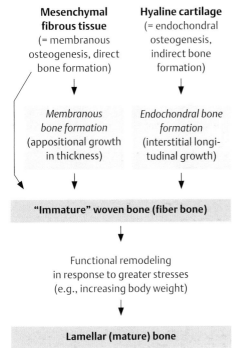

"Immature" woven bone (fiber bone)

↓

Functional remodeling
in response to greater stresses
(e.g., increasing body weight)

↓

Lamellar (mature) bone

D Development of an osteon (after Hees)

The process of functional remodeling (see upper left page) begins with the invasion of blood vessels and accompanying osteoclasts ("bone-eating cells") into woven bone. They burrow through the woven bone like a drill, cutting a vascularized channel (resorption canal or cavity) which is equal in diameter to the future osteon.

a Longitudinal section through a resorption canal.
b Cross section at the level of the resorption canal.
c Transformation zone: osteoprogenitor cells (a kind of precursor for bone-forming cells) are transformed into osteoblasts.
d Osteogenic zone (osteoblasts produce bony lamellae).
e Newly formed osteon.

E Types of bone development (osteogenesis)

Note: Most bones are formed by *indirect* osteogenesis (the few exceptions include the clavicle and certain bones of the calvaria). But portions of these bones still develop from the direct transformation of mesenchyme, i.e., by *direct* osteogenesis.

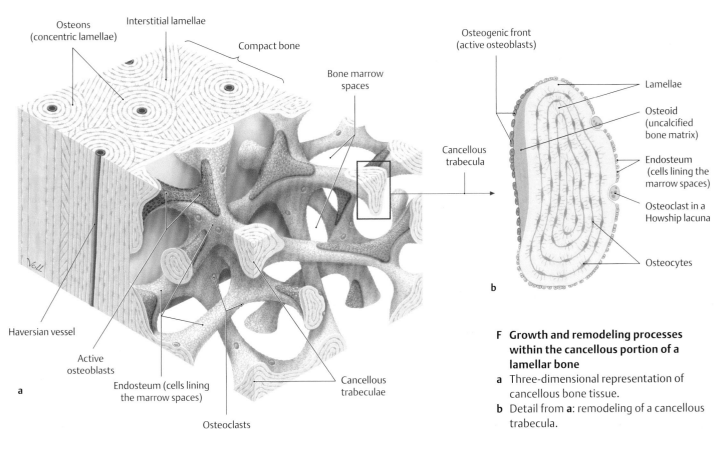

F Growth and remodeling processes within the cancellous portion of a lamellar bone

a Three-dimensional representation of cancellous bone tissue.
b Detail from **a**: remodeling of a cancellous trabecula.

1.8 Ossification of the Limbs

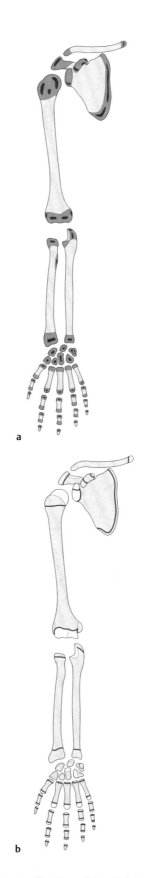

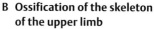

a

b

B Ossification of the skeleton of the upper limb

a Location of the epi- and apophyseal ossification centers.

b Location of the epi- and apophyseal plates.

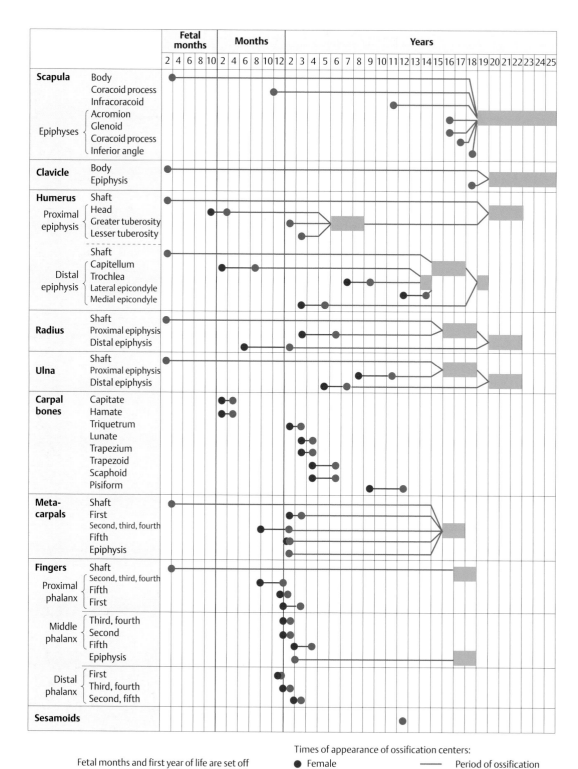

Times of appearance of ossification centers:
- ● Female
- ● Male
- —— Period of ossification
- ▨ Period of synostosis

A Fetal months and first year of life are set off from the rest of the table.

A and C Timetable of regional bone growth in the upper limb (A) and lower limb (C)
(From Niethard: *Kinderorthopädie* (Pediatric Orthopedics). Thieme, Stuttgart 1997)
The current stage of skeletal development, and thus the individual skeletal age, can be estimated from the times of appearance of the ossification centers. *Primary ossification centers*, which generally appear in the shaft region of bones *during the fetal period* (diaphyseal ossification), are distinguished from *secondary ossification centers*, which form *after birth* within the cartilaginous epiphysis and apophysis (epi- and

apophyseal ossification). Longitudinal growth ceases with the closure of the epiphyseal plate (synostosis). The greater tuberosity of the humerus, for example, begins to ossify at two years of age. A period of synostosis follows from six to eight years of age, and after that the greater tuberosity shows only external, appositional growth. With the cessation of longitudinal growth, the ossification centers disappear and are no longer visible on x-ray films. The relationship between maturation and the appearance of secondary ossification centers is most clearly demonstrated in the bones of the carpus (see also **B**). The eight car-

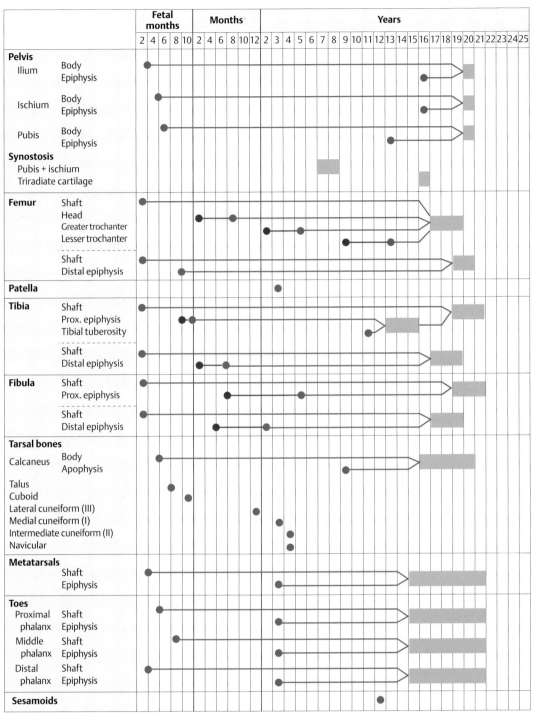

		Fetal months				Months						Years																								
		2	4	6	8	10	2	4	6	8	10	12	2	3	4	5	6	7	8	9	10	11	12	13	14	15	16	17	18	19	20	21	22	23	24	25
Pelvis																																				
Ilium	Body																																			
	Epiphysis																																			
Ischium	Body																																			
	Epiphysis																																			
Pubis	Body																																			
	Epiphysis																																			
Synostosis																																				
Pubis + ischium																																				
Triradiate cartilage																																				
Femur	Shaft																																			
	Head																																			
	Greater trochanter																																			
	Lesser trochanter																																			
	Shaft																																			
	Distal epiphysis																																			
Patella																																				
Tibia	Shaft																																			
	Prox. epiphysis																																			
	Tibial tuberosity																																			
	Shaft																																			
	Distal epiphysis																																			
Fibula	Shaft																																			
	Prox. epiphysis																																			
	Shaft																																			
	Distal epiphysis																																			
Tarsal bones																																				
Calcaneus	Body																																			
	Apophysis																																			
Talus																																				
Cuboid																																				
Lateral cuneiform (III)																																				
Medial cuneiform (I)																																				
Intermediate cuneiform (II)																																				
Navicular																																				
Metatarsals	Shaft																																			
	Epiphysis																																			
Toes																																				
Proximal phalanx	Shaft																																			
	Epiphysis																																			
Middle phalanx	Shaft																																			
	Epiphysis																																			
Distal phalanx	Shaft																																			
	Epiphysis																																			
Sesamoids																																				

Times of appearance of ossification centers:
- ● Female —— Period of ossification
- ● Male ▨ Period of synostosis

C Fetal months and first year of life are set off from the rest of the table.

pal bones ossify gradually over a period of approximately nine years. The first ossification center is that of the capitate bone, which appears during the first year of life; the last is that of the pisiform bone, which ossifies at nine years of age. It is standard practice to use the left or nondominant hand for radiographic examinations. The skeletal age reflects the biological maturity of the organism more than chronological age. The estimation of skeletal age, and thus of growth potential, is of key importance, for example, in the prognosis and treatment of orthopedic diseases and deformities in children. Also, given the relationship that exists between skeletal maturity and body height, the definitive adult height can usually be predicted with reasonable accuracy after six years of age based on the skeletal age and longitudinal measurements.

D Ossification of the skeleton of the lower limb

a Location of the epi- and apophyseal ossification centers.

b Location of the epi- and apophyseal plates.

1.9   Development and Position of the Limbs

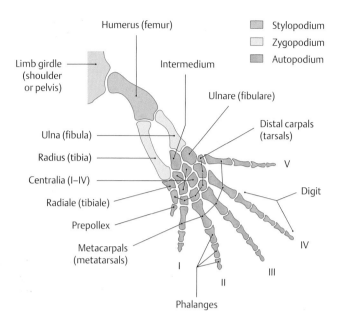

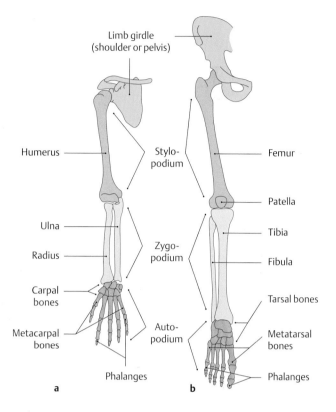

A Basic skeletal structure of a five-ray (pentadactyl) tetrapod limb
(after Romer)

Both the forelimb and hindlimb of a free-ranging terrestrial vertebrate have the same basic, three-part structure consisting of a proximal, middle, and distal segment (called the *stylopodium*, *zygopodium*, and *autopodium*). The elbow or knee joint is placed between the stylopodium, which consists of a single bone (humerus or femur), and the zygopodium, which consists of two bones (the radius and ulna or the tibia and fibula). The five-ray autopodium (hand or foot) is also made up of proximal, middle, and distal units (called the *basipodium*, *metapodium,* and *acropodium*; see **C**). Additionally, there are some vertebrate classes that depart from this basic structure by showing a reduction or fusion of various bony units.

B Basic skeletal structure of the human limbs
Anterior view. **a** Right upper limb, **b** right lower limb.

The skeletal elements of the human upper and lower limbs have been colored to show how they are homologous with the tetrapod limb segments shown in **A** (stylo-, zygo-, and autopodium). Congenital malformations such as polydactyly or syndactyly (the presence of supernumerary fingers or toes or their fusion) are not uncommon.

C Bony constituents of the pentadactyl tetrapod limb

Segments	Paired forelimbs	Paired hindlimbs
Limb girdle	Shoulder girdle – Scapula and clavicle	Pelvic girdle – Hip bone
Free limbs		
Stylopodium	Arm (brachium) – Humerus	Thigh (femur) – Femur
Zygopodium	Forearm (antebrachium) – Radius – Ulna	Leg (crus) – Tibia – Fibula
Autopodium	Hand	Foot
– Basipodium	Carpus – Proximal row: radiale, intermedium, ulnare – Central group: centralia I–IV – Distal row: carpals I–V	Tarsus – Proximal row: tibiale, intermedium, fibulare – Central group: centralia I–IV – Distal row: tarsals I–V
– Metapodium	Metacarpus – Metacarpals I–V	Metatarsus – Metatarsals I–V
– Acropodium	Fingers – Digits I–V (with different numbers of phalanges)	Toes – Digits I–V (with different numbers of phalanges)

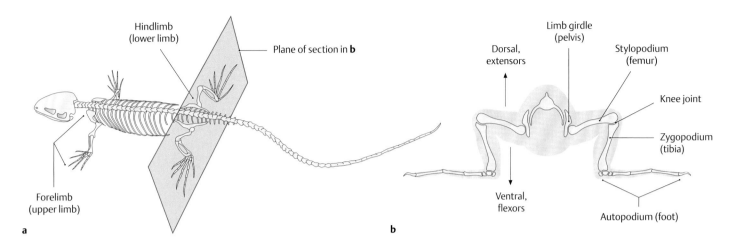

a

b

D Limb positions in a primitive terrestrial tetrapod (the lizard *Lacerta viridis*)

a Dorsal view, **b** cross section at the level of the hindlimbs.

In amphibian and reptilian tetrapods (e.g., salamanders, turtles, and lizards), the trunk is slung between the limbs and frequently touches the ground. The limbs are set almost at right angles to the body, so that the arm and thigh are nearly horizontal and the elbow and knee point outward. The radius and ulna and the tibia and fibula are flexed at right angles at the elbow and knee. The volar surface of the hand and the plantar surface of the foot are in contact with the ground. The axes of all the joints are directed parallel to the spinal column (see **E**).

Note that the *extensor* muscles are placed *dorsally*, while the *flexor* muscles are *ventral*. Thus, the location of the extensors and flexors relative to the bone does not change with evolution—the bone merely assumes a different alignment (see also **F**).

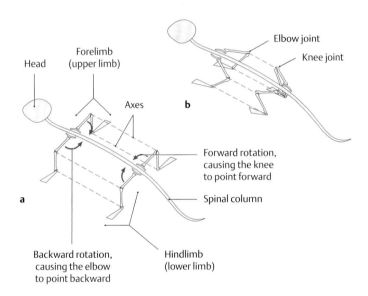

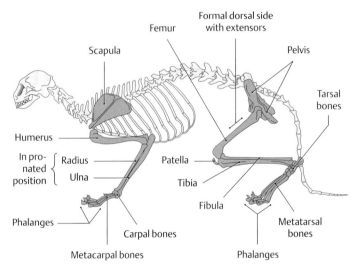

E Rotation of the limbs in mammalian evolution

a Before rotation, **b** after rotation.

An important feature of mammalian evolution involved *rotation* of the tetrapod limb. The limb was reoriented, placed parallel to the body, and moved closer to or beneath the body. This improved locomotion and supported the body more efficiently. The hindlimb rotated *forward* (with the knee pointing cephalad) while the forelimb rotated *backward* against the body (the elbow pointing caudad). As a result, both sets of limbs assumed a sagittal orientation under or alongside the trunk (see **F**).

F Skeleton of a cat (*Felis catus*)

Left lateral view. In order for the volar surfaces of the forelimbs to rest on the ground despite the backward angulation of the elbows, the forearm bones must cross to a pronated position. In the hindlimbs, there is no need for pronation of the leg bones because the thigh is rotated forward.

This arrangement of the skeletal elements in the various limb segments is essentially preserved in humans. Because the lower limb has been rotated forward, the *former dorsal side* of this limb faces *forward* in a human standing upright. As a result, the extensors of the thigh and leg (the genetically "dorsal" muscles) are on the anterior side of the limb, placed in front of the corresponding limb bones. This is one reason why the terms "anterior" and "posterior" are preferred over "dorsal" and "ventral" in the human lower limb. By contrast, the extensors and flexors of the arm and forearm have maintained their original dorsal and ventral positions, respectively.

2.1 The Human Body (Proportions, Surface Areas, and Body Weights)

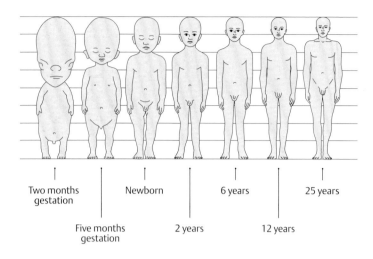

Two months gestation | Five months gestation | Newborn | 2 years | 6 years | 12 years | 25 years

A Change in body proportions during growth
While the head height in embryos at two months' gestation is equal to approximately half the total body length, it measures approximately one-fourth of the body length in newborns, one-sixth in a six-year-old child, and one-eighth in an adult.

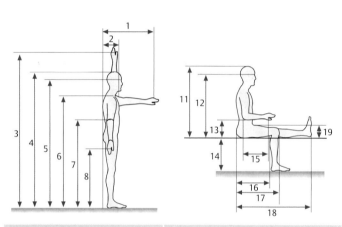

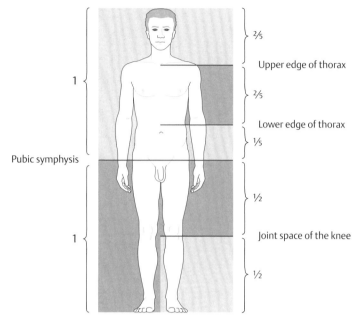

Upper edge of thorax — ²⁄₅
Lower edge of thorax — ²⁄₅
¹⁄₅
Pubic symphysis
½
Joint space of the knee
½

B Normal body proportions
In an adult, the midpoint of the total body height lies approximately at the level of the pubic symphysis, i.e., there is a 1:1 ratio of upper to lower body height at that level. The pelvis accounts for one-fifth of the upper body height, the thorax for two-fifths, and the head and neck for two-fifths. The lower body height is distributed equally between the thigh and leg (plus heel) at the joint space of the knee.

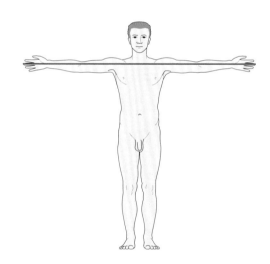

C Span of the outstretched arms
The arm span from fingertip to fingertip (= 1 fathom) is slightly *greater* than the body height (approximately 103 % in women and 106 % in men).

Measurements (in cm)	Male			Female		
	5th	50th	95th	5th	50th	95th
1 Forward reach	66.2	72.2	78.7	61.6	69.0	76.2
2 AP body thickness	23.2	27.6	31.8	23.8	28.5	35.7
3 Overhead reach (with both arms)	191.0	205.1	221.0	174.8	187.0	200.0
4 Body height	162.9	173.3	184.1	151.0	161.9	172.5
5 Ocular height	150.9	161.3	172.1	140.2	150.2	159.6
6 Shoulder height	134.9	144.5	154.2	123.4	133.9	143.6
7 Elbow-to-floor distance	102.1	109.6	117.9	95.7	103.0	110.0
8 Hand-to-floor distance	72.8	76.7	82.8	66.4	73.8	80.3
9 Shoulder width	31.0	34.4	36.8	31.4	35.8	40.5
10 Hip width, standing	36.7	39.8	42.8	32.3	35.5	38.8
11 Sitting body height (trunk height)	84.9	90.7	96.2	80.5	85.7	91.4
12 Ocular height while sitting	73.9	79.0	84.4	68.0	73.5	78.5
13 Elbow to sitting surface	19.3	23.0	28.0	19.1	23.3	27.8
14 Height of leg and foot (height of sitting surface)	39.9	44.2	48.0	35.1	39.5	43.4
15 Elbow to gripping axis	32.7	36.2	38.9	29.2	32.2	36.4
16 Sitting depth	45.2	50.0	55.2	42.6	48.4	53.2
17 Buttock–knee length	55.4	59.9	64.5	53.0	58.7	63.1
18 Buttock–leg length	96.4	103.5	112.5	95.5	104.4	112.6
19 Thigh height	11.7	13.6	15.7	11.8	14.4	17.3
20 Width above the elbow	39.9	45.1	51.2	37.0	45.6	54.4
21 Hip width, sitting	32.5	36.2	39.1	34.0	38.7	45.1

D Selected body measurements in the standing and sitting human being (unclothed, 16–60 years of age)
The percentile values indicate what percentage in a population group are below the value stated for a particular body measurement. For example, the 95th percentile for body height in males 16–60 years of age is 184.1 cm, meaning that 95 % of this population group are shorter than 184.1 cm, and 5 % are taller.

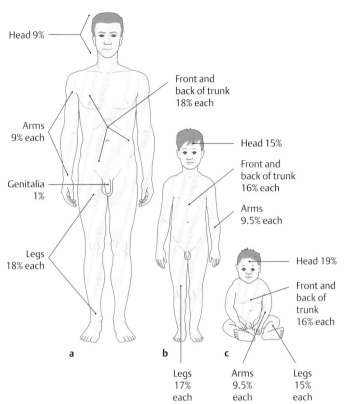

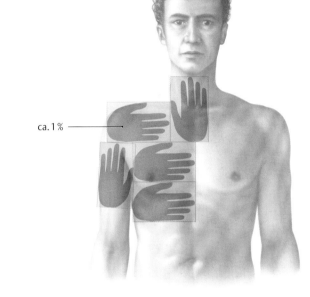

E Distribution of body surface area in adults, children, and infants

According to the "rule of nines" described by Wallace (1950), the body surface area of adults over about 15 years of age (**a**) can be divided into units that are a *multiple* of 9%: the head and each arm account for 9% each, the front and back of the trunk and each leg account for 18% (2 × 9) each, and the external genitalia comprise 1%. In children (**b**) and infants (**c**), the rule of nines must be adjusted for age.

Note: The rule of nines can be used in burn victims to provide a quick approximation of the area of skin that has been burned.

F Hand area rule

The percentage of the body surface affected by burns can be accurately estimated with the hand area rule, which states that the area of the patient's hand is approximately 1% of the patient's own total body surface area. The hand rule also applies to children, whose hands and total surface area are both proportionately smaller than in adults.

G Dependence of relative body surface area (skin surface area) on age, and consequences

For progressively larger solid bodies, the surface area increases as the square of the radius, but the volume increases as the cube of the body's radius. Because of this basic geometrical relationship, smaller animals generally have a larger relative surface area than larger animals. A higher ratio of surface area to volume causes smaller animals to radiate relatively more body heat. As a result, small animals like mice and children tend to have a higher metabolic rate than larger animals like elephants and human adults.

Age	Body weight (kg)	Body surface area (cm²)	Body surface area over body weight (cm²/kg)
Newborn	3.4	2100	617.6
Six months	7.5	3500	466.7
One year	9.3	4100	440.9
Four years	15.5	6500	419.4
Ten years	30.5	10500	344.3
Adult	70.0	18100	258.6

Height in meters

	1,48	1,52	1,56	1,60	1,64	1,68	1,72	1,76	1,80	1,84	1,88	1,92	1,96	2,00
120	55 53	52 51	49 48	47 46	45 44	43 42	41 40	39 38	37 36	35 35	34 33	33 32	31 31	30
118	54 52	51 50	48 47	46 45	44 43	42 41	40 39	38 37	36 36	35 34	33 33	32 31	31 30	30
116	53 52	50 49	48 46	45 44	43 42	41 40	39 38	37 36	35 34	34 33	32 32	31 31	30 30	29
114	52 51	49 48	47 46	45 43	42 41	40 39	39 38	37 36	35 34	34 33	32 32	31 30	30 29	29
112	51 50	48 47	46 45	44 43	42 41	40 39	38 37	36 35	35 34	33 32	32 31	30 30	29 29	28
110	50 49	48 46	45 44	43 42	41 40	39 38	37 36	36 35	34 33	33 32	32 31	30 30	29 28	28
108	49 48	47 46	44 43	42 41	40 39	38 37	37 36	35 34	33 33	32 31	31 30	29 29	28 28	27
106	48 47	46 45	44 42	41 40	39 38	38 37	36 35	34 33	33 32	31 31	30 29	29 28	28 27	27
104	47 46	45 44	43 42	41 40	39 38	37 36	35 34	34 33	32 31	31 30	29 29	28 28	27 27	26
102	47 45	44 43	42 41	40 39	38 37	36 35	34 34	33 32	31 31	30 29	29 28	28 27	27 26	26
100	46 44	43 42	41 40	39 38	37 36	35 35	34 33	32 32	31 30	30 29	28 28	27 27	26 26	25
98	45 44	42 41	40 39	38 37	36 36	35 34	33 32	32 31	30 30	29 28	28 27	27 26	26 25	25
96	44 43	42 40	39 38	38 37	36 35	34 33	33 32	31 30	30 29	28 28	27 27	26 26	25 24	24
94	43 42	41 40	39 38	37 36	35 34	33 33	32 31	30 30	29 28	28 27	27 26	25 25	24 24	24
92	42 41	40 39	38 37	36 35	34 33	33 32	31 30	30 29	28 28	27 26	26 25	25 24	24 23	23
90	41 40	39 38	37 36	35 34	33 33	32 31	30 30	29 28	28 27	26 26	25 24	24 23	23 23	23
88	40 39	38 37	36 35	34 34	33 32	31 30	30 29	28 28	27 26	26 25	24 24	23 23	23 22	22
86	39 38	37 36	35 34	34 33	32 31	30 30	29 28	28 27	26 26	25 24	24 23	23 22	22 22	22
84	38 37	36 35	34 34	33 32	31 30	30 29	28 27	27 26	26 25	24 24	23 23	22 22	21 21	21
82	37 36	35 35	34 33	32 31	30 30	29 28	28 27	26 26	25 24	24 23	23 22	22 21	21 21	21
80	37 36	35 34	33 32	31 30	30 29	28 28	27 26	26 25	25 24	23 23	22 22	21 21	20 20	20
78	36 35	34 33	32 31	30 30	29 28	28 27	26 26	25 25	24 24	23 22	22 21	21 20	20 20	20
76	35 34	33 32	31 30	30 29	28 28	27 26	26 25	25 24	24 23	23 22	22 21	20 20	19 19	19
74	34 33	32 31	30 30	29 28	28 27	26 26	25 24	24 23	23 22	22 21	21 20	20 19	19 19	19
72	33 32	31 30	30 29	28 27	27 26	26 25	24 24	23 23	22 22	21 21	20 20	19 19	18 18	18
70	32 31	30 30	29 28	27 27	26 25	25 24	24 23	23 22	22 21	21 20	20 19	19 18	18 18	18
68	31 30	29 29	28 27	27 26	25 25	24 24	23 22	22 21	21 20	20 19	19 18	18 17	17 17	17
66	30 29	29 28	27 26	26 25	25 24	23 23	22 22	21 21	20 20	19 19	18 18	17 17	17 16	17
64	29 28	28 27	26 26	25 24	24 23	23 22	22 21	21 20	20 19	19 18	18 17	17 16	16 16	16
62	28 28	27 26	26 25	24 24	23 22	22 21	21 20	20 19	19 18	18 17	17 16	16 16	15 15	16
60	27 27	26 25	24 23	23 22	22 21	21 20	20 19	19 18	18 17	17 16	16 16	15 15	15 14	15
58	26 26	25 24	24 23	23 22	21 21	20 20	19 19	18 18	18 17	17 16	16 15	15 15	14 14	15
56	26 25	24 24	23 22	22 21	20 20	19 19	18 18	18 17	17 16	16 16	15 15	15 14	14 14	14
54	25 24	23 23	22 22	21 21	20 20	19 19	18 18	17 17	17 16	16 15	15 15	14 14	14 13	14
52	24 23	23 22	21 20	20 19	19 18	18 17	17 17	16 16	15 15	15 14	14 14	14 13	13 13	13
50	23 22	22 21	21 20	20 19	19 18	18 17	17 16	16 15	15 15	14 14	14 13	13 13	13	13
48	22 21	21 20	20 19	19 18	18 17	17 17	16 16	15 15	15 14	14 14	13 13	13 12	12 12	

▮ Extremely obese ▮ Obese ▮ Overweight ▯ Normal ▯ Underweight

Weight in kilograms (vertical axis label)

H Body mass index

In anthropometry, the body mass index (BMI) has become the international standard for evaluating body weight because it correlates relatively well with total body fat. BMI is defined as the body weight in kilograms divided by the square of the height in meters:

$$BMI = \frac{kg}{m^2}$$

2.2 The Structural Design of the Human Body

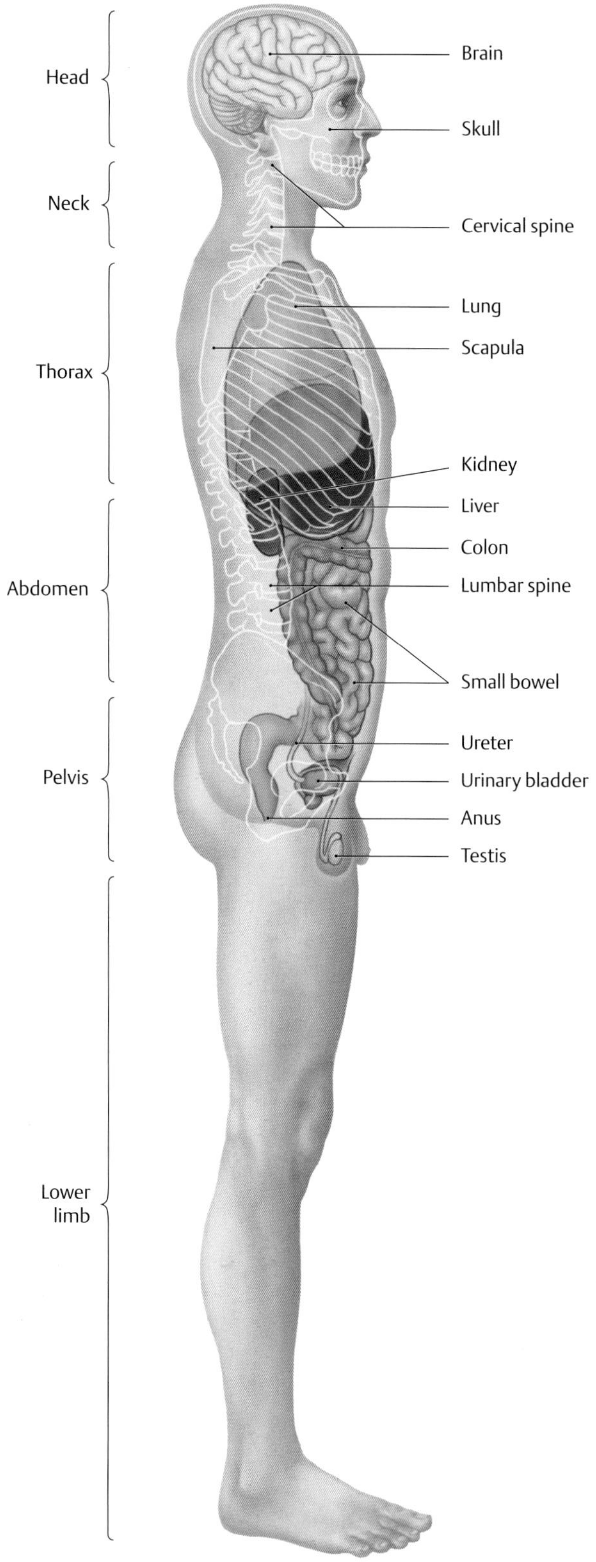
Head
Neck
Thorax
Abdomen
Pelvis
Lower limb
Brain
Skull
Cervical spine
Lung
Scapula
Kidney
Liver
Colon
Lumbar spine
Small bowel
Ureter
Urinary bladder
Anus
Testis

A Location of the internal organs
Lateral view.

B Regional subdivisions of the body

Head

Neck

Trunk
- Thorax (chest)
- Abdomen
- Pelvis

Upper limb
- Shoulder girdle
- Free upper limb

Lower limb
- Pelvic girdle
- Free lower limb

C Functional subdivision by organ systems

Locomotor system (musculoskeletal system)
- Skeleton and skeletal connections (passive part)
- Striated skeletal musculature (active part)

Viscera
- Cardiovascular system
- Hemolymphatic system
- Endocrine system
- Respiratory system
- Digestive system
- Urinary system
- Male and female reproductive system

Nervous system
- Central and peripheral nervous system
- Sensory organs

The skin and its appendages

D Serous cavities and connective-tissue spaces
Organs and organ systems are embedded either in serous cavities or in connective-tissue spaces of varying size. A serous cavity is a fully enclosed potential space that is lined by a shiny membrane (serosa) and contains a small amount of fluid. The serosa consists of two layers that are *usually* apposed (both layers are not *necessarily* in direct contact, as in the abdominal cavity): a visceral layer that directly invests the organ, and a parietal layer that lines the wall of the serous cavity.

Serous cavities
- Thoracic cavity (chest cavity) with:
  - the pleural cavity
  - the pericardial cavity
- Abdominopelvic cavity with:
  - the peritoneal cavity
  - the pelvic cavity

Connective-tissue spaces
- Space between the middle and deep layers of cervical fascia
- Mediastinum
- Extraperitoneal space with:
  - the retroperitoneal space (retroperitoneum) and
  - the subperitoneal space
- Bursa and synovial cavities

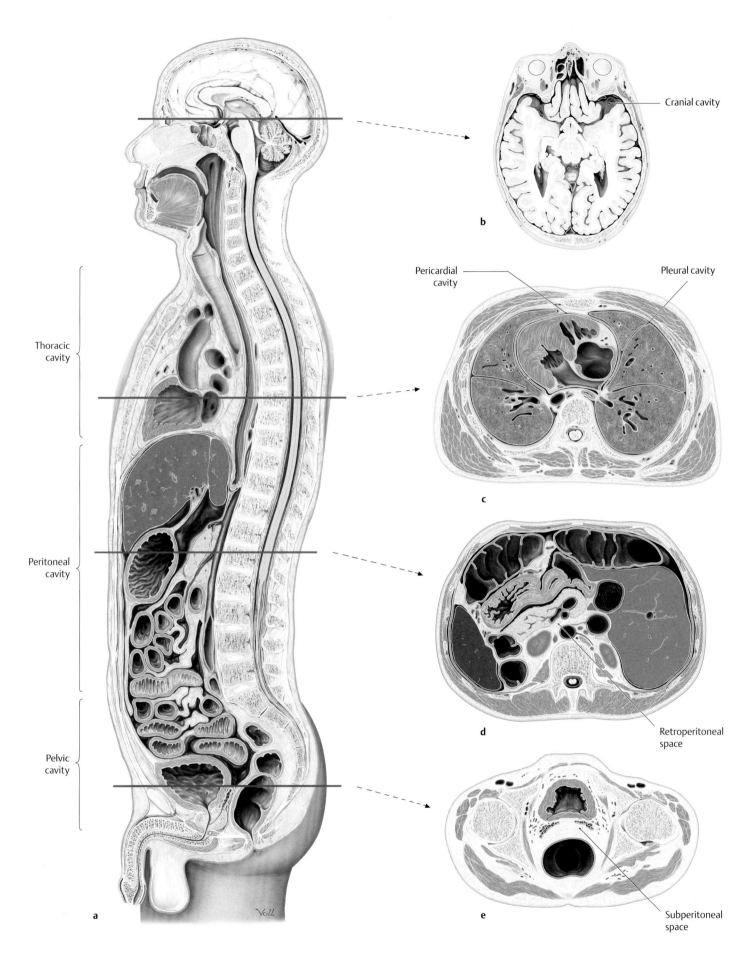

E Selected planes of section through the human body

a Midsagittal section

b Cross section at the level of the head

c Cross section through the thorax

d Cross section through the abdomen

e Cross section through the lesser pelvis (see also Cardinal Planes and Axes, p. 25)

3.1 Terms of Location and Direction, Cardinal Planes and Axes

A General terms of location and direction

Upper body (head, neck, and trunk)	
Cranial	Pertaining to, or located toward the head)
Cephalad	Directed toward the head
Caudal	Pertaining to, or located toward the tail
Caudad	Directed toward the tail
Anterior	Pertaining to, or located toward, the front
	Synonym: Ventral (used for all animals)
Posterior	Pertaining to, or located toward, the back
	Synonym: Dorsal (used for all animals)
Superior	Upper or above
Inferior	Lower or below
Medius	Located in the middle
Flexor	Pertaining to a flexor muscle or surface
Extensor	Pertaining to an extensor muscle or surface
Axial	Pertaining to the axis of a structure
Transverse	Situated at right angles to the long axis of a structure
Longitudinal	Parallel to the long axis of a structure
Horizontal	Parallel to the plane of the horizon
Vertical	Perpendicular to the plane of the horizon
Medial	Toward the median plane
Lateral	Away from the medial plane (toward the side)
Median	Situated in the median plane or midline
Central	Situated at the center or interior of the body
Peripheral	Situated away from the center
Superficial	Situated near the surface
Deep	Situated deep beneath the surface
External	Outer or lateral
Internal	Inner or medial
Apical	Pertaining to the tip or apex
Basal	Pertaining to the bottom or base
Occipital	Pertaining to the back of the head
Temporal	Pertaining to the lateral region of the head (the temple)
Sagittal	Situated parallel to the sagittal suture
Coronal	Situated parallel to the coronal suture (pertaining to the crown of the head)
Rostral	Situated toward the nose or brow
Frontal	Pertaining to the forehead
Basilar	Pertaining to the skull base

Limbs	
Proximal	Close to or toward the trunk
Distal	Away from the trunk (toward the end of the limb)
Radial	Pertaining to the radius or the lateral side of the forearm
Ulnar	Pertaining to the ulna or the medial side of the forearm
Tibial	Pertaining to the tibia or the medial side of the leg
Fibular	Pertaining to the fibula or the lateral side of the leg
Palmar (volar)	Pertaining to the palm of the hand
Plantar	Pertaining to the sole of the foot
Dorsal	Pertaining to the back of the hand or top of the foot

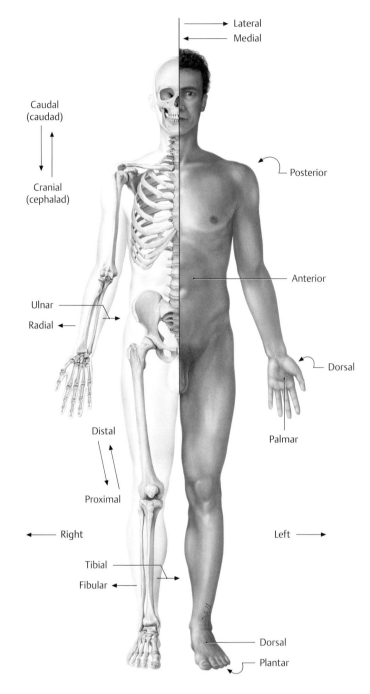

B The anatomical body position
The gaze is directed forward, the hands are supinated. The *right* half of the body is shown in light shading to demonstrate the skeleton.
Note that the designations "left" and "right" always refer to the patient.

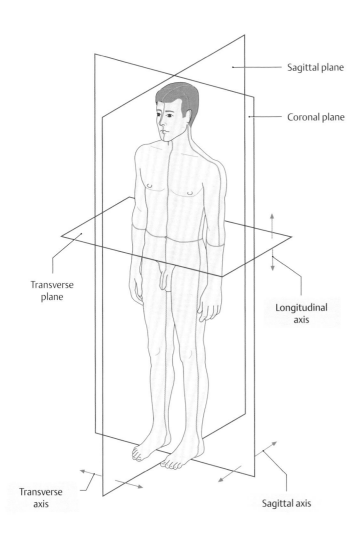

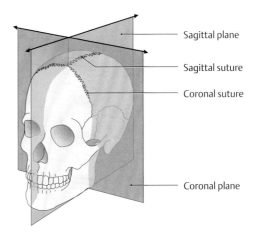

D Coronal and sagittal planes in the skull
The coronal plane is named for the fact that it is parallel to the coronal suture, just as the sagittal plane is parallel to the sagittal suture. The cranial sutures serve as directional indicators, "sagittal" meaning in the direction of the sagittal suture, "coronal" in the direction of the coronal suture.

C Cardinal planes and axes in the human body (neutral position, left anterolateral view)
Although any number of planes and axes can be drawn through the human body, it is standard practice to designate *three cardinal planes and axes*. They are perpendicular to one another and are based on the three spatial coordinates.

The cardinal body planes:
• **Sagittal plane:** Any *vertical* plane that is parallel to the sagittal suture of the skull, passing through the body from front to back. The *midsagittal plane* (= median plane) divides the body into equal left and right halves.
• **Coronal plane (frontal plane):** Any plane that is *parallel to the forehead* or to the coronal suture of the skull. In the standing position, it passes vertically through the body from side to side.
• **Transverse plane (axial plane):** Any *horizontal*, cross-sectional plane that divides the body into upper and lower portions. It is perpendicular to the longitudinal body axis.

The cardinal body axes:
• **Vertical or longitudinal axis:** In the standing position, this axis runs through the body *craniocaudally* and is perpendicular to the ground. It lies at the intersection of the coronal and sagittal planes.
• **Sagittal axis:** This axis runs *anteroposteriorly* from the front to back surface of the body (or from back to front) and lies at the intersection of the sagittal and transverse planes.
• **Transverse or horizontal axis:** This axis runs from side to side and lies at the intersection of the coronal and transverse planes.

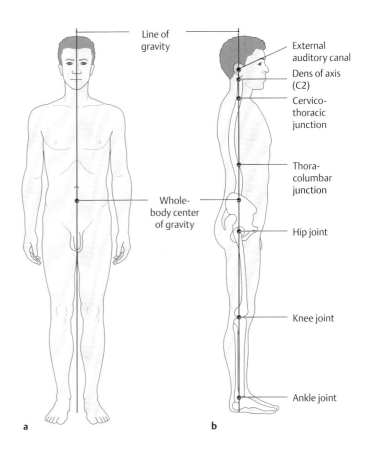

E The whole-body center of gravity and the line of gravity
a Anterior view. The line of gravity is directed vertically along the midsagittal plane, passing through the whole-body center of gravity below the sacral promontory at the level of the second sacral vertebra.
b Lateral view. The line of gravity passes through the external auditory canal, the dens of the axis (second cervical vertebra), the anatomical and functional junctions within the spinal column, the whole-body center of gravity, and through the hip, knee, and ankle joints (after Kummer).

3.2 Body Surface Anatomy

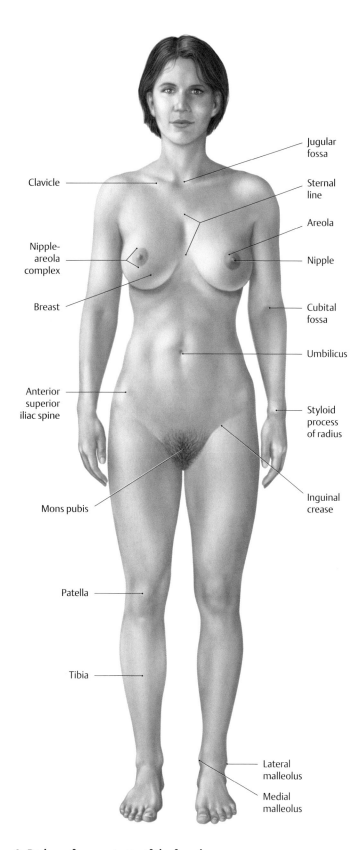

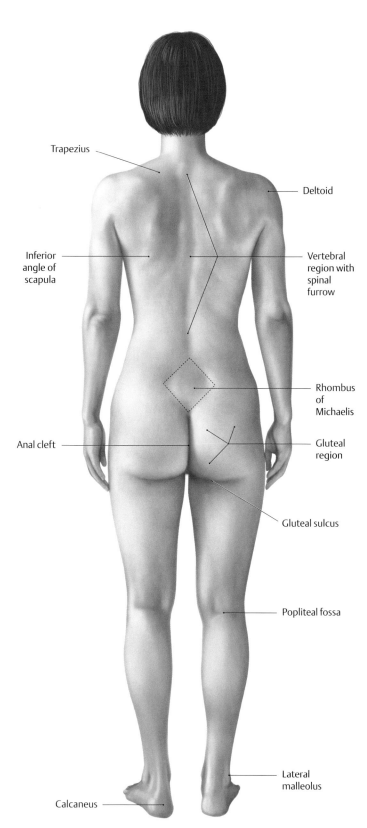

Clavicle

Nipple-areola complex

Breast

Anterior superior iliac spine

Mons pubis

Patella

Tibia

Jugular fossa

Sternal line

Areola

Nipple

Cubital fossa

Umbilicus

Styloid process of radius

Inguinal crease

Lateral malleolus

Medial malleolus

Trapezius

Inferior angle of scapula

Anal cleft

Calcaneus

Deltoid

Vertebral region with spinal furrow

Rhombus of Michaelis

Gluteal region

Gluteal sulcus

Popliteal fossa

Lateral malleolus

A Body surface anatomy of the female
Anterior view. Body surface anatomy deals with the surface anatomy of the living subject. It plays an important role in classic methods of examination (inspection, palpation, percussion, auscultation, function testing), and so it has particular significance in clinical examination courses. To avoid repetition, identical structures such as the olecranon have not been labeled on both the female and male bodies.

B Body surface anatomy of the female
Posterior view.

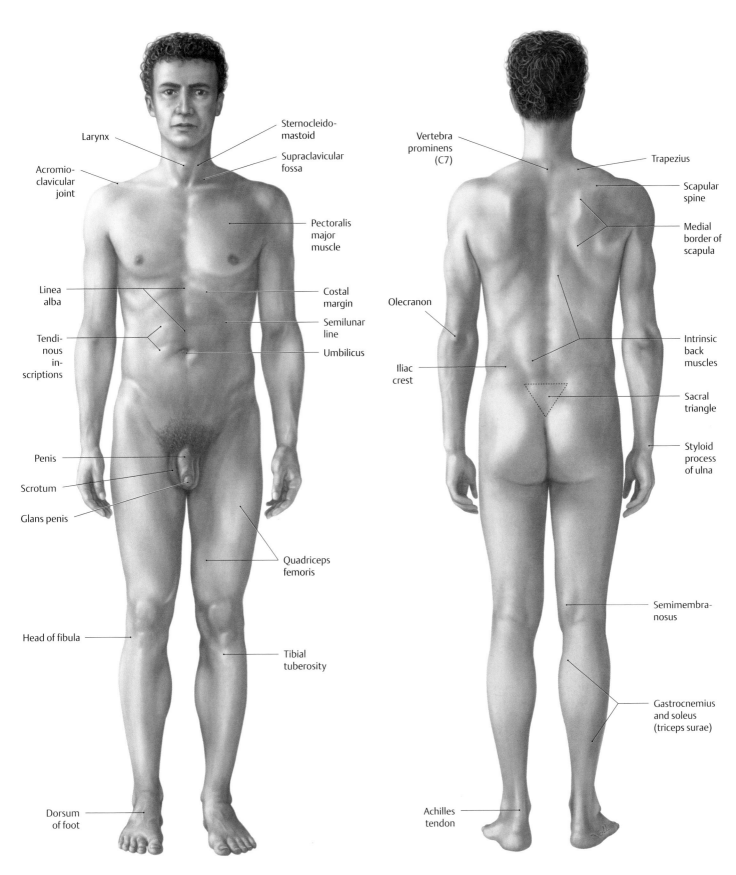

Larynx

Acromio-
clavicular
joint

Linea
alba

Tendi-
nous
in-
scriptions

Penis

Scrotum

Glans penis

Head of fibula

Dorsum
of foot

Sternocleido-
mastoid

Supraclavicular
fossa

Pectoralis
major
muscle

Costal
margin

Semilunar
line

Umbilicus

Quadriceps
femoris

Tibial
tuberosity

Vertebra
prominens
(C7)

Olecranon

Iliac
crest

Achilles
tendon

Trapezius

Scapular
spine

Medial
border of
scapula

Intrinsic
back
muscles

Sacral
triangle

Styloid
process
of ulna

Semimembra-
nosus

Gastrocnemius
and soleus
(triceps surae)

C Body surface anatomy of the male
Anterior view.

D Body surface anatomy of the male
Posterior view.

3.3   Body Surface Contours and Palpable Bony Prominences

Palpable bony prominences are important landmarks for anatomical orientation in the skeleton, as it is not always possible to palpate articulating skeletal structures (e.g., the hip joint). In these cases the examiner must rely on palpable bony prominences as an indirect guide to the location of the inaccessible structure.

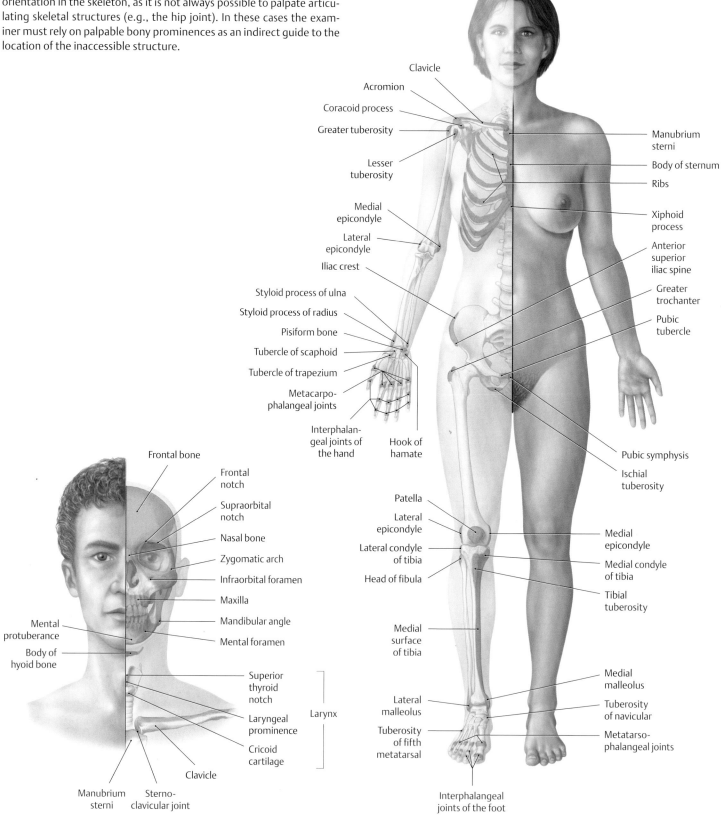

A Surface contours and palpable bony prominences of the face and neck
Anterior view.

B Surface contours and palpable bony prominences of the trunk and upper and lower limbs in the female
Anterior view.

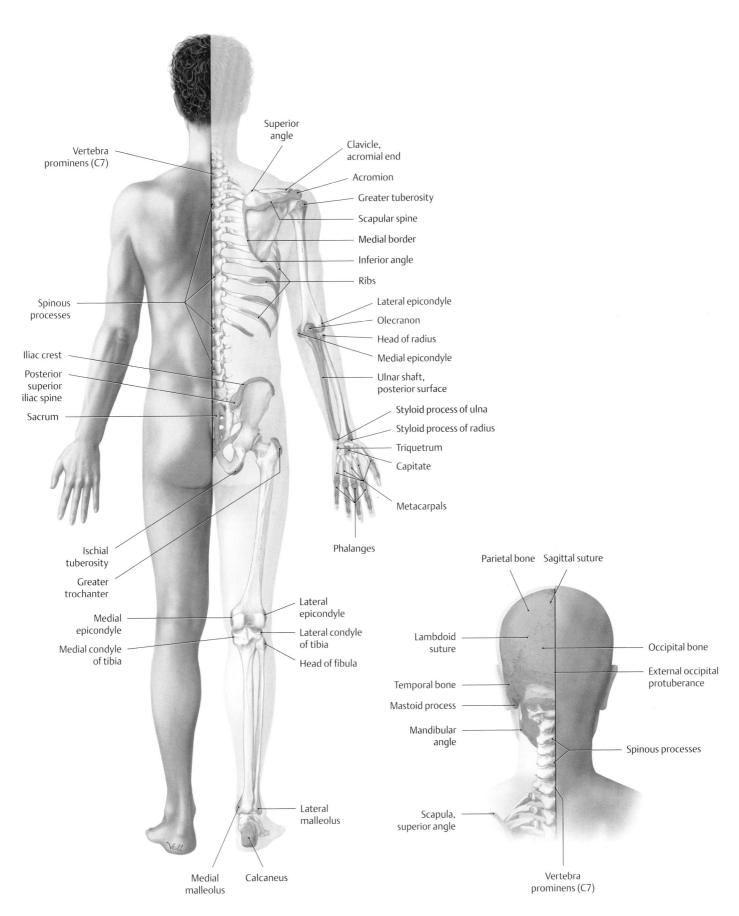

Vertebra prominens (C7)

Superior angle

Clavicle, acromial end

Acromion

Greater tuberosity

Scapular spine

Medial border

Inferior angle

Ribs

Lateral epicondyle

Olecranon

Head of radius

Medial epicondyle

Spinous processes

Ulnar shaft, posterior surface

Iliac crest

Posterior superior iliac spine

Styloid process of ulna

Styloid process of radius

Triquetrum

Capitate

Sacrum

Metacarpals

Ischial tuberosity

Phalanges

Parietal bone   Sagittal suture

Greater trochanter

Medial epicondyle

Lambdoid suture

Occipital bone

Lateral epicondyle

Lateral condyle of tibia

Head of fibula

External occipital protuberance

Medial condyle of tibia

Temporal bone

Mastoid process

Spinous processes

Mandibular angle

Lateral malleolus

Scapula, superior angle

Medial malleolus   Calcaneus

Vertebra prominens (C7)

C Surface contours and palpable bony prominences of the trunk and upper and lower limbs in the male
Posterior view.

D Surface contours and palpable bony prominences of the face and neck
Posterior view.

3.4 Landmarks and Reference Lines on the Human Body

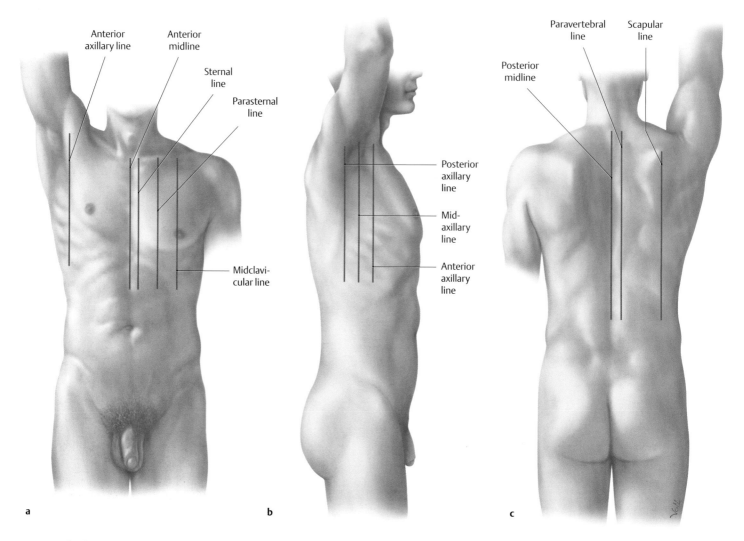

A Vertical reference lines on the trunk
a Anterior view, **b** right lateral view, **c** posterior view.

Anterior midline	Anterior trunk midline passing through the center of the sternum
Sternal line	Line along the sternal margin
Parasternal line	Line midway between the sternal line and midclavicular line
Midclavicular line	Line through the midpoint of the clavicle (often identical to the nipple line)
Anterior axillary line	Line at the level of the anterior axillary fold (pectoralis major muscle)
Midaxillary line	Line midway between the anterior and posterior axillary lines
Posterior axillary line	Line at the level of the posterior axillary fold (latissimus dorsi muscle)
Posterior midline	Posterior trunk midline at the level of the spinous processes
Paravertebral line	Line at the level of the transverse processes
Scapular line	Line through the inferior angle of the scapula

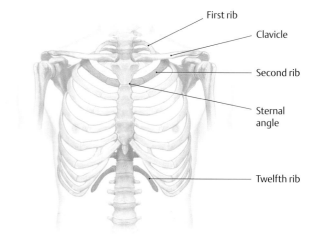

B "Rib counting" for anatomical orientation in the thorax
The first rib is covered by the clavicle. The first palpable rib is the second rib, and therefore the count begins at that level. The second rib attaches to the sternum at the level of the sternal angle. At the lower end of the rib cage, it is best to start at the twelfth rib, which is palpable only in its posterior portion.

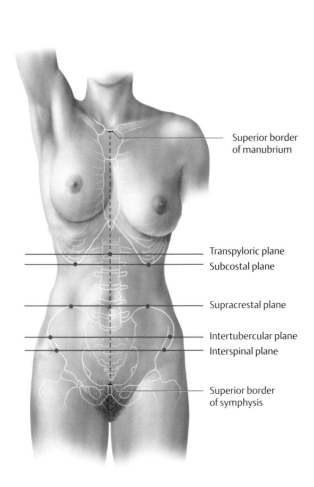

Superior border of manubrium

Transpyloric plane
Subcostal plane

Supracrestal plane

Intertubercular plane
Interspinal plane

Superior border of symphysis

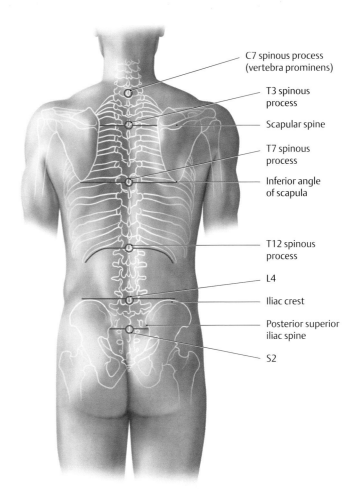

C7 spinous process (vertebra prominens)

T3 spinous process

Scapular spine

T7 spinous process

Inferior angle of scapula

T12 spinous process

L4

Iliac crest

Posterior superior iliac spine

S2

C Standard transverse planes through the abdominal cavity
(see also p. 171)
Anterior view.

Transpyloric plane	Transverse plane midway between the superior borders of the symphysis and manubrium
Subcostal plane	Plane at the lowest level of the costal margin (inferior margin of the tenth costal cartilage)
Supracrestal plane	Plane passing through the summits of the iliac crests
Intertubercular plane	Plane at the level of the iliac tubercles (the iliac tubercle lies approximately 5 cm posterolateral to the anterior superior iliac spine)
Interspinal plane	Plane at the level of the anterior superior iliac spines

D Spinous processes that provide useful posterior landmarks
Posterior view.

C7 spinous process	Vertebra prominens (the projecting spinous process of C7 is clearly visible and palpable)
T3 spinous process	At the level of the line connecting the two scapular spines
T7 spinous process	At the level of the line connecting the inferior angles of both scapulae
T12 spinous process	Just below the twelfth rib
L4 spinous process	At the level of the line connecting the summits of the iliac crests
S2 spinous process	At the level of the line connecting the posterior superior iliac spines (recognized by small skin depressions directly over the iliac spines)

E Lithotomy position (supine with the legs, hips, and knees flexed and the thighs abducted)
The position of choice for proctological examinations. Clock-face notation is used for anatomical orientation (e.g., to describe the location of a lesion):

- Top = toward the pubis = 12 o'clock
- Bottom = toward the sacrum = 6 o'clock
- Right = 3 o'clock
- Left = 9 o'clock

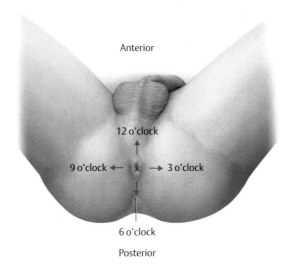

Anterior

12 o'clock

9 o'clock ← → 3 o'clock

6 o'clock

Posterior

31

3.5 Body Regions (Regional Anatomy)

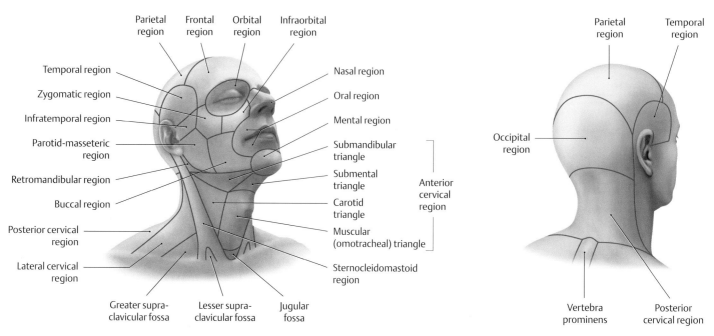

A Regions of the head and neck
Right anterolateral view.

B Regions of the head and neck
Right posterolateral view.

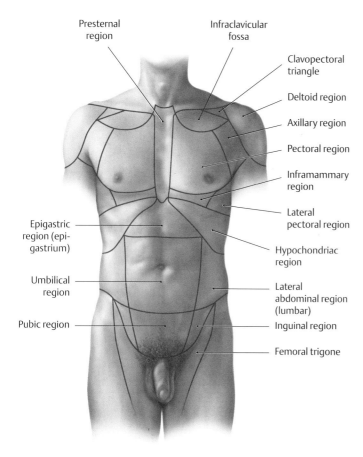

C Regions of the thorax and abdomen
Anterior view.

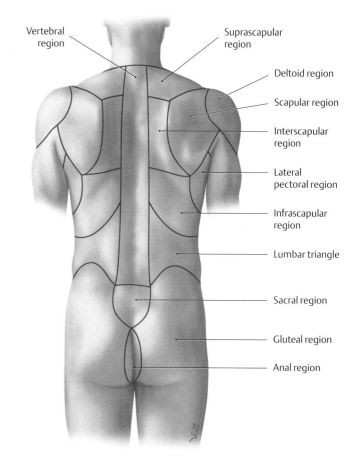

D Regions of the back and buttocks
Posterior view.

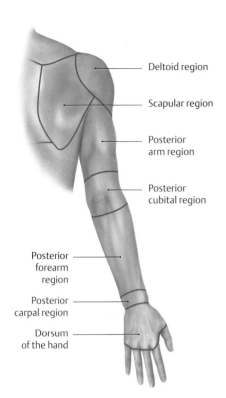

Deltoid region

Scapular region

Posterior arm region

Posterior cubital region

Posterior forearm region

Posterior carpal region

Dorsum of the hand

E Regions of the upper limb
Posterior view.

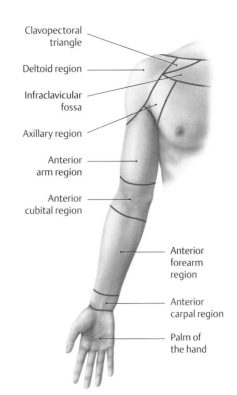

Clavopectoral triangle

Deltoid region

Infraclavicular fossa

Axillary region

Anterior arm region

Anterior cubital region

Anterior forearm region

Anterior carpal region

Palm of the hand

F Regions of the upper limb
Anterior view.

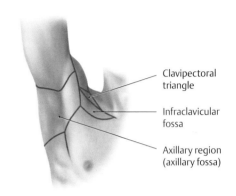

Clavipectoral triangle

Infraclavicular fossa

Axillary region (axillary fossa)

G Regions about the axilla
Anterior view.

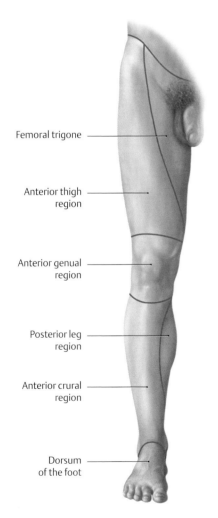

Femoral trigone

Anterior thigh region

Anterior genual region

Posterior leg region

Anterior crural region

Dorsum of the foot

H Regions of the lower limb
Anterior view.

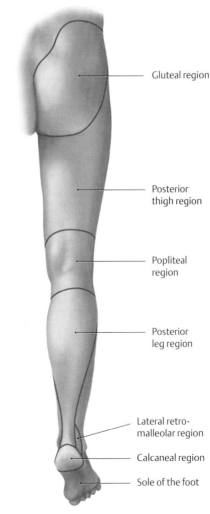

Gluteal region

Posterior thigh region

Popliteal region

Posterior leg region

Lateral retromalleolar region

Calcaneal region

Sole of the foot

J Regions of the lower limb
Posterior view.

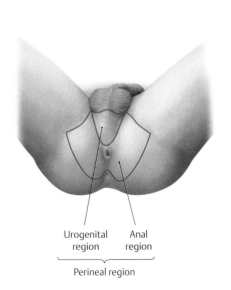

Urogenital region

Anal region

Perineal region

K Perineal region (lithotomy position)

33

4.1 The Bony Skeleton and the Structure of Tubular Bones

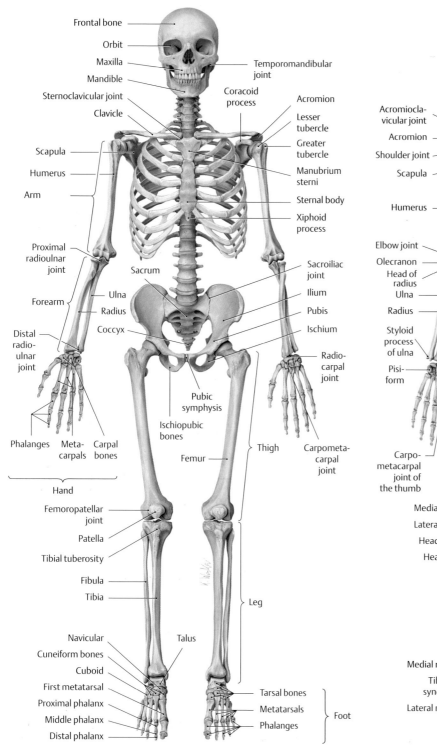

A Human skeleton from the anterior view
The left forearm is pronated, and both feet are in plantar flexion.

B Human skeleton from the posterior view
The left forearm is pronated, and both feet are in plantar flexion.

C Types of bone

- **Long bones,** e.g., tubular bones of the limbs
- **Short bones,** e.g., carpal and tarsal bones
- **Flat bones,** e.g., scapula, ilium, and bones of the calvaria
- **Irregular bones, e.g. vertebrae** anomalous, supernumerary bones not consistently present, as in the skull base

- **Pneumatic bones** (containing air-filled spaces), e.g., bones of the facial skeleton and paranasal sinuses
- **Sesamoid bones** (bones incorporated in tendons), e.g., the patella
- **Accessory bones** (anomalous, supernumerary bones), as in the calvaria and foot (generally result from the failure of fusion of certain adjacent ossification centers)

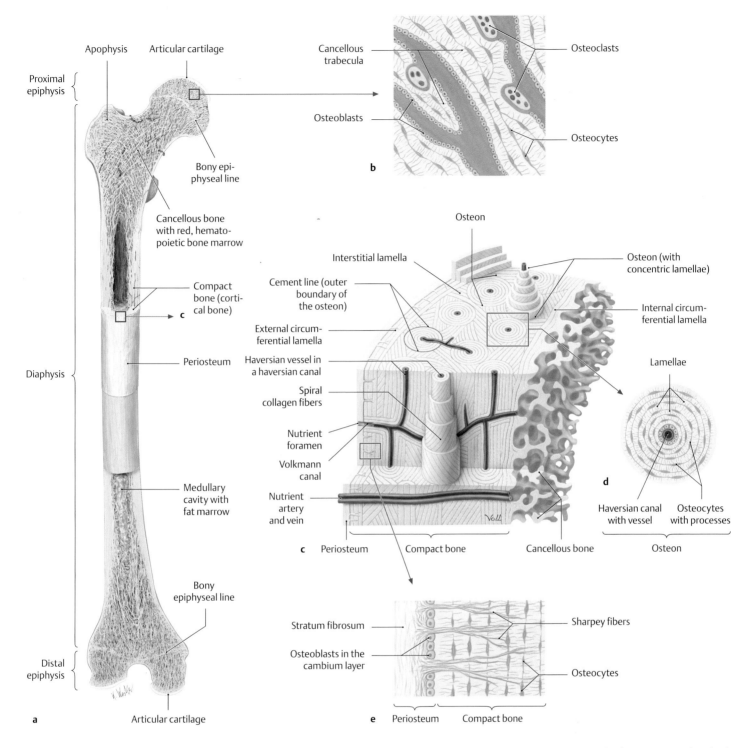

a
- Apophysis
- Articular cartilage
- Proximal epiphysis
- Bony epiphyseal line
- Cancellous bone with red, hematopoietic bone marrow
- Compact bone (cortical bone)
- c
- Periosteum
- Diaphysis
- Medullary cavity with fat marrow
- Bony epiphyseal line
- Distal epiphysis
- Articular cartilage

b
- Cancellous trabecula
- Osteoblasts
- Osteoclasts
- Osteocytes

c
- Osteon
- Interstitial lamella
- Cement line (outer boundary of the osteon)
- External circumferential lamella
- Haversian vessel in a haversian canal
- Spiral collagen fibers
- Nutrient foramen
- Volkmann canal
- Nutrient artery and vein
- Periosteum
- Compact bone
- Osteon (with concentric lamellae)
- Internal circumferential lamella
- Cancellous bone

d
- Lamellae
- Haversian canal with vessel
- Osteocytes with processes
- Osteon

e
- Stratum fibrosum
- Osteoblasts in the cambium layer
- Sharpey fibers
- Osteocytes
- Periosteum
- Compact bone

D Structure of a typical tubular bone, illustrated for the femur

a Coronal saw cuts have been made through the proximal and distal parts of an adult femur (without sectioning the midshaft region).

b Detail from **a**: The sectioned areas display the lamellar architecture ("lamellar bone") of the cancellous trabeculae. The lamellae are arranged in contiguous plates, similar to plywood. Since the cancellous trabeculae do not have an actual vascular supply and are nourished by diffusion from the adjacent medullary cavity, the trabeculae attain a thickness of only about 200–300 μm.

c Detail from **a**: Three-dimensional representation of compact bone, whose structural units consist of vascularized osteons approximately

1 cm long and 250–350 μm in diameter. The haversian canals, which tend to run longitudinally in the bone, are connected to one another by short transverse and oblique Volkmann canals and also to the vessels of the periosteum and medullary cavity.

d Detail from **c**, demonstrating the microstructure of an osteon. The haversian canal at the center is surrounded by approximately 5–20 concentric lamellar systems composed of osteocytes and extracellular matrix. The osteocytes are interconnected by numerous fine cytoplasmic processes.

e Detail from **c**, showing the structure of the periosteum.

4.2 Continuous and Discontinuous Joints: Synarthroses and Diarthroses

A Different types of bone-to-bone connections

False joints	True joints	
(= continuous bone connections in which the intervening tissue consists of fibrous connective tissue, cartilage, or bone): • Low to moderate mobility	(= discontinuous connections in which the bones are separated by a joint space): • Mobility is variable, depending on the attached ligaments	
Synarthroses • Syndesmoses (fibrous joints) • Synchondroses (cartilaginous joints) (If the intervening tissue is mostly fibrocartilage, the joint is called a symphysis, e.g., the pubic symphysis.) • Synostoses (sites of bony fusion) (Because a synostosis is immobile, it is no longer classified as a synarthrosis in the strict sense.)	**Diarthroses** Classified according to various criteria: (see p. 38) • Shape and arrangement of the articular surfaces • Number of joint axes • Number of degrees of freedom	**Amphiarthroses** "Stiff joints" whose mobility is greatly limited by strong ligaments (e.g., the sacroiliac joint and proximal tibiofibular joint)

Ankylosis = abnormal bony fixation of a true joint
Arthrodesis = surgical fusion of a joint for therapeutic reasons
Pseudarthrosis (nonunion) = "false joint" due to abnormal fracture healing

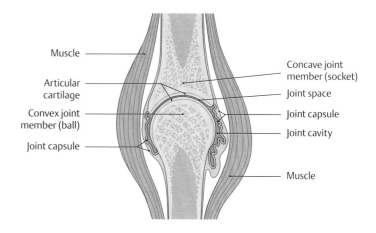

B Structure of a true (synovial) joint
True joints have the following characteristics:

* Joint space
* Articular surfaces covered by hyaline cartilage
* Joint cavity
* Closed joint capsule
* Ligaments and muscles acting as primary joint stabilizers

Some joints also contain **intra-articular structures** that help the joint to function: menisci (e.g., in the knee joint), articular disk (e.g., in the temporomandibular joint), articular labrum (e.g., in the shoulder joint), and intra-articular ligaments (e.g., the cruciform ligaments of the knee).

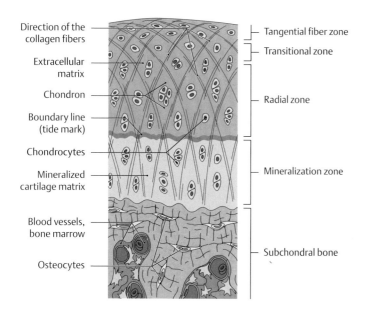

C Structure of articular cartilage (after Kristic)
Articulating bone surfaces are covered by a layer of *hyaline cartilage* of variable thickness (exceptions are the temporomandibular and sternoclavicular joints, which are covered by *fibrocartilage*). The thickness of the articular cartilage depends largely on the magnitude of the joint stresses, ranging from 1–2 mm in the phalangeal joints and 2–4 mm in the hip joint to 5–7 mm in the femoropatellar joint.

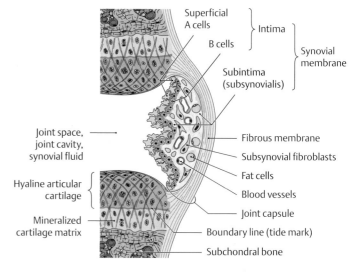

D Structure of the joint capsule
The joint space is shown greatly widened in the diagram to exhibit its features more clearly. The synovial fluid, produced mainly by type B synoviocytes, is a very viscous intra-articular fluid with a high content of hyaluronic acid. The synovial fluid performs three main functions:

* It nourishes the articular cartilage through diffusion and convection.
* It lubricates the articular surfaces to reduce friction.
* It cushions shocks by evenly distributing compressive forces.

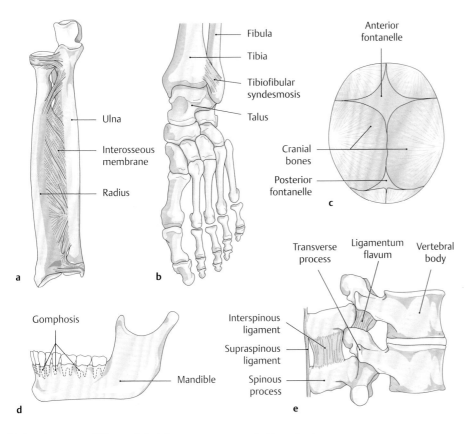

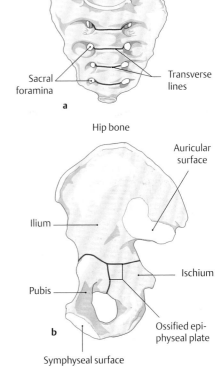

E Syndesmoses (fibrous joints)
a Interosseous membrane.
b Tibiofibular syndesmosis.
c Fontanelles.

d Gomphosis.
e Ligamentum flavum, interspinous ligament and supraspinous ligament.

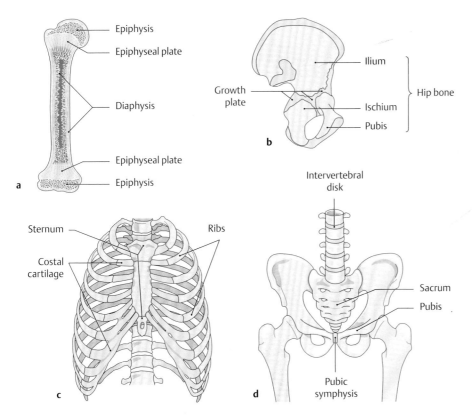

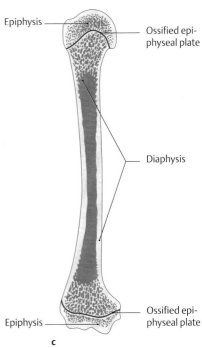

F Synchondroses (cartilaginous joints)
a Epiphyseal plates prior to closure.
b Hip bone before closure of the growth plates.

c Costal cartilage.
d Pubic symphysis and intervertebral disks (intervertebral symphysis).

G Synostoses (sites of bony fusion)
a Sacrum (fused sacral vertebrae).
b Hip bone (fusion of the ilium, ischium, and pubis).
c Closed and ossified epiphyseal plates.

4.3 Basic Principles of Joint Mechanics

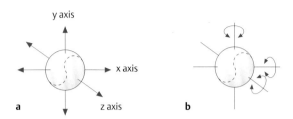

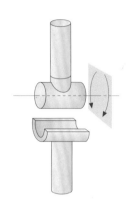

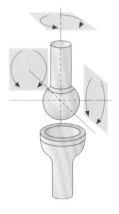

A Degrees of freedom, illustrated for the possible movements of a tennis ball in space

a Three degrees of freedom in *translation* (one each *along* the x, y, and z axes).

b Three degrees of freedom in *rotation* (one each *around* the x, y, and z axes).

With its similarity to a tennis ball, the spheroidal joint (see **Da**) has the greatest freedom of movement.

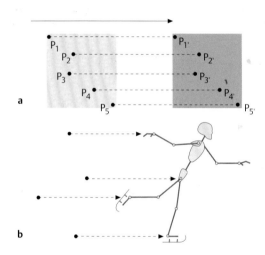

a Spheroidal joint
This type of joint has three mutually perpendicular axes of motion, resulting in six primary movements (example: hip joint).

b Hinge joint
This joint has one axis of motion, resulting in two primary movements (example: parts of the elbow joint).

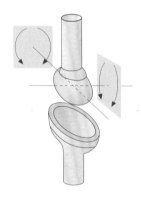

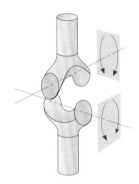

B Translation
Translation means that a body is sliding on a straight or curved path *without rotating*. As a result, all points on the moving body travel an *equal distance* in the same direction.

a All the points move on parallel lines.
b The gliding ice skater illustrates movement in translation.

c Ellipsoid joint
This joint is biaxial and has four primary movements (example: the radiocarpal joint).

d Saddle joint
This is a biaxial joint with four primary movements (example: the carpometacarpal joint of the thumb).

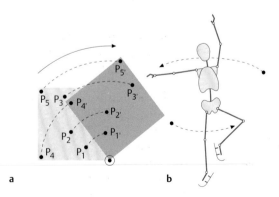

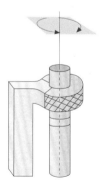

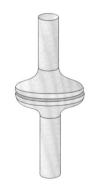

e Pivot joint
This is a uniaxial joint with two primary movements (example: the proximal radioulnar joint).

f Plane joint
The only movement allowed is a translation (sliding) of one member on the other (example: vertebral facet joint).

C Rotation
When a body is rotating, different points on the body move on concentric circles and travel *different distances*.

a All the points move on circular arcs.
b The spinning ice skater illustrates movement in rotation.

D The classification of joints by shape
The arrows indicate the direction in which the skeletal elements can move around the axis or axes of the joint. *Amphiarthroses* (not shown here) are "stiff" because their mobility is greatly restricted by the shape of their articular surfaces and by tight ligaments (examples are the proximal tibiofibular joint and sacroiliac joint).

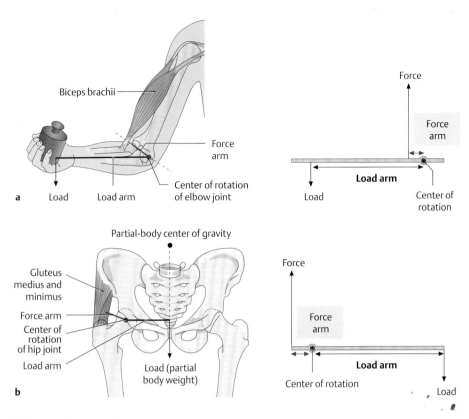

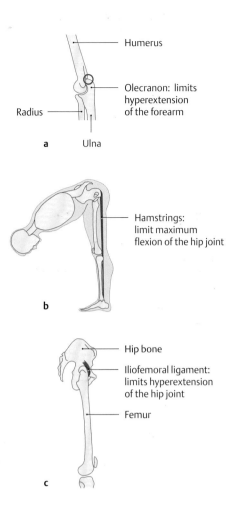

E One- and two-arm levers

a One-arm lever (elbow joint), **b** two-arm lever (hip joint).

Joint mechanics is based on the principles of the lever. The amount of force that a muscle can transmit to a joint depends on the length of the associated lever arm. This depends on the perpendicular distance from the muscle and its tendon to the center of rotation (= *force arm*) and is opposed by the force of the *load arm*. In the case of the elbow joint in **a**, the load arm is the distance from the joint axis (center of rotation) to the load. The *magnitude of each of the three active forces* is determined by multiplying the force by the force arm and the load by the load arm. This product is called the *torque* (= moment of rotational force) because the active forces produce a rotational movement of the associated lever. If the product of the load times the load arm equals the product of the force times the force arm, both torques are identical and the joint is at rest. The lever in **a** is classified as a *one-arm lever* because the muscular force and load act *on the same side* – in this case to the left of the center of joint rotation. The lever in **b** is a *two-arm lever* because the muscular force acts to the left of the center of joint rotation while the force of the body weight acts to the right of the joint center.

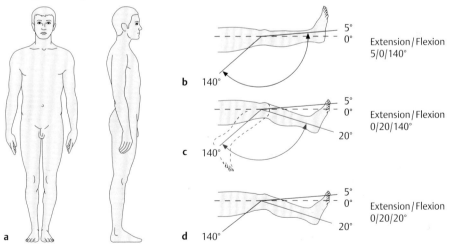

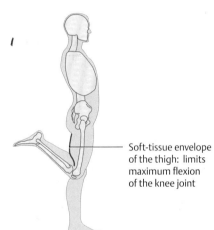

F Constraints to joint motion

The range of joint motion depends not only on the shape of the bony joint members (see **D**, left) but also on the muscles, ligaments, and soft-tissue envelope that surround the joint. Accordingly, all of these factors determine the total range of joint motion:

a Bony constraint
b Muscular constraint
c Ligamentous constraint
d Soft-tissue constraint

G The neutral-zero method

The "neutral-zero method" is a standardized method for measuring the range of joint motion.

a Zero-degree starting position, viewed from the anterior and lateral aspects.
b Range of motion of a normal knee joint.
c Limitation of motion caused by a flexion contracture.
d Ankylosis of the knee joint in 20° of flexion.

5.1 The Skeletal Muscles

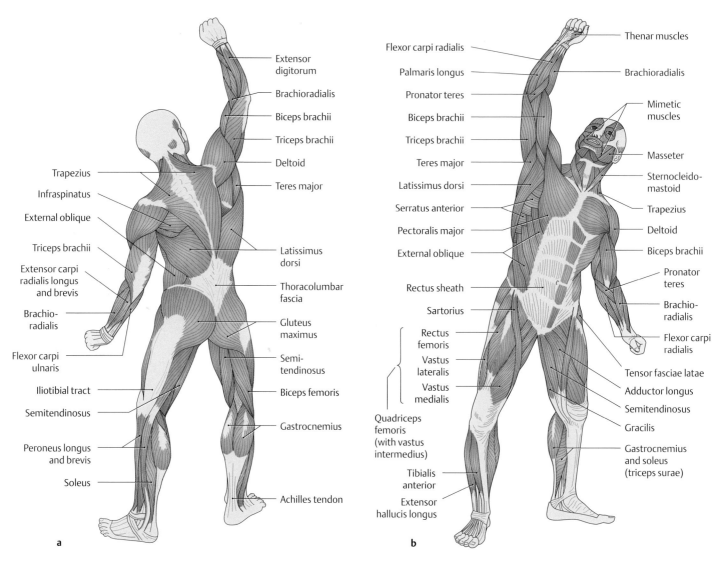

A Postural muscles and muscles of movement
a Posterolateral view, **b** anterolateral view (drawings made from a Somso model).

B Postural muscles and muscles of movement: characteristics and examples

The voluntary skeletal muscles are classified functionally into two broad groups: postural muscles (tonic muscles) and muscles of movement (phasic muscles).

	Postural muscles (red muscles)	Muscles of movement (white muscles)
Charac-teristics:	• Phylogenetically older • Predominantly slow-twitch fibers (type 1 fibers, approximately 100 ms) • Function best in endurance • Fatigue slowly • Large motor units • Rich in myoglobin • Abundant mitochondria • Energy derived from oxidative (aerobic) metabolism • Little glycogen (PAS-negative) • Relatively highly vascularized • Prone to shortening (increased resting tonus) and require regular stretching	• Phylogenetically more recent • Predominantly fast-twitch fibers (type 2 fibers, approximately 30 ms) • Brief periods of intense activity • Fatigue more rapidly • Small motor units • Scant myoglobin • Few mitochondria • Energy derived mainly from anaerobic glycolysis • Abundant glycogen (PAS-positive) • Much smaller capillary supply • Prone to atrophy and require regular strengthening
Examples:	Intercostal muscles, masticatory muscles, trapezius (descending part), hamstrings, iliopsoas, adductors, rectus femoris, soleus, erector spinae (mainly the cervical and lumbar part)	Biceps brachii, vastus lateralis and medialis, tibialis anterior, serratus anterior, gluteus maximus, gastrocnemius

Studies have shown that athletes who engage in sports involving intense bursts of muscular activity (e.g., sprinters) have more white (fast-twitch) fibers, while endurance athletes (e.g., marathon runners) have more red (slow-twitch) fibers (Pette and Staron 2001).

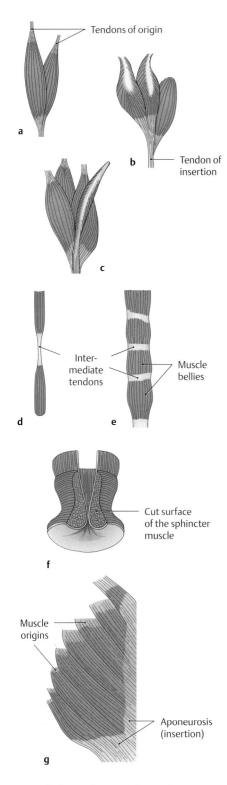

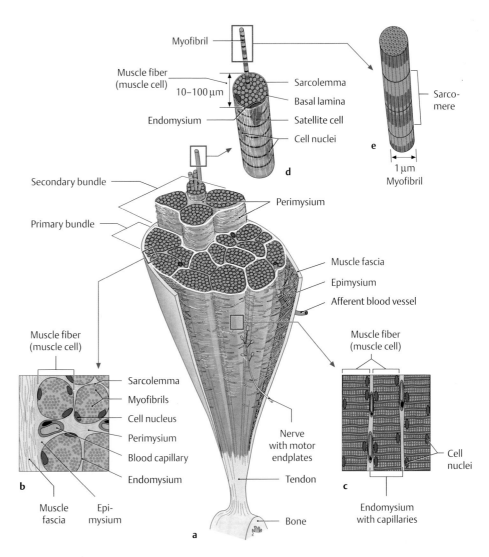

D Structure of a skeletal muscle
a Cross section of a skeletal muscle.
b Detail from **a** (cross section).
c Detail from **a** (longitudinal section).

d Structure of a muscle fiber (= muscle cell).
e Structure of a myofibril.

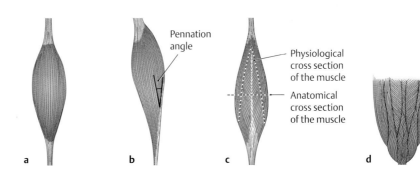

C Morphological forms of muscles
a Two heads = bicipital
(e.g., the biceps brachii).
b Three heads = tricipital
(e.g., the triceps surae).
c Four heads = quadricipital
(e.g., the quadriceps femoris).
d Two bellies = digastric
(e.g., the digastric muscle).
e Multiple bellies = multigastric
(e.g., the rectus abdominis).
f Radial (e.g., the external anal sphincter).
g Flat (e.g., the external oblique).

E Arrangement of muscle fibers and the pennation angle
Muscle fibers may have a parallel arrangement or may show varying degrees of obliquity, or pennation, at their attachment.
a Muscle with parallel fibers (fusiform muscle), **b** unipennate muscle, **c** bipennate muscle, **d** multipennate muscle.
In contrast to parallel muscles, whose fibers are approximately parallel to the "line of pull" of the tendon, pennate muscles converge toward the tendon at a certain angle called the *pennation angle*. While the muscle fibers are shorter due to their oblique attachment to the tendon, their total physiological cross section is increased (see **c**) because more muscle fibers can radiate into the tendon at once. This increased total cross section also enables the muscle to generate more force. The more complex the pennation pattern of the muscle, the greater the total physiological cross section and the greater the force the muscle can exert.
Note: The physiological cross section is perpendicular to the cross sections of the muscle fibers, whereas the anatomical cross section is measured at the thickest part of the muscle.

41

5.2 The Tendons and Mechanisms That Assist Muscle Function

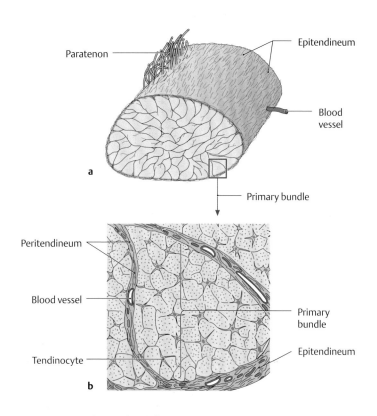

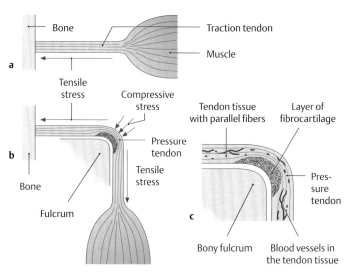

A Structure of a tendon (after Kristic)

a The tendon is connected to its surroundings by the loose, richly vascularized paratenon.

b Detail from **a**: The individual primary bundles are surrounded by peritendineum and are grouped into the actual tendon by the epitendineum. The function of a tendon is to transmit force from the muscle to the bone.

B Pressure tendons and traction tendons

a Traction tendons are subject to tensile stresses and consist of strong connective tissue with parallel fibers.

b Pressure tendons are strained by pressure and change their direction by running around the bone (unlike traction tendons). They consist of fibrocartilage on the side in contact with the bone, which acts as a fulcrum.

c Detail from **b**: The fibrocartilage layer in the compressed area, unlike the strong connective tissue in a traction tendon, is not vascularized.

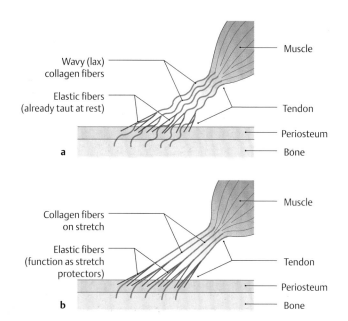

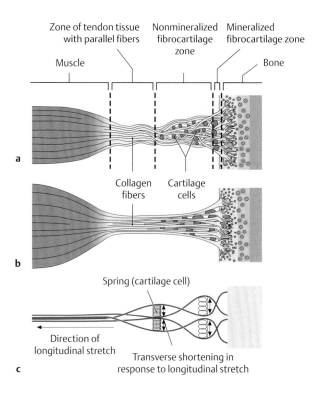

C Structure and function of a periosteal diaphyseal tendon insertion

a Tendon in the lax condition.

b Tendon on stretch.

D Structure and function of a chondral apophyseal tendon insertion

a Tendon in the lax condition (muscle relaxed).

b Tendon on stretch (muscle contracted).

c The principle of stretch protection: Cartilage cells in the nonmineralized fibrocartilage zone act like taut springs to resist transverse shortening.

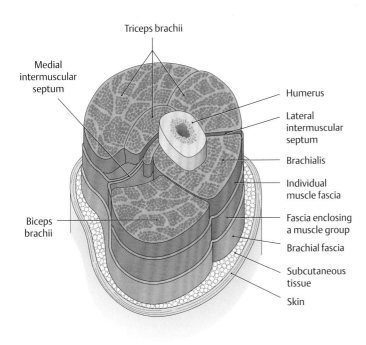

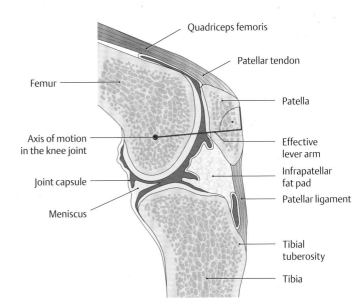

E Muscle fasciae

Proximal view. Cross section through the middle third of the right arm. Muscle fasciae (fibrous sheaths enclosing muscle) are composed of tough collagenous connective tissue. They help to maintain the shape and position of muscles and permit adjacent muscles or muscle groups to glide past each other with relatively little friction (less friction means less loss of force).

F Structure of a tendon sheath (synovial sheath)

Tendon sheaths serve to protect and facilitate the gliding of tendons that run directly on bone. The wall structure of the sheath, consisting of an outer fibrous membrane and an inner synovial membrane, resembles that of a joint capsule. The inner layer of the synovial membrane is firmly attached to the tendon, while its outer layer is attached to the fibrous membrane of the tendon sheath. The space between the two layers is filled with synovial fluid. The mesotendineum (sometimes referred to as *vincula brevia* and *longa* in different locations) transmits blood vessels to the tendon.

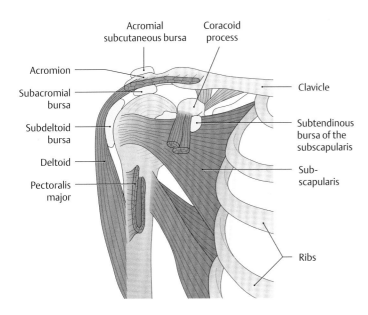

G Synovial bursae in the shoulder region

Right shoulder viewed from the anterior aspect, with some of the muscles removed. Bursae are pouchlike structures of varying size, usually flattened, that contain synovial fluid. Their wall structure is similar to that of a joint capsule. The bursae may become inflamed (*bursitis*), causing severe pain.

H Functional significance of sesamoid bones

Sagittal section through a knee joint. Sesamoid bones are bones that are embedded in tendons and protect the tendons from excessive friction. Their occurrence is variable, so everyone does not have an equal number of sesamoid bones. Their main functional role is to *lengthen the effective lever arm of a mus*cle, increasing its mechanical efficiency. The diagram illustrates this principle for the patella, which is the largest sesamoid bone in the body. The patella significantly lengthens the effective lever arm, represented by a perpendicular line from the joint axis to the tendon of insertion of the quadriceps femoris.

6.1 Overview of the Human Cardiovascular System

A Schematic representation of the circulatory system

Special circulatory organs are needed to transport and distribute the blood, ensuring that it is made accessible to all the cells in the body. These organs consist of the heart and vascular system (blood vessels and lymphatics). The **system of blood vessels** consists of arteries, capillaries, and veins. The *arteries* carry the blood from the heart and distribute it throughout the body. The *veins* return the blood to the heart. The exchange of gases, nutrients, and waste products takes place in the *capillary* region. All blood vessels leading away from the heart are called arteries and all vessels leading toward the heart are called veins, regardless of their oxygen content (the umbilical vein, for example, carries oxygen-rich blood). The blood flow in this closed vascular system is maintained by the **pumping action of the heart**. The **lymphatic system** runs parallel to the venous system. It originates with blind-ended vessels in the capillary region, collects the *extracellular* fluid that is deposited there, and returns it to the venous blood through *lymphatic vessels*. *Lymph nodes* are interposed along these pathways to filter the lymph. Functionally, the circulatory system is divided into two main circuits:

- **The pulmonary circulation:** *Deoxygenated venous blood* from the upper and lower body regions is returned through the superior and inferior vena cava to the *right* atrium. It then enters the *right* ventricle, which pumps it through the pulmonary arteries to the lungs.
- **The systemic circulation:** *Oxygen-enriched blood* from the lungs returns through the pulmonary veins to the *left* atrium. From the left atrium it enters the *left* ventricle, which pumps the blood through the aorta into the systemic circulation. A special part of the systemic circuit is the **portal circulation,** which includes two successive capillary beds. *Before* venous blood returns to the inferior vena cava from the capillary beds of the unpaired abdominal organs (stomach, bowel, pancreas, and spleen), it is carried by the portal vein to the capillary bed of the liver. This ensures that nutrient-rich blood from the digestive organs undergoes numerous filtering and metabolic processes in the liver before it is returned to the inferior vena cava via the hepatic veins.

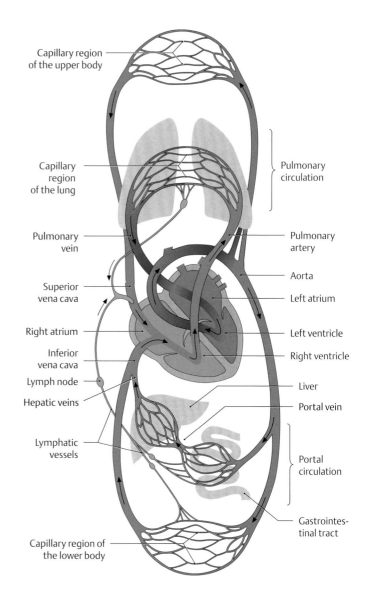

B Basic functional diagram of the circulatory system

(no distinction is made between the systemic and pulmonary systems in the diagram; after Klinke, Silbernagl)

Blood is transported through the circulatory system along a *pressure gradient* created by the different pressure levels in the arterial and venous systems. While the average blood pressure in the *arterial high-pressure system* is approximately 100 mmHg (13.3 N), the pressure in the *venous low-pressure system* generally does not exceed 20 mmHg (2.6 N). The two systems meet in the capillary region of the terminal vascular bed, where metabolic exchange takes place. When the heart expels blood during systole, the *arteries surrounding the heart* (*elastic*-type arteries) can temporarily expand to accommodate the ejected blood volume. During the diastole that follows, the vessel lumen undergoes an *elastic recoil* that transforms the intermittently ejected blood volumes into continuous flow. *Arteries distant from the heart* (*muscular*-type arteries) can actively expand (*vasodilation*) and contract (*vasoconstriction*), providing a very effective means of controlling vascular resistance and regulating local blood flow. The veins are also called *capacitance vessels* because of the high volume of blood contained within the veins. They can accommodate 80 % of the total blood volume and thus serve an important reservoir function.

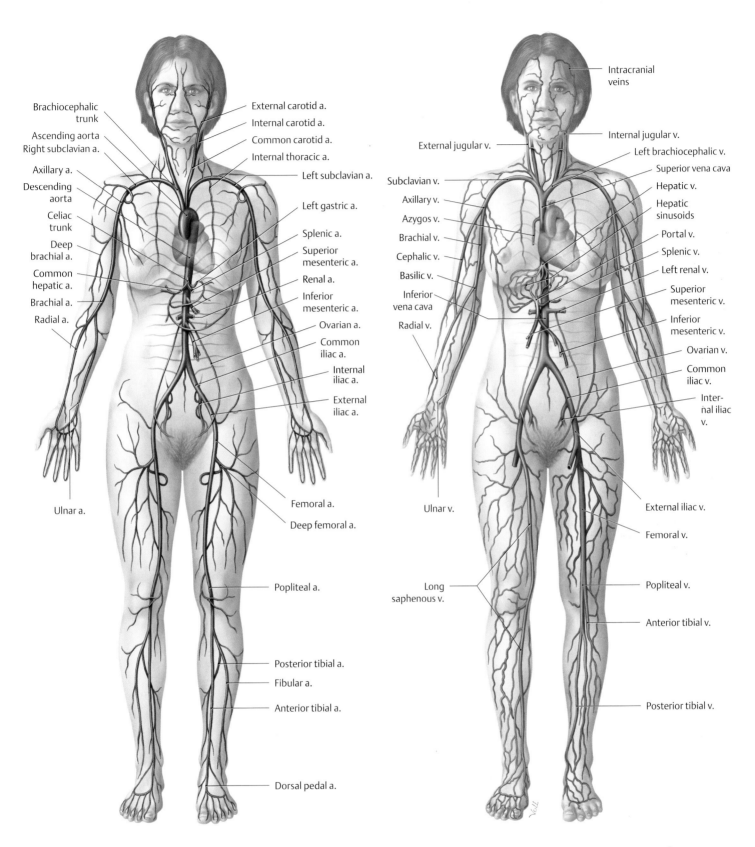

Brachiocephalic trunk

Ascending aorta
Right subclavian a.

Axillary a.

Descending aorta

Celiac trunk

Deep brachial a.

Common hepatic a.

Brachial a.

Radial a.

Ulnar a.

External carotid a.

Internal carotid a.

Common carotid a.

Internal thoracic a.

Left subclavian a.

Left gastric a.

Splenic a.

Superior mesenteric a.

Renal a.

Inferior mesenteric a.

Ovarian a.

Common iliac a.

Internal iliac a.

External iliac a.

Femoral a.

Deep femoral a.

Popliteal a.

Posterior tibial a.

Fibular a.

Anterior tibial a.

Dorsal pedal a.

External jugular v.

Subclavian v.

Axillary v.

Azygos v.

Brachial v.

Cephalic v.

Basilic v.

Inferior vena cava

Radial v.

Ulnar v.

Long saphenous v.

Intracranial veins

Internal jugular v.

Left brachiocephalic v.

Superior vena cava

Hepatic v.

Hepatic sinusoids

Portal v.

Splenic v.

Left renal v.

Superior mesenteric v.

Inferior mesenteric v.

Ovarian v.

Common iliac v.

Internal iliac v.

External iliac v.

Femoral v.

Popliteal v.

Anterior tibial v.

Posterior tibial v.

C Overview of the principal arteries in the systemic circulation

D Overview of the principal veins in the systemic circulation

The venous system is comprised of superficial veins, deep veins, and also perforator veins, which interconnect the superficial and deep venous systems.

Note the portal circulation (portal vein), which carries nutrient-rich blood (shown here in purple) from the digestive organs directly to the liver (compare with the left side of **A**).

6.2   The Structure of Arteries and Veins

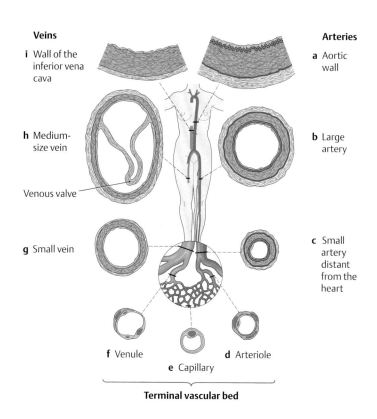

Veins

i Wall of the inferior vena cava

h Medium-size vein

Venous valve

g Small vein

f Venule

e Capillary

d Arteriole

Terminal vascular bed

Arteries

a Aortic wall

b Large artery

c Small artery distant from the heart

A Structure of the blood vessels in different regions of the systemic circulation

Consistent with changing demands, the vessels in different regions of the systemic circulation (high- and low-pressure systems, microcirculation) show significant local structural differences despite a basic similarity in the arrangement of their wall layers. Whereas a relatively high internal pressure prevails throughout the *arterial system*, and the arterial vessels have correspondingly thick walls, the *veins* have a considerably lower intravascular pressure, resulting in thinner walls and larger lumi-

B Organization of the blood vessel system

Arteries (high-pressure system = supply function)

- Elastic-type arteries
- Muscular-type arteries

Terminal vascular bed (microcirculation = exchange function)

- Arterioles
- Capillaries
- Venules

Veins (low-pressure system = reservoir function)

- Small and medium-size veins (with valves)
- Large venous trunks

	Arteries		Terminal vascular bed		Veins	
	Aorta	Small artery	Arteriole	Venule	Vein	Vena cava
Wall thickness (w)	2.5 mm	1 mm	20 μm	5 μm	0.5 mm	1.5 mm
Luminal radius (r_i)	12.5 mm	2 mm	20 μm	20 μm	2.5 mm	15 mm

nal diameters than in the arteries. In the terminal vascular bed, on the other hand, the vessel wall layers are reduced to permit the exchange of gases, fluids, and other substances.
a–c Arteries, **d–f** terminal vascular bed, **g–i** veins. **a** Close-up view of the aortic wall (elastic-type artery). **b,c** Large and small arteries distant from the heart (muscular-type arteries). **d** Arteriole. **e** Capillary. **f** Venule. **g,h** Small and medium-size veins (some with venous valves). **i** Close-up view of the wall of the inferior vena cava.

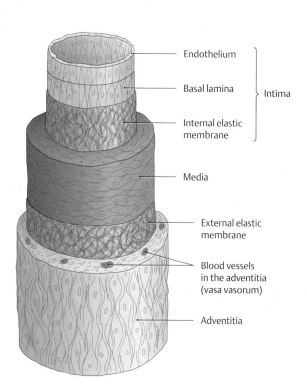

Endothelium

Basal lamina

Internal elastic membrane

Intima

Media

External elastic membrane

Blood vessels in the adventitia (vasa vasorum)

Adventitia

C Wall structure of a blood vessel, illustrated for a muscular-type artery

The wall of a blood vessel basically consists of *three layers*: the *intima*, *media*, and *adventitia*. The three-layered structure is clearly apparent in the walls of arteries and is less conspicuous in veins (see **D**).

- The **intima** consists of a layer of spindle-shaped endothelial cells that are aligned along the vessel axis and rest upon a basement membrane and a thin layer of subendothelial connective tissue. In muscular-type arteries, the intima is consistently separated from the media by an internal elastic membrane.
- The **media** consists of an approximately circular arrangement of smooth muscle cells, elastic and collagenous fibers, and proteoglycans. Muscular-type arteries may have an external elastic membrane that separates the media from the adventitia.
- The **adventitia**, like the intima, is composed of longitudinally aligned elements, mostly connective tissue. The adventitia of veins may additionally contain smooth muscle. The adventitia transmits autonomic nerves to the muscle of the vessel wall and, especially in larger vessels, it also transmits the vasa vasorum, which supply blood to the outer third of the vessel wall.

Specific functions can be assigned to all three layers: The intima is concerned with the exchange of gases, fluids, and other substances through the vessel wall. The media regulates blood flow, and the adventitia integrates the blood vessel into its surroundings.

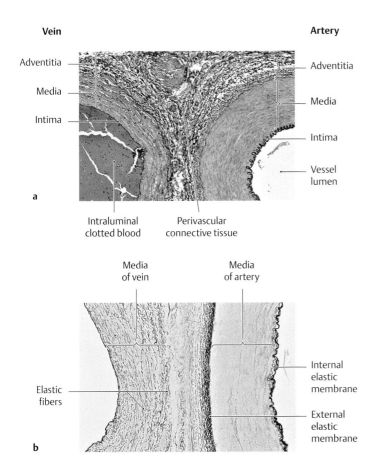

Vein — **Artery**

Adventitia

Media

Intima

a

Intraluminal clotted blood — Perivascular connective tissue

Adventitia

Media

Intima

Vessel lumen

Media of vein — Media of artery

Elastic fibers

Internal elastic membrane

External elastic membrane

b

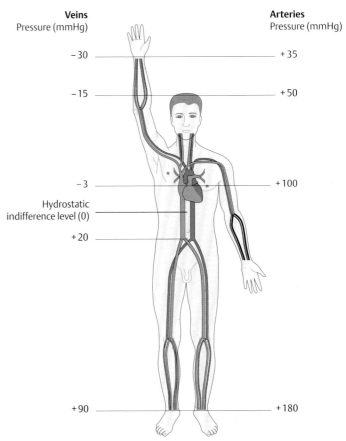

Veins
Pressure (mmHg)

Arteries
Pressure (mmHg)

− 30 —— + 35

− 15 —— + 50

− 3 —— + 100

Hydrostatic indifference level (0)

+ 20

+ 90 —— + 180

D Differences in the wall structure of arteries and veins

Wall sections from a muscular-type artery and an accompanying vein. Comparison of tissue cross sections treated with different stains. **a** H&E-resorcin-fuchsin stain of the posterior tibial artery and vein. **b** Resorcin-fuchsin stain of the femoral artery and vein.

Note the characteristic structural differences in the media: While the arterial media consists of densely packed layers of smooth muscle cells, the venous media contains a far greater amount of connective tissue elements (collagenous and elastic fibers), giving it a much looser structure. The veins also lack a conspicuous layered structure and an internal elastic membrane (from Lüllmann-Rauch: *Histologie*, 1st ed. Thieme, Stuttgart 2003).

E Arterial and venous pressure changes in the standing position

Changing from a recumbent to a standing position radically alters the pressure relationships in the circulatory system. The hydrostatic effects of this change cause the pressure to rise sharply in the lower parts of the body, while the pressures in the upper body decrease (the pressures remain unchanged at the "hydrostatic indifference level" just below the diaphragm). Along with the hydrostatic pressure changes, approximately 500 mL of blood volume is shifted into the lower limb veins. This rise of venous pressure greatly increases the transmural pressure in the lower limb veins, while the pressure in the head and neck veins may fall so low that the veins collapse. This explains why analogous veins in the lower and upper body regions have wall layers of different thickness, i.e., the veins on the dorsum of the foot are much more muscular than on the dorsum of the hand. The wall of the inferior vena cava, however, is paper-thin due to the low venous pressures at that level.

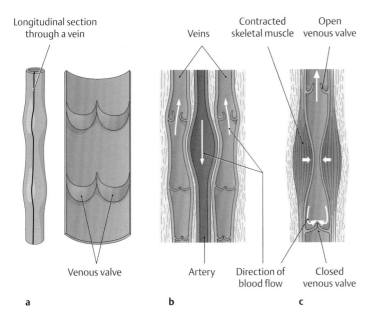

Longitudinal section through a vein

Veins

Contracted skeletal muscle

Open venous valve

Venous valve

Artery

Direction of blood flow

Closed venous valve

a — b — c

F Venous return to the heart

The following factors promote the return of venous blood to the heart: **a** opening and closing of the venous valves, **b** arteriovenous coupling (the pulse wave in the artery is transmitted to the accompanying vein), and **c** the muscle pump.

Venous return is also aided by the "suction effect" of the heart, i.e., the negative pressure produced when the valve plane moves toward the cardiac apex during systole. A lack of muscular movement due to prolonged standing or sitting, for example, can cause the damming back of venous blood, leading to a raised intravascular pressure and incompetence of the venous valves. This can result in edema, varicose veins, and circulatory impairment.

6.3   The Terminal Vascular Bed

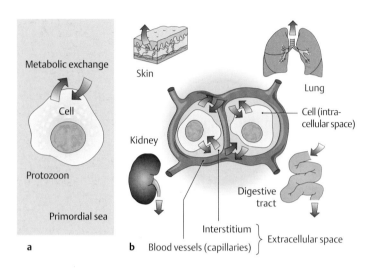

a   **b**

A   The milieu in which a cell lives (after Silbernagl, Despopoulos)
a   Protozoan: The first single-cell organisms lived in an environment, the primordial sea, which provided a milieu of constant composition. The internal and external milieu were the same, and so neither of them changed during metabolism.
b   Human: The cells of a multicellular organism are bathed by extracellular fluid, whose volume is substantially smaller than the intracellular volume. The extra- and intracellular fluids also have a different composition. In this situation the internal milieu would change very quickly if the intercellular space (interstitium) were not linked via the bloodstream to organs such as the lung, kidneys, and digestive tract, which absorb nutrients and excrete metabolic products. Nutrients absorbed from the bowel are distributed to the cells of the various organs (interstitium of the capillary beds) via the bloodstream. The blood also transports the metabolic products of the cells to the organs that are responsible for their excretion (e.g., the lungs and kidneys).

B   Characteristics of different vascular regions (after Silbernagl, Despopoulos)
The terminal vascular bed is the site of the microcirculation and therefore is the site where gases, fluids, and other substances are exchanged. It consists of:

- an *afferent arterial limb* (precapillary arterioles),
- the *capillary bed* itself, and
- an *efferent venous limb* (postcapillary venules).

The smallest vessels, the capillaries, consist only of an endothelial layer and a basal lamina to which pericytes may be externally attached (contrast with the more complex structure of large vessels, p. 46). Owing to the extensive branching of the vessels in the capillary bed, the total vascular cross section is greatly increased (approximately 800 times) while the flow velocity is correspondingly reduced (from 50 cm/s in the aorta to 0.05 cm/s in the capillaries). With an average capillary length of 0.5 mm, a time of approximately 1 second is available for metabolic exchange. The increased vascular resistance in the arterioles and capillaries caused by contact of the blood with the large endothelial surface area (increased friction) lowers the blood pressure and eliminates pressure spikes. Thus the capillaries provide ideal conditions for exchange processes to occur between the blood and the interstitial fluid that bathes the body's cells.

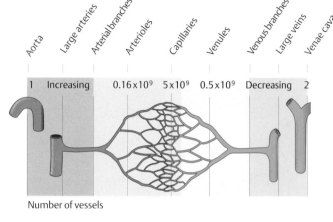

Number of vessels

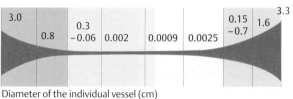

Diameter of the individual vessel (cm)

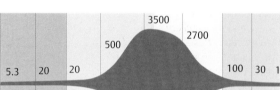

Total cross-sectional area (cm²)

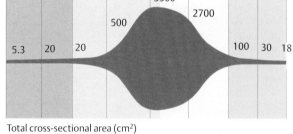

Flow velocity (cm/s)

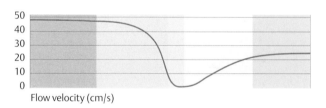

Intravascular pressure (mmHg)

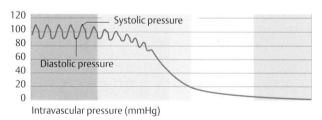

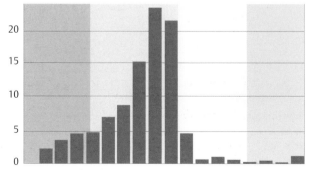

Percentage of total resistance

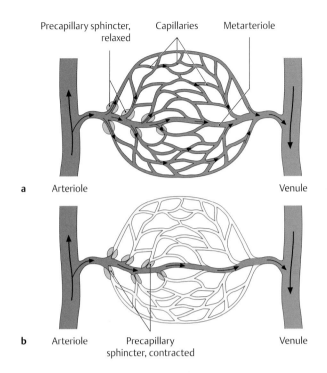

a Arteriole — Venule

b Arteriole — Precapillary sphincter, contracted — Venule

C Blood flow in the capillary bed

a Sphincter relaxed, **b** sphincter contracted.

Precapillary sphincters, with their circular array of muscle cells, are located at the junction of the metarterioles and capillaries and regulate blood flow within the capillary network. When the sphincters contract, the branching capillaries are closed and the capillary bed is unperfused except for the metarterioles (e.g., only about 25–35% of all capillaries are perfused under resting conditions). The arterioles and venules may also be interconnected by shunts called *arteriovenous anastomoses*.

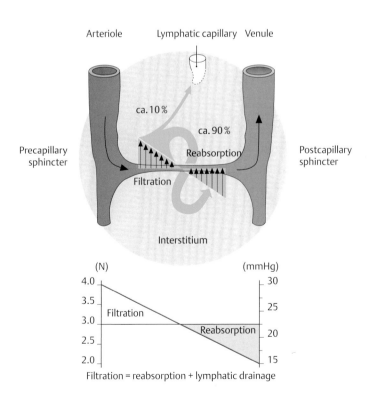

Filtration = reabsorption + lymphatic drainage

E Mechanism of fluid exchange in a capillary (after Silbernagl, Despopoulos)

Fluid exchange between capillaries and the surrounding tissue (interstitium) is regulated by a changing pressure gradient between the blood pressure in the capillaries (hydrostatic pressure) and the intra-

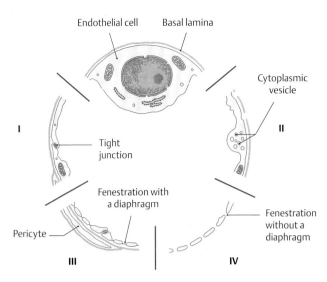

D Different forms of capillary endothelial cells (scheme of ultrastructural features)

Capillaries range from 5 to 15 μm in diameter and consist of endothelial cells, basal lamina, and external pericytes. Pericytes have various properties and functions, including a role in vascular development and angiogenesis. The individual endothelial cells are connected to one another by adhesion contacts, tight junctions, and gap junctions, largely preventing any metabolic exchange between individual endothelial cells. The endothelia of different capillaries have varying degrees of permeability, and several types of endothelium are distinguished on that basis:

I Closed endothelium without fenestrations and with a continuous basal lamina (e.g., nervous system)
II Closed endothelium with pinocytotic activity (e.g., cardiac and skeletal muscle)
III Endothelial cells fenestrated by a diaphragm (e.g., gastrointestinal tract)
IV Endothelial cells with intercellular gaps (large fenestrations) and without a continuous basal lamina (e.g., liver)

vascular colloid osmotic pressure. The driving force behind the fluid exchange is the hydrostatic blood pressure. The pressure at the arterial end of the capillary is 35 mmHg (= 4.6 N), which is 10 mmHg *higher* than the colloid osmotic pressure of approximately 25 mmHg (= 3.3 N). This positive pressure differential makes it possible for fluid as well as dissolved particles to filter out of the capillaries and into the surrounding tissue. These relationships are reversed at the venous end of the capillary—there, the hydrostatic blood pressure falls to approximately 15 mmHg (2.0 N) while the colloid osmotic pressure remains essentially unchanged at about 25 mmHg. As a result of this, the hydrostatic pressure on the *venous side of the capillary* is 10 mmHg *lower* than the colloid osmotic pressure (15–25 = –10 mmHg), causing fluid with its solute particles to flow back into the vessel (*reabsorption*).

Of the 20 liters of fluid that leave the capillaries each day, only about 18 liters (90%) are reabsorbed. Approximately 2 liters (10%) of the filtered volume are removed by lymphatic vessels in the form of lymph. If this fluid exchange does not occur in the manner described, edema may develop (i.e., a persistent accumulation of fluids in the interstitium). The reasons for this may include an *elevated hydrostatic pressure* (due to blood pooling on the venous side of the capillaries) or a *decreased colloid osmotic pressure* (due to a decrease in plasma proteins). In both cases there is an imbalance of fluid exchange, allowing fluid to accumulate in the tissue, known as edema.

7.1   The Human Lymphatic System

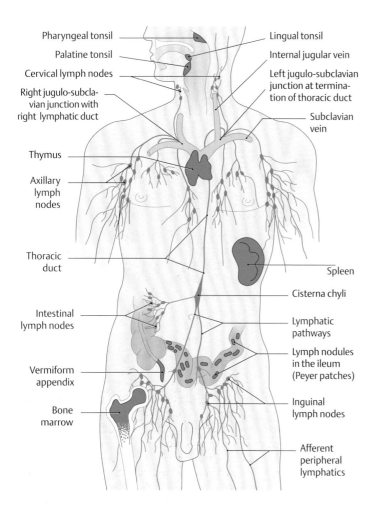

Pharyngeal tonsil
Palatine tonsil
Cervical lymph nodes
Right jugulo-subcla-vian junction with right lymphatic duct
Thymus
Axillary lymph nodes
Thoracic duct
Intestinal lymph nodes
Vermiform appendix
Bone marrow

Lingual tonsil
Internal jugular vein
Left jugulo-subclavian junction at termina-tion of thoracic duct
Subclavian vein
Spleen
Cisterna chyli
Lymphatic pathways
Lymph nodes in the ileum (Peyer patches)
Inguinal lymph nodes
Afferent peripheral lymphatics

A The human lymphatic system

This system includes the lymphatic vessels and the lymphatic organs (immune organs, see **B**). The **lymphatic vascular system** runs parallel to the venous system and performs several functions:

* Its primary function is to clear the interstitial spaces of tissue fluid and substances that cannot be reabsorbed in the venous capillary bed. The composition of the lymph varies in different regions and is similar to that of the surrounding interstitial fluid.
* It carries away food lipids (chylomicrons) that are absorbed in the bowel.
* It returns lymphocytes from the lymphatic organs to the blood.

The lymphatic vascular system consists of:

* *lymphatic capillaries*, which begin peripherally as blind-ended vessels;
* the *lymphatic vessels* and interposed *lymph nodes*; and
* the *major lymphatic trunks* (thoracic duct and right lymphatic duct).

The lymphatic capillaries collect fluid from the interstitium and trans-port it via the lymphatic vessels and lymph nodes to the major lymphatic trunks. The fluid reenters the venous system from these trunks at the junctions of the left and right subclavian and internal jugular veins. The lymph drained from three body quadrants enters the left jugulo-subcla-vian venous junction, while only lymph from the right upper quadrant enters the right jugulo-subclavian venous junction.

The **lymphatic organs** are part of the specific immune system and, as such, are situated at likely portals of entry for infectious microorgan-isms. The spleen is the only immune organ that is directly integrated into the bloodstream.

B Primary and secondary lymphatic organs

The functions of the lymphatic organs include mounting a specific immune response. A distinction is drawn between primary and second-ary lymphatic organs. The primary lymphatic organs are concerned with the production, maturation, and selection of immune cells. The second-ary lymphatic organs are subsequently populated by the immunocom-petent lymphocytes and are sites for various processes such as antigen presentation, lymphocyte proliferation, and antibody formation.

* **Primary lymphatic organs:**
  – Thymus (selection of T-lymphocytes)
  – Bone marrow (selection of B-lymphocytes)
* **Secondary lymphatic organs:**
  – Spleen
  – Lymph nodes
  – Mucosa-associated lymphatic tissue (MALT) and the pharyngeal lymphatic (Waldeyer's) ring—the pharyngeal, palatine, and lingual tonsils.
  – Bronchus-associated lymphatic tissue (BALT)
  – Gut-associated lymphatic tissue (GALT), such as Peyer plaques and the vermiform appendix

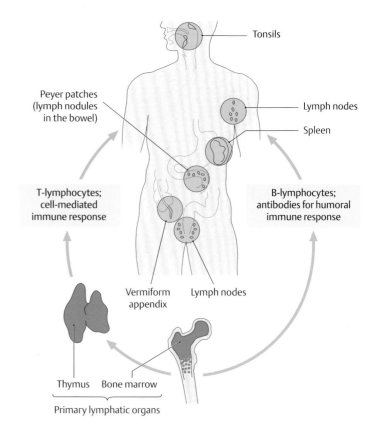

Tonsils
Peyer patches (lymph nodes in the bowel)
Lymph nodes
Spleen
T-lymphocytes; cell-mediated immune response
B-lymphocytes; antibodies for humoral immune response
Vermiform appendix
Lymph nodes
Thymus   Bone marrow
Primary lymphatic organs

C Organization of the lymphatic vascular system (after Kubik)

Three compartments can be distinguished in the lymphatic vascular system based on **topographical** and **functional** criteria:

1. A superficial system → drains the skin and subcutaneous tissue.
2. A deep system → drains lymph from the muscles, joints, tendon sheaths, and nerves.
3. An organ-specific system → drains the organs and shows organ-specific differences.

A system of **perforator vessels** interconnects the superficial and deep systems, conveying lymphatic fluid toward the surface from deeper tissues.

The lymphatic vascular system can be subdivided into *four different regions* based on the **histologic structure of the vessel walls**:

1. Lymphatic capillaries,
2. Precollectors,
3. Collectors,
4. Lymphatic trunks.

Lymphatic capillaries and precollectors are also known as *initial lymphatics*.

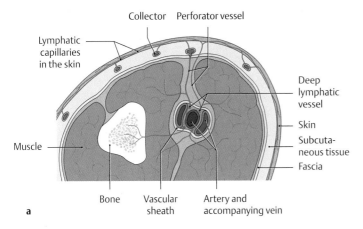

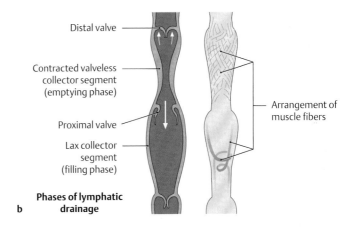

Phases of lymphatic drainage

D Organization and structure of the different lymphatic regions (after Kubik)

a Lymphatics in the skin and muscles.
b Detail from **a**, showing the structure and function of a collector segment.

Both the superficial and deep lymphatics originate with the extremely thin-walled **lymphatic capillaries**, which are approximately 50 μm in diameter. Their endothelium is bounded by an incomplete basal lamina, and they are attached by collagenous "anchoring filaments" to elastic fibers and collagen fibers in their surroundings. The network of lymphatic capillaries opens into larger **precollectors** approximately

100 μm in diameter. Unlike the lymphatic capillaries, these vessels contain valve cusps and their wall is reinforced by a layer of connective tissue. They open into **collectors**, which also contain valves and have a transverse diameter of 150–600 μm. Like the larger lymphatic vessels and the lymphatic trunks, the collectors have a venous-type wall structure divided indistinctly into an intima (endothelium and basement membrane), a smooth-muscle media, and a fibrous adventitia. *Lymph transport* is effected by series of rhythmic contractile waves (10–12/min) that are generated in the smooth-muscle, valveless collector segments. The *direction* of lymph flow is controlled by closing the distal valves and opening the proximal valves of the precollectors and collectors.

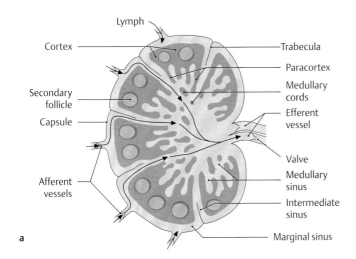

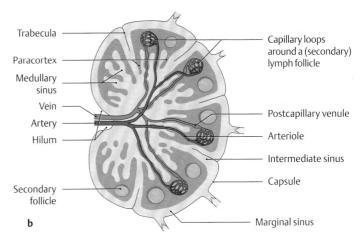

E Structure of a lymph node

a Lymph circulation, **b** blood supply to the lymph node.
Lymph nodes are small filtering stations located in the course of lymphatic vessels and are components of the specific immune response (they contain T- and B-lymphocytes). *Regional lymph nodes* are distinguished from the *collecting lymph nodes* that receive lymph from multiple regional nodes. The lymph enters the lymph node through multiple afferent vessels. As the fluid passes along the various lymph sinuses to the efferent vessels, it comes into contact with the lymph node tissue over a broad surface area. From outside to inside, a lymph node con-

sists of the cortex, paracortex, and medulla. The numerous secondary follicles in the *cortex* form the *B-lymphocyte region*, and the lymphocyte-rich areas between and below the secondary follicles are the *T-lymphocyte regions (paracortex)*. Lymphocytes leave the bloodstream in the high-endothelial postcapillary venules of the T-lymphocyte region; then, after differentiating, they leave the lymph node with the draining lymph via efferent lymph vessels, which often become the afferent vessel of another lymph node of a lymph node group.

7.2 Exocrine and Endocrine Glands

A Development and classification of glands

Glands are epithelial aggregations of highly specialized single cells (goblet cells, multicellular intraepithelial glands) or of larger cell groups that have migrated to deeper levels. Their function is to synthesize and release secretions. Glands fall into two main categories:

- **Exocrine glands** (e.g., salivary glands, sweat glands): These glands release their secretion *externally* to the skin or mucosa, either directly or through excretory ducts.
- **Endocrine glands:** Their secretions (in this case hormonal messengers) are released *internally*, i.e., into the bloodstream, lymphatics, or intercellular spaces. Endocrine glands do not have excretory ducts (see **F** for mechanisms of hormone release). Once released into the bloodstream, the hormones are distributed throughout the body and are transported to their target cells, where they bind to specific receptors and exert their effect.

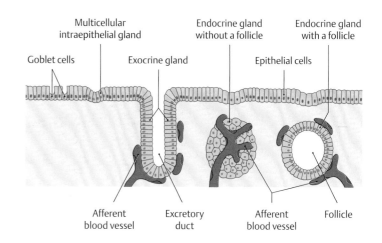

B Mechanisms by which exocrine glands release their secretions

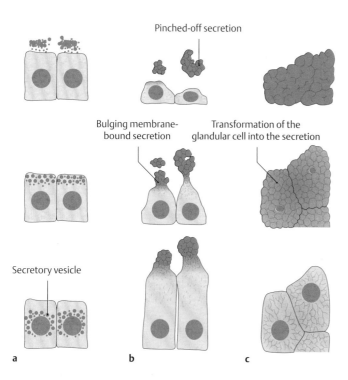

(light-microscopic scale)
a Exocytosis: In this mechanism, the secretion is released *without an enclosing membrane* (merocrine or eccrine secretion). The membrane-bound vesicles containing the secretion fuse with the apical cell membrane and discharge their contents to the outside with no loss of membranous material (the secretory mechanism of most glands, see also **C**).
b Apocytosis: The membrane-bound vesicles form a bulge in the apical cell membrane and are finally *pinched off* by it (apocrine secretion). The pinched-off secretory products are enclosed within a membrane. This mechanism is necessary in the secretion of fats. The membrane encloses the fats and keeps them emulsified (e.g., scent glands, mammary glands).
c Holocytosis: In this mechanism the *entire glandular cell disintegrates and becomes the secretory product* (holocrine secretion). As a result, the glandular cells must be constantly replaced by a basal regenerative cell layer (e.g., sebaceous glands in the skin).

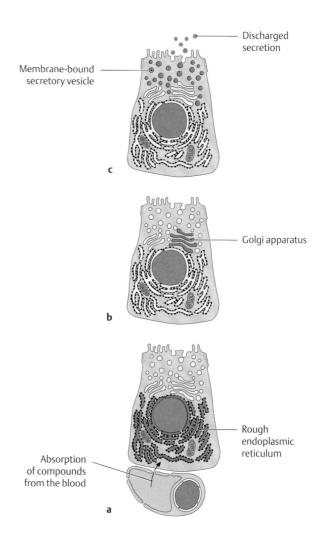

C Production and release of secretions by exocytosis (electron-microscopic scale)

After the glandular cell has absorbed essential compounds from the blood and synthesized necessary materials such as secretory proteins in the rough endoplasmic reticulum (**a**), the secretions are transported by the Golgi apparatus (**b**) to the apical part of the cell, where they are discharged by exocytosis (**c**).

D Principal sites where hormones and hormonelike substances are formed

Hormones are vitally important chemical messengers that enable cells to communicate with one another. Usually, very small amounts of these messengers act on metabolic processes in their target cells. Different hormones can be classified on the basis of their:

- site of formation,
- site of action,
- mechanism of action, or
- chemical structure.

Examples are steroid hormones (e.g., testosterone, aldosterone), amino acid derivatives (e.g., epinephrine, norepinephrine, dopamine, serotonin), peptide hormones (e.g., insulin, glucagon), and fatty acid derivatives (e.g., prostaglandins).

Principal sites of formation	Hormones and hormonelike substances
Classic endocrine hormonal glands	
Pituitary gland (anterior and posterior lobes)	ACTH (adrenocorticotropic hormone, corticotropin) TSH (thyroid-stimulating hormone, thyrotropin) FSH (follicle-stimulating hormone, follitropin) LH (luteinizing hormone, lutropin) STH (somatotropic hormone, somatotropin) MSH (melanocyte-stimulating hormone, melanotropin) PRL (prolactin) ADH (antidiuretic hormone or vasopressin) Oxytocin (formed in the hypothalamus and secreted by the posterior pituitary)
Pineal gland	Melatonin
Thyroid gland	Thyroxine (T_4) and triiodothyronine (T_3)
C cells of the thyroid gland	Calcitonin
Parathyroid glands	Parathormone
Adrenal glands	Mineralocorticoids and glucocorticoids Androgens Epinephrine and norepinephrine
Pancreatic islet cells (Langerhans cells)	Insulin, glucagon, somatostatin, and pancreatic polypeptide
Ovary	Estrogens and progestins
Testis	Androgens (mainly testosterone)
Placenta	Chorionic gonadotropin, progesterone
Hormone-producing tissues and single cells	
Central and autonomic nervous system	Neuronal transmitters
Parts of the diencephalon (e.g., the hypothalamus)	Releasing and inhibitory hormones (liberins and statins)
System of gastrointestinal cells in the GI tract	Gastrin, cholecystokinin, secretin
Cardiac atria	Atrial natriuretic peptide
Kidney	Erythropoietin, renin
Liver	Angiotensinogen, somatomedins
Immune organs	Thymus hormones, cytokins, lymphokines
Tissue hormones	Eicosanoids, prostaglandins, histamine, bradykinin

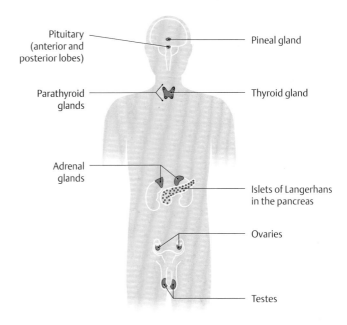

E Overview of the human endocrine glands

The diffuse or disseminated endocrine cell system (individual endocrine cells dispersed among the cells of the surface epithelium) in the gastrointestinal tract is not shown.

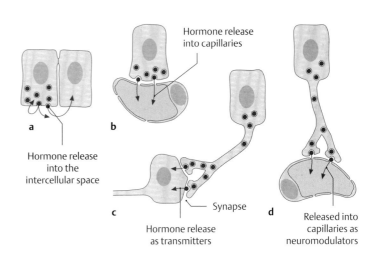

F Types of hormone-mediated information transmission

The endocrine system is closely linked to the autonomic nervous system and immune system in terms of its biological tasks. It functions as a kind of wireless communication system that coordinates the functions of target tissues and target organs, which may be located at distant sites.

a **Paracrine and autocrine secretion:** The hormones are not released into the bloodstream but into the intercellular space. Hence they act only in close proximity to their site of synthesis.

b **Endocrine secretion:** The hormones are synthesized and released into the bloodstream (fenestrated capillaries).

c **Neurocrine secretion:** Hormones of the neurocrine system (neurotransmitters) act in the form of synaptic transmitter substances and are concerned with local information transmission.

d **Neurosecretion:** Hormones or neuromodulators (neurohormones) are produced in specialized nerve cells and released to blood vessels in neurohemal regions (e.g., the pituitary). This enables them to act on distant organs.

8.1 Development of the Central Nervous System (CNS)

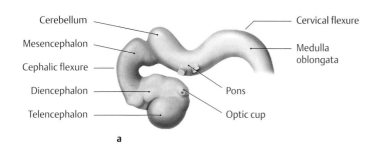

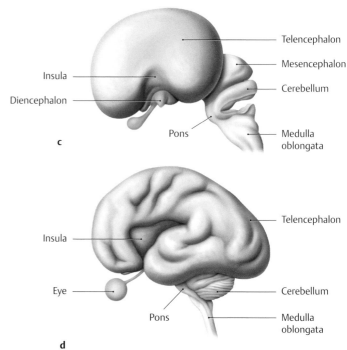

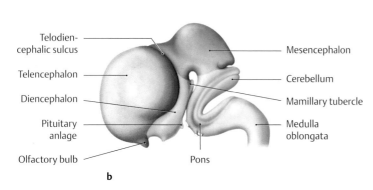

A Development of the brain

a Embryo with a greatest length (GL, see p. 4) of 10 mm, *at the beginning of the second month of development.* Even at this stage we can see the differentiation of the neural tube into segments that will generate various brain regions (see **C**):

- Medulla oblongata (gray)
- Pons (gray)
- Cerebellum (light blue)
- Midbrain (mesencephalon, dark blue)
- Interbrain (diencephalon, yellow)
- Forebrain (telencephalon, red)

Note: The telencephalon grows over all the other brain structures as development proceeds.

b Embryo with a GL of 27 mm, *near the end of the second month of development* (end of the embryonic period). The olfactory bulb is developing from the telencephalon, part of the pituitary anlage (*neurohypophysis*) from the diencephalon.

c Fetus with a GL of 53 mm, in approximately the *third month of development.* By this time the telencephalon has begun to overgrow the other brain areas. The insula is still on the surface but will subsequently be covered by the cerebral hemispheres (compare with **d**).

d Fetus with a crown-rump length (CRL, see p. 4) of 27 cm (270 mm), in approximately the *seventh month of development.* The brain has begun to develop conspicuous gyri and sulci.

B Brain vesicles and their derivatives

The cranial end of the neural tube expands to form three primary brain vesicles: the forebrain (prosencephalon), the midbrain (mesencephalon), and the hindbrain (rhombencephalon). The forebrain (telencephalon) and interbrain (diencephalon) develop from the prosencephalon. The mesencephalon gives rise to the superior and inferior colliculi and related structures. The rhombencephalon differentiates into the pons, cerebellum, and medulla oblongata. The pons and cerebellum are also known collectively as the metencephalon. Some important structures of the adult brain are listed at far right to illustrate the derivatives of the brain vesicles. They can be traced back in the diagram to their developmental precursors.

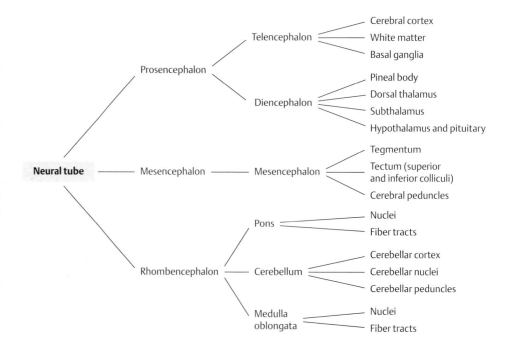

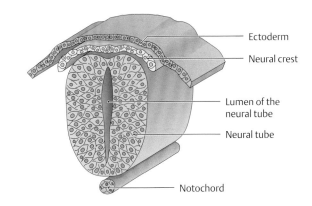

Ectoderm

Neural crest

Lumen of the
neural tube

Neural tube

Notochord

C Development of the nervous system: cross section through the neural tube, neural crest, and dorsal ectoderm

During development, the neural groove folds away from the overlying dorsal ectoderm and closes to form the *neural tube*. Cells migrate from the lateral portions of the neural groove to form the *neural crest* on each side. The *central* nervous system (brain and spinal cord) develops from the neural *tube* while the *peripheral* nervous system develops from derivatives of the neural *crest* (see p. 56).

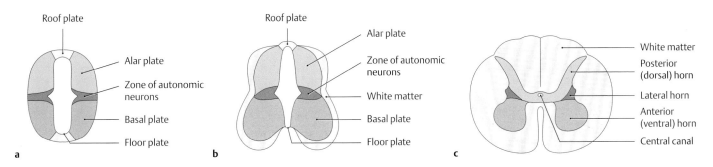

Roof plate

Alar plate

Zone of autonomic
neurons

Basal plate

Floor plate

a

Roof plate

Alar plate

Zone of autonomic
neurons

White matter

Basal plate

Floor plate

b

White matter

Posterior
(dorsal) horn

Lateral horn

Anterior
(ventral) horn

Central canal

c

D Differentiation of the neural tube in the spinal cord region during development

Cross section, cranial view.
a Early neural tube, **b** intermediate stage, **c** adult spinal cord.
The neurons that form in the *basal plate* are *efferent* (motor) neurons, while those that form in the *alar plate* are *afferent* (sensory) neurons.

The area between them—the future thoracic, lumbar and sacral cord—is another zone that gives rise to preganglionic autonomic neurons. The roof plate and floor plate do not form neurons. A knowledge of how these neuron populations are distributed is helpful in understanding the structure of the hindbrain (rhombencephalon, see **E**).

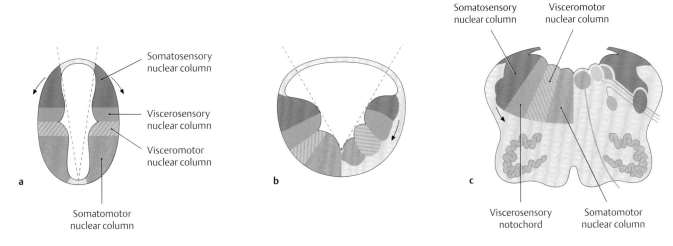

Somatosensory
nuclear column

Viscerosensory
nuclear column

Visceromotor
nuclear column

a

Somatomotor
nuclear column

b

Somatosensory
nuclear column

Visceromotor
nuclear column

c

Viscerosensory
notochord

Somatomotor
nuclear column

E Embryonic migratory movements of neuron populations and their effect on the location of the cranial nerve nuclei

Cross section, cranial view. (Visual aid: If we compare the spinal cord to a book, it would be closed in **a** and open in **b** and **c**.)

a In the **initial stage** the motor neurons are ventral and the sensory neurons are dorsal. The arrows indicate the directions of migration.
b In the **early embryonic stage,** the neurons of the alar plate migrate laterally and ventrally.

c In the adult brain (medulla oblongata and pons, derivatives of the rhombencephalon) we can distinguish **four nuclear columns** (after His and Herrick) that contain functionally distinct cranial nerve nuclei (from medial to lateral):

1. Somatomotor column (lilac)
2. Visceromotor column (orange and green stripes)
3. Viscerosensory column (light blue)
4. Somatosensory column (dark blue)

8.2 Neural Crest Derivatives and the Development of the Peripheral Nervous System (PNS)

A Development of the neural crest cells

At three weeks' development, the notochord induces surface ectoderm in the medial embryonic disk to thicken and form the neural plate (neuroectoderm). The neural plate differentiates to form the primordia of the nervous system. Neural folds are raised on each side of the neural plate, and a median groove develops between them—the neural groove. This groove subsequently deepens and closes to form the neural tube, which sinks below the ectoderm. Portions of the folds that do not contribute to neural tube formation differentiate to form the neural crest. While neural crest cells in the future head region start to migrate even before the neural tube is closed, crest migration in the trunk is delayed until tube closure. Cells destined to form the neural crest detach from the ectoderm at the fusing margins of the neural tube and undergo an *epithelio-mesenchymal transition*, diving into underlying mesoderm, where they begin a long and tortuous migration. As the neural tube differentiates into the central nervous system, migrating neural crest cells settle in different locations and develop into sensory and autonomic ganglia, endocrine glands, melanocytes, cartilage, and other structures (see **B** and **C**) (after Wolpert).

B Main migratory pathways and derivatives of the neural crest

(after Christ and Wachtler)

Neural crest cells originated in different regions have different migration paths and fates. Those from cranial levels contribute to cartilage and bone in the head and neck, and to cranial parasympathetic ganglia (see **C**). Those from thoracolumbar levels do not become skeletal cells, but generate peripheral neurons, endocrine cells, melanocytes, and Schwann cells. This diagram shows the migration of the neural crest cells *in the trunk of the early embryo* (four weeks' development, see p. 7). They follow three **main migratory pathways**:

① Dorsolateral pathway (melanoblasts, which differentiate into melanocytes)
② Ventrolateral pathway (ganglioblasts, which differentiate into sensory nerve cells in the dorsal root [spinal] ganglia)
③ Ventral pathway (cells differentiate into neurons and associated cells of the paravertebral sympathetic ganglia; into chromaffin cells of the adrenal medulla; and into autonomic plexuses in the gastrointestinal tract)

Thus, the neural crest can develop into a variety of seemingly unrelated *nonneuronal* cells as well as peripheral ganglion cells. These unusual characteristics of the neural crest—its pluripotential capacity and wide-ranging migration—have consequences when its differentiation or migration is defective. Disruption of neural crest development may deprive organs of their autonomic innervation (Hirschsprung disease). Tumors derived from neural crest cells tend to be highly malignant and difficult to treat. (See **D**.)

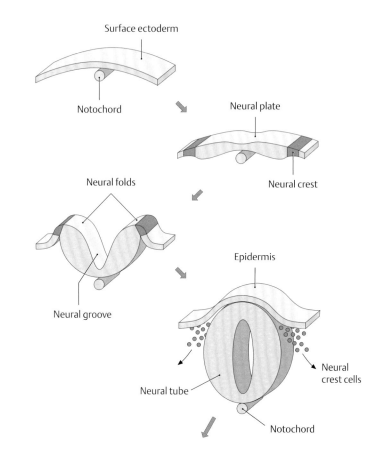

Surface ectoderm
Notochord
Neural plate
Neural folds
Neural crest
Neural groove
Epidermis
Neural tube
Neural crest cells
Notochord

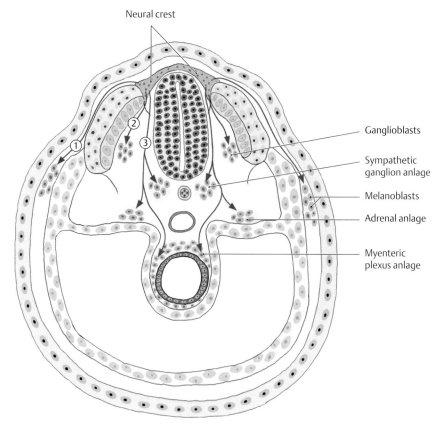

Neural crest
Ganglioblasts
Sympathetic ganglion anlage
Melanoblasts
Adrenal anlage
Myenteric plexus anlage

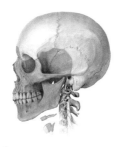
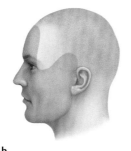

a   b

C Neural crest derivatives in the head and neck region
Besides the equivalents of the structures named in **B** (such as melano-cytes), other structures in the head and neck region that originate from the cranial neural crest include skeletal, cartilaginous, and desmal mus-cles.

a Cranial neural crest derivatives in the adult skeleton: facial bones, hyoid bone, portions of the thyroid cartilage.
b Most of the facial skin is derived from the neural crest.

**D Diseases of neural crest derivatives
(selected examples)**

Neural crest	Disease
Parasympathetic visceral ganglia	Neuroblastoma (malignant childhood tumor)
Enteric nervous system	Hirschsprung disease (aganglionic colon)
Glial cells (Schwann cells, satellite cells)	Neurofibromatosis (Recklinghausen disease)
Melanocytes	Malignant melanoma, albinism
Adrenal medulla	Pheochromocytoma (adrenal gland tumor)
Endocrine cells of the lung and heart	Carcinoids (malignant tumors with endocrine activity)
Parafollicular cells (C cells) of the thyroid gland	Medullary thyroid carcinoma

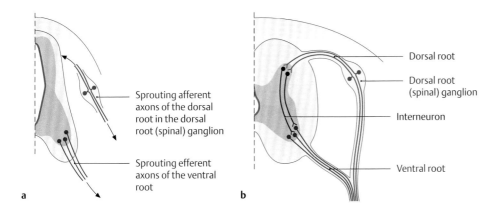

Sprouting afferent axons of the dorsal root in the dorsal root (spinal) ganglion

Sprouting efferent axons of the ventral root

a

Dorsal root

Dorsal root (spinal) ganglion

Interneuron

Ventral root

b

E Development of a peripheral nerve
Afferent (blue) and efferent (red) axons sprout *separately* from the neuron somata during early development (**a**). Primary afferent (sensory) neurons develop in the dorsal root (spinal) ganglion, and primary motor neurons develop from the basal plate of the spinal cord (**b**). *Interneurons* (black), which connect sensory ganglion and motor neurons, develop later.

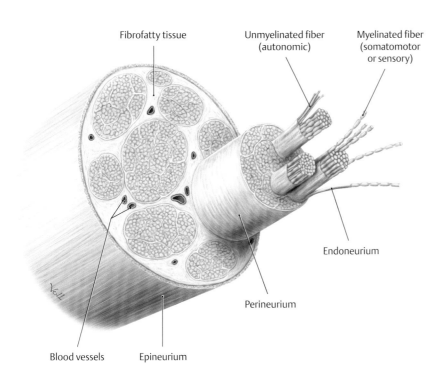

Fibrofatty tissue

Unmyelinated fiber (autonomic)

Myelinated fiber (somatomotor or sensory)

Endoneurium

Perineurium

Blood vessels   Epineurium

F Structure of a peripheral nerve
A peripheral nerve consists entirely of axons (also called neurites) and sheath tissue (Schwann cells, fibroblasts, blood vessels). The axons transmit information either from the periphery to the CNS (*afferents*) or in the opposite direction from the CNS to the periphery (*efferents*). Axons may be myelinated or unmyelinated. The latter have a much slower conduction velocity and are usually fibers of the autonomic nervous system (see p. 73). Among the investing layers of the nerve, the *perineurium* ensheaths the nerve fascicles and provides an important tissue barrier (see p. 71)

57

8.3 Topography and Structure of the Nervous System

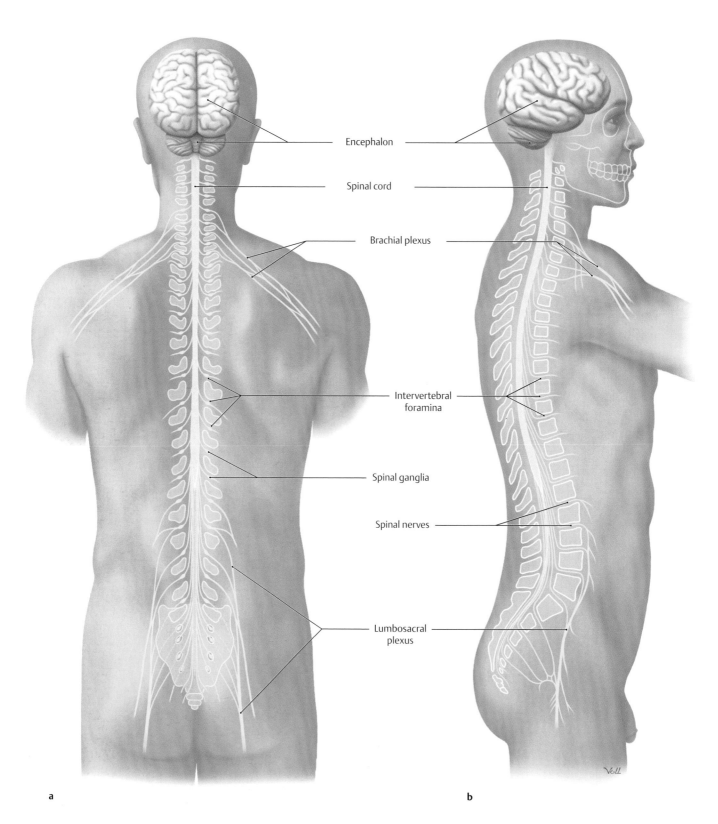

a

b

A Topography of the nervous system
a Posterior view, **b** right lateral view.
The *central nervous system* (CNS), consisting of the brain (encephalon) and spinal cord, is shown in pink. The *peripheral nervous system* (PNS), consisting of nerves and ganglia, is shown in yellow. The nerves arising from the spinal cord leave their bony canal through the *intervertebral foramina* and are distributed to their target organs. The *spinal nerves* are formed in the foramina by the union of their dorsal (posterior) roots and ventral (anterior) roots (see p. 63). The small *spinal ganglion* in the intervertebral foramen appears as a slight swelling of the dorsal root (visible only in the posterior view; its function is described on p. 64).
In the limbs, the ventral rami of the spinal nerves come together to form plexuses. These plexuses then give rise to the peripheral nerves that supply the limbs.

Labels in figure:
Encephalon
Spinal cord
Brachial plexus
Intervertebral foramina
Spinal ganglia
Spinal nerves
Lumbosacral plexus

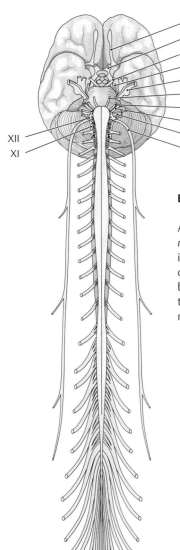

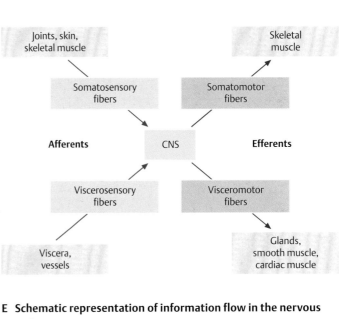

B Spinal nerves and cranial nerves

Anterior view. *Thirty-one pairs of spinal nerves* arise from the spinal cord in the *PNS*, compared with *12 pairs of cranial nerves* that arise from the brain. The cranial nerve pairs are traditionally designated by Roman numerals.

D Terms of location and direction in the CNS

Midsagittal section, right lateral view.
Note two important axes:

① The almost vertical brainstem axis (corresponds approximately to the body axis).
② The horizontal axis through the diencephalon and telencephalon.

Keep these reference axes in mind when using directional terms in the CNS!

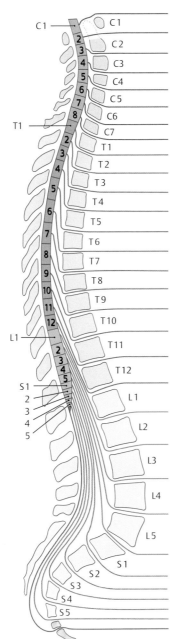

C Location and designation of spinal cord segments in relation to the spinal canal

Right lateral view. The longitudinal growth of the spinal cord lags behind that of the spinal column, with the result that the cord extends only about to the level of the first lumbar vertebra (L 1).
Note that there are seven cervical vertebrae (C 1–C 7) but eight pairs of cervical nerves (C 1–C 8).
The highest pair of cervical nerves exit the spinal canal superior to the first cervical vertebra. The remaining pairs of cervical nerves, like all the other spinal nerve pairs, exit inferior to the cervical vertebral body. The pair of coccygeal nerves (gray) has no clinical importance.

E Schematic representation of information flow in the nervous system

The information encoded in nerve fibers is transmitted either *to the CNS* (brain and spinal cord) or *from the CNS* to the periphery (PNS, including the peripheral parts of the autonomic nervous system, see p. 72). Fibers that carry information to the CNS are called afferent fibers or *afferents* for short; fibers that carry signals away from the CNS are called efferent fibers or *efferents*.

8.4 Cells of the Nervous System

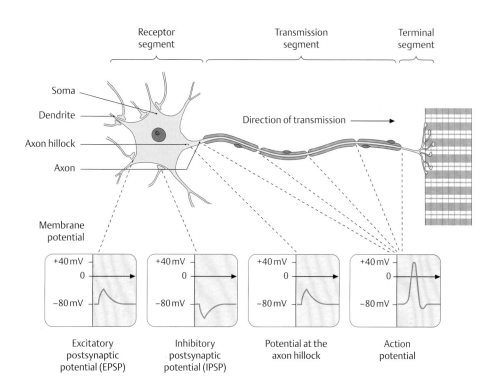

A The nerve cell (neuron)

The neuron is the smallest functional unit of the nervous system. Neurons communicate with other nerve cells through synapses. The *synapses that end at nerve cells* usually do so at dendrites (as seen here). The transmitter substance that is released at the synapses to act on the dendrite membrane may have an *excitatory* or *inhibitory* action, meaning that the transmitter either increases or decreases the local action potential at the nerve cell membrane. All of the excitatory and inhibitory potentials of a nerve cell are integrated in the axon hillock. If the excitatory potentials predominate, the stimulus exceeds the excitation threshold of the neuron, causing the axon to fire (transmit an impulse) according to the all-or-nothing rule.

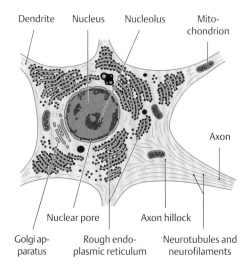

B Electron microscopy of the neuron

Neurons are rich in *rough endoplasmic reticulum* (protein synthesis, active metabolism). This endoplasmic reticulum (known also as *Nissl substance*) is easily demonstrated by light microscopy using cationic dyes, which bind to the phosphodiester backbone of the ribosomal RNAs. The distribution pattern of the Nissl substance is used in neuropathology to evaluate the functional integrity of neurons. Neurotubules and neurofilaments are referred to collectively as *neurofibrils* in light microsopy, as they are too fine to be identified as separate structures under a light microscope. Neurofibrils can be demonstrated in light microscopy by impregnating the nerve tissue with silver salts. This is of interest in neuropathology because the clumping of neurofibrils is an important histological feature of Alzheimer disease.

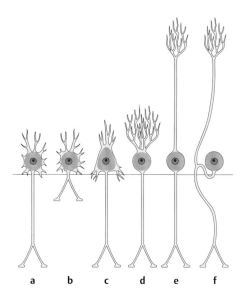

C Basic forms of the neuron and its functionally adapted variants

The horizontal line marks the region of the axon hillock, which represents the initial segment of the axon. (The structure of a peripheral nerve, consisting only of axons and sheath tissue, is shown on p. 57.)

a Multipolar neuron (multiple dendrites) with a *long* axon (= long transmission path). Examples are projection neurons such as alpha motor neurons in the spinal cord.

b Multipolar neuron with a short axon (= short transmission path). Examples are interneurons like those in the gray matter of the brain and spinal cord.

c Pyramidal cell: Dendrites are present only at the apex and base of the *tridentate* cell body, and the axon is long. Examples are efferent neurons of the cerebral motor cortex.

d Purkinje cell: An elaborately branched dendritic tree arises from a circumscribed site on the cell body. The Purkinje cell receives many synaptic contacts from afferents to the cerebellum and is also the efferent cell of the cerebellar cortex.

e Bipolar neuron: The dendrite branches in the periphery. Examples are bipolar cells of the retina.

f Pseudounipolar neuron: The dendrite and axon are not separated by a cell body. An example is the primary afferent (= first sensory) neuron in the spinal ganglion (see p. 63).

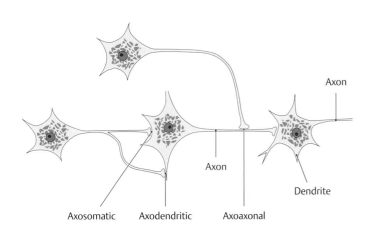

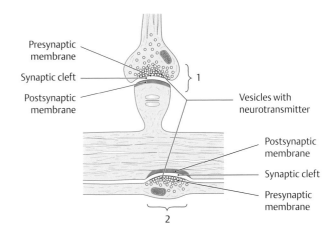

D Synaptic patterns in a small group of neurons

Axons can terminate at various sites on the target neuron and form synapses there. The synaptic patterns are described as axodendritic, axosomatic, or axoaxonal. Axodendritic synapses are the most common (see also **A**).

E Electron microscopy of synapses in the CNS

Synapses are the functional connection between two neurons. They consist of a presynaptic membrane, a synaptic cleft, and a postsynaptic membrane. In a *spine synapse* (1), the presynaptic knob (bouton) is in contact with a specialized protuberance (spine) of the target neuron. The side-by-side synapse of an axon with the flat surface of a target neuron is called a parallel contact or *bouton en passage* (2). The vesicles in the presynaptic expansion contain the neurotransmitters that are released into the synaptic cleft by exocytosis when the axon fires. From there the neurotransmitters diffuse to the postsynaptic membrane, where their receptors are located. A variety of drugs and toxins act upon synaptic transmission (antidepressants, muscle relaxants, toxic gases, botulinum toxin).

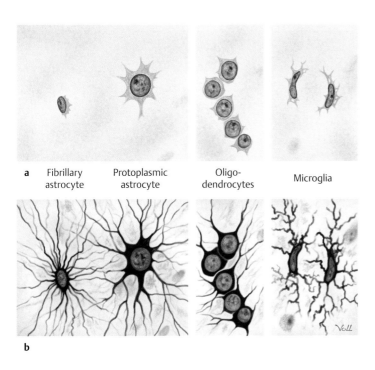

a Fibrillary astrocyte   Protoplasmic astrocyte   Oligo-dendrocytes   Microglia

b

F Cells of the neuroglia in the CNS

Neuroglial cells surround the neurons, providing them with structural and functional support (see **G**). Various staining methods are available in light microscopy for selectively demonstrating different portions of the neuroglial cells:

a Cell nuclei demonstrated with a basic stain.
b Cell body demonstrated by silver impregnation.

G Summary: cells of the CNS and PNS and their functional importance

Type of cell	Function
Neurons (CNS and PNS)	1. Impulse formation 2. Impulse conduction 3. Information processing
Glial cells	
Astrocytes (CNS only)	1. Maintain a constant internal milieu in the CNS 2. Contribute to the structure of the blood–brain barrier (see p. 71) 3. Phagocytize dead synapses 4. Form scar tissue in the CNS (e.g., in multiple sclerosis or following a stroke)
Microglial cells (CNS only)	Phagocytosis ("macrophages of the brain")
Oligodendrocytes (CNS only)	Myelin sheath formation in the CNS
Schwann cells (PNS only)	Myelin sheath formation in the PNS
Satellite cells (PNS only)	Modified Schwann cells; surround the cell body of neurons in PNS ganglia

8.5   Structure of a Spinal Cord Segment

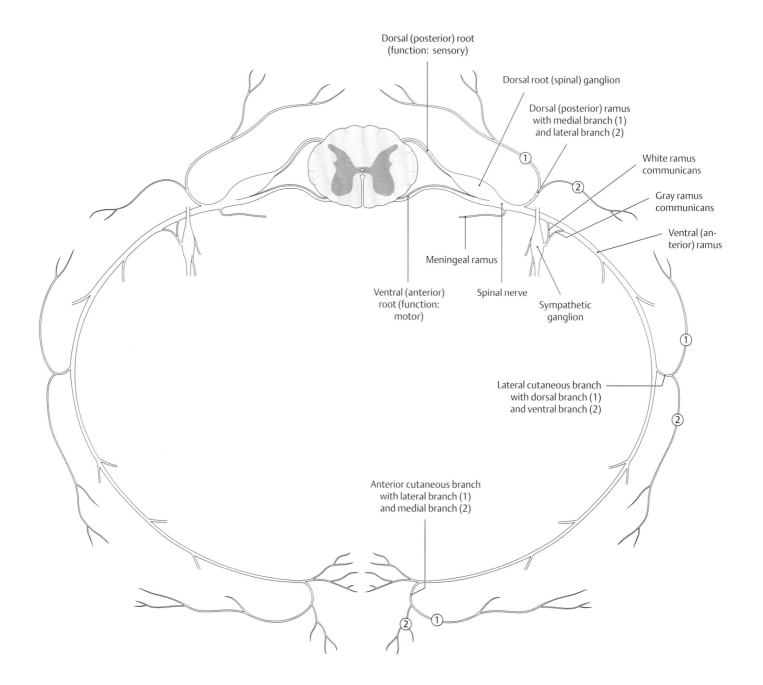

Dorsal (posterior) root
(function: sensory)

Dorsal root (spinal) ganglion

Dorsal (posterior) ramus
with medial branch (1)
and lateral branch (2)

White ramus
communicans

Gray ramus
communicans

Ventral (an-
terior) ramus

Meningeal ramus

Ventral (anterior)
root (function:
motor)

Spinal nerve

Sympathetic
ganglion

Lateral cutaneous branch
with dorsal branch (1)
and ventral branch (2)

Anterior cutaneous branch
with lateral branch (1)
and medial branch (2)

A Structure of a spinal cord segment with its spinal nerve
Superior view. The spinal cord is made up of 31 consecutive segments arranged one above the other (see **B**). A *ventral root (anterior root)* and a *dorsal root (posterior root)* emerge from the sides of each segment. The *ventral* root consists of *efferent* (motor) fibers, while the *dorsal* root consists of *afferent* (sensory) fibers. Both roots from one segment unite in the intervertebral foramen to form the *spinal nerve*. The afferent (sensory) fibers and efferent (motor) fibers intermingle at this junction, so that the branches into which the spinal nerve divides (see below) contain motor *and* sensory elements (except for the meningeal ramus, which is purely sensory). This division into branches (rami) occurs shortly after the dorsal and ventral roots unite to form the spinal nerve. Consequently, the spinal nerve itself is only about 1 cm long.

The principal branches of the spinal nerve have the following functions:

- The ventral ramus innervates the anterior and lateral body wall and the limbs.
- The dorsal ramus innervates the skin of the back and the intrinsic back muscles.
- The meningeal ramus reenters the spinal canal, providing sensory innervation to the spinal membranes and other structures.
- The white ramus communicans carries white (= myelinated) fibers *to* the ganglion of the sympathetic trunk.
- The gray ramus communicans carries gray (= unmyelinated) fibers *from* the sympathetic ganglion back to the spinal nerve (the functional significance of this is described on p. 73). The dorsal and ventral rami of the spinal nerves subdivide into further branches.

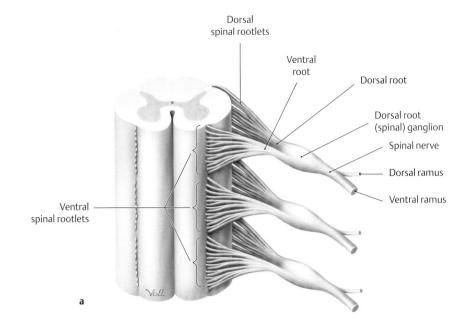

B Spinal cord segment

a Anterior view, demonstrating the stacked arrangement of the spinal cord segments. The spinal nerves and their roots are pictured only on the left side.

b Anterior view, demonstrating the spatial extent of one segment along the spinal cord. The diagram illustrates the vertical arrangement of the spinal "rootlets" (root filaments), which combine to form the ventral and dorsal roots of the associated spinal nerve.

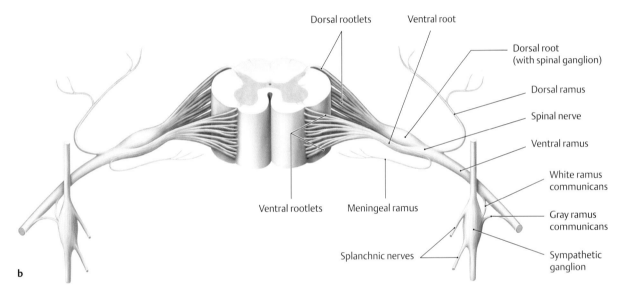

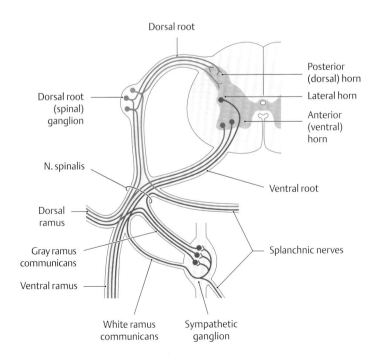

C Topographical and functional organization of a spinal cord segment

- The *afferent fibers* from the skin, muscles, and joints (somato*sensory*, blue) and from the viscera (viscero*sensory*, green) pass through the *dorsal root* into the spinal cord and terminate in the posterior horn. Both fibers arise from pseudounipolar cells in the dorsal root (spinal) ganglion.

- The *efferent fibers* for the skeletal musculature (somato*motor*, red) and for the viscera (viscero*motor*, brown) pass through the *ventral root* to the corresponding end organs, which consist of the skeletal muscles and the smooth muscle of the internal organs. The fibers differ in their origin: Fibers for the skeletal muscles originate in the anterior horn of the spinal cord, and fibers for the viscera originate in the lateral horn. The axons of somatic motor neurons in the ventral horn synapse directly upon skeletal muscle fibers (p. 68). Visceral motor neurons in the lateral horn, however, provide indirect innervation to most of their target organs. Their axons form synapses with autonomic neurons in larger discrete sympathetic ganglia or in scattered clusters embedded in the visceral organs (p. 73).

63

8.6 Sensory Innervation: An Overview

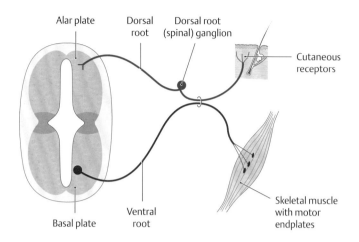

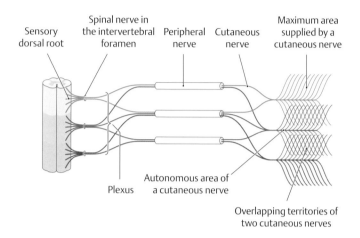

A Embryological origins of the topographical and functional anatomy of a spinal cord segment

The afferent fibers (e.g., from cutaneous receptors) pass through the *dorsal root* into the posterior horn of the spinal cord, which is derived embryologically from the alar plate. The efferent fibers arise from neurons located in the anterior horn of the spinal cord, which is a derivative of the basal plate. They leave the spinal cord by the *ventral root* and are distributed to their target organ, such as a skeletal muscle.

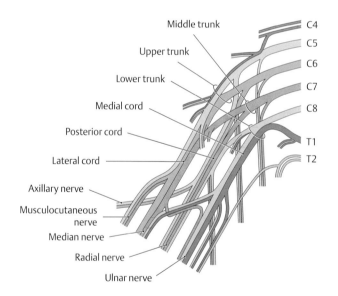

C Plexus formation, illustrated for the brachial plexus

The period of embryonic development is characterized by a migration and intermixing of ventral muscle primordia in the *limbs*. As the muscles migrate to the limbs, they take their segmental innervation with them, resulting in a complex intermingling of axons (plexus formation). Since only the ventral muscle primordia migrate into the limbs, only the ventral rami of the spinal nerves are intermixed. A prime example of this process is the brachial plexus. The ventral rami from segments C 5 through T 1 that form the roots of the plexus are shown in different colors. First the C 5 and C 6 roots unite to form the *upper trunk* of the plexus. The fibers from C 7 form the *middle trunk*, and the fibers from C 8 and T 1 unite to form the *lower trunk*. The anterior branches of the upper and middle trunks then unite to form the *lateral cord*, while the anterior branch of the lower trunk forms the *medial cord* and the posterior branches of all three trunks combine to form the *posterior cord*. Finally, the cords of the brachial plexus give rise to the major nerves that supply the arm and shoulder.

B Course of sensory fibers from the dorsal root to the dermatome

Sensory fibers pass from the *dorsal root* to the intervertebral foramen, where they unite with motor fibers to form the spinal nerve. The sensory fibers are then distributed to the ventral and dorsal rami of the spinal nerve. The simple segmental arrangement of the sensory territories that occurs on the trunk is not found in the limbs (see **D**). This results from the migratory movements of various muscular and cutaneous anlages (precursors or primordia) during the development of the limbs. Because these anlages carry their segmental innervation with them, the sensory fibers from different segments become intermingled in the limbs (plexus formation, see **C**). After fibers have been exchanged in the plexus, the fibers in peripheral nerves are distributed to their destinations, their terminal portions often consisting entirely of sensory cutaneous nerves. The area of skin that is innervated by one spinal cord segment is called a *dermatome*. The dermatomes of adjacent spinal cord segments are often located so close together that their territories broadly overlap. This explains why the clinically detectable area of sensory loss caused by a segmental nerve lesion may be considerably smaller than the dermatome itself. The area that receives all of its sensory supply from one cutaneous nerve is called the *autonomous area* of that nerve. When a segmental nerve lesion occurs, the cutaneous nerves from the two adjacent spinal cord segments are still available to supply at least the peripheral part of the affected skin area.

This helps in understanding the difference between *radicular (= segmental)* and *peripheral sensory innervation*. When a nerve root becomes damaged (e.g., due to a herniated intervertebral disk), the resulting sensory loss will follow a radicular innervation pattern (see p. 66). But when a peripheral nerve is damaged (e.g., due to a limb injury), the sensory loss will conform to a peripheral innervation pattern (see p. 67).

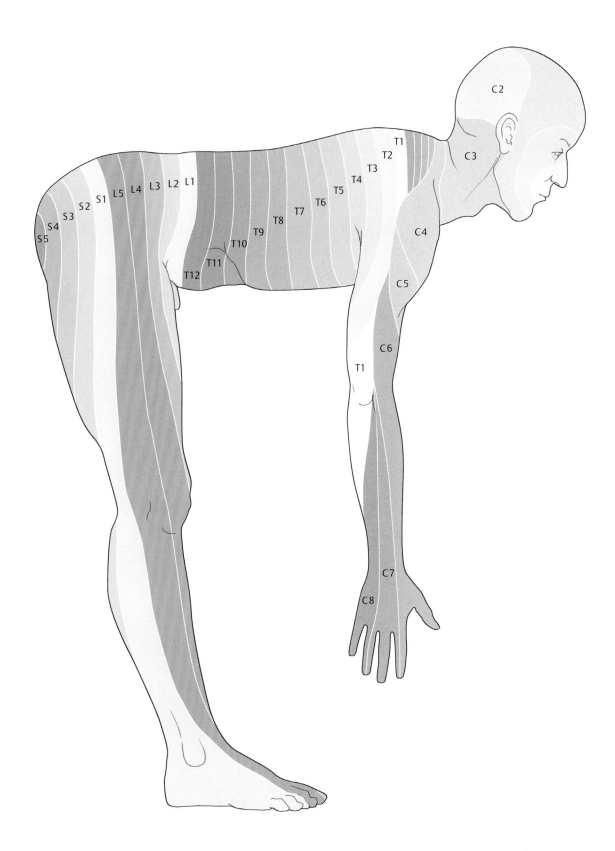

D Simplified scheme for learning the dermatomes
The distribution of dermatomes on the human limbs results from the sprouting of the limb buds that occurs during embryonic development. When the limbs are positioned at right angles to the body as in a quadruped, it is easier to appreciate the pattern of dermatomic innervation (after Mumenthaler).

8.7 Sensory Innervation: Dermatomes and Cutaneous Nerve Territories

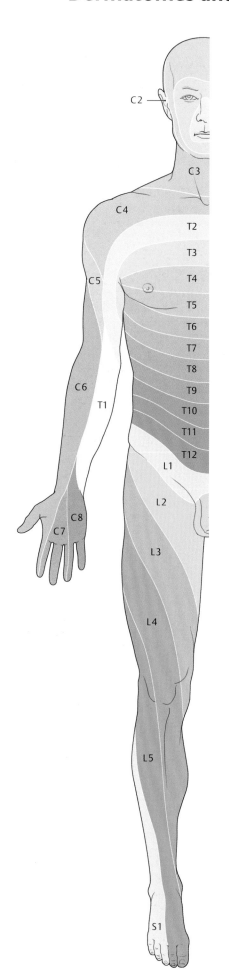

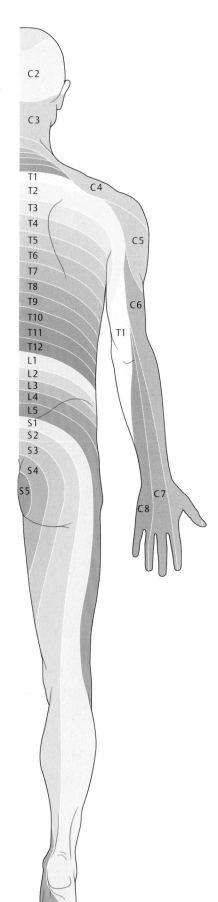

A Pattern of radicular (segmental) sensory innervation

The skin area supplied by a dorsal spinal nerve root is called a *dermatome*. Because the C1 segment consists entirely of motor fibers, it lacks a corresponding sensory field. A knowledge of radicular innervation is very important clinically. For example, when a herniated intervertebral disk is impinging on a sensory root, it will cause sensory losses in the affected dermatome. The area of sensory loss can then be used to locate the level of the lesion: Which intervertebral disk is affected? In a patient with shingles (herpes zoster inflammation of a spinal ganglion), the dermatome supplied by that ganglion will be affected (after Mumenthaler).

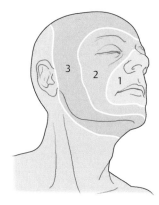

B Pattern of nuclear sensory innervation in the head region

The head receives its sensory innervation from the trigeminal nerve (cranial nerve V). A lesion of the sensory nucleus of the trigeminal nerve within the brain (= central lesion) causes an onion-skin pattern of sensory alteration along the concentric *Sölder lines* that encircle the mouth and nostrils. The pattern of these lines corresponds to the distribution of the neurons in the sensory nucleus of the trigeminal nerve (somatotopic organization, i.e., certain groups of neurons in the CNS are linked to certain territories in the periphery). Territory 1 is supplied by the cranial nuclear column, territory 2 by the middle column, and territory 3 by the caudal column. This pattern of sensory loss is like that associated with radicular neuropathy affecting a peripheral nerve.

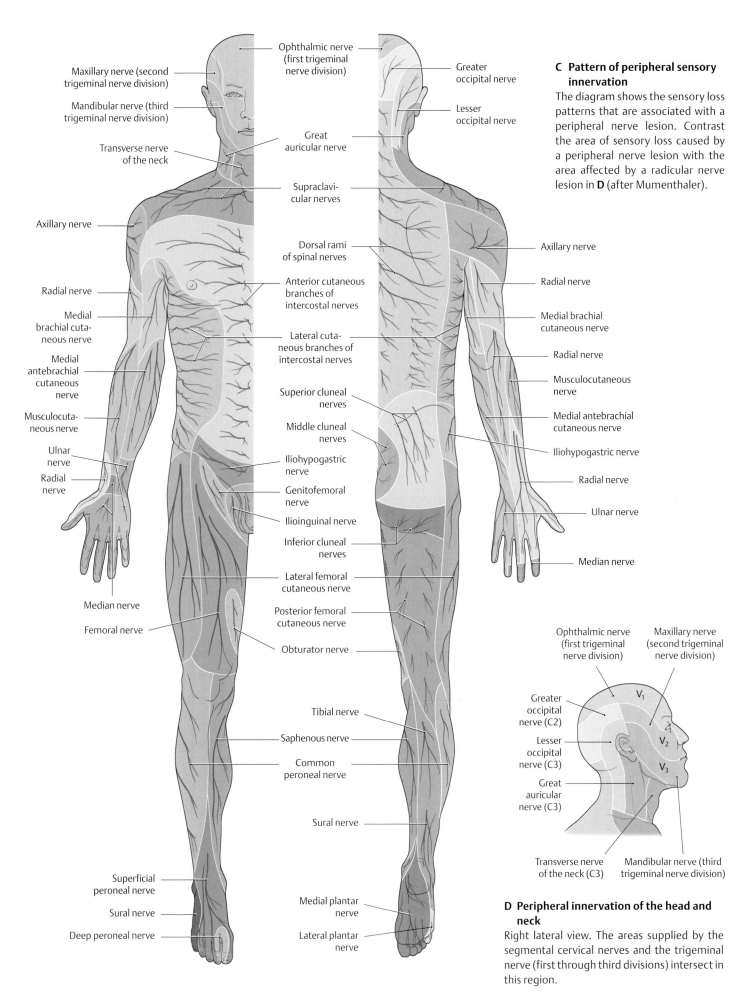

Maxillary nerve (second trigeminal nerve division)

Mandibular nerve (third trigeminal nerve division)

Transverse nerve of the neck

Axillary nerve

Radial nerve

Medial brachial cutaneous nerve

Medial antebrachial cutaneous nerve

Musculocutaneous nerve

Ulnar nerve

Radial nerve

Median nerve

Femoral nerve

Superficial peroneal nerve

Sural nerve

Deep peroneal nerve

Ophthalmic nerve (first trigeminal nerve division)

Great auricular nerve

Supraclavicular nerves

Dorsal rami of spinal nerves

Anterior cutaneous branches of intercostal nerves

Lateral cutaneous branches of intercostal nerves

Superior cluneal nerves

Middle cluneal nerves

Iliohypogastric nerve

Genitofemoral nerve

Ilioinguinal nerve

Inferior cluneal nerves

Lateral femoral cutaneous nerve

Posterior femoral cutaneous nerve

Obturator nerve

Tibial nerve

Saphenous nerve

Common peroneal nerve

Sural nerve

Medial plantar nerve

Lateral plantar nerve

Greater occipital nerve

Lesser occipital nerve

Axillary nerve

Radial nerve

Medial brachial cutaneous nerve

Radial nerve

Musculocutaneous nerve

Medial antebrachial cutaneous nerve

Iliohypogastric nerve

Radial nerve

Ulnar nerve

Median nerve

C Pattern of peripheral sensory innervation

The diagram shows the sensory loss patterns that are associated with a peripheral nerve lesion. Contrast the area of sensory loss caused by a peripheral nerve lesion with the area affected by a radicular nerve lesion in **D** (after Mumenthaler).

Ophthalmic nerve (first trigeminal nerve division)

Maxillary nerve (second trigeminal nerve division)

Greater occipital nerve (C2)

Lesser occipital nerve (C3)

Great auricular nerve (C3)

V_1

V_2

V_3

Transverse nerve of the neck (C3)

Mandibular nerve (third trigeminal nerve division)

D Peripheral innervation of the head and neck

Right lateral view. The areas supplied by the segmental cervical nerves and the trigeminal nerve (first through third divisions) intersect in this region.

67

8.8 Motor Innervation

A Simplified scheme of motor innervation

The simplest common path of motor innervation originates in the primary cerebral motor cortex. Large neurons (dark red) contribute axons to bundles collected into massive *corticospinal* tracts. Many axons pass uninterrupted to the spinal cord, where they synapse upon motor neurons in the ventral horn (orange). In the brainstem the bundles of corticospinal axons are designated *pyramids* or *pyramidal tracts*. In the medulla oblongata, most corticospinal axons cross the midline in the *pyramidal decussation* and continue on the opposite side. Axons from motor neurons in the ventral horn of the spinal cord exit in *ventral roots* (p. 62) and reach their targets, skeletal muscles, via peripheral nerves, where they synapse directly at *neuromuscular junctions*.

The typical spinal motor neuron receives inputs from multiple sources. The simplest local circuit involves afferent (sensory) synapses from fibers from dorsal root (spinal) ganglion cells (blue). Although most afferent information is relayed to spinal motor neurons through multiple intermediate *interneurons*, some sensory input—particularly from tendon stretch receptors—is transmitted directly via a single synapse, as depicted. This chain of connections is called a *reflex arc*. One such arc produces the knee-jerk or patellar tendon reflex.

This pattern of motor connections is responsible for two fundamental principles in the diagnosis of neurological disorders. Because of their positions in the pathway, the cerebral cortical cells are referred to as *upper motor neurons*, those in the spinal cord as *lower motor neurons*. Damage to lower motor neurons or their axons leads to denervation of muscles, with *flaccid paralysis* and eventual muscle atrophy. In contrast, interruption of corticospinal axons or destruction of the upper motor neurons themselves, resulting, for instance, from a cerebral infarction (stroke), leads to a loss of voluntary control over the lower motor neurons. With such an upper motor neuron lesion, the lower motor neuron is controlled solely by local spinal circuits. Local reflexes remain or are enhanced, but muscles show sustained contractions and increased tone, with *spastic paralysis*.

The second fundamental correlation between the anatomy of the motor pathway and neurological diagnosis involves the crossing of corticospinal axons in the pyramidal decussation. Upper motor lesions that occur above (cranial to) this decussation will produce spastic paralysis on the *contralateral* side of the body; lesions in corticospinal axons below (caudal to) this point will cause spastic paralysis on the same side as (*ipsilateral* to) the lesion.

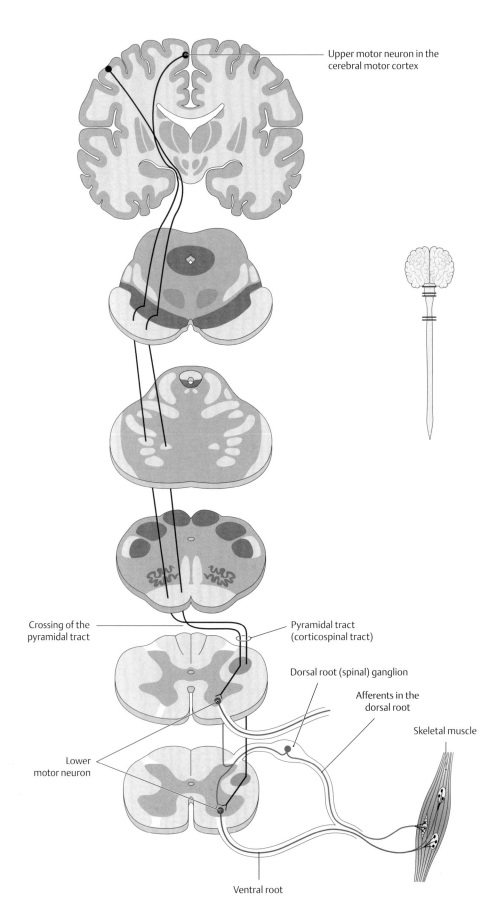

Upper motor neuron in the cerebral motor cortex

Crossing of the pyramidal tract

Pyramidal tract (corticospinal tract)

Dorsal root (spinal) ganglion

Afferents in the dorsal root

Skeletal muscle

Lower motor neuron

Ventral root

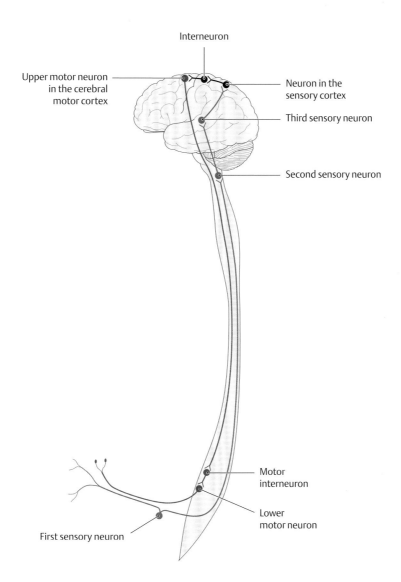

Interneuron

Upper motor neuron
in the cerebral
motor cortex

Neuron in the
sensory cortex

Third sensory neuron

Second sensory neuron

Motor
interneuron

Lower
motor neuron

First sensory neuron

B Neural circuit for sensory and motor innervation
Left lateral view. Information processing in the CNS is actually more complex than shown in **A** because motor innervation is influenced by afferents of a kind not illustrated here (= sensorimotor circuit). Although a great many neurons are active at each step in the circuit, the diagram shows only one at each level. Sensory information, encoded as electrical impulses, enters the spinal cord through a primary afferent neuron (first sensory neuron) whose cell body is in the spinal ganglion (afferent neurons shown in blue). The information is relayed synaptically to the second and third afferent (sensory) neurons, which transfer it to the sensory cortex (black). Associative neurons (interneurons, black) transmit the information to the upper motor neuron in the cerebral motor cortex, where the information is modified by many associated inputs. The cortical motor neuron (upper motor neuron) redirects the information to the spinal cord, where it reaches the spinal (lower) motor neuron, either directly or via interneurons and additional synaptic relays. Finally, the lower motor neuron in the spinal cord transmits the impulses to the voluntary skeletal muscle. Corticospinal projections are most direct and numerous for lower motor neurons that innervate muscles, like those in the human hand, which are often under fine control and coordinated cognitive direction. Other motor pathways, not depicted here, are more important for controlling posture and balance. Because the axons in some of these other pathways are not in the corticospinal and pyramidal tracts, they are sometimes referred to as *extrapyramidal*.

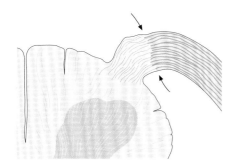

C Obersteiner–Redlich zone in a dorsal root
The Obersteiner–Redlich zone marks the morphological junction between the CNS and PNS (arrow). Oligodendrocytes in the CNS form a myelin sheath around the axons only as far as this zone, which is located just past the emergence of the dorsal root from the spinal cord. The myelin sheaths in the PNS are formed by Schwann cells (see p. 70 for details). The myelin is so thin at these sites that the fibers appear almost unmyelinated. This creates a site of predilection for immunological diseases such as the immune reactions that occur in the late stages of syphilis.

8.9 Differences between the Central and Peripheral Nervous Systems

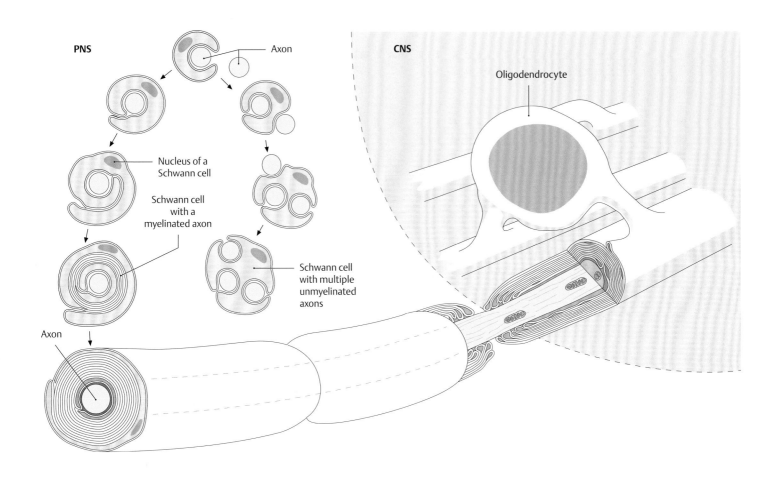

A Myelination differences in the PNS and CNS

The purpose of myelination is to provide the axons with electrical insulation, which significantly increases the nerve conduction velocity. The very lipid-rich membranes of myelinating cells are wrapped around the axons to produce this insulation. Schwann cells (left) myelinate the axons in the *PNS*, while oligodendrocytes (right) form the myelin in the *CNS*.

Note: In the *CNS*, one oligodendrocyte *always* wraps around *multiple* axons. In the *PNS*, one Schwann cell *may* ensheath *multiple* axons if the peripheral nerve is *unmyelinated*. If the peripheral nerve is *myelinated*, one Schwann cell *always* wraps around *one* axon.

Owing to this improved insulation, the nerve conduction velocity is higher in myelinated nerves than in unmyelinated nerves. Myelinated fibers occur in areas where fast reaction speeds are needed (muscular contractions), while unmyelinated fibers occur in areas that do not require rapid information transfer, as in the transmission of visceral pain. Because of the different cell types, myelin has a different composition in the CNS and PNS. This difference in myelination is also important clinically. An example is multiple sclerosis, in which the oligodendrocytes are damaged but the Schwann cells are not, so that the central myelin sheaths are disrupted while the peripheral myelin sheaths remain intact.

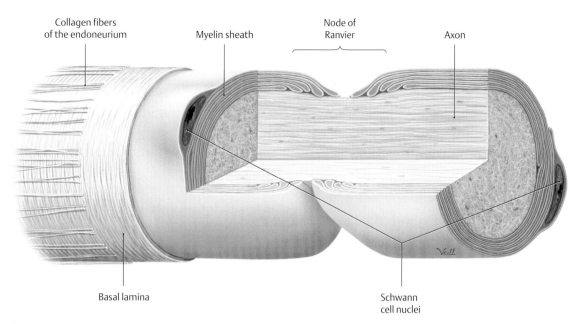

B Structure of a node of Ranvier in the PNS
In the PNS, the *node of Ranvier* is the site where two Schwann cells come together. That site is marked by a small gap in the myelin sheath, which forms the morphological basis for *saltatory nerve conduction*, allowing impulses to be transmitted at a higher velocity.

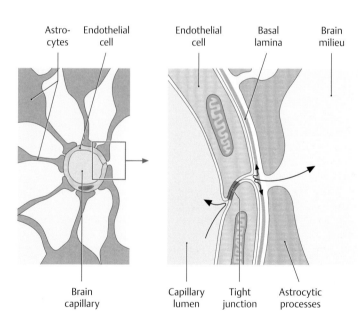

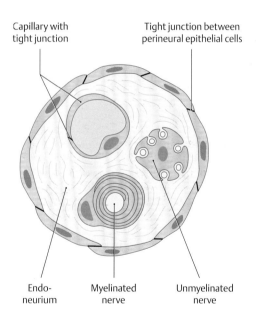

C Structure of the blood–brain barrier in the CNS
Besides the type of myelination, there is also a difference in tissue barriers between the CNS and PNS. The CNS is isolated from surrounding tissues by the blood–brain barrier. The components of the blood–brain barrier include: (1) most importantly, a continuous capillary endothelial cell layer, sealed by tight junctions; (2) a continuous basal lamina surrounding the endothelial cells; and (3) enveloping astrocytic processes surrounding the brain capillary. This barrier serves to exclude macromolecules, as well as many small molecules that are not actively transported by the endothelial cells, thus protecting the delicate environment of the central nervous system. The barrier is vulnerable, however, to lipid-soluble molecules that can traverse the endothelial cell membranes. The perineurial sheath creates a similar barrier in the PNS (see **D**).

D Structure of the perineurial sheath in the PNS
The perineurial sheath, like the blood–brain barrier, is formed by tight junctions between the epithelium-like fibroblasts (perineurial cells; the perineurium is described on p. 57). It isolates the milieu of the axon from that of the surrounding endoneural space (endoneurium), thereby preventing harmful substances from invading the axon. This tissue barrier must be surmounted by drugs that are designed to act on the axon, such as local anesthetic agents.

8.10 The Autonomic Nervous System

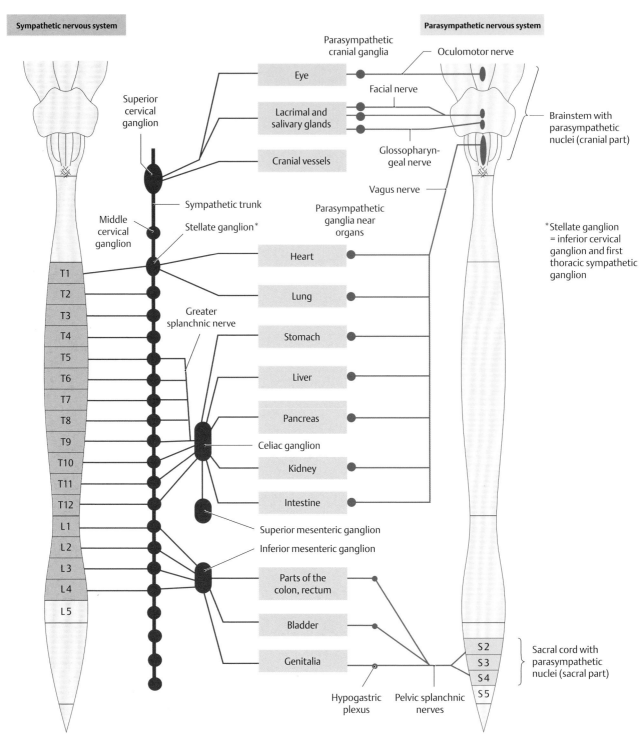

Sympathetic nervous system

Parasympathetic nervous system

Parasympathetic cranial ganglia

Oculomotor nerve

Eye

Facial nerve

Superior cervical ganglion

Lacrimal and salivary glands

Cranial vessels

Glossopharyn-geal nerve

Brainstem with parasympathetic nuclei (cranial part)

Vagus nerve

Sympathetic trunk

Parasympathetic ganglia near organs

Middle cervical ganglion

Stellate ganglion*

*Stellate ganglion = inferior cervical ganglion and first thoracic sympathetic ganglion

Heart

T1

T2

Lung

T3

Greater splanchnic nerve

T4

Stomach

T5

T6

Liver

T7

T8

Pancreas

T9

Celiac ganglion

T10

Kidney

T11

T12

Intestine

L1

Superior mesenteric ganglion

L2

Inferior mesenteric ganglion

L3

L4

Parts of the colon, rectum

L5

Bladder

S2

Sacral cord with parasympathetic nuclei (sacral part)

Genitalia

S3

S4

S5

Hypogastric plexus

Pelvic splanchnic nerves

A Structure of the autonomic nervous system
The system of motor innervation of skeletal muscle is complemented by the *autonomic nervous system*, with two divisions: sympathetic (red) and parasympathetic (blue). Both divisions have a two-neuron path between the CNS and their targets: a *preganglionic* CNS neuron, and a ganglion cell in the PNS that is close to the target. The preganglionic neurons of the sympathetic system are in the lateral horns of the cervical, thoracic, and lumbar spinal cord. Their axons exit the CNS via the ventral roots and synapse in sympathetic ganglia in bilateral *paraverte-bral* chains (*sympathetic trunks*), or as single midline *prevertebral ganglia* (see **E**). Axons from these ganglion cells course in unmyelinated bundles on blood vessels or in peripheral nerves to their targets. The pregangli-onic neurons of the parasympathetic system are located in the brain-

stem and sacral spinal cord. Their axons exit the CNS via cranial and pel-vic splanchnic nerves to synapse with parasympathetic ganglion cells. In the head, these cells are in discrete ganglia associated with the cranial nerves. In other locations the parasympathetic ganglion cells are in tiny clusters embedded in their target tissues. The sympathetic and para-sympathetic systems regulate blood flow, secretions, and organ func-tion; the two divisions often act in antagonistic ways on the same tar-get (see **B**). Although this basic dichotomy of visceral motor activity was identified early, by Langley (1905) and others, it has been shown more recently that autonomic control of various organs, particularly in the gastrointestinal and urogenital tracts, is highly sophisticated, depen-dent upon feedback from local visceral afferents that relay pain and stretch information, etc., through complex local circuits.

B Synopsis of the sympathetic and parasympathetic nervous systems

1. The sympathetic nervous system can be considered the excitatory part of the autonomic nervous system that prepares the body for a "fight or flight" response.
2. The parasympathetic nervous system is the part of the autonomic nervous system that coordinates the "rest and digest" responses of the body.
3. Although there are separate control centers for the two divisions in the brainstem and spinal cord, they have close anatomical and functional ties in the periphery.
4. The principal transmitter at the target organ is *acetylcholine* in the parasympathetic nervous system and *norepinephrine* in the sympathetic nervous organ.
5. Stimulation of the sympathetic and parasympathetic nervous systems produces the following different effects on specific organs:

Organ	Sympathetic nervous system	Parasympathetic nervous system
Eye	Pupillary dilation	Pupillary constriction and increased curvature of the lens
Salivary glands	Decreased salivation (scant, viscous)	Increased salivation (copious, watery)
Heart	Elevation of the heart rate	Slowing of the heart rate
Lungs	Decreased bronchial secretions and bronchial dilation	Increased bronchial secretions and bronchial constriction
Gastrointestinal tract	Decreased secretions and motor activity	Increased secretions and motor activity
Pancreas	Decreased secretion from the endocrine part of the gland	Increased secretion
Male sex organs	Ejaculation	Erection
Skin	Vasoconstriction, sweat secretion, piloerection	No effect

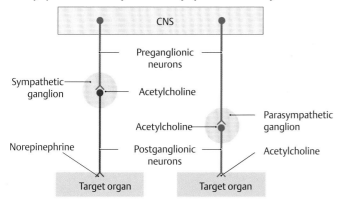

C Circuit diagram of the autonomic nervous system

The synapse of the central, preganglionic neuron uses *acetylcholine* as a transmitter in both the sympathetic *and* parasympathetic nervous systems (cholinergic neuron, shown in blue). In the sympathetic nervous system, the transmitter changes to *norepinephrine* at the synapse of the postganglionic neuron with the target organ (adrenergic neuron, shown in red), while the parasympathetic system continues to use acetylcholine at that level.

Note: Various types of receptors for acetylcholine (= neurotransmitter sensors) are located in the membrane of the target cells. As a result, acetylcholine can produce a range of effects depending on the receptor type.

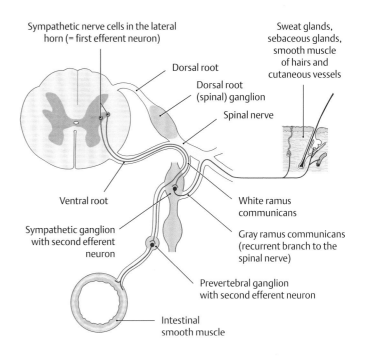

D Distribution of sympathetic fibers in the periphery

Some sympathetic fibers in the periphery (e.g., in the trunk region) "hitchhike" on spinal nerves to reach their destinations. The synapse of the first with the second efferent neuron (red) may occur at three locations (see **E**).

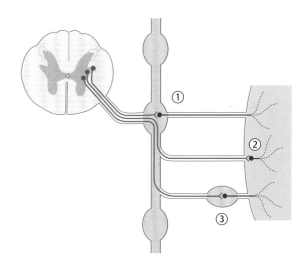

E Location of synapses in the autonomic nervous system

Acetylcholine is the transmitter for both the first and second neurons in the parasympathetic system, but the sympathetic system switches to norepinephrine for the second neuron. Synapses of the first, preganglionic cholinergic neuron (blue) with the second neuron (red) may be located in three different sites:

① In discrete bilateral clusters of postganglionic neurons (autonomic ganglia). In the sympathetic system, these synapses are in the paravertebral ganglia on either side of the vertebral column. In the cranial part of the parasympathetic system, the synapses are in paired cranial parasympathetic ganglia (see **A**).
② In the target organ, on small clusters of embedded ganglion cells (parasympathetic system only). In the adrenal gland, preganglionic cholinergic sympathetic fibers synapse directly on adrenal medullary (endocrine) cells (embryologically related to sympathetic neurons [see pp. 56–57]).
③ In unpaired prevertebral ganglia (celiac and mesenteric), located in front of the vertebral column, in close proximity to the abdominal aorta (sympathetic system only).

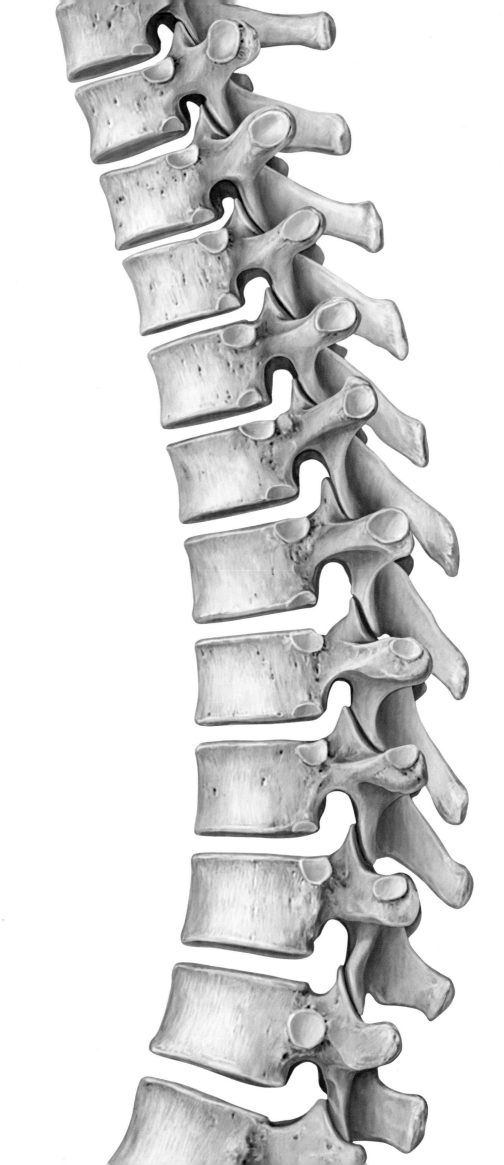

Trunk Wall

1.1 The Skeleton of the Trunk

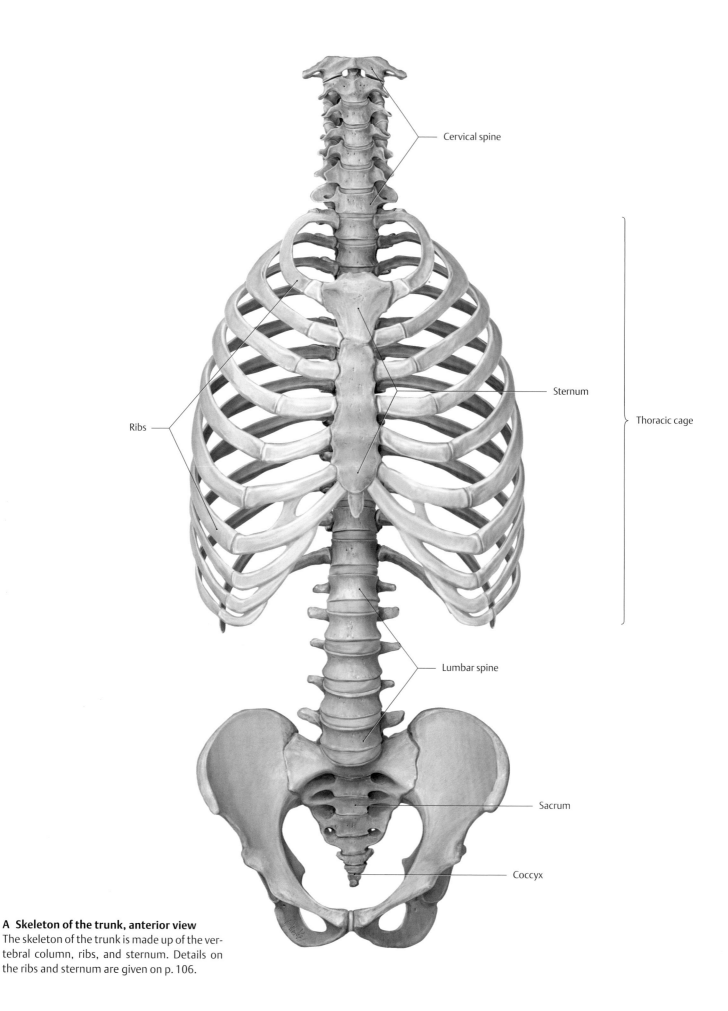

Cervical spine

Sternum

Thoracic cage

Ribs

Lumbar spine

Sacrum

Coccyx

A Skeleton of the trunk, anterior view
The skeleton of the trunk is made up of the vertebral column, ribs, and sternum. Details on the ribs and sternum are given on p. 106.

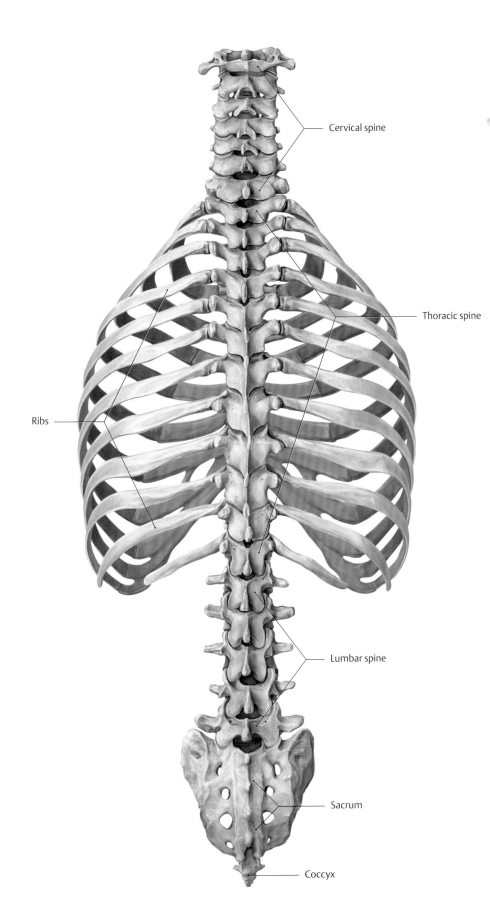

Cervical spine

Thoracic spine

Ribs

Lumbar spine

Sacrum

Coccyx

B Skeleton of the trunk, posterior view

Spinous process of C7 (vertebra prominens)

Spinous process of T3; scapular spine

Spinous process of T7; inferior scapular angle

Spinous process of T12; twelfth rib

Spinous process of L4; iliac crest

C The spinous processes as anatomical landmarks

Posterior view. The spinous processes of the vertebrae appear as variable prominences beneath the skin and provide important landmarks during the physical examination. With few exceptions, they are easily palpated.

- The spinous process of the seventh cervical vertebra, located at the junction of the cervical and thoracic spine. Usually it is the most prominent of the spinous processes, causing the seventh cervical vertebra to be known also as the *vertebra prominens*.
- The spinous process of the third thoracic vertebra, located on a horizontal line connecting the scapular spines.
- The spinous process of the seventh thoracic vertebra, located at the level of the inferior angles of the scapulae.
- The spinous process of the twelfth thoracic vertebra, located slightly below the attachment of the last rib.
- The spinous process of the fourth lumbar vertebra, located on a horizontal line connecting the highest points of the iliac crests.

Note: The spinous processes of the thoracic vertebrae are angled downward (see p. 86), and so the spinous process of the fifth thoracic vertebra, for example, is at the level of the sixth thoracic vertebral body.

1.2   The Bony Spinal Column

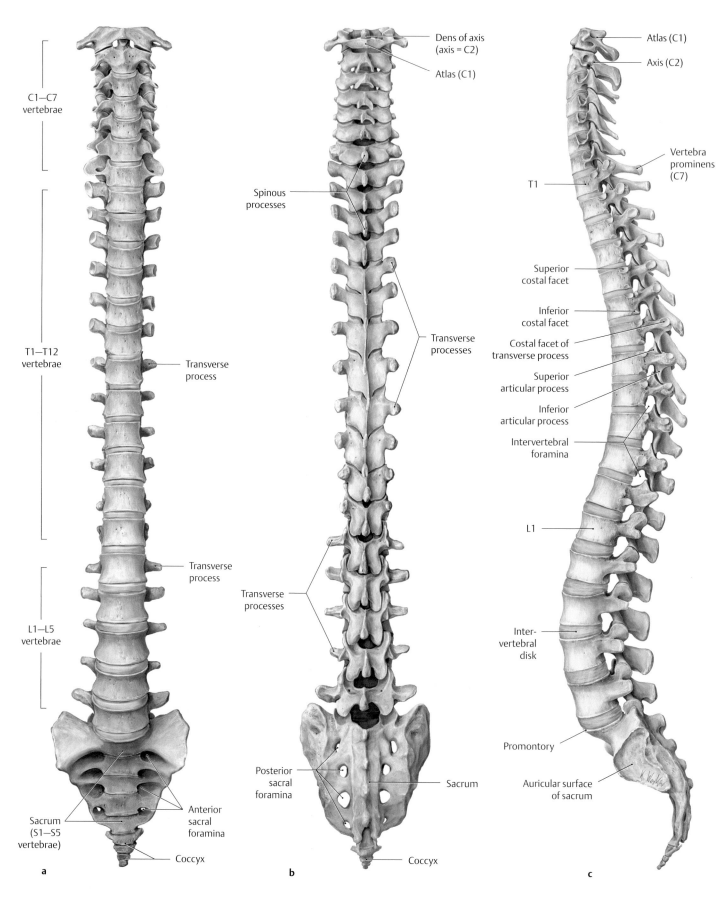

C1—C7
vertebrae

T1—T12
vertebrae

L1—L5
vertebrae

Transverse
process

Transverse
process

Sacrum
(S1—S5
vertebrae)

Anterior
sacral
foramina

Coccyx

a

Spinous
processes

Transverse
processes

Transverse
processes

Posterior
sacral
foramina

Sacrum

Coccyx

b

Dens of axis
(axis = C2)

Atlas (C1)

Atlas (C1)

Axis (C2)

Vertebra
prominens
(C7)

T1

Superior
costal facet

Inferior
costal facet

Costal facet of
transverse process

Superior
articular process

Inferior
articular process

Intervertebral
foramina

L1

Inter-
vertebral
disk

Promontory

Auricular surface
of sacrum

c

A The bony spinal column
a Anterior view, **b** posterior view, **c** left lateral view.

Note that, phylogenetically, the transverse processes of the lumbar vertebrae are rudimentary ribs. They are often known as costal processes therefore (see also p. 82).

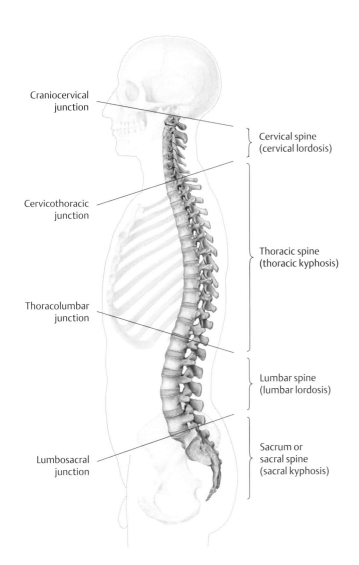

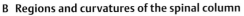

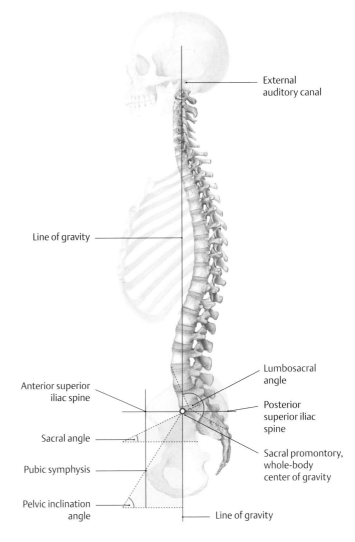

B Regions and curvatures of the spinal column

Left lateral view. The spinal column of an adult is divided into four regions and presents four characteristic curvatures in the sagittal plane. These curves are the result of human adaptation to upright bipedal locomotion, acting as springs to cushion axial loads. The following regions and curvatures are distinguished in the craniocaudal direction:

- Cervical spine – cervical lordosis
- Thoracic spine – thoracic kyphosis
- Lumbar spine – lumbar lordosis
- Sacral spine – sacral kyphosis

The cervical, thoracic, and lumbar regions of the spinal column are also known collectively as the *presacral spine*. The transitional areas between the different regions are of clinical importance because they are potential sites for spinal disorders (e.g., herniated disks). Occasionally the vertebrae in these transitional areas have an atypical morphology which identifies them as *transitional vertebrae*. This is particularly common at the lumbosacral junction, where *sacralization* or *lumbarization* may be seen, depending on the appearance of the atypical vertebra. With lumbarization, the first sacral vertebra is not fused to the sacrum and constitutes an extra lumbar vertebra. With sacralization, there are only four lumbar vertebrae, the fifth being "sacralized" by fusion to the sacrum. These *assimilation disorders* are often unilateral (hemilumbarization, hemisacralization).

C Integration of the spinal column into the pelvic girdle

Skeleton of the trunk with the skull and pelvic girdle, left lateral view. Normally the spinal column is curved and integrated into the pelvic girdle in such a way that characteristic angles are formed between certain imaginary lines and axes. These angles and lines are useful in the radiographic evaluation of positional abnormalities and deformities of the spine and trunk.

Lumbosacral angle: angle formed by the axes of the L 5 and S 1 vertebrae, averaging 143°. It results from the fact that the sacrum is a fixed component of the pelvic ring (see p. 112) and thus contributes little to straightening the vertebral column. The result is a characteristic sharp angle at the junction of the presacral part of the spinal column with the sacrum.

Sacral angle: angle between the horizontal plane and the superior surface of the sacrum, averaging approximately 30°.

Pelvic inclination angle: angle formed by the pelvic inlet plane (connecting the sacral promontory to the upper border of the symphysis) with the horizontal. It measures approximately 60° in upright stance. The pelvic inclination angle increases or decreases as the pelvis is tilted forward or backward (see p. 131). With an ideal pelvic position in upright stance, the anterior and posterior superior iliac spines are at the same horizontal level while the anterior superior iliac spine is directly above the pubic symphysis. By knowing this, the examiner can easily evaluate the position of the pelvis by using palpable bony landmarks.

Line of gravity: The line of gravity passes through landmarks that include the external auditory canal, the dens of the axis (C 2), the functional-anatomical transition points in the spinal column (between lordosis and kyphosis), and the whole-body center of gravity just anterior to the sacral promontory.

79

1.3 Development of the Spinal Column

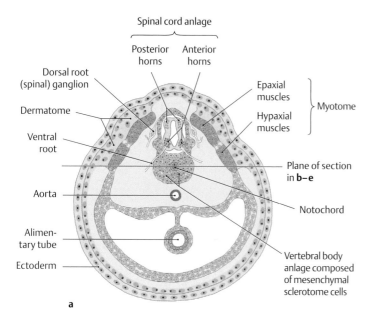

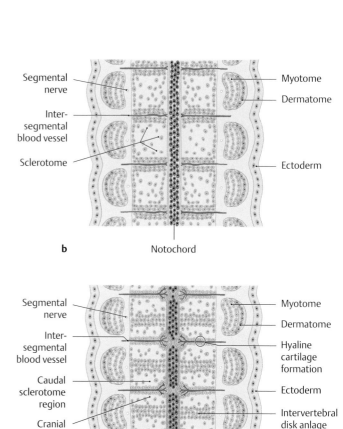

b Notochord

c Notochord sheath / Notochord (notochord segment)

d Notochord sheath / Remnant of notochord (notochord segment)

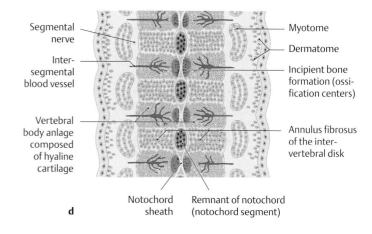

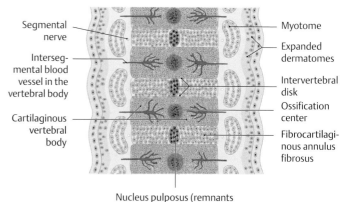

e Nucleus pulposus (remnants of notochord segments)

A Development of the spinal column (weeks 4–10)

a Schematic cross section, **b–e** schematic coronal sections (the plane of section in **b–e** is indicated in **a**).

a, b The former somites have differentiated into the myotome, dermatome, and sclerotome. The sclerotome cells separate from the other cells at four weeks, migrate toward the notochord, and form a cluster of mesenchymal cells around the notochord (anlage of the future spinal column).

c Adjacent cranial and caudal sclerotome segments above and below the intersegmental vessels join together and begin to chondrify in the sixth week, displacing the notochord material superiorly and inferiorly (notochord segments).

d The intervertebral disks with their nucleus pulposus and anulus fibrosus develop between the rudimentary vertebral bodies. Ossification begins at the center of the vertebral bodies in the eighth week of development.

e By fusion of the caudal and cranial sclerotome segments, the segmentally arranged mytomes interconnect the processes of two adjacent vertebral anlages, bridging the gap across the intervertebral disks. This is how the *motion segments* are formed (see p. 100). The segmental spinal nerve courses at the level of the future intervertebral foramen, and the intersegmental vessels become the *nutrient vessels* of the vertebral bodies (week 10).

Clinical aspects: If the neural tube or the dorsal portions of the vertebral arches fail to close normally during embryonic development, the result is *spina bifida*—a cleft spine. In this anomaly the spinal column is open posteriorly and the spinous processes are absent (the various forms and manifestations are described in textbooks of embryology). Usually there is a bilateral defect in the vertebral arches (generally affecting the L 4 and L 5 region), known as *spondylolysis*. This defect may be congenital or acquired (e.g., due to trauma). Acquired cases are common in sports that pose a risk of vertebral arch fractures (javelin throwing, gymnastics, high jumping). If the associated intervertebral disk is also damaged, the vertebral body will begin to slip forward (*spondylolisthesis*). In cases of *congenital spondylolysis* (which are associated with varying degrees of spondylolisthesis), the slippage progresses slowly during growth, and the condition tends to stabilize after 20 years of age.

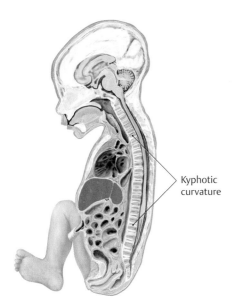

Kyphotic curvature

B Neonatal kyphosis
Midsagittal section through a newborn, left lateral view. Owing to the curved intrauterine position of the fetus, the newborn has a "kyphotic" spinal curvature with no lordotic straightening of the cervical and lumbar spine (after Rohen, Yokochi, Lütjen-Drecoll).

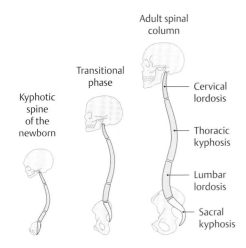

Adult spinal column

Transitional phase

Kyphotic spine of the newborn

Cervical lordosis

Thoracic kyphosis

Lumbar lordosis

Sacral kyphosis

C Straightening of the spine during normal development (after Debrunner)
The characteristic curvatures of the adult spine are only partially present in the newborn (compare with **B**) and appear only during the course of postnatal development. First cervical lordosis develops to balance the head in response to the growing strength of the posterior neck muscles. Lumbar lordosis develops later as the child learns to sit, stand, and walk. The degree of lordosis increases until the legs can be fully extended at the hips, and it finally becomes stable during puberty. A similar transformation of the spinal column is observed in the phylogenetic transition from quadrupedal to bipedal locomotion.

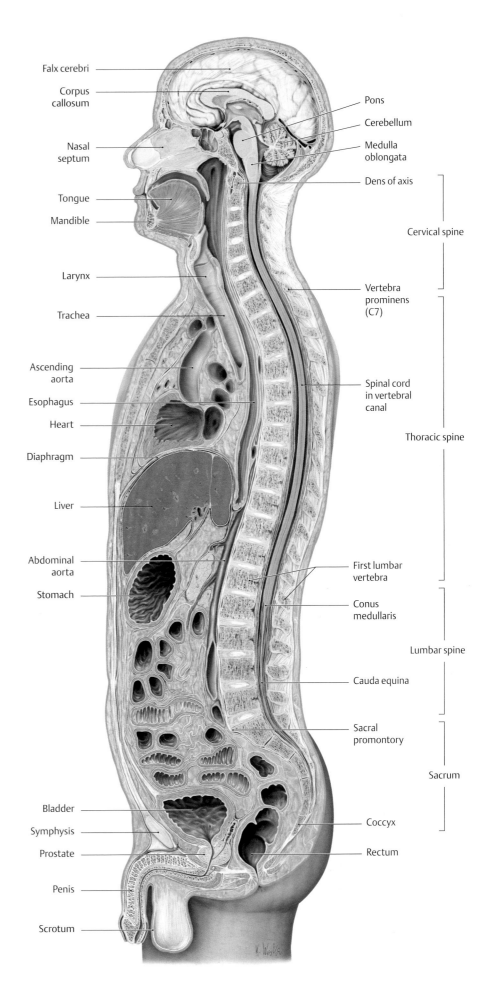

Falx cerebri

Corpus callosum

Nasal septum

Tongue

Mandible

Larynx

Trachea

Ascending aorta

Esophagus

Heart

Diaphragm

Liver

Abdominal aorta

Stomach

Bladder

Symphysis

Prostate

Penis

Scrotum

Pons

Cerebellum

Medulla oblongata

Dens of axis

Cervical spine

Vertebra prominens (C7)

Spinal cord in vertebral canal

Thoracic spine

First lumbar vertebra

Conus medullaris

Lumbar spine

Cauda equina

Sacral promontory

Sacrum

Coccyx

Rectum

D Physiological curvatures of the adult spinal column

Midsagittal section through an adult male, left lateral view.

1.4 The Structure of a Vertebra

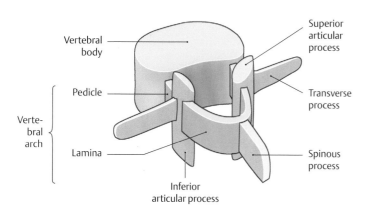

A Structural elements of a vertebra

Left posterosuperior view. All vertebrae except the atlas and axis (see p. 84) consist of the same basic structural elements:

- A vertebral body
- A vertebral arch
- A spinous process
- Two transverse processes (called costal processes in the lumbar vertebrae)
- Four articular processes

The processes give attachment to muscles and ligaments, and the bodies of the thoracic vertebrae have costovertebral joints. The vertebral bodies and arches enclose the vertebral foramen, and all of the vertebral foramina together constitute the vertebral (spinal) canal.

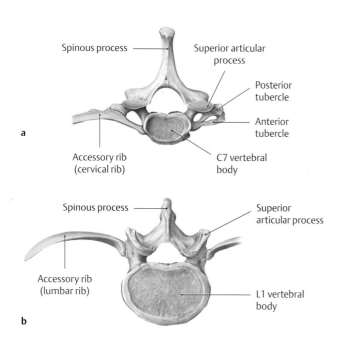

B Accessory ribs

Superior view. **a** Cervical rib, **b** lumbar rib.

The presence of anomalous cervical ribs can narrow the scalene interval, causing compression of the brachial plexus and subclavian artery (scalenus syndrome or cervical rib syndrome, see also p. 317). An accessory lumbar rib, on the other hand, has no adverse clinical effects.

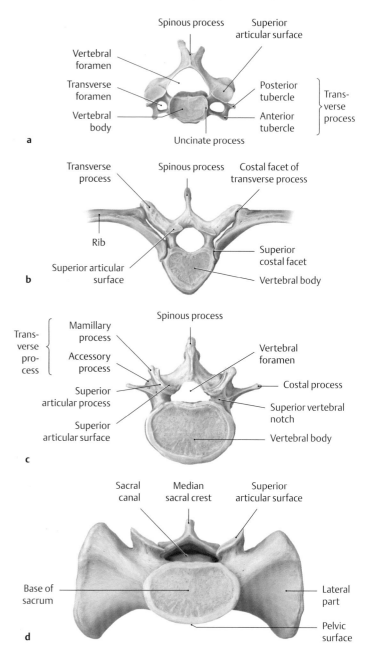

C Costal elements in different regions of the spinal column

Superior view. The shape and configuration of the vertebrae are closely related to the development of the ribs and their rudiments (indicated here by color shading).

- **a** Cervical vertebrae: Here the rudimentary rib forms a process called the anterior tubercle. It unites with the posterior tubercle to form the transverse foramen.
- **b** Thoracic vertebrae: Because these vertebrae give attachment to the ribs, their bodies and transverse processes bear corresponding cartilage-covered articular surfaces (costal facets on the transverse processes, also superior and inferior costal facets).
- **c** Lumbar vertebrae: The costal elements in the lumbar spine take the form of "transverse processes," which are much larger than in the cervical spine. Because of their size, they are also known as costal processes.
- **d** Sacrum: Here the rudimentary rib forms the anterior portion of the lateral part of the sacral vertebra. It is fused to the transverse processes.

D Typical vertebrae from different regions of the spinal column

Superior and left lateral view.

a, b First cervical vertebra (atlas).
c, d Second cervical vertebra (axis).
e, f Fourth cervical vertebra.
g, h Sixth thoracic vertebra.
i, j Fourth lumbar vertebra.
k, l Sacrum.

The vertebrae in different regions of the spinal column differ not only in their size but also in their special features. While the vertebral *bodies* gradually become larger from superior to inferior to accommodate the increasing stresses imposed by the gravity and body weight, the vertebral *foramina* gradually become smaller to match the decreasing diameter of the spinal cord. The arrangement of the vertebral arches and adjacent processes also varies at different levels in the spine (for details see pp. 85, 87, and 89).

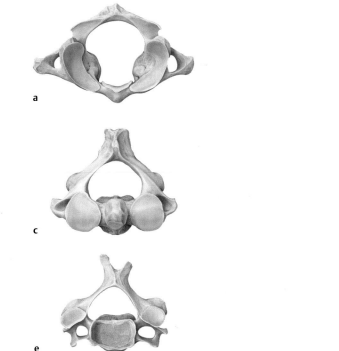

a

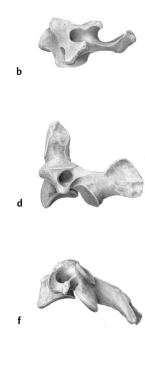

b

c

d

e

f

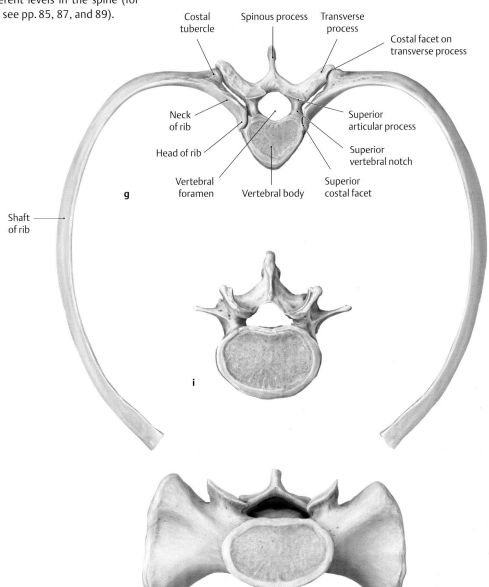

Costal tubercle

Spinous process

Transverse process

Costal facet on transverse process

Neck of rib

Superior articular process

Head of rib

Superior vertebral notch

Vertebral foramen

Vertebral body

Superior costal facet

Shaft of rib

g

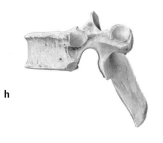

h

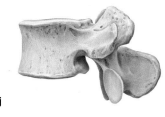

j

i

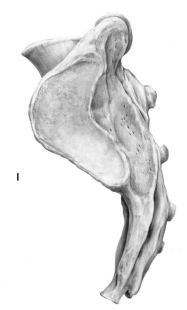

l

k

1.5   The Cervical Spine

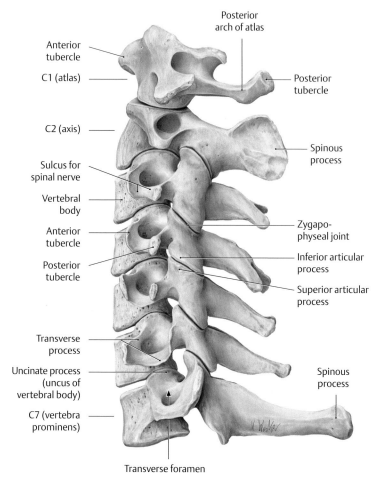

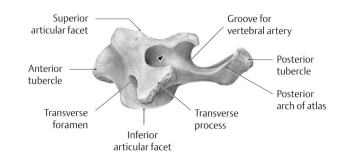

a   First cervical vertebra (atlas)

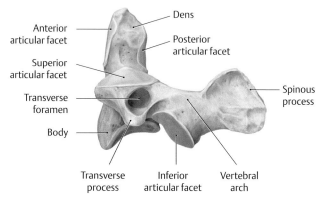

b   Second cervical vertebra (axis)

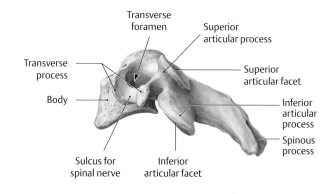

c   Fourth cervical vertebra

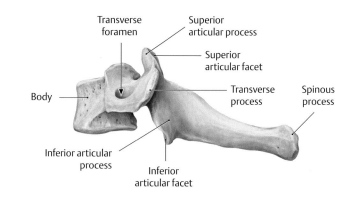

d   Seventh cervical vertebra (vertebra prominens)

B   Cervical vertebrae, left lateral view

A   Cervical spine, left lateral view

Of the cervical vertebrae, which number seven in all, the **first and second cervical vertebrae** (C1 and C2, atlas and axis) differ most conspicuously from the common vertebral morphology. They are specialized for bearing the weight of the head and allowing the head to move in all directions, similar to a ball-and-socket joint. Each of the **remaining five cervical vertebrae** (C3–C7) has a relatively small body, which presents a more or less square shape when viewed from above, and a large, triangular vertebral foramen (see **Cc**). The superior and inferior surfaces of the vertebral bodies are saddle-shaped, the superior surfaces bearing lateral uncinate processes that do not appear until about the tenth year of life (see p. 102). The transverse process consists of an anterior and a posterior bar, which terminate laterally in two small tubercles (anterior and posterior tubercles). These bars enclose the transverse foramen, through which the vertebral artery ascends from the C6 to the C1 level. The superior surface of the transverse process of the first three cervical vertebrae bears a broad, deep notch (spinal nerve sulcus), in which lies the emerging spinal nerve at that level. The superior and inferior articular processes are broad and flat. Their articular surfaces are flat and are inclined approximately 45° from the horizontal plane. The spinous processes of the third through sixth cervical vertebrae are short and bifid. The spinous process of the seventh cervical vertebra is longer and thicker than the others and is the first of the spinous processes that is distinctly palpable through the skin (vertebra prominens).

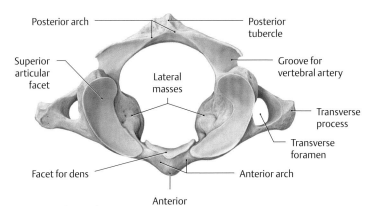

Posterior arch — Posterior tubercle

Superior articular facet

Lateral masses

Groove for vertebral artery

Transverse process

Transverse foramen

Facet for dens — Anterior arch

Anterior tubercle

a First cervical vertebra (atlas)

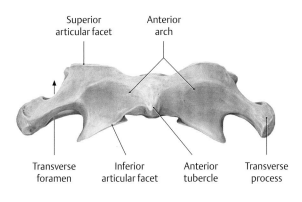

Superior articular facet — Anterior arch

Transverse foramen — Inferior articular facet — Anterior tubercle — Transverse process

a First cervical vertebra (atlas)

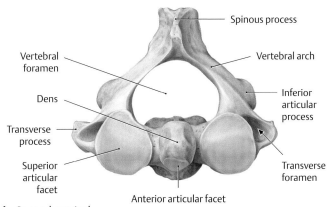

Spinous process

Vertebral foramen

Vertebral arch

Dens

Inferior articular process

Transverse process

Superior articular facet

Transverse foramen

Anterior articular facet

b Second cervical vertebra (axis)

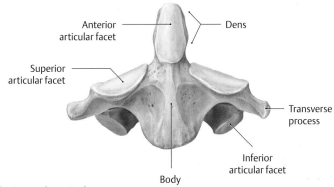

Anterior articular facet — Dens

Superior articular facet

Transverse process

Inferior articular facet

Body

b Second cervical vertebra (axis)

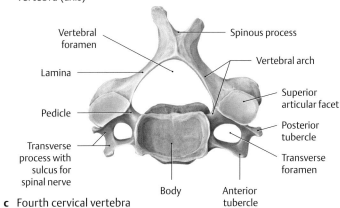

Vertebral foramen — Spinous process

Lamina — Vertebral arch

Pedicle — Superior articular facet

Transverse process with sulcus for spinal nerve

Posterior tubercle

Transverse foramen

Body — Anterior tubercle

c Fourth cervical vertebra

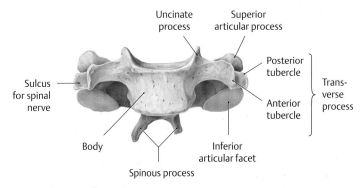

Uncinate process — Superior articular process

Sulcus for spinal nerve

Posterior tubercle

Trans-verse process

Anterior tubercle

Body

Inferior articular facet

Spinous process

c Fourth cervical vertebra

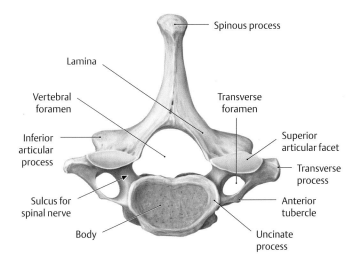

Spinous process

Lamina

Vertebral foramen

Transverse foramen

Inferior articular process

Superior articular facet

Transverse process

Sulcus for spinal nerve

Anterior tubercle

Body

Uncinate process

d Seventh cervical vertebra (vertebra prominens)

C Cervical vertebrae, superior view

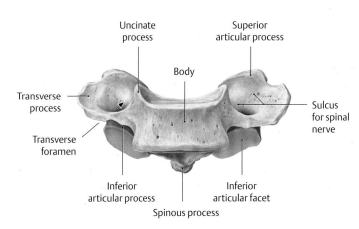

Uncinate process — Superior articular process

Body

Transverse process

Sulcus for spinal nerve

Transverse foramen

Inferior articular process

Inferior articular facet

Spinous process

d Seventh cervical vertebra (vertebra prominens)

D Cervical vertebrae, anterior view

85

1.6 The Thoracic Spine

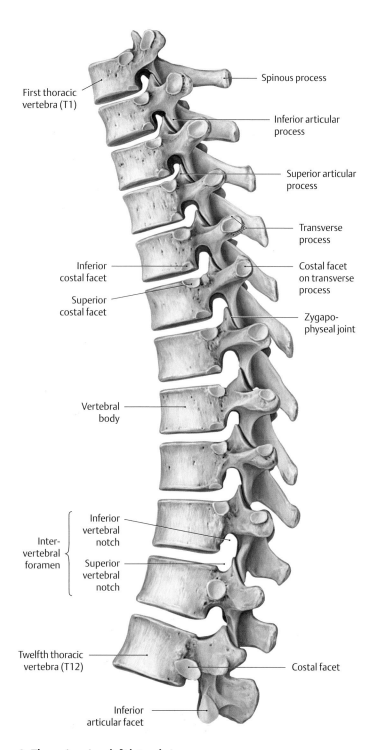

A Thoracic spine, left lateral view

The thoracic vertebral bodies gradually become taller and broader from superior to inferior, the lower vertebral bodies assuming a transverse oval shape like that of the lumbar vertebrae. The vertebral foramen is roughly circular and is smaller than in the cervical and lumbar vertebrae. The endplates are rounded and triangular. The spinous processes are long and angled sharply inferiorly, creating an overlapping arrangement that interlinks the thoracic vertebrae. The facets of the *inferior* articular processes are directed anteriorly, while the facets of the *superior* articular processes face posterior so that they can articulate with the inferior facets to form the zygapophyseal or facet joints (p. 100). Another special feature of the thoracic vertebrae is that their transverse processes are angled posterior to allow for articulations of the ribs.

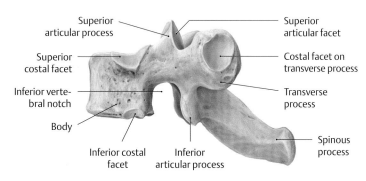

a Second thoracic vertebra

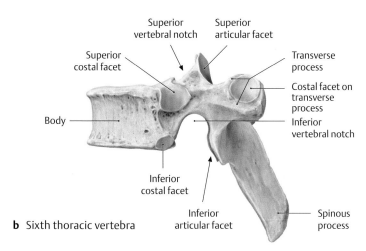

b Sixth thoracic vertebra

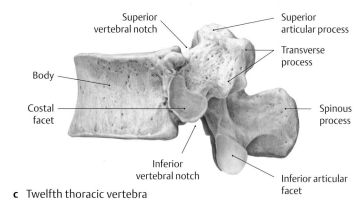

c Twelfth thoracic vertebra

B Thoracic vertebrae, left lateral view

The costal facets are cartilage-covered surfaces which articulate with the corresponding ribs (see p. 111). The bodies of the first through ninth thoracic vertebrae (T1–T9) bear two articular facets on each side —a superior costal facet and an inferior costal facet—such that two adjacent vertebrae combine to articulate with the head of a rib. Thus a given numbered rib articulates with its own numbered vertebra and the vertebra above. Exceptions to this scheme are ribs 1, 11, and 12, which articulate only with the vertebral body of the same number. The body of the tenth thoracic vertebra has only superior articular facets, and the tenth rib articulates with the ninth and tenth thoracic vertebrae. As mentioned, the transverse processes of the thoracic vertebrae (except for T11 and T12) also bear articular facets for the ribs.

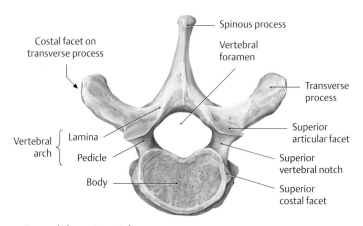

a Second thoracic vertebra

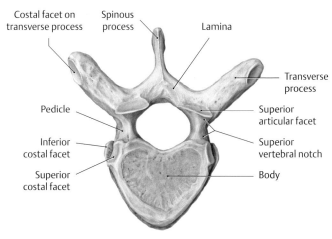

b Sixth thoracic vertebra

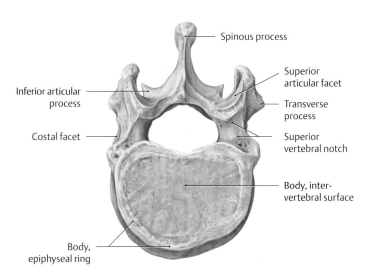

c Twelfth thoracic vertebra

C Thoracic vertebrae, superior view
The laminae and pedicles make up the vertebral arch.

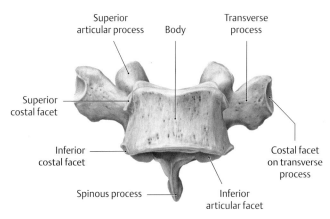

a Second thoracic vertebra

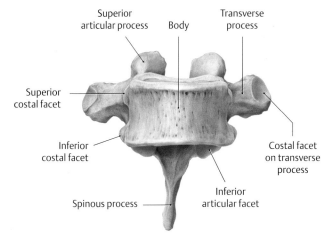

b Sixth thoracic vertebra

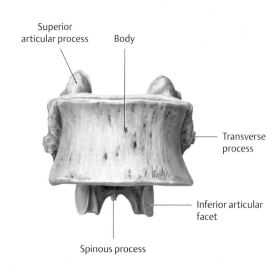

c Twelfth thoracic vertebra

D Thoracic vertebrae, anterior view

87

1.7 The Lumbar Spine

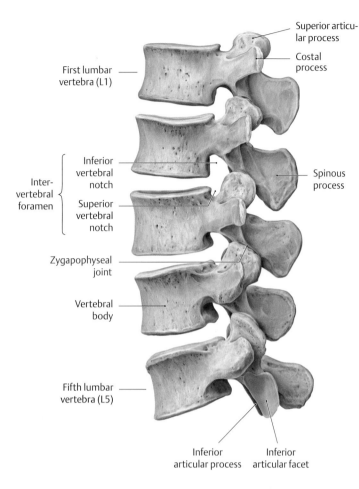

A Lumbar spine, left lateral view
The bodies of the lumbar vertebrae are large and have a transverse oval shape when viewed from above (see **C**). The massive vertebral arches enclose an almost triangular vertebral foramen, and they unite posteriorly to form a thick spinous process that is flattened on each side. The "transverse processes" of the lumbar vertebrae correspond phylogenetically to rudimentary ribs (see p. 82). Thus they are more accurately termed costal processes and are not homologous with the transverse processes of the other vertebrae. The thick costal process is fused with the actual transverse process, which is a small, pointed eminence located at the root of each costal process (accessory process, see **Cb**). The relatively massive superior and inferior articular processes bear slightly inclined articular facets that have a vertical, almost sagittal orientation. The articular facets of the superior articular processes are slightly concave and face medially, while those of the inferior articular processes are slightly convex and face laterally. The mamillary processes on the lateral surfaces of the superior articular processes serve as origins and insertions for the intrinsic back muscles (see **Bb** and **Ca**).

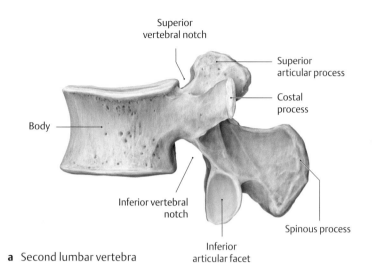

a Second lumbar vertebra

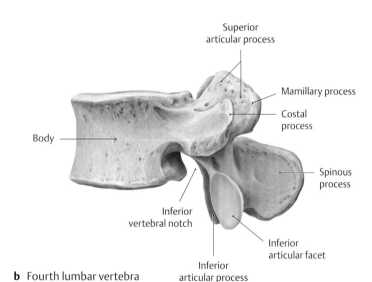

b Fourth lumbar vertebra

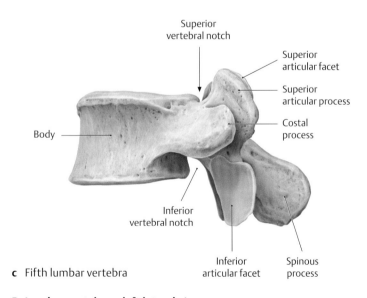

c Fifth lumbar vertebra

B Lumbar vertebrae, left lateral view

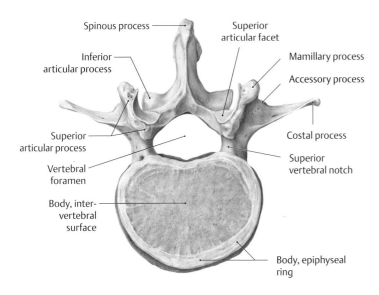

Spinous process
Inferior articular process
Superior articular process
Vertebral foramen
Body, inter-vertebral surface
Superior articular facet
Mamillary process
Accessory process
Costal process
Superior vertebral notch
Body, epiphyseal ring

a Second lumbar vertebra

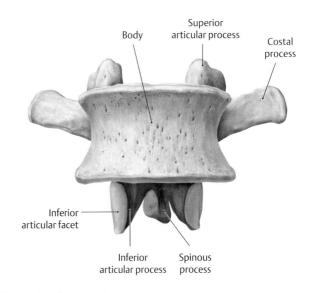

Body
Superior articular process
Costal process
Inferior articular facet
Inferior articular process
Spinous process

a Second lumbar vertebra

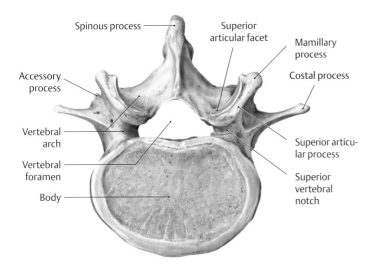

Spinous process
Accessory process
Vertebral arch
Vertebral foramen
Body
Superior articular facet
Mamillary process
Costal process
Superior articular process
Superior vertebral notch

b Fourth lumbar vertebra

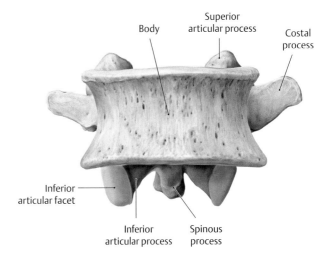

Body
Superior articular process
Costal process
Inferior articular facet
Inferior articular process
Spinous process

b Fourth lumbar vertebra

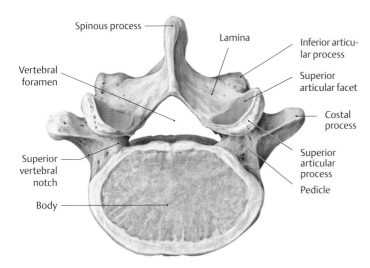

Spinous process
Vertebral foramen
Superior vertebral notch
Body
Lamina
Inferior articular process
Superior articular facet
Costal process
Superior articular process
Pedicle

c Fifth lumbar vertebra

C Lumbar vertebrae, superior view

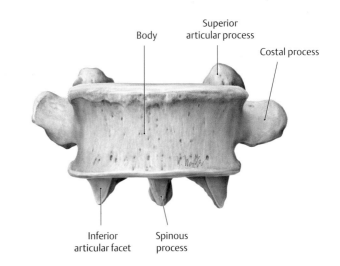

Body
Superior articular process
Costal process
Inferior articular facet
Spinous process

c Fifth lumbar vertebra

D Lumbar vertebrae, anterior view

89

1.8   The Sacrum and Coccyx

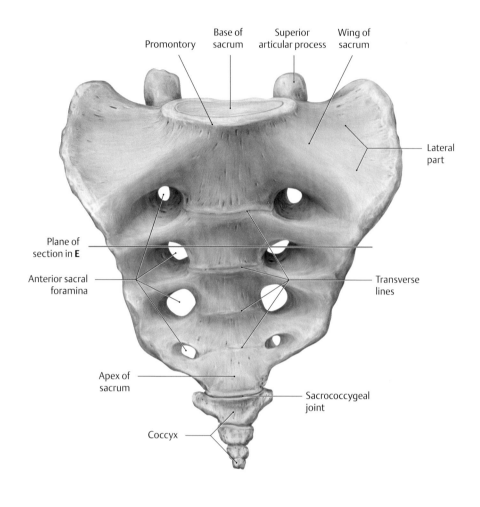

A Sacrum and coccyx, anterior (pelvic) view

The sacrum at birth is composed of five separate sacral vertebrae. Postnatally they fuse to form a single bone that is flattened anteroposteriorly and has a triangular shape when viewed from the front. The *base of the sacrum,* located at the superior end of the bone, articulates with the body of the fifth lumbar vertebra by a wedge-shaped intervertebral disk. The *apex of the sacrum* is at the inferior end of the bone and articulates with the coccyx. The anterior or *pelvic surface* of the sacrum is concave in both the sagittal and transverse planes (see **C**). Between the anterior sacral foramina are four transverse ridges (transverse lines), which mark the sites of fusion between the five sacral vertebrae. The coccyx consists of three or four rudimentary vertebrae. Only the first coccygeal vertebra exhibits some of the typical structural elements of a fully formed vertebra. It has two small coccygeal cornua representing the superior articular processes, in addition to two rudimentary transverse processes. A cartilaginous disk usually connects the base of the coccyx to the apex of the sacrum (sacrococcygeal joint). This joint allows passive forward and backward motion of the coccyx, increasing the anteroposterior diameter of the pelvic outlet during childbirth (see p. 115).

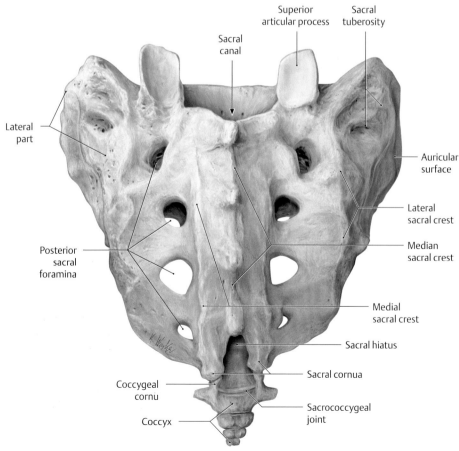

B Sacrum and coccyx, posterior (dorsal) view

The fused spinous processes form a jagged bony ridge on the convex dorsal surface of the sacrum, the *median sacral crest.* This ridge is flanked on each side by the paired *medial sacral crests,* formed by fusion of the articular processes. The medial crests are continuous below with the rudimentary inferior articular processes of the fifth sacral vertebra (the sacral cornua); they are continuous above with the two superior articular processes which face posteriorly. Between the sacral cornua is an aperture, the sacral hiatus, which is formed by the incomplete vertebral arch of the fifth sacral vertebrae and provides access to the sacral canal (e.g., for anesthesia). Lateral to the posterior sacral foramina are another pair of longitudinal ridges, the *lateral sacral crests,* formed by the fused transverse processes. The bony union of the transverse processes with the rudimentary ribs forms the thick *lateral* parts of the sacral wing which flank the body of the sacrum. Each lateral part bears an ear-shaped ("auricular") surface that articulates with the ilium (see **C**).

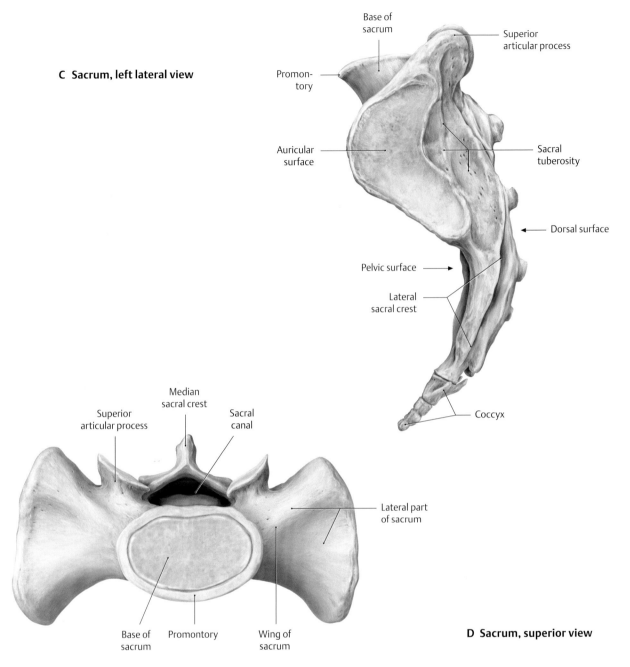

C Sacrum, left lateral view

Base of sacrum

Superior articular process

Promon- tory

Auricular surface

Sacral tuberosity

Dorsal surface

Pelvic surface

Lateral sacral crest

Coccyx

Superior articular process

Median sacral crest

Sacral canal

Lateral part of sacrum

Base of sacrum

Promontory

Wing of sacrum

D Sacrum, superior view

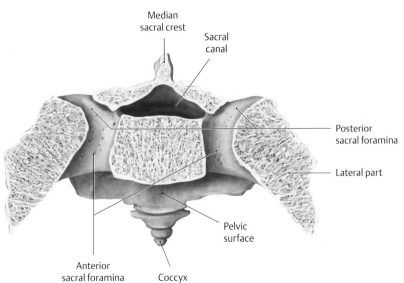

Median sacral crest

Sacral canal

Posterior sacral foramina

Lateral part

Pelvic surface

Anterior sacral foramina

Coccyx

E Transverse section through the sacrum
Superior view (the level of the section is shown in **A**). Fusion of the upper four sacral verte- brae creates four T-shaped bony canals at the level of the intervertebral foramina on each side, providing sites of emergence for the first through fourth sacral nerves. The correspond- ing ventral and dorsal rami of the spinal nerves exit the bony canals through the anterior and posterior sacral foramina (see p. 477).

1.9 The Intervertebral Disk: Structure and Function

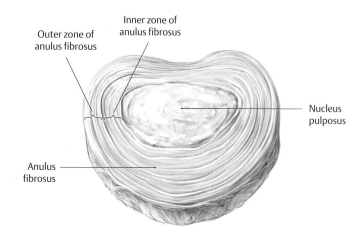

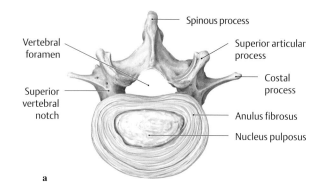

a

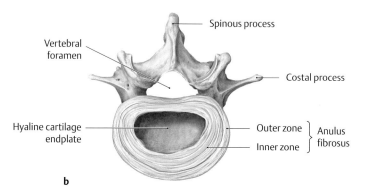

b

A Structure of an intervertebral disk

Isolated lumbar intervertebral disk, anterosuperior view.

The intervertebral disk consists of an external fibrous ring, the *anulus fibrosus,* and a gelatinous core, the *nucleus pulposus.* The anulus fibrosus consists of an outer zone and an inner zone. The outer zone is a fibrous sheath that possesses high tensile strength and is made up of concentric laminae of type I collagen fibers. Its fiber systems crisscross due to their varying obliquity and interconnect the marginal ridges of two adjacent vertebrae (see **B**), to which they are attached. At the junction with the inner zone of the anulus fibrosus, the tough fibrous tissue of the outer zone blends with a fibrocartilaginous tissue whose type II collagen fibers are attached to the hyaline cartilage endplates of the vertebral bodies (see **Da** and **Ea**).

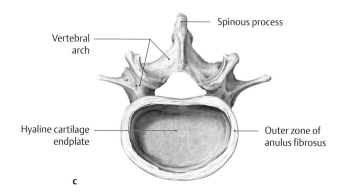

c

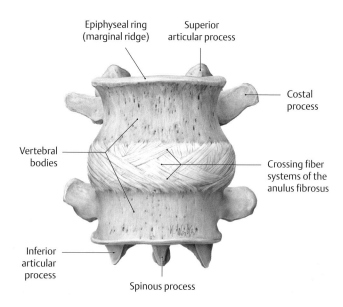

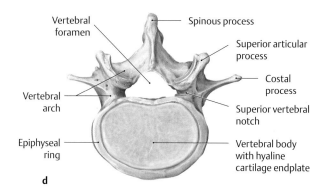

d

B Outer zone of the anulus fibrosus

Intervertebral disk between the third and fourth lumbar vertebrae, anterior view.

The connective-tissue fiber bundles in the outer zone of the anulus fibrosus cross one another at various angles, interconnecting the bony marginal ridges of two adjacent vertebral bodies.

C Main structural components of an intervertebral disk

Fourth lumbar vertebra with its associated upper disk, superior view.

a Intervertebral disk with the anulus fibrosus and nucleus pulposus.
b Anulus fibrosus (with the nucleus pulposus removed).
c Outer zone of the anulus fibrosus (with the inner zone removed).
d Hyaline cartilage endplate within the bony marginal ridge (entire intervertebral disk removed).

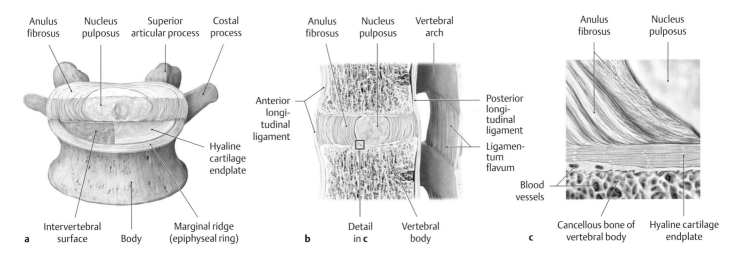

a

| Anulus fibrosus | Nucleus pulposus | Superior articular process | Costal process |

Hyaline cartilage endplate

| Intervertebral surface | Body | Marginal ridge (epiphyseal ring) |

b

| Anulus fibrosus | Nucleus pulposus | Vertebral arch |

Anterior longitudinal ligament

Posterior longitudinal ligament

Ligamentum flavum

Blood vessels

| Detail in **c** | Vertebral body |

c

| Anulus fibrosus | Nucleus pulposus |

| Cancellous bone of vertebral body | Hyaline cartilage endplate |

D Position of the intervertebral disk in the motion segment

a Hyaline cartilage endplate, anterosuperior view (the anterior half of the disk and right half of the endplate have been removed).

b Sagittal section through a motion segment (see p.100), left lateral view.

c Detail from **b.**

Except for the outer zone of the anulus fibrosus, the entire disk is in contact superiorly and inferiorly with the hyaline cartilage layer of the adjacent vertebral endplates. The subchondral, bony portion of the endplate consists of compact bone (intervertebral surface) permeated by myriad pores (see **c**) through which the vessels in the bone marrow spaces of the vertebral bodies can supply nutrients to the disk tissue.

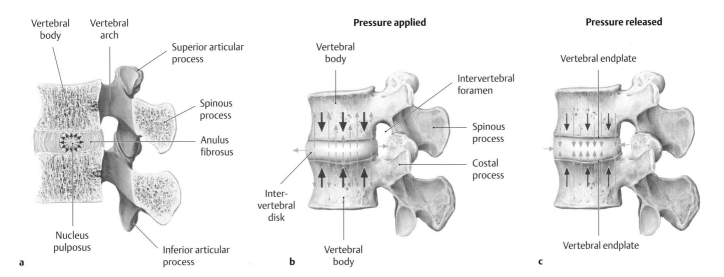

a

| Vertebral body | Vertebral arch |

Superior articular process

Spinous process

Anulus fibrosus

Nucleus pulposus

Inferior articular process

Pressure applied

Vertebral body

Intervertebral foramen

Spinous process

Costal process

Intervertebral disk

b Vertebral body

Pressure released

Vertebral endplate

Vertebral endplate

c

E Load-dependent fluid shifts in the intervertebral disk

a The nucleus pulposus functions as a "water cushion" to absorb transient axial loads on the intervertebral disk. Mechanically, the disk represents a hydrostatic system that is resilient under pressure. It is composed of a tension-resistant sheath (the anulus fibrosus) and a watery, incompressible core, the nucleus pulposus. This core consists of 80–85 % water, which it can reversibly bind in its paucicellular, gelatinous, mucoviscous tissue (owing to its high content of glycosaminoglycans). The nucleus pulposus is under a very high hydrostatic pressure, particularly when acted upon by gravity and other forces. This pressure can be absorbed by the adjacent cartilaginous endplates and also by the anulus fibrosus (which transforms compressive forces into tensile forces). In this way the nucleus pulposus functions as a "water cushion" or hydraulic press between two adjacent vertebral bodies. Combined with the anulus fibrosus, it acts as an effective shock absorber that can distribute pressures uniformly over the adjacent vertebral endplates.

b Fluid outflow from the intervertebral disk (green arrows) in response to a sustained pressure load (thick red arrows). While transient loads are cushioned by the shock-absorber function of the nucleus pulposus and anulus fibrosus (see **a**), sustained loads cause a gradual but permanent outflow of fluid from the disk. The turgor and height of the disk are reduced, while the endplates and eventually the bony vertebral elements move closer together (see p.105 for further details on disk degeneration).

c Fluid uptake by the intervertebral disk (green arrows) when pressure is released (thin red arrows). The process described in **b** is reversed when the pressure on the disk is released, and the height of the disk increases. This increase is caused by fluid uptake from the subchondral blood vessels in the bone marrow spaces, which are instrumental in disk nutrition (see **Dc**). As a result of pressure-dependent fluid shifts (convection) in the intervertebral disks, the overall body height decreases temporarily by approximately 1 % (1.5–2.0 cm) relative to the initial body height during the course of the day.

A The ligaments of the spinal column at the level of the thoracolumbar junction (T11–L3)

Left lateral view. The two uppermost thoracic vertebrae have been sectioned in the midsagittal plane.

B The ligaments of the spinal column

The ligaments of the spinal column bind the vertebrae securely to one another and enable the spine to withstand high mechanical loads and shearing stresses. The ligaments are subdivided into vertebral *body* ligaments and vertebral *arch* ligaments.

Vertebral body ligaments
• Anterior longitudinal ligament
• Posterior longitudinal ligament

Vertebral arch ligaments
• Ligamenta flava
• Interspinous ligaments
• Supraspinous ligament
• Nuchal ligament*
• Intertransverse ligaments

* The sagittally oriented nuchal ligament runs between the external occipital protuberance and the seventh cervical vertebra; it corresponds to a supraspinal ligament that is broadened superiorly (see p. 97).

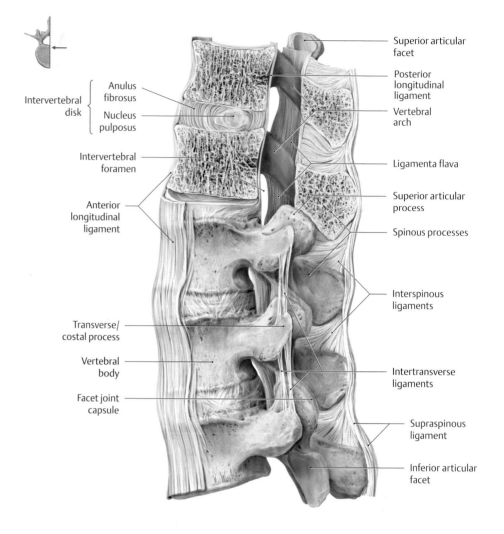

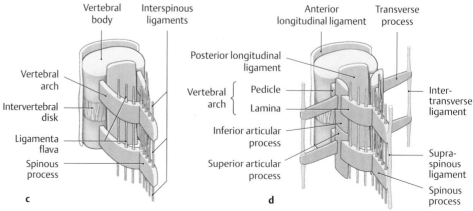

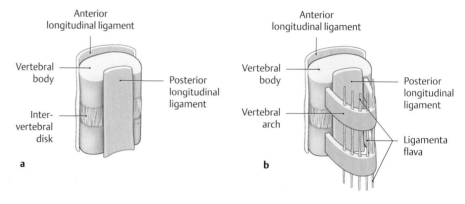

C Schematic representation of the vertebral body and vertebral arch ligaments

Viewed obliquely from the left posterior view.

a Vertebral body ligaments.
b–d Vertebral arch ligaments.

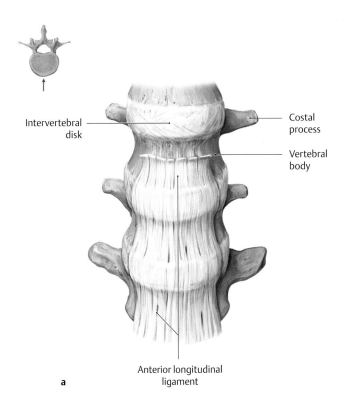

Intervertebral disk

Costal process

Vertebral body

Anterior longitudinal ligament

a

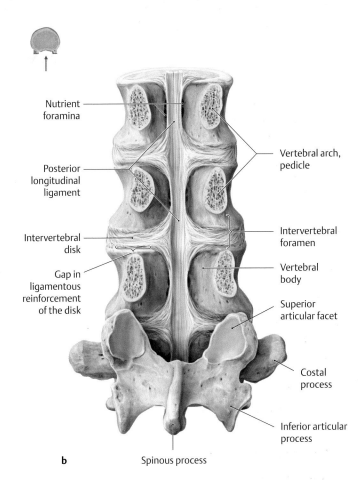

Nutrient foramina

Posterior longitudinal ligament

Intervertebral disk

Gap in ligamentous reinforcement of the disk

Vertebral arch, pedicle

Intervertebral foramen

Vertebral body

Superior articular facet

Costal process

Inferior articular process

b

Spinous process

D The ligaments surrounding the lumbar spine

a Anterior longitudinal ligament, anterior view.

b Posterior longitudinal ligament, posterior view after removal of the vertebral arches at the pedicular level.

c Ligamenta flava and intertransverse ligaments, anterior view (after removal of the L 2–L 4 vertebral bodies). (The other vertebral arch ligaments are not visible in this view.)

The **anterior longitudinal ligament** runs broadly on the anterior side of the vertebral bodies, extending from the skull base to the sacrum. Its deep fibers bind adjacent vertebral bodies together while its superficial fibers span multiple segments. Its collagenous fibers are attached firmly to the vertebral bodies but have only a loose attachment to the intervertebral disks. The thinner **posterior longitudinal ligament** descends from the clivus along the posterior view of the vertebral bodies, passing into the sacral canal. The portion over the vertebral bodies is narrow and is attached to their superior and inferior margins. The ligament broadens at the levels of the intervertebral disks, to which it is firmly attached by tapered lateral extensions. Despite the attachment of the ligament to the anulus fibrosus of the intervertebral disks (not seen clearly here, being hidden by the posterior longitudinal ligament), a large portion of the intervertebral disk has no ligamentous reinforcement, especially laterally (predisposing to lateral disk herniation, see p.105). Both longitudinal ligaments contribute to maintaining the normal curvature of the spinal column. The **ligamenta flava** consist mainly of elastic fibers, which give these ligaments their characteristic yellow color. They are thick, powerful ligaments that connect the laminae of adjacent vertebral arches and reinforce the wall of the vertebral canal posterior to the intervertebral foramina (see **A**). When the spinal column is erect, the ligamenta flava are under tension and help the back muscles to stabilize the spine in the sagittal plane. They also act as checkreins to limit forward flexion of the spinal column, thereby helping to maintain the position of the flexed spine. The tips of the transverse processes are connected on each side by the **intertransverse ligaments,** which serve to limit rocking movements of one vertebra upon another.

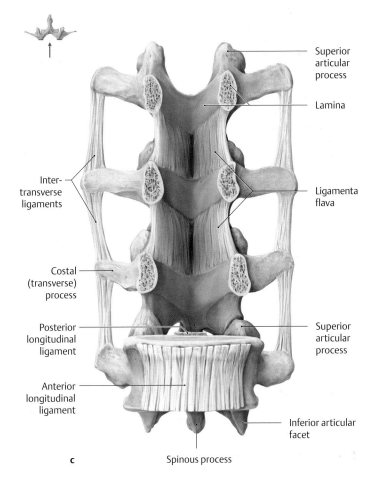

Superior articular process

Lamina

Intertransverse ligaments

Ligamenta flava

Costal (transverse) process

Posterior longitudinal ligament

Superior articular process

Anterior longitudinal ligament

Inferior articular facet

c

Spinous process

95

1.11 Overview of the Ligaments of the Cervical Spine

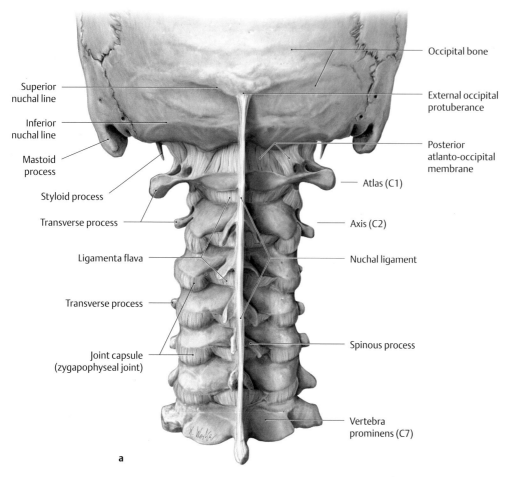

- Superior nuchal line
- Inferior nuchal line
- Mastoid process
- Styloid process
- Transverse process
- Ligamenta flava
- Transverse process
- Joint capsule (zygapophyseal joint)
- Occipital bone
- External occipital protuberance
- Posterior atlanto-occipital membrane
- Atlas (C1)
- Axis (C2)
- Nuchal ligament
- Spinous process
- Vertebra prominens (C7)

a

A The ligaments of the cervical spine
a Posterior view.
b Anterior view after removal of the anterior skull base (see p. 98 for the ligaments of the upper cervical spine, especially the craniovertebral joints).

b → ← a

B The craniovertebral joints

The craniovertebral joints are the articulations between the atlas (C1) and occipital bone (atlanto-occipital joints) and between the atlas and axis (C2, atlantoaxial joints). While these joints, which number six in all, are anatomically distinct, they are mechanically interlinked and comprise a functional unit (see p. 101).

Atlanto-occipital joints

Paired joints where the oval, slightly concave superior articular facets of the atlas articulate with the convex occipital condyles.

Atlantoaxial joints

- *Lateral atlantoaxial joint* = paired articulation between the inferior articular facets of the atlas and the superior articular facets of the axis
- *Median atlantoaxial joint* = unpaired articulation (comprising an anterior and posterior compartment) between the dens of the axis, the fovea of the atlas, and the cartilage-covered anterior surface of the transverse ligament of the atlas (see p. 99)

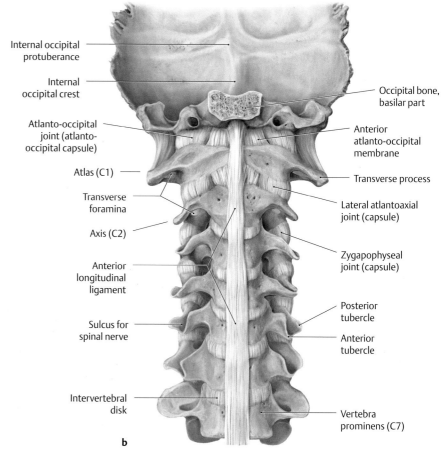

- Internal occipital protuberance
- Internal occipital crest
- Atlanto-occipital joint (atlanto-occipital capsule)
- Atlas (C1)
- Transverse foramina
- Axis (C2)
- Anterior longitudinal ligament
- Sulcus for spinal nerve
- Intervertebral disk
- Occipital bone, basilar part
- Anterior atlanto-occipital membrane
- Transverse process
- Lateral atlantoaxial joint (capsule)
- Zygapophyseal joint (capsule)
- Posterior tubercle
- Anterior tubercle
- Vertebra prominens (C7)

b

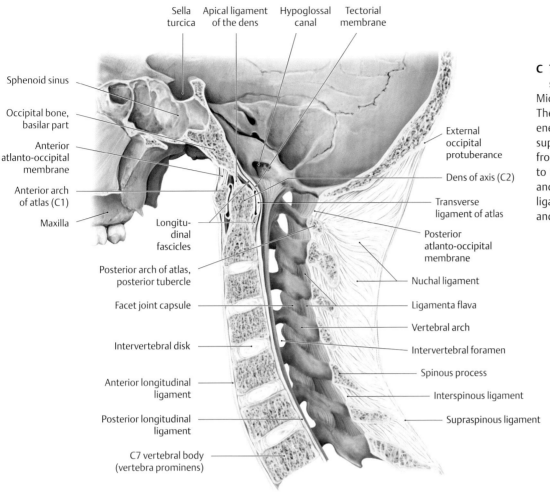

Sella turcica · Apical ligament of the dens · Hypoglossal canal · Tectorial membrane

Sphenoid sinus

Occipital bone, basilar part

Anterior atlanto-occipital membrane

Anterior arch of atlas (C1)

Maxilla

Longitudinal fascicles

Posterior arch of atlas, posterior tubercle

Facet joint capsule

Intervertebral disk

Anterior longitudinal ligament

Posterior longitudinal ligament

C7 vertebral body (vertebra prominens)

External occipital protuberance

Dens of axis (C2)

Transverse ligament of atlas

Posterior atlanto-occipital membrane

Nuchal ligament

Ligamenta flava

Vertebral arch

Intervertebral foramen

Spinous process

Interspinous ligament

Supraspinous ligament

C The ligaments of the cervical spine: nuchal ligament

Midsagittal section, left lateral view. The nuchal ligament is the broadened, sagittally oriented part of the supraspinous ligament that extends from the vertebra prominens (C1) to the external occipital protuberance (see **A**; see also p. 98 for the ligaments of the atlanto-occipital and atlantoaxial joints).

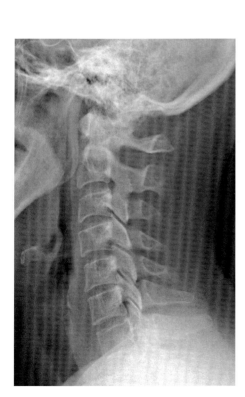

D Plain lateral radiograph of the cervical spine

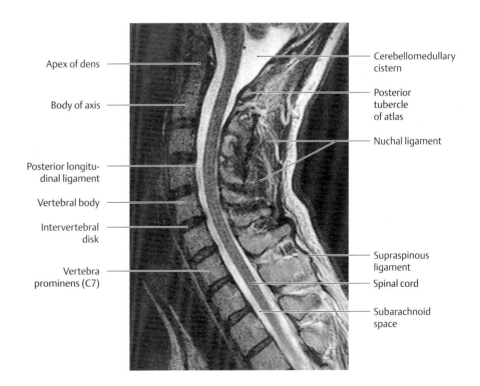

Apex of dens

Body of axis

Posterior longitudinal ligament

Vertebral body

Intervertebral disk

Vertebra prominens (C7)

Cerebellomedullary cistern

Posterior tubercle of atlas

Nuchal ligament

Supraspinous ligament

Spinal cord

Subarachnoid space

E Magnetic resonance image of the cervical spine

Midsagittal section, left lateral view, T2-weighted TSE sequence. (from Vahlensieck u. Reiser: MRT des Bewegungsapparates, 2. ed. Thieme, Stuttgart 2001).

1.12 The Ligaments of the Upper Cervical Spine (Atlanto-occipital and Atlantoaxial Joints)

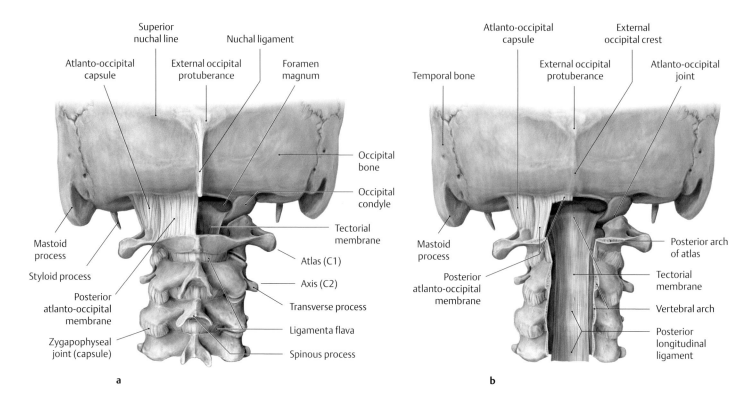

a

b

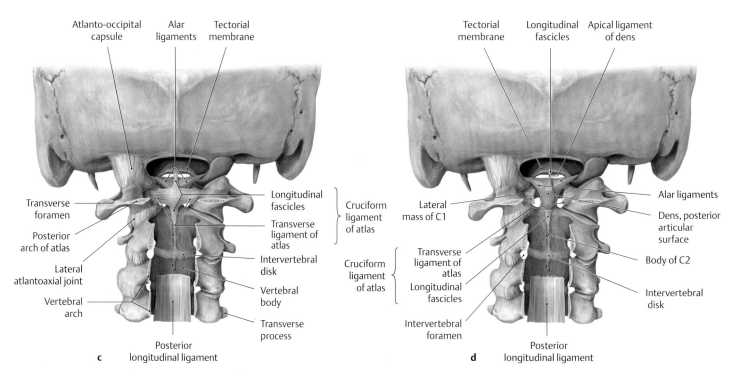

c

d

A The ligaments of the craniovertebral joints
Skull and upper cervical spine, posterior view.

a The posterior atlanto-occipital membrane—the "ligamentum flavum" between the atlas and occipital bone (see p. 94)—stretches from the posterior arch of the atlas to the posterior rim of the foramen magnum. This membrane has been removed on the right side.

b With the vertebral canal opened and the spinal cord removed, the tectorial membrane, a broadened expansion of the posterior longitudinal ligament, is seen to form the anterior boundary of the vertebral canal at the level of the craniovertebral joints.

c With the tectorial membrane removed, the cruciform ligament of the atlas can be seen. The transverse ligament of the atlas forms the thick horizontal bar of the cross, and the longitudinal fascicles form the thinner vertical bar.

d The transverse ligament of the atlas and longitudinal fascicles have been partially removed to demonstrate the paired alar ligaments, which extend from the lateral surfaces of the dens to the corresponding inner surfaces of the occipital condyles, and the unpaired apical ligament of the dens, which passes from the tip of the dens to the anterior rim of the foramen magnum.

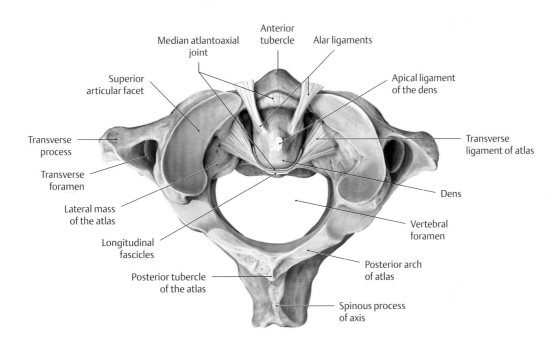

B The ligaments of the median atlantoaxial joint
Atlas and axis, superior view. (The fovea, while part of the median atlantoaxial joint, is hidden by the joint capsule.)

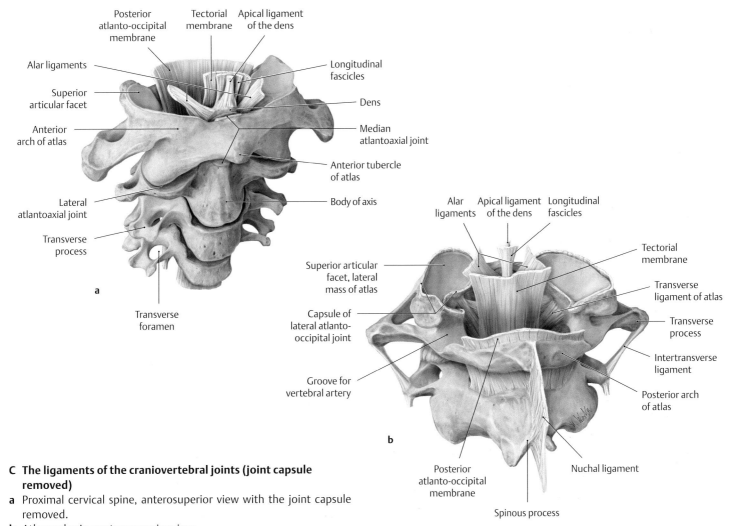

C The ligaments of the craniovertebral joints (joint capsule removed)
a Proximal cervical spine, anterosuperior view with the joint capsule removed.
b Atlas and axis, posterosuperior view.

1.13 The Intervertebral Facet Joints, Motion Segments, and Range of Motion in Different Spinal Regions

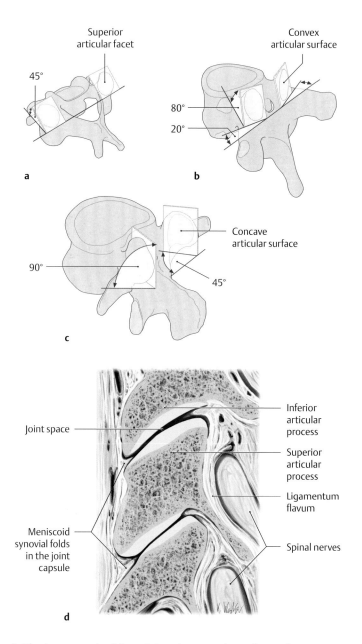

a

b

c

d

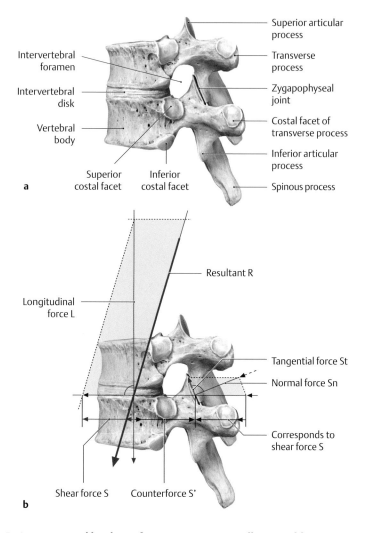

a

b

A The intervertebral facet joints (zygapophyseal joints)

The diagrams show the position of the articular surfaces of the intervertebral facet joints in different regions of the spinal column, shown from the left posterosuperior view: **a** cervical spine, **b** thoracic spine, **c** lumbar spine. Panel **d** is a sagittal section through the facet joints at the level of the third, fourth, and fifth cervical vertebrae, shown from the lateral view (drawing based on a specimen from the Anatomical Collection at Kiel University).

The paired facet joints are true synovial joints formed by the articular processes of the vertebral arches (see p. 82). Their articular surfaces, called **facets,** show varying degrees of inclination from the horizontal (and vertical) in different spinal regions and are therefore specialized for certain directions and ranges of motion (the movements that can occur in different spinal regions are shown in **D**). The **joint capsule** of the facet joints is inserted into the margins of the articular facets and is often firmly attached to the ligamentum flavum (see **d**). The joint capsule tends to be broad and lax in the cervical spine but is considerably narrower in the thoracic and lumbar regions. Almost all the intervertebral joints contain *meniscoid synovial folds,* which form a crescent-shaped projection into the joint space. The folds consist of some loose but mostly firm connective tissue that has a rich vascular supply. The function of these folds is to fill the spaces around the articular surfaces (**d**).

B Structure and loading of a motion segment, illustrated for two thoracic vertebrae

Lateral view. "Motion segment" is the term applied to the articular and muscular connection between two adjacent vertebrae (**a**). It consists of the intervertebral disk, the paired intervertebral facet joints (zygapophyseal joints), and the associated ligaments and muscles (not depicted here). For clinical purposes, the motion segment is also considered to include the contents of the intervertebral foramina (nerves and blood vessels, see pp. 162 and 168) and the contents of the vertebral canal. In all, the spinal column contains 25 of these motion segments, which constitute distinct functional and morphological units. However, because of the interdependence of these units, abnormalities in a circumscribed portion of the spinal column tend to affect the other spinal segments as well. Each of these motion segments is subjected to certain loads that can be represented as applied forces (**b**): a forward-directed *shear force* and a downward-directed *longitudinal force,* which combine to give the resultant force R. The longitudinal force acts on the vertebral body and intervertebral disk, while the shear force is absorbed mainly by the ligaments and facet joints (counterforce S'). The shear force can be subdivided into a normal force (Sn) and a tangential force (St). Because the shearing forces are not perpendicular to the articular surfaces of the facet joints, these surfaces are loaded by the axially directed *normal force* (Sn), which is weaker than the original shear force. Displacement of the vertebrae by the upward-directed *tangential force* (St) is prevented by the ligaments and intrinsic back muscles (after Kummer).

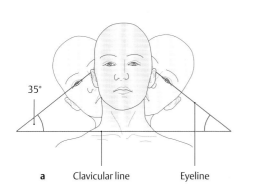

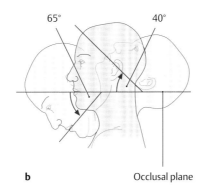

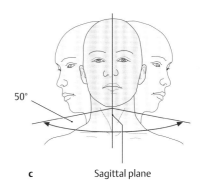

| a | Clavicular line | Eyeline | b | Occlusal plane | c | Sagittal plane |

C Total range of motion of the cervical spine
a Lateral flexion, **b** flexion/extension, **c** rotation.

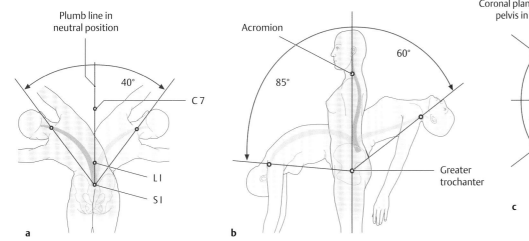

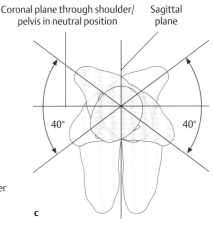

D Total range of motion of the thoracic and lumbar spine
a Lateral flexion, **b** flexion/extension, **c** rotation.
The clinical examination, particularly function testing, is of key importance in examinations of the spine. Because the total range of spinal motion is comprised of the movements of a total of 25 motion segments, generally the examiner can detect only movement disorders that affect individual regions. For example, clinical testing can show clear evidence of ankylosis affecting particular spinal segments. The examiner makes use of standard reference lines (e.g., the clavicular line or occlusal plane) in determining whether the range of spinal motion is normal or decreased.

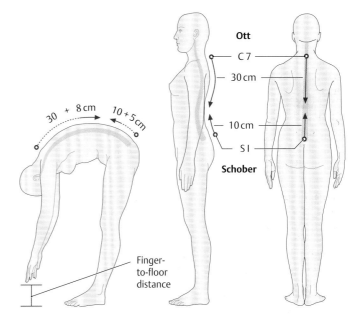

E Average ranges of motion in different spinal regions (degrees)

	Cervical spine			Tho-racic spine	Lum-bar spine	Cervical + thoracic + lumbar
	A-o joint	A-a joint	Entire cervical spine			
Flexion	20	—	65	35	50	150
Extension	10	—	40	25	35	100
Lateral flexion*	5	—	35	20	20	75
Rotation*	—	35	50	35	5	90

A-o joint = Atlanto-occipital joint
A-a joint = Atlantoaxial joint   * To each side

F Measurement of the range of thoracic and lumbar spinal flexion by the method of Schober and Ott
In the method of Schober and Ott, the patient stands erect while the examiner marks the S1 spinous process and a second point 10 cm higher. When the patient bends as far forward as possible, the distance between the two skin markings will increase to approximately 15 (10 + 5) cm (range of motion of the lumbar spine). The thoracic range of motion is determined by measuring 30 cm down from the spinous process of the C7 vertebra (vertebra prominens) and marking that point on the skin. When the patient bends forward, the distance between the markings may increase by up to 8 cm. An alternative method is to measure the smallest finger-to-floor distance (FFD) with the knees extended.

1.14 The Uncovertebral Joints of the Cervical Spine

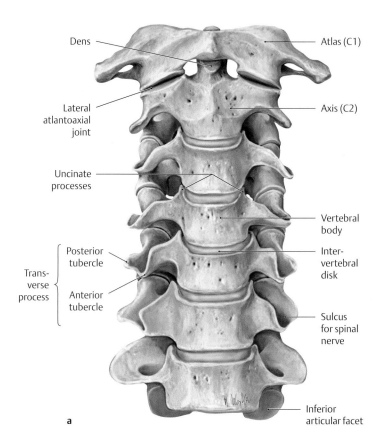

a

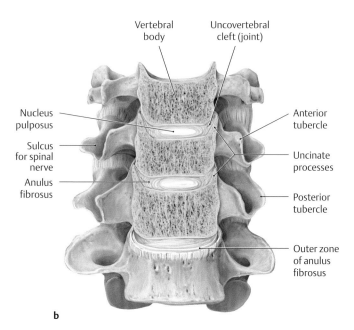

b

A The uncovertebral joints in a young adult
Cervical spine of an 18-year-old man, anterior view.

a The upper endplates of the C3 through C7 vertebral bodies have lateral projections (uncinate processes) that develop during childhood. Starting at about 10 years of age, the uncinate processes gradually come into contact with the oblique, crescent-shaped margin on the undersurface of the next higher vertebral body. This results in the formation of lateral clefts (uncovertebral clefts or joints, see **b**) in the outer portions of the intervertebral disks.

b C4 through C7 vertebrae. The bodies of the C4–C6 vertebrae have been sectioned in the coronal plane to demonstrate more clearly the uncovertebral joints or clefts. These clefts are bounded laterally by a connective tissue structure, a kind of joint capsule, which causes them to resemble true joint spaces. These clefts or fissures in the intervertebral disk were first described by the anatomist Hubert von Luschka in 1858, who called them "*lateral hemiarthroses.*" He interpreted them as primary mechanisms designed to enhance the flexibility of the cervical spine and confer a functional advantage (drawings based on specimens from the Anatomical Collection at Kiel University).

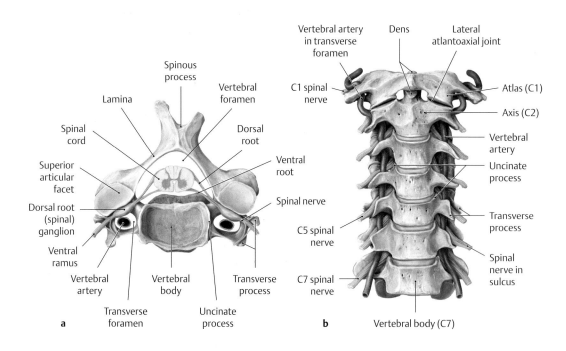

a

b

B Topographic relationship of the spinal nerve and vertebral artery to the uncinate process
a Fourth cervical vertebra with spinal cord, spinal roots, spinal nerves, and vertebral arteries, superior view.
b Cervical spine with both vertebral arteries and the emerging spinal nerves, anterior view.

Note the course of the vertebral artery through the transverse foramina and the course of the spinal nerve at the level of the intervertebral foramina. Given their close proximity, both the artery and nerve may be compressed by osteophytes (bony outgrowths) caused by uncovertebral arthrosis (see **D**).

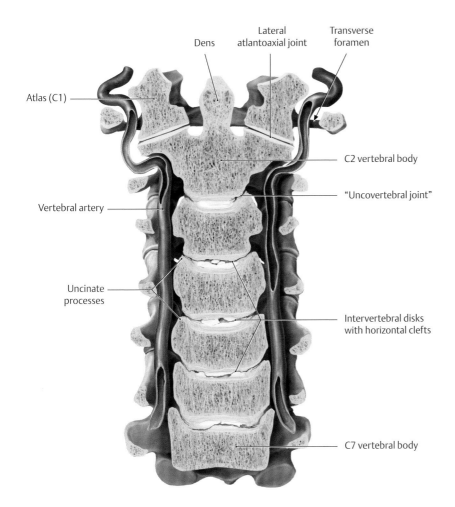

Atlas (C1)

Dens

Lateral atlantoaxial joint

Transverse foramen

C2 vertebral body

"Uncovertebral joint"

Vertebral artery

Uncinate processes

Intervertebral disks with horizontal clefts

C7 vertebral body

C Degenerative changes in the cervical spine (uncovertebral arthrosis)

Coronal section through the cervical spine of a 35-year-old man, anterior view. *Note* the course of the vertebral arteries on both sides of the vertebral bodies.

The development of the uncovertebral joints at approximately 10 years of age initiates a process of cleft formation in the intervertebral disks. This process spreads toward the center of the disk with aging, eventually resulting in the formation of complete transverse clefts that subdivide the intervertebral disks into two slabs of roughly equal thickness. The result is a progressive degenerative process marked by flattening of the disks and consequent instability of the motion segments (drawing based on specimens from the Anatomical Collection at Kiel University).

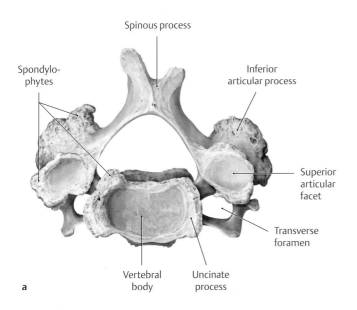

Spinous process

Spondylo-phytes

Inferior articular process

Superior articular facet

Transverse foramen

Vertebral body

Uncinate process

a

Vertebral body

Superior vertebral notch

Superior articular process

Zygapophyseal joint (facet joint)

Spondylo-phytes

Intervertebral foramen

Uncovertebral joint

Sulcus for spinal nerve

Spinous process

b

D Advanced uncovertebral arthrosis of the cervical spine

a Fourth cervical vertebra, superior view.

b Fourth and fifth cervical vertebrae, lateral view (drawings based on specimens from the Anatomical Collection at Kiel University).

The uncovertebral joints undergo degenerative changes comparable to those seen in other joints, including the formation of osteophytes (called spondylophytes when they occur on vertebral bodies). These sites of new bone formation serve to distribute the imposed forces over a larger area, thereby reducing the pressure on the joint. With progres-

sive destabilization of the corresponding motion segment, the facet joints undergo osteoarthritic changes leading to osteophyte formation. Osteophytes of the uncovertebral joints have major clinical importance because of their relation to the intervertebral foramen and vertebral artery (uncovertebral arthrosis). They cause a gradually progressive narrowing of the intervertebral foramen, with increasing compression of the spinal nerve and often of the vertebral artery as well (see **C**). Meanwhile the spinal canal itself may become significantly narrowed (spinal stenosis) by the same process.

1.15 Degenerative Changes in the Lumbar Spine

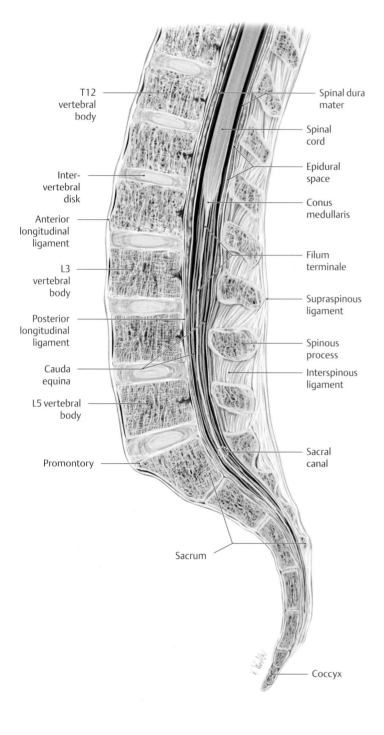

A Midsagittal section through the lower part of the spinal column
Left lateral view.
Note: The caudal end of the spinal cord, the conus medullaris, terminates at the level of the first or second lumbar vertebra. The spinal cord and spinal canal are approximately the same length until the 12th week of prenatal development, so that each pair of spinal nerves emerges through the intervertebral foramen at the level of the nerves. With further growth, however, the vertebral column lengthens more rapidly than the spinal cord, resulting in an increasing cephalad displacement of the cona medullaris. At birth the cona medullaris has already reached the level of the third lumbar vertebra, and it continues its gradual upward shift until about the 10th year of life. Because of these disparate growth rates, the spinal roots run obliquely downward from their segment of origin in the cord to reach their corresponding intervertebral foramen. The spinal roots that descend from the lower end of the cord are collectively termed the *cauda equina* ("horse's tail"). Because the membranes that enclose the spinal cord (the meninges) extend into the sacral canal, a needle can be safely introduced into the subarachnoid space below the conus medullaris to sample cerebrospinal fluid without injuring the cord *(lumbar puncture)*. This site is also used for *lumbar spinal anesthesia* to block both the afferent nerve roots (for analgesia) and the efferent nerve roots (for muscular paralysis) that supply the pelvic region and lower limbs.

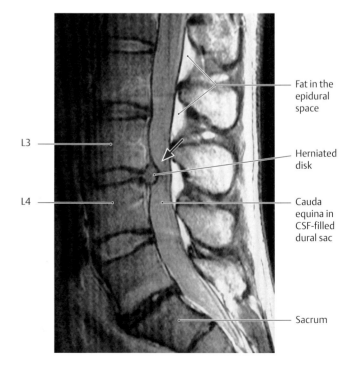

B Posterior disk herniation in the lumbar spine
Midsagittal T2-weighted magnetic resonance image of the lumbar spine, left lateral view (from Vahlensieck u. Reiser: MRT des Bewegungsapparates, 2. ed. Thieme, Stuttgart 2001). The image shows a conspicuous herniated disk at the L3–L4 level (red arrow), which protrudes posteriorly (transligamentous herniation). The dural sac at that level is deeply indented (see **Cb**).

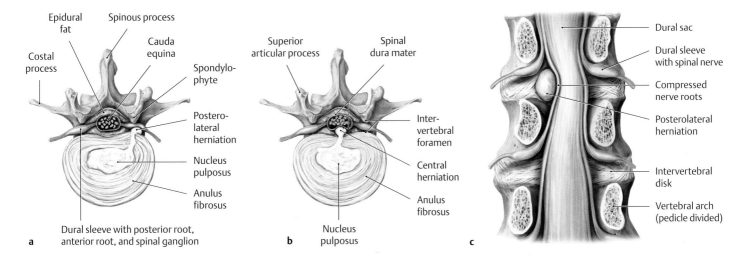

C Lumbar disk herniation
a Posterolateral herniation, superior view
b Posterior herniation, superior view
c Posterolateral herniation, posterior view (the vertebral arches have been removed to demonstrate the lumbar dural sac and corresponding nerve roots)

With aging, the intervertebral disk tissue undergoes regressive changes in which the water content of the disk decreases and, with it, the turgor of the disk. As a result of this, the disks become thinner (see p. 93), often leading to a loss of stability in the motion segment (see **Da**). As the stress resistance of the anulus fibrosus (the "outer sheath" of the disk)

also declines with age, providing less effective containment, the tissue of the nucleus pulposus may protrude through weak spots under loading. The initial step in this process is a disk protrusion. If the fibrous ring of the anulus eventually ruptures completely, the nucleus pulposus can prolapse through the defect, resulting in a herniated or "ruptured" disk. The herniated material may compress the contents of the intervertebral foramen (nerve roots and blood vessels). A posterolateral herniation generally compresses the subjacent nerve root (**c**), causing pain and paralysis that affect caudally adjacent dermatomes and corresponding muscles.

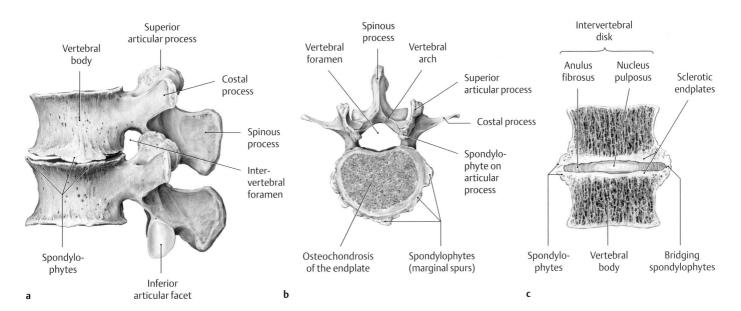

D Spondylophytes involving a spinal motion segment
a Third and fourth lumbar vertebrae, lateral view (intervertebral disk removed).
b Fourth lumbar vertebra, superior view.
c Coronal section through the third and fourth lumbar vertebrae.

The degeneration of intervertebral disk material is usually accompanied by reactive changes in the bone (aimed at increasing the load-bearing surface area and reducing stresses on the joint). The overall effect of these changes is to stabilize the motion segment. The principle of these processes is similar to that involved in osteoarthritis of the joints

in the limbs. Typically the changes begin with marginal spurring of the vertebral bodies (osteophytes = spondylophytes, **a**), narrowing of the intervertebral disk space (chondrosis, **b**), and sclerosis of the vertebral endplates (osteochondrosis, **c**). Similar changes also take place in the facet joints (spondylarthrosis). Further progression may lead to the formation of "bridging osteophytes" as adjacent marginal spurs grow together and create a bony ankylosis across the motion segment (**c**). However, the body of the vertebra may be the principal focus of deterioration in the geriatric spine. Progressive osteoporosis and the associated loss of bony stability may culminate in vertebral body collapse and deformity.

1.16 The Thoracic Skeleton

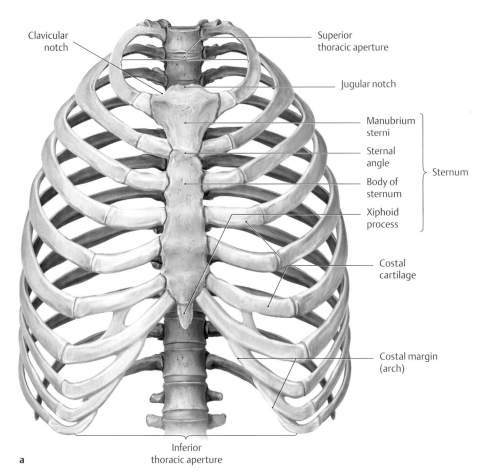

Clavicular notch

Superior thoracic aperture

Jugular notch

Manubrium sterni

Sternal angle

Body of sternum

Xiphoid process

Sternum

Costal cartilage

Costal margin (arch)

a

Inferior thoracic aperture

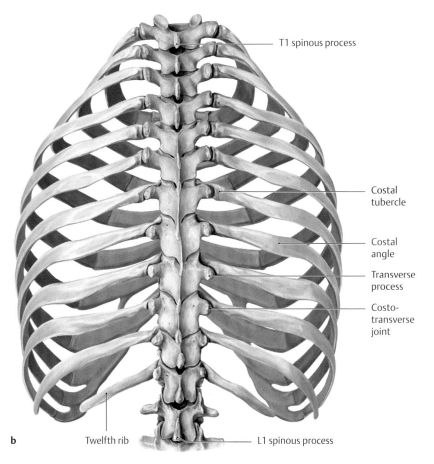

T1 spinous process

Costal tubercle

Costal angle

Transverse process

Costo-transverse joint

b

Twelfth rib

L1 spinous process

A Thoracic skeleton

a Anterior view, **b** posterior view.

The thoracic skeleton (thoracic cage, thorax) consists of the vertebral column, the twelve pairs of ribs, and the sternum. These structures are movably interconnected by ligaments, true joints, and synchondroses. Tension is imparted to the thorax by the intercostal muscles. The thoracic cage encloses the chest cavity and has a superior aperture (the thoracic inlet) and an inferior aperture (the thoracic outlet). Its shape is subject to marked variations relating to age and gender. The ribs of an infant have very little obliquity and are approximately horizontal. With increasing age, the ribs incline downward while the thoracic cage becomes flattened anteroposteriorly. This is associated with a decrease in the size of the thoracic outlet. Generally the female thorax is narrower and shorter than in the male. From a functional standpoint, the thoracic skeleton and its muscular wall structures form a rugged, stable enclosure which permits the respiratory excursions that are necessary for normal breathing. This is clearly apparent in patients with severe chest injuries such as multiple rib fractures due to blunt trauma, where instability of the chest wall leads to paradoxical respiration: the affected side of the rib cage moves inward during inspiration and outward during expiration. This results in a *pendelluft* effect (from the German *Pendel,* pendulum, and *Luft,* air): air streams back and forth between the lungs, leading to increased dead space ventilation, decreased alveolar gas exchange, and respiratory failure. Patients thus affected generally require intubation.

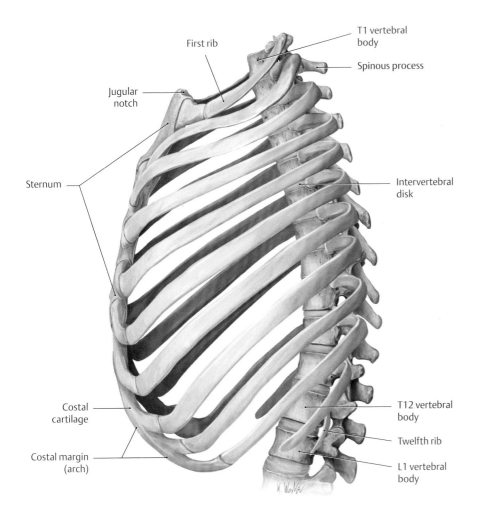

B Thoracic skeleton, lateral view

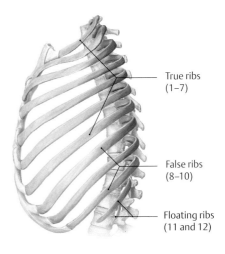

C True, false, and floating ribs
Lateral view. Each of the twelve pairs of ribs is bilaterally symmetrical, but the shapes of the ribs vary at different levels. The first seven pairs of ribs, called the *true ribs,* are normally connected anteriorly to the sternum. Of the remaining five, called the *false ribs,* the eighth, ninth, and tenth ribs are joined to the cartilage of the rib directly above, contributing to the structure of the costal margin (arch) (see **Aa**). The last two pairs of "false" ribs, called the *floating ribs,* usually terminate freely between the muscles of the lateral abdominal wall.

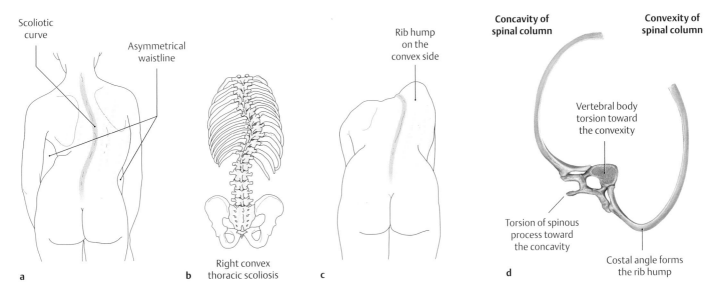

D Lateral curvature of the spinal column (scoliosis)
a, b Posterior view. Scoliosis most commonly presents as a *right convex* curve of the spinal column at the level of the T8–T9 vertebrae (**b**). It is manifested by a typical postural deformity in upright stance (**a**).

c, d When a patient with right convex scoliosis bends forward, a typical rib hump appears on the convex side of the curve (**c**). This happens because the adjacent ribs also occupy an abnormal position due to torsion of the vertebral bodies (**d**, superior view).

1.17 The Sternum and Ribs

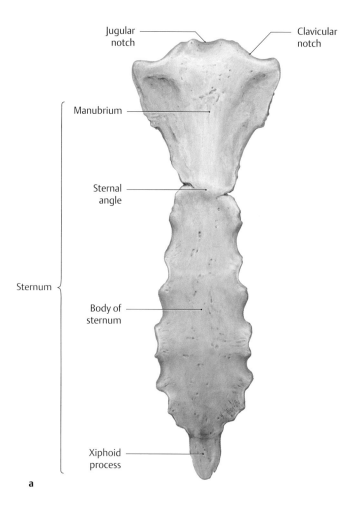

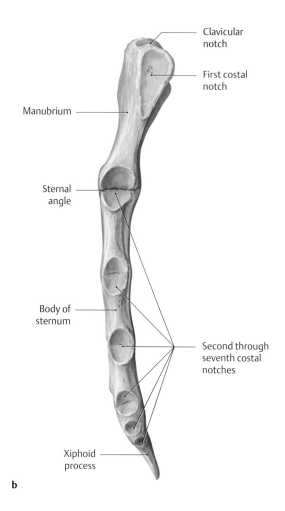

a

b

A The sternum

a Anterior view.
b Lateral view.

The sternum is a flattened bone, slightly convex anteriorly, with multiple indentations along its lateral borders (costal notches). The adult sternum consists of three bony parts:

- The manubrium
- The body of the sternum
- The xiphoid process

The manubrium, body, and xiphoid process in adolescents and young adults are connected to one another by cartilaginous plates (manubriosternal synchondrosis and xiphosternal synchondrosis), which gradually ossify with increasing age. The fully ossified, mature adult form is depicted here. The depression in the superior border of the manubrium (jugular notch) is clearly palpable through the skin and marks the inferior margin of the jugular fossa. On each side of the jugular notch is a depression for articulation with the clavicle on that side (clavicular notch), and just below that is a shallow concavity (first costal notch) for the synchondrosis with the first rib. At the junction of the sternal manubrium and body is an articular facet for the second rib (second costal notch). At that site the manubrium is usually angled slightly backward in relation to the body of the sternum (sternal angle). The lateral borders of the sternal body bear additional costal notches that articulate with the third through seventh costal cartilages, the notches for the sixth and seventh costal cartilages being placed very close together. The sometimes bifid and perforated xiphoid process itself is devoid of costal attachments and is highly variable in its form. Frequently the xiphoid process is still cartilaginous in adults.

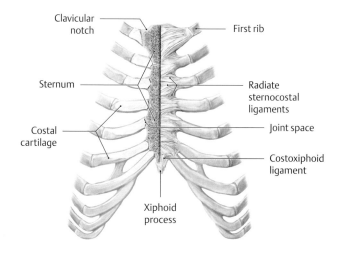

B The sternocostal joints

Anterior view (the right half of the sternum has been sectioned frontally to show the sternocostal joints). The connections between the costal cartilages for the first through seventh ribs and the costal notches of the sternum consist partly of synchondroses and partly of true joints. Generally a joint space is found only at the second through fifth ribs, while the first, sixth, and seventh ribs are attached to the sternum by synchondroses. In the true joints as well as the synchondroses, ligaments (radiate sternocostal ligaments) radiate from the perichondrium of the costal cartilage to the anterior surface of the sternum, where they blend with the periosteum to form a dense fibrous membrane (the sternal membrane).

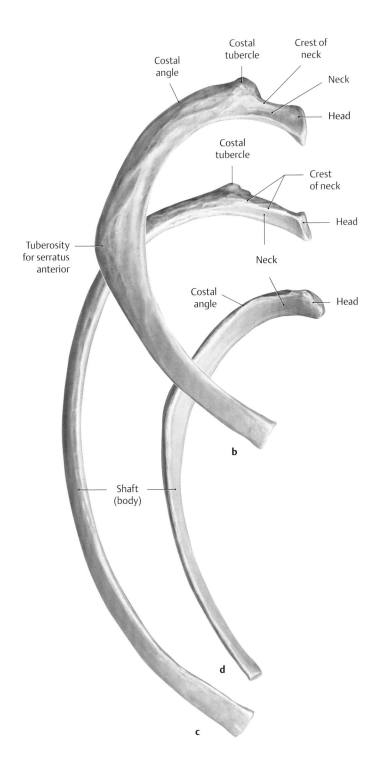

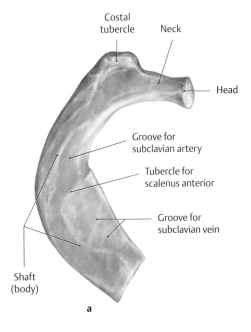

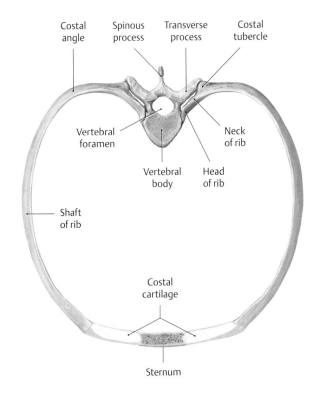

C Variable size and shape of the ribs

a First rib, **b** second rib, **c** fifth rib, **d** eleventh rib (all are right ribs, viewed from above).

The neck of the rib extends from the head of the rib to the costal tubercle. Except on the first rib, the neck bears a sharp superior ridge (crest of the neck of the rib). Lateral to the costal tubercle is the shaft (body) of the rib, which curves forward to form the costal angle. The shafts of the second through twelfth ribs in particular show irregular curvatures (on the flat and on the edges) and are also twisted about their long axis. Because of this torsion, the external surfaces of the ribs face slightly downward at their vertebral end and slightly upward at their anterior end. Normally the first and twelfth ribs are the shortest while the seventh rib is the longest. The costal cartilage increases in length from the first to the seventh rib and shortens again past the eighth rib. Every rib except the first, eleventh, and twelfth has a groove along its inferior border (costal groove) that affords some protection for the intercostal vessels and nerves (see p. 145).

D Segments of the rib and structure of a thoracic segment

Sixth pair of ribs, superior view. Each rib consists of a bony part (costal bone) and a cartilaginous part (costal cartilage). The bony part consists of the following segments, starting from its vertebral end:

- Head
- Neck
- Costal tubercle
- Shaft (body), which includes the costal angle

1.18 The Costovertebral Joints and Thoracic Movements

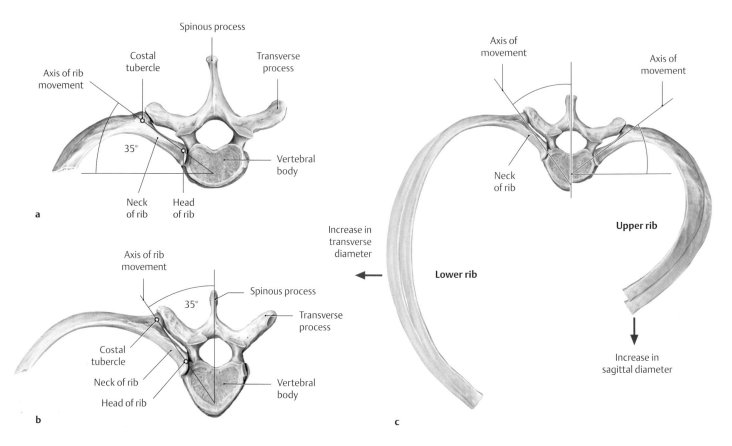

A Axes for movements of the costovertebral joints and ribs
(after Kapandji)
Superior view.

a Axis of upper rib movements.
b Axis of lower rib movements.
c Direction of rib movements (see **C** for the costovertebral joints).

The axes of rib movements are directed parallel to the necks of the ribs. The axes for the upper ribs are closer to the coronal plane (**a**), while those for the lower ribs are closer to the sagittal plane (**b**). For this reason, a rib excursion in the upper part of the rib cage mainly increases the sagittal thoracic diameter while a lower rib excursion increases the transverse diameter (see **B**).

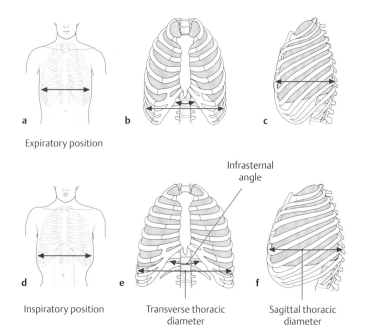

B Movements of the rib cage during costal or chest breathing (sternocostal breathing)

Respiration (ventilation) is effected through changes in the thoracic volume. The increase in thoracic volume that is necessary for inspiration can be accomplished in two ways:

1. By lowering the diaphragm (costodiaphragmatic breathing or abdominal breathing, see p.134)
2. By elevating the ribs (sternocostal breathing, also known as costal or chest breathing)

While breathing at rest is almost entirely abdominal, respiration during physical effort is augmented by chest breathing with the intercostal muscles and the auxiliary muscles of respiration. The drawings illustrate the thoracic volume changes that occur during *chest or costal breathing,* in which the thoracic volume decreases and increases in both the coronal and sagittal planes. Panels **a–c** show the *decrease* in the transverse and sagittal chest diameters at end-expiration, and **d–f** show the *increase* at end-inspiration.

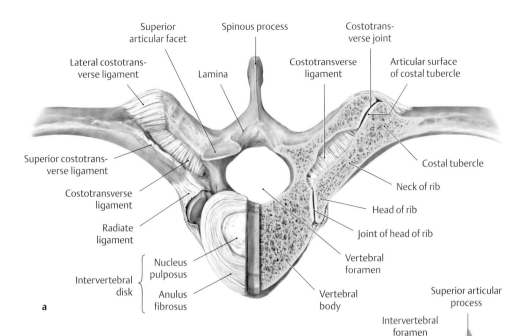

Superior articular facet · Spinous process · Costotransverse joint

Lateral costotransverse ligament · Lamina · Costotransverse ligament · Articular surface of costal tubercle

Superior costotransverse ligament

Costotransverse ligament

Radiate ligament

Intervertebral disk { Nucleus pulposus / Anulus fibrosus

Costal tubercle

Neck of rib

Head of rib

Joint of head of rib

Vertebral foramen

Vertebral body

a

C Ligaments of the costovertebral joints

The costovertebral joints are the joints by which the ribs articulate with the vertebrae. They consist of two types: the joints of the heads of the ribs and the costotransverse joints. Though morphologically distinct, these different joint types are functionally interrelated.

a Articulation of the eighth rib with the eighth thoracic vertebra, superior view (the joint of the head of the rib and costotransverse joint on the left side have been transversely sectioned).

b The fifth through eighth thoracic vertebrae and associated ribs (seventh and eighth ribs), left lateral view (the joint of the head of the seventh rib has been transversely sectioned).

Joint of the head of the rib: This joint consists of two articular surfaces:

1. An articular facet on the head of the rib
2. A costal facet on the vertebral body

The articular facets on the head of the second through tenth ribs (defined by the crest of the rib head) articulate with the fossa formed by the superior and inferior costal facets on two adjacent vertebral bodies and the intervertebral disk between them. The intra-articular ligament, which extends from the crest of the rib head to the intervertebral disk, separates the joint cavity of the second through tenth rib heads into two compartments. By contrast, the heads of the first, eleventh, and twelfth ribs each articulate with only one thoracic vertebral body (see **A**, p. 86). In all the joints of the heads of the ribs, the joint capsule is reinforced by the *radiate ligament.*

Costotransverse joint: In the costotransverse joints of the first through tenth ribs, the artic-

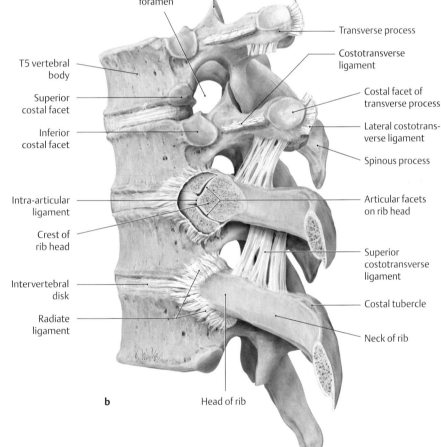

Intervertebral foramen · Superior articular process

T5 vertebral body

Superior costal facet

Inferior costal facet

Intra-articular ligament

Crest of rib head

Intervertebral disk

Radiate ligament

Transverse process

Costotransverse ligament

Costal facet of transverse process

Lateral costotransverse ligament

Spinous process

Articular facets on rib head

Superior costotransverse ligament

Costal tubercle

Neck of rib

b · Head of rib

ular surface of the costal tubercle articulates with the costal facet on the transverse process of the corresponding thoracic vertebra. The eleventh and twelfth ribs do not have a costotransverse joint because their transverse processes do not have articular facets (see **A**, p. 86). Three ligaments stabilize the costotransverse joint and also strengthen the joint capsule:

1. The lateral costotransverse ligament (from the tip of the transverse process to the costal tubercle)
2. The costotransverse ligament (between the neck of the rib and the transverse process)
3. The superior costotransverse ligament (between the neck of the rib and the transverse process of the vertebra above it)

1.19 The Bony Pelvis

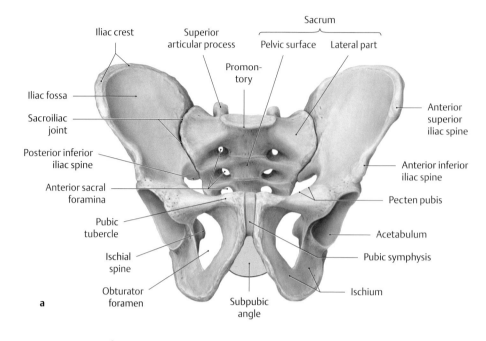

Iliac crest

Superior articular process

Sacrum

Pelvic surface   Lateral part

Promontory

Iliac fossa

Sacroiliac joint

Posterior inferior iliac spine

Anterior sacral foramina

Pubic tubercle

Ischial spine

Obturator foramen

Subpubic angle

Anterior superior iliac spine

Anterior inferior iliac spine

Pecten pubis

Acetabulum

Pubic symphysis

Ischium

a

A The male pelvis
a Anterior view.
b Posterior view.
c Superior view.

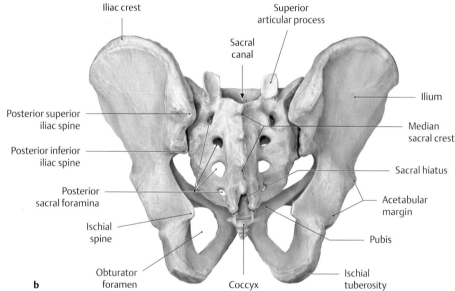

Iliac crest

Superior articular process

Sacral canal

Posterior superior iliac spine

Posterior inferior iliac spine

Posterior sacral foramina

Ischial spine

Obturator foramen

Coccyx

Ilium

Median sacral crest

Sacral hiatus

Acetabular margin

Pubis

Ischial tuberosity

b

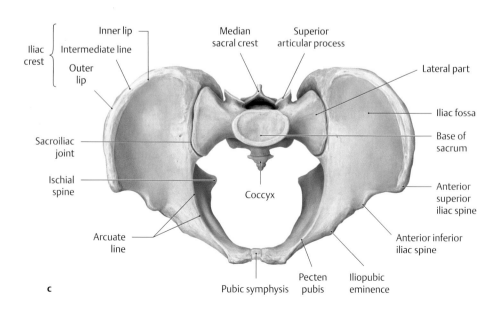

Iliac crest

Inner lip

Intermediate line

Outer lip

Median sacral crest

Superior articular process

Lateral part

Iliac fossa

Base of sacrum

Sacroiliac joint

Ischial spine

Coccyx

Arcuate line

Pubic symphysis

Pecten pubis

Iliopubic eminence

Anterior superior iliac spine

Anterior inferior iliac spine

c

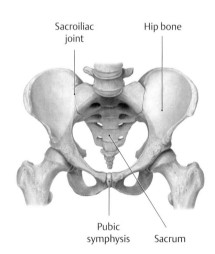

Sacroiliac joint

Hip bone

Pubic symphysis

Sacrum

B The pelvic girdle and pelvic ring
Anterosuperior view. The pelvic girdle consists of the two hip bones (coxal bones). The sacroiliac joints and the cartilaginous pubic symphysis unite the bony parts of the pelvic girdle with the sacrum to form a stable ring called the pelvic ring (indicated by color shading). It allows very little mobility, because stability throughout the pelvic ring is an important prerequisite for transmitting the trunk load to the lower limbs.

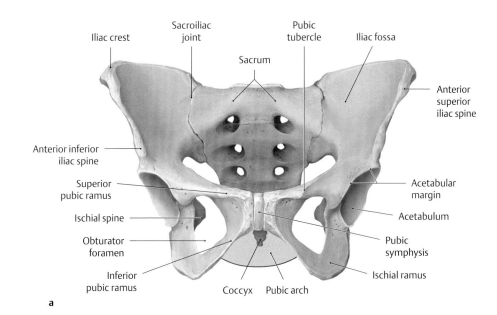

C The female pelvis
a Anterior view.
b Posterior view.
c Superior view.

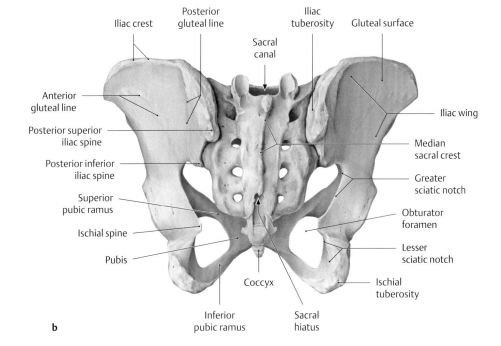

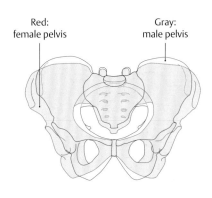

Red: female pelvis

Gray: male pelvis

D Gender-specific features of the pelvis
Anterosuperior view. A male and female pelvis have been superimposed to illustrate the gender-specific differences. Comparison reveals that the female pelvis is larger and broader than the male pelvis, while the latter is taller, narrower, and more massive than the female pelvis. The inlet of the female pelvis is larger and has an almost oval shape, while the sacral promontory shows a greater projection in the male pelvis (**Cc**). Sex differences are also noted in the angle between the inferior pubic rami, which is acute in men (70°) but significantly larger in women (almost 90–100°). Accordingly, this angle is called the subpubic angle in men and the pubic arch in women (see **D**, p.115). The sacrum also exhibits differences between the sexes. In women the sacrum is angled at the level of the third and fourth vertebrae (see p.90), while in men it presents a uniform curvature.

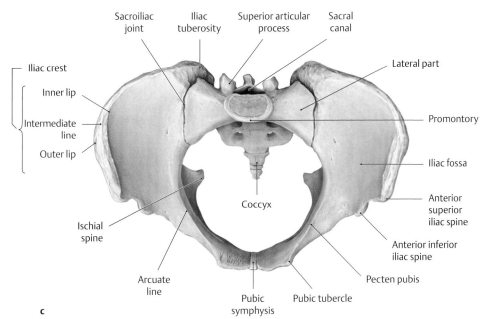

113

1.20 The Pelvic Ligaments and Pelvic Measurements

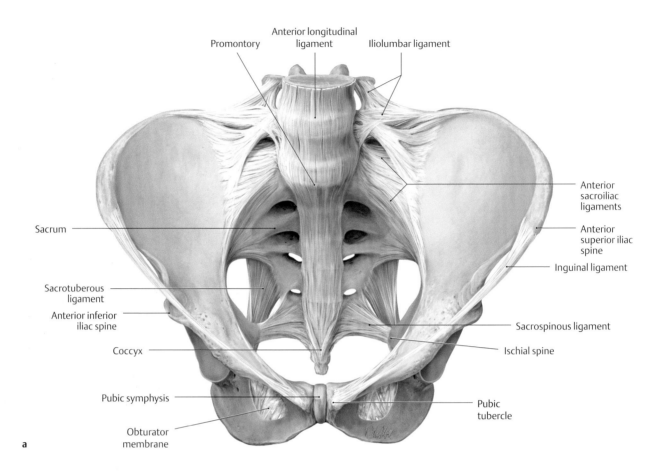

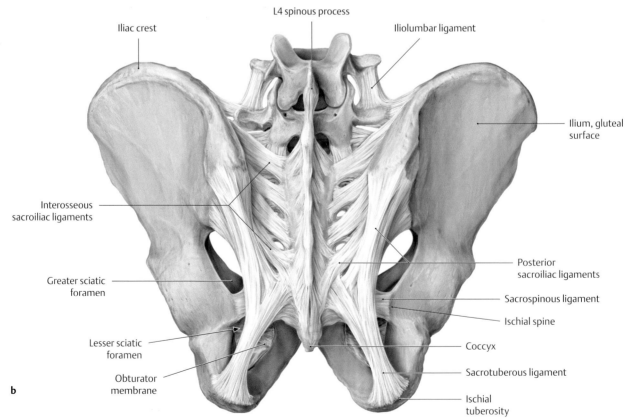

A Ligaments of the male pelvis

a Anterosuperior view.

b Posterior view.

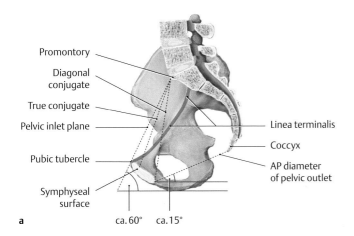

Promontory
Diagonal conjugate
True conjugate
Pelvic inlet plane
Pubic tubercle
Symphyseal surface

Linea terminalis
Coccyx
AP diameter of pelvic outlet

a   ca. 60°   ca. 15°

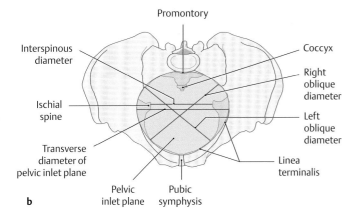

Promontory

Interspinous diameter

Ischial spine

Transverse diameter of pelvic inlet plane

Coccyx
Right oblique diameter
Left oblique diameter
Linea terminalis

Pelvic inlet plane   Pubic symphysis

b

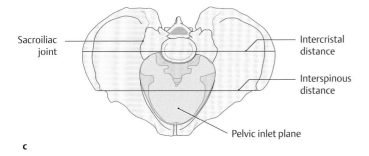

Sacroiliac joint

Intercristal distance

Interspinous distance

Pelvic inlet plane

c

B Internal and external pelvic measurements
a Right half of a female pelvis, medial view.
b Female pelvis, superior view.
c Male pelvis, superior view.

The linea terminalis is marked in red in **a**. The pelvic inlet plane is color-shaded in **b** and **c**.

C Internal and external pelvic measurements, linea terminalis, and pelvic inlet plane

The internal and external pelvic measurements provide direct or indirect information on the size and shape of the bony boundaries of the lesser pelvis. Because the lesser pelvis functions as the birth canal, the internal and external pelvic dimensions have special practical significance in obstetrics, determining whether the pelvic cavity is broad enough to allow for a vaginal delivery. A particularly important measurement is the true conjugate of the pelvic inlet (the obstetric conjugate), which is the smallest anteroposterior dimension of the lesser pelvis. With *pelvimetry,* a method of measuring pelvic dimensions, potential obstructions to labor can be identified prior to the delivery. Generally the measurements are performed by transvaginal sonography. Some pelvic dimensions, such as the diagonal conjugate, can be accurately determined by bimanual examination.

Internal pelvic measurements in women (see **Ba** and **Bb**)

- True conjugate = 11 cm (distance from the sacral promontory to the posterior border of the symphysis)
- Diagonal conjugate = 12.5–13 cm (distance from the sacral promontory to the lower border of the symphysis)
- AP diameter of the pelvic outlet = 9 (+2) cm (distance from the lower border of the symphysis to the tip of the coccyx)
- Transverse diameter of the pelvic inlet plane = 13 cm (greatest distance between the lineae terminales)
- Interspinous diameter = 11 cm (distance between the ischial spines)
- Right (I) and left (II) oblique diameter = 12 cm (distance from the sacroiliac joint at the level of the linea terminalis to the iliopectineal eminence on the opposite side)

External pelvic measurements in men (see **Bc**)

- Interspinous distance = 25–26 cm (distance between the anterior superior iliac spines)
- Intercristal distance = 28–29 cm (greatest distance between the left and right iliac crests in the coronal plane)
- External conjugate = 20–21 cm (distance from the upper border of the symphysis to the spinous process of the L5 vertebra)

Linea terminalis (see **B**)

Boundary line between the greater and lesser pelvis, consists of the pubic symphysis and crest + pecten pubis + the arcuate line and sacral promontory.

Pelvic inlet plane (see **Bb** and **Bc**)

Plane through the pelvic inlet at the level of the linea terminalis, below which is the lesser pelvis

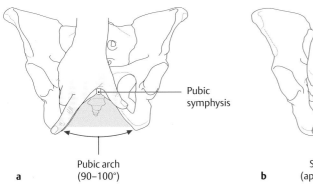

Pubic symphysis

Pubic arch
(90–100°)

a

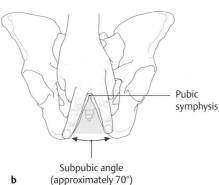

Pubic symphysis

Subpubic angle
(approximately 70°)

b

D Lower pubic angle
Anterior view.

a Female pelvis: pubic arch.
b Male pelvis: subpubic angle.

1.21 The Sacroiliac Joint

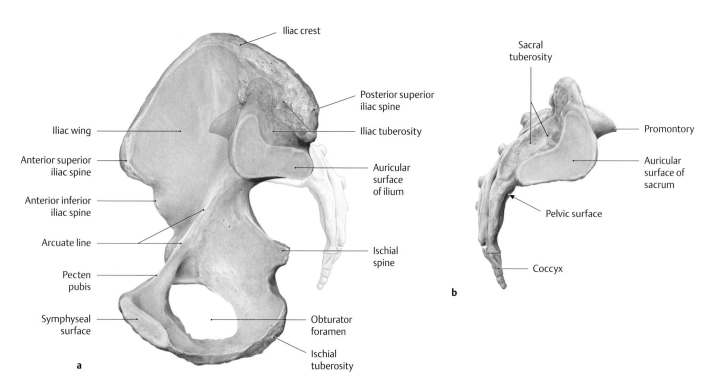

a

b

A Articular surfaces of the sacroiliac joint

a Auricular surface of the ilium, right hip bone, medial view (the sacrum is transparent in this view).

b Auricular surface of the sacrum, right lateral view.

The two ear-shaped articular surfaces of the ilium and sacrum (auricular surfaces) are brought together at the sacroiliac joint. The auricular sur-

face of the ilium is slightly notched at its center, and there is a reciprocal ridge on the articular surface of the ilium. The shape and size of both articular surfaces show considerable individual variation—more so than in other joints. Their cartilaginous covering is generally irregular, the articular cartilage on the sacral side being approximately twice as thick as on the iliac side.

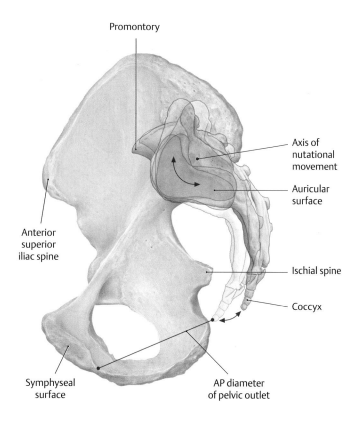

B Nutation in the sacroiliac joint

Right half of pelvis, medial view. Movements in the sacroiliac joints alter the width of the pelvic ring and thus have practical importance in obstetrics. The amplitude of the movements is greatly limited by tight ligaments and varies considerably in different individuals and between the sexes. Basically, very slight rotational and translational movements can be distinguished in the joints. Nutation, as shown here, is a rotational or "tilting" movement of the sacrum about an axis located at the attachments of the interosseous sacroiliac ligaments. With *anterior rotation of the sacrum*, the promontory moves forward and downward while the coccyx moves upward and backward, thereby increasing the AP diameter of the pelvic outlet. With *posterior rotation of the sacrum*, the AP diameter of the pelvic inlet plane increases while the AP diameter of the pelvic outlet is decreased.

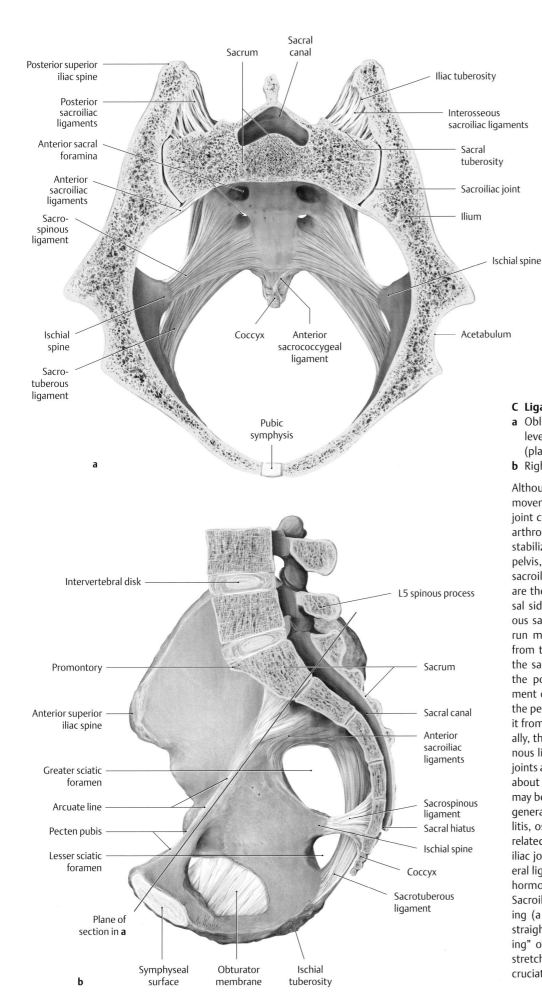

a

Posterior superior iliac spine

Posterior sacroiliac ligaments

Anterior sacral foramina

Anterior sacroiliac ligaments

Sacro-spinous ligament

Ischial spine

Sacro-tuberous ligament

Sacrum

Sacral canal

Iliac tuberosity

Interosseous sacroiliac ligaments

Sacral tuberosity

Sacroiliac joint

Ilium

Ischial spine

Acetabulum

Coccyx

Anterior sacrococcygeal ligament

Pubic symphysis

b

Intervertebral disk

Promontory

Anterior superior iliac spine

Greater sciatic foramen

Arcuate line

Pecten pubis

Lesser sciatic foramen

Plane of section in **a**

Symphyseal surface

Obturator membrane

Ischial tuberosity

L5 spinous process

Sacrum

Sacral canal

Anterior sacroiliac ligaments

Sacrospinous ligament

Sacral hiatus

Ischial spine

Coccyx

Sacrotuberous ligament

C Ligaments of the sacroiliac joint

a Oblique section through the pelvis at the level of the pelvic inlet plane, superior view (plane of section indicated in **b**).

b Right half of pelvis, medial view.

Although the sacroiliac joint is a true joint, its movements are greatly restricted by a tight joint capsule and powerful ligaments (amphiarthrosis). The anterior sacroiliac ligaments stabilize the joint on the anterior side of the pelvis, while the interosseous and posterior sacroiliac ligaments and iliolumbar ligaments are the main stabilizing elements on the dorsal side (see p.114). The powerful interosseous sacroiliac ligaments are deep bands that run medially just behind the sacroiliac joint from the iliac tuberosity to the tuberosity of the sacrum. They are completely covered by the posterior sacroiliac ligaments. The ligament complex helps to anchor the sacrum in the pelvic ring during upright stance and keep it from sliding into the pelvic cavity. Additionally, the sacrotuberous ligament and sacrospinous ligament (see **b**) stabilize both sacroiliac joints and prevent posterior tilting of the pelvis about the transverse axis. *Sacroiliac joint pain* may be caused by chronic inflammatory or degenerative changes (e.g., ankylosing spondylitis, osteoarthritis) or by trauma (e.g., sport-related injuries). Hypermobility of the sacroiliac joint may also develop as a result of general ligamentous weakness or a pregnancy- or hormone-related laxity of the ligaments.

Sacroiliac dysfunction may include joint locking (a sudden force like that occurring in a straight-legged jump may cause a "wedging" of the sacrum with joint locking). This stretches the joint capsule and can cause excruciating pain during most body movements.

117

2.1 The Muscles of the Trunk Wall, Their Origin and Function

Overview of the Trunk Wall Muscles

The muscles of the trunk wall in the strict sense consist of the intrinsic back muscles and the musculature of the chest and abdominal wall. In the broad sense, they include the muscles of the pelvic floor (which form the caudal boundary of the abdominal and pelvic cavity) and the diaphragm (which separates the thoracic and abdominal cavities). Besides the actual (primary) muscles of the trunk wall, the back and thorax also contain muscles of the shoulder girdle and upper limb whose origins

have migrated onto the trunk during the course of phylogenetic development (*nonintrinsic back and thoracic muscles*). Examples are the *thoracohumeral muscles* anteriorly, the *spinohumeral* muscles laterally and posteriorly, and the *spinocostal* muscles. Other muscles that have migrated to the trunk, such as the trapezius, are derived from the mesenchyme of the branchial arches (branchial musculature). They are innervated by cranial nerves (the trapezius by the accessory nerve) and were incorporated secondarily into the locomotor apparatus (see p. 258 ff.).

A Trunk wall muscles in the strict sense

Intrinsic back muscles

Lateral tract
- Sacrospinal system
  - Iliocostalis
  - Longissimus
- Spinotransverse system
  - Splenius
- Intertransverse system
  - Intertransversarii
  - Levatores costarum

Medial tract
- Spinal system
  - Interspinales
  - Spinalis
- Transversospinal system
  - Rotatores breves and longi
  - Multifidus
  - Semispinalis

Short nuchal and craniovertebral joint muscles (capitis and suboccipital muscles) *
- Rectus capitis posterior major
- Rectus capitis posterior minor
- Obliquus capitis superior
- Obliquus capitis inferior

Prevertebral neck muscles (belong topographically to the group of deep neck muscles but act mainly on the cervical spine)

- Longus capitis
- Longus colli
- Rectus capitis lateralis
- Rectus capitis anterior

Muscles of the thoracic cage (chest wall muscles)

- Intercostal muscles
- Transversus thoracis
- Subcostal muscles
- Scaleni (belong topographically to the group of deep neck muscles but are functionally related to thoracic breathing)

Muscles of the abdominal wall

Lateral (oblique) abdominal muscles
- External oblique
- Internal oblique
- Transversus abdominis

Anterior (straight) abdominal muscles
- Rectus abdominis
- Pyramidalis

Posterior (deep) abdominal muscles
- Quadratus lumborum
- Psoas major (belongs functionally to the hip muscles, see p. 422)

B Trunk wall muscles in the broad sense

Pelvic floor muscles

Pelvic diaphragm
- Levator ani muscle
  - Puborectalis
  - Pubococcygeus
  - Iliococcygeus
  - Eoccygeus

Urogenital diaphragm
- Deep transverse perineal
- Sphincter urethrae

Sphincters and erectile muscles of the urogenital and intestinal tract
- External anal sphincter
- Bulbospongiosus
- Ischiocavernosus
- Superficial transverse perineal

Diaphragm

- Costal part
- Lumbar part
- Sternal part

C Muscles that migrated secondarily to the trunk wall
(described in the chapter on the Upper Limb, p. 208)

Spinocostal muscles

- Serratus posterior superior
- Serratus posterior inferior

Spinohumeral muscles between the trunk and shoulder girdle

- Rhomboid major and minor
- Levator scapulae
- Serratus anterior
- Subclavius
- Pectoralis minor
- Trapezius

Spinohumeral muscles between the trunk and arm

- Latissimus dorsi

Thoracohumeral muscles

- Pectoralis major

---

* The suboccipital muscles in the strict sense are the short or deep nuchal muscles that are counted among the intrinsic back muscles (criterion: innervated by a dorsal ramus). The rectus capitis anterior and lateralis muscles are *not* classified as intrinsic back muscles because they are supplied by ventral rami, even though they are also suboccipital in their location.

Origin of the Trunk Wall Muscles

The striated muscles of the trunk wall (including the muscles of the diaphragm and pelvic floor), like the limb muscles, develop embryologically from the myotomes of the somites (see p.6) and are therefore called the *somatic muscles.* In all, approximately 42 to 44 pairs of segmental somites are formed in the paraxial mesoderm between the 20th and 30th weeks of development. Five occipital, 7 cervical, 12 thoracic, 5 lumbar, 5 sacral, and 8–10 coccygeal somites are formed in a craniocaudal sequence (see **D**). Some of these somites regress with further development, particularly the first occipital somites and most of the coccygeal somites, so that the number of original somites is greater than the number of subsequent vertebral segments. The boundary between the head and neck runs through the fifth pair of occipital somites. At the end of the sixth week of development, the somite myotomes migrate in the dorsoventral direction and become separated into a dorsal part (epimere or epaxial muscles) and a ventral part (hypomere or hypaxial muscles) (**E**). While the epaxial muscles develop into intrinsic (local) back muscles and retain their original location, the hypomere develops into the anterolateral muscles of the chest and abdominal wall and the limb musculature (**F**). As the myotomes become segregated, the spinal nerves undergo a corresponding division into a *dorsal ramus* for the epaxial muscles and a *ventral ramus* for the hypaxial muscles (see **Ea**). The original segmental (metameric) arrangement of the trunk muscles mostly disappears with further development. It persists only in the deep layers of the intrinsic back muscles (e.g., the rotator, interspinal, and intertransverse muscles) and the thoracic muscles (e.g., the internal and external intercostal muscles), while the superficial portions of the myotomes fuse together to form long, continuous muscles ("polymerization") in which only the neurovascular supply still exhibits the original segmental arrangement (see **F**).

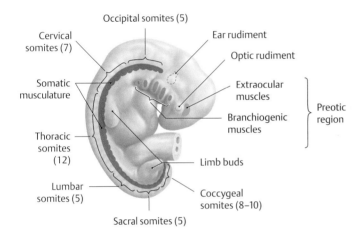

D Somites in a five-week-old human embryo

Right lateral view. The somites formed from the paraxial mesoderm are classified as *preotic* (shown in blue and green) or *postotic* (shown in red), meaning that they are located cranial or caudal to the ear rudiment. The somatic muscles develop from postotic somites. Segmentation into different somites is not observed in the preotic region, which contains the rudiments for the branchiogenic pharyngeal arch muscles and the extraocular muscles. The structures in this region are innervated by cranial nerves (after Boyd, Hamilton, and Mossmann, quoted in Starck).

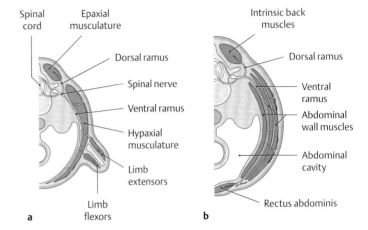

E Transverse sections through a six-week-old human embryo

a Transverse section at the level of a limb bud.
b Transverse section through the abdominal wall.

Muscle precursor cells with replicative capacity located at the level of the limb buds migrate from the myotomes into the limb buds, and the myotome that remains in these regions develops into intrinsic back muscles. With further growth of the limb bud, the muscle tissue differentiates into a dorsal rudiment (blastema) for the extensor muscles and a ventral rudiment for the flexor muscles of the upper and lower limbs (see p.18). As in the hypomere, the limb muscles are innervated by ventral spinal nerve rami (brachial plexus and lumbosacral plexus, see pp. 314 and 470).
Note the different innervation of the epaxial muscles (dorsal ramus) and hypaxial muscles (ventral ramus).

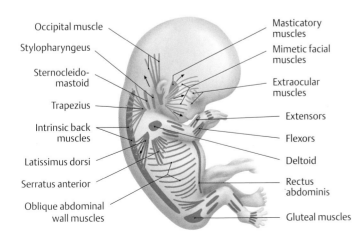

F Diagram of the principal muscle groups in an eight-week-old human embryo

Right lateral view. Red = somatic muscles, blue = branchiogenic (branchial arch) muscles, green = extraocular muscles (after Boyd, Hamilton, and Mossmann, quoted in Starck).

2.2 The Intrinsic Back Muscles: Lateral Tract

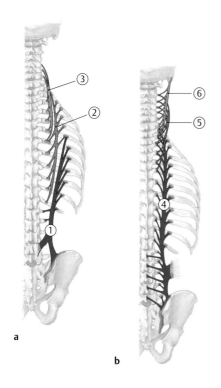

a

b

A Lateral tract: schematic of the sacrospinal system

a Iliocostalis muscles.
b Longissimus muscles.

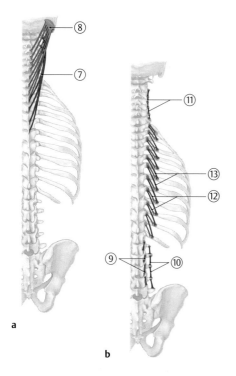

a

b

B Lateral tract: schematic of the spinotransverse and intertransverse system

a Splenius muscles.
b Intertransversarii and levatores costarum.

Iliocostalis muscles   (*see p. 121, opposite, lower right)

Origin:	① Iliocostalis lumborum: sacrum, iliac crest, thoracolumbar fascia
	② Iliocostalis thoracis: 7th–12th ribs
	③ Iliocostalis cervicis: 3rd–7th ribs
Insertion:	• Iliocostalis lumborum: 6th–12th ribs, deep layer of thoracolumbar fascia, transverse processes of upper lumbar vertebrae
	• Iliocostalis thoracis: 1st–6th ribs
	• Iliocostalis cervicis: transverse processes of C4–C6 vertebrae
Action:	Entire muscle: bilateral contraction extends the spine, unilateral contraction bends the spine laterally to the same side
Innervation:	Lateral branches of dorsal rami of spinal nerves C8–L1

Longissimus muscles

Origin:	④ Longissimus thoracis: sacrum, iliac crest (common tendon of origin with iliocostalis), spinous processes of lumbar vertebrae, transverse processes of lower thoracic vertebrae
	⑤ Longissimus cervicis: transverse processes of T1–T6 vertebrae
	⑥ Longissimus capitis: transverse processes of T1–T3 vertebrae and transverse and articular processes of C4–C7 vertebrae
Insertion:	• Longissimus thoracis: 2nd–12th ribs, costal processes of lumbar vertebrae, transverse processes of thoracic vertebrae
	• Longissimus cervicis: transverse processes of C2–C5 vertebrae
	• Longissimus capitis: mastoid process of occipital bone
Action:	• Entire muscle: bilateral contraction extends the spine, unilateral contraction bends the spine laterally to the same side
	• Longissimus capitis: bilateral contraction extends the head, unilateral contraction flexes and rotates the head to the same side
Innervation:	Lateral branches of dorsal rami of spinal nerves C1–L5

Splenius muscles

Origin:	⑦ Splenius cervicis: spinous processes of the T3–T6 vertebrae
	⑧ Splenius capitis: spinous processes of the C3–T3 vertebrae
Insertion:	• Splenius cervicis: transverse processes of C1 and C2
	• Splenius capitis: lateral superior nuchal line, mastoid process
Action:	Entire muscle: bilateral contraction extends the cervical spine and head, unilateral contraction flexes and rotates the head to the same side
Innervation:	Lateral branches of dorsal rami of spinal nerves C1–C6

Intertransversarii

Origin and insertion:	⑨ Intertransversarii mediales lumborum: course between adjacent mamillary processes of all lumbar vertebrae
	⑩ Intertransversarii laterales lumborum: course between adjacent costal processes of all lumbar vertebrae
	⑪ Intertransversarii posteriores cervicis: course between adjacent pubic tubercles of the C2–C7 vertebrae
	• Intertransversarii anteriores cervicis: course between adjacent anterior tubercles of the C2–C7 vertebrae
Action:	• Bilateral contraction stabilizes and extends the cervical and lumbar spine
	• Unilateral contraction bends the cervical and lumbar spine laterally to the same side
Innervation:	Dorsal rami of the spinal nerves except for intertransversarii laterales lumborum and intertransversarii anteriores cervicis (ventral rami of the spinal nerves)

Levatores costarum

Origin:	⑫ Levatores costarum breves: transverse processes of the C7 and T1–T11 vertebrae
	⑬ Levatores costarum longi: transverse processes of the C7 and T1–T11 vertebrae
Insertion:	• Levatores costarum breves: costal angle of the next lower rib
	• Levatores costarum longi: costal angle of next higher rib
Action:	• Bilateral contraction extends the thoracic spine
	• Unilateral contraction bends the thoracic spine to the same side, rotates it to the opposite side
Innervation:	Both dorsal and ventral rami of the spinal nerves

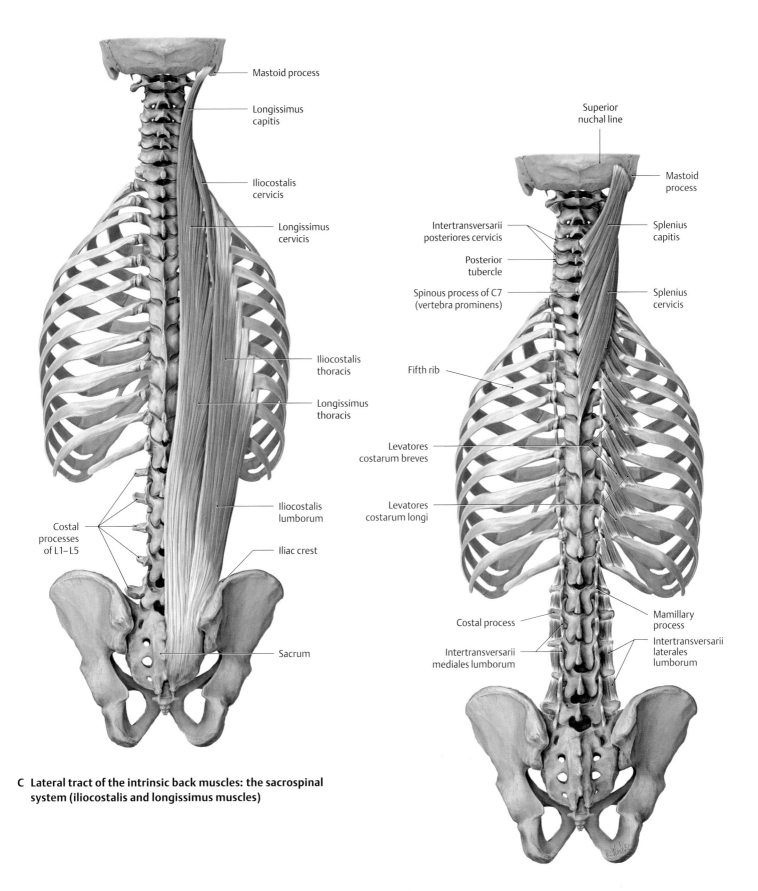

C Lateral tract of the intrinsic back muscles: the sacrospinal system (iliocostalis and longissimus muscles)

D Lateral tract of the intrinsic back muscles: the spinotransverse system (splenius muscle) and intertransverse system (intertransversarii and levatores costarum muscles)

* The structures named in the tables at left are not all labeled in the drawings above, as they may not all be visible in the perspectives shown. The schematic diagrams at left, along with the tables, are intended to give a systematic overview of the muscles and their actions. The drawings on the right-hand page are intended to display the muscles as they would appear in a dissection.

2.3 The Intrinsic Back Muscles: Medial Tract

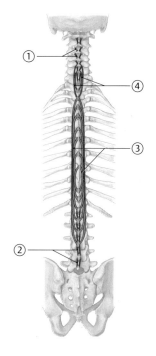

Interspinales muscles

Origin and insertion:
① Interspinales cervicis: course between the spinous processes of the cervical vertebrae
② Interspinales lumborum: course between the spinous processes of the lumbar vertebrae

Action: Extends the cervical and lumbar spine

Innervation: Dorsal rami of the spinal nerves

Spinalis muscles

Origin:
③ Spinalis thoracis: lateral surface of the spinous processes of the T10–T12 and L1–L3 vertebrae
④ Spinalis cervicis: spinous processes of the T1–T2 and C5–C7 vertebrae

Insertion:
• Spinalis thoracis: lateral surface of the spinous processes of the T2–T8 vertebrae
• Spinalis cervicis: spinous processes of the C2–C5 vertebrae

Action:
• Bilateral contraction extends the cervical and thoracic spine
• Unilateral contraction bends the cervical and thoracic spine to the same side

Innervation: Dorsal rami of the spinal nerves

A Medial tract of the intrinsic back muscles: schematic of the spinal system
The interspinales and spinalis muscles.

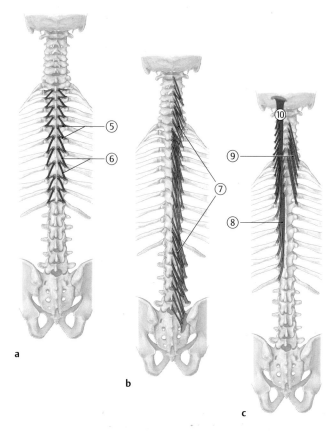

Rotatores breves and longi

Origin and insertion:
⑤ Rotatores breves: course between the transverse process and next higher spinous process of all cervical vertebrae
⑥ Rotatores longi: course between the transverse process and next higher spinous process of all cervical vertebrae

Action:
• Bilateral contraction extends the thoracic spine
• Unilateral contraction rotates it to the opposite side

Innervation: Dorsal rami of the spinal nerves

⑦ Multifidus

Origin and insertion:
Courses between the transverse and spinous process (skipping 2–4 vertebrae) of all cervical vertebrae (C2 to the sacrum); most fully developed in the lumbar spine

Action:
• Bilateral contraction extends the spine
• Unilateral contraction flexes to the same side and rotates to the opposite side

Innervation: Dorsal rami of the spinal nerves

Semispinalis

Origin:
⑧ Semispinalis thoracis: transverse processes of the T6–T12 vertebrae
⑨ Semispinalis cervicis: transverse processes of the T1–T6 vertebrae
⑩ Semispinalis capitis: transverse processes of the C3–T6 vertebrae

Insertion:
• Semispinalis thoracis: spinous processes of the C6–T4 vertebrae
• Semispinalis cervicis: spinous processes of the C2–C7 vertebrae
• Semispinalis capitis: occipital bone between the superior nuchal line and inferior nuchal line

Action:
• Bilateral contraction extends the thoracic spine, cervical spine, and head (stabilizes the craniovertebral joints)
• Unilateral contraction bends the head, cervical spine, and thoracic spine to the same side and rotates them to the opposite side

Innervation: Dorsal rami of the spinal nerves

B Medial tract of the intrinsic back muscles: schematic of the transversospinal system
a Rotatores breves and longi.
b Multifidus.
c Semispinalis.

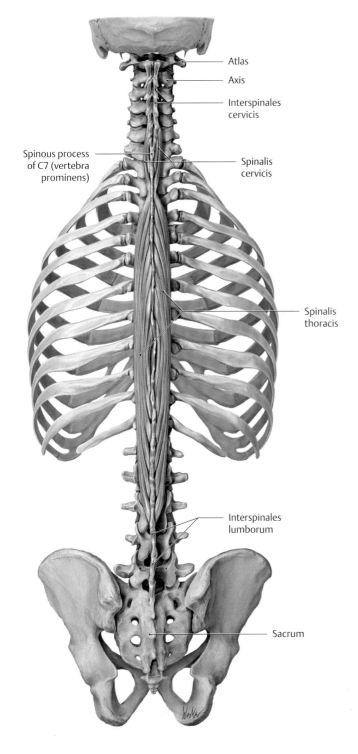

C Medial tract of the intrinsic back muscles: the spinal system (interspinales and spinalis)

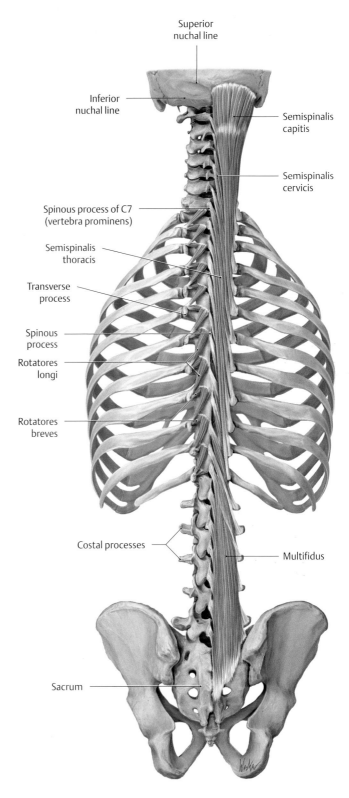

D Medial tract of the intrinsic back muscles: the transversospinal system (rotatores breves and longi, multifidus, and semispinalis)

123

2.4   The Intrinsic Back Muscles: The Short Nuchal and Craniovertebral Joint Muscles and the Prevertebral Muscle

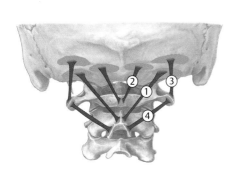

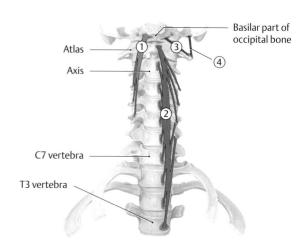

A Schematic of the short nuchal and craniovertebral joint muscles (suboccipital muscles): recti capitis posterior major and minor and obliquii capitis superior and inferior

B Schematic of the prevertebral neck muscles (colli and cervicis muscles): longi capitis and colli and recti capitis anterior and lateralis

① **Rectus capitis posterior major**

Origin:	Spinous process of the axis
Insertion:	Middle third of the inferior nuchal line
Action:	• Bilateral contraction extends the head
	• Unilateral contraction rotates the head to the same side
Innervation:	Dorsal ramus of C1 (suboccipital nerve)

② **Rectus capitis posterior minor**

Origin:	Posterior tubercle of the atlas
Insertion:	Inner third of the inferior nuchal line
Action:	• Bilateral contraction extends the head
	• Unilateral contraction rotates the head to the same side
Innervation:	Dorsal ramus of C1 (suboccipital nerve)

③ **Obliquus capitis superior**

Origin:	Transverse process of the atlas
Insertion:	Above the insertion of the rectus capitis posterior major
Action:	• Bilateral contraction extends the head
	• Unilateral contraction tilts the head to the same side and rotates it to the opposite side
Innervation:	Dorsal ramus of C1 (suboccipital nerve)

④ **Obliquus capitis inferior**

Origin:	Spinous process of the axis
Insertion:	Transverse process of the atlas
Action:	• Bilateral contraction extends the head
	• Unilateral contraction rotates the head to the same side
Innervation:	Dorsal ramus of C1 (suboccipital nerve)

① **Longus capitis**

Origin:	Anterior tubercle of the transverse processes of the C3–C6 vertebrae
Insertion:	Basilar part of the occipital bone
Action:	• Unilateral: tilts and slightly rotates the head to the same side
	• Bilateral: flexes the head
Innervation:	Direct branches from the cervical plexus (C1–C4)

② **Longus colli (cervicis)**

Origin:	• Vertical (medial) part: anterior sides of the C5–C7 and T1–T3 vertebral bodies
	• Superior oblique part: anterior tubercle of the transverse processes of the C3–C5 vertebrae
	• Inferior oblique part: anterior sides of the T1–T3 vertebral bodies
Insertion:	• Vertical part: anterior sides of the C2–C4 vertebrae
	• Superior oblique part: anterior tubercle of the atlas
	• Inferior oblique part: anterior tubercle of the transverse processes of the C5 and C6 vertebrae
Action:	• Unilateral: tilts and rotates the cervical spine to the same side
	• Bilateral: flexes the cervical spine
Innervation:	Direct branches from the cervical plexus (C2–C6)

③ **Rectus capitis anterior**

Origin:	Lateral mass of the atlas
Insertion:	Basilar part of the occipital bone
Action:	• Unilateral: lateral flexion at the atlanto-occipital joint
	• Bilateral: flexion at the atlanto-occipital joint
Innervation:	Ventral ramus of the C1 nerve

④ **Rectus capitis lateralis**

Origin:	Transverse process of the atlas
Insertion:	Basilar part of the occipital bone (lateral to the occipital condyles)
Action:	• Unilateral: lateral flexion at the atlanto-occipital joint
	• Bilateral: flexion at the atlanto-occipital joint
Innervation:	Ventral ramus of the C1 nerve

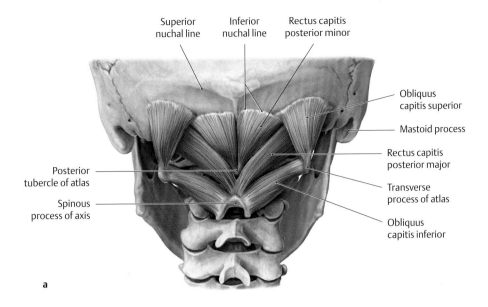

Superior nuchal line — Inferior nuchal line — Rectus capitis posterior minor

Obliquus capitis superior

Mastoid process

Rectus capitis posterior major

Transverse process of atlas

Obliquus capitis inferior

Posterior tubercle of atlas

Spinous process of axis

a

C The short nuchal and craniovertebral joint muscles: recti capitis posterior and obliquii capitis

a Posterior view, **b** lateral view.

In a strict sense, the short nuchal muscles consist only of the muscles innervated by the dorsal ramus of the first spinal nerve (suboccipital nerve). They include representatives of the lateral tract (obliquus capitis inferior) and the medial tract (obliquus capitis superior and rectus capitis posterior major and minor). The anterior group of short nuchal muscles (recti capitis lateralis and anterior) is innervated by the ventral rami, placing them among the prevertebral muscles (see **D**).

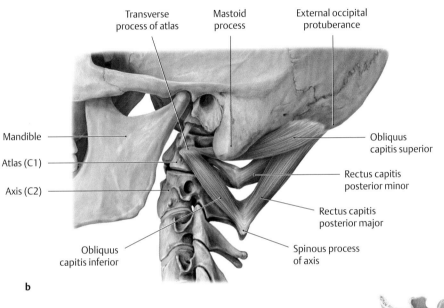

Transverse process of atlas — Mastoid process — External occipital protuberance

Obliquus capitis superior

Rectus capitis posterior minor

Rectus capitis posterior major

Mandible

Atlas (C1)

Axis (C2)

Obliquus capitis inferior

Spinous process of axis

b

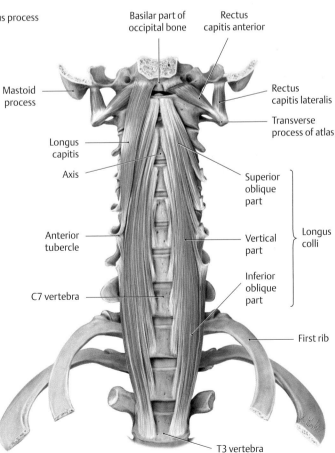

Basilar part of occipital bone — Rectus capitis anterior

Mastoid process

Rectus capitis lateralis

Transverse process of atlas

Longus capitis

Axis

Superior oblique part

Anterior tubercle

Vertical part

Longus colli

Inferior oblique part

C7 vertebra

First rib

T3 vertebra

D The prevertebral muscles: longus capitis, longus colli, and recti capitis anterior and lateralis

Anterior view after removal of the cervical viscera. The longus capitis muscle has been partially removed on the left side.

125

2.5 The Muscles of the Abdominal Wall: Lateral and Oblique Muscles

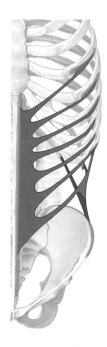

A Schematic of the external oblique (obliquus externus abdominis)

External oblique

Origin:	Outer surface of the 5th–12th ribs
Insertion:	• Outer lip of the iliac crest
	• Anterior layer of the rectus sheath, linea alba
Action:	• Unilateral: bends the trunk to the same side, rotates the trunk to the opposite side
	• Bilateral: flexes the trunk, straightens the pelvis, active in expiration, maintenance of abdominal tone (abdominal press)
Innervation:	Intercostal nerves (T5–T12), iliohypogastric nerve

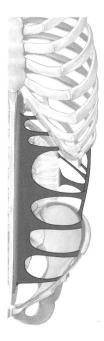

C Schematic of the transversus abdominis

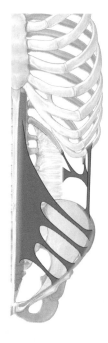

B Schematic of the internal oblique (obliquus internus abdominis)

Internal oblique

Origin:	Deep layer of the thoracolumbar fascia, intermediate line of the iliac crest, anterior superior iliac spine, lateral half of the inguinal ligament
Insertion:	• Lower borders of the 10th–12th ribs
	• Anterior and posterior layers of the rectus sheath, linea alba
	• Junction with the cremaster muscle
Action:	• Unilateral: bends the trunk to the same side, rotates the trunk to the same side
	• Bilateral: flexes the trunk, straightens the pelvis, active in expiration, maintenance of abdominal tone (abdominal press)
Innervation:	• Intercostal nerves (T8–T12), iliohypogastric nerve, ilioinguinal nerve
	• Cremaster muscle (genital branch of genitofemoral nerve)

Transversus abdominis

Origin:	• Inner surfaces of the 7th–12th costal cartilages
	• Deep layer of the thoracolumbar fascia
	• Inner lip of the iliac crest, anterior superior iliac spine
	• Lateral part of the inguinal ligament
Insertion:	Posterior layer of the rectus sheath, linea alba
Action:	• Unilateral: rotates the trunk to the same side
	• Bilateral: active in expiration, maintenance of abdominal tone (abdominal press)
Innervation:	Intercostal nerves (T5–T12), iliohypogastric nerve, ilioinguinal and genitofemoral nerves

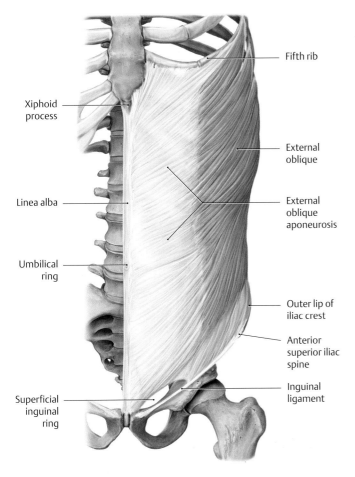

Xiphoid process
Linea alba
Umbilical ring
Superficial inguinal ring

Fifth rib
External oblique
External oblique aponeurosis
Outer lip of iliac crest
Anterior superior iliac spine
Inguinal ligament

D External oblique
Left side, anterior view.

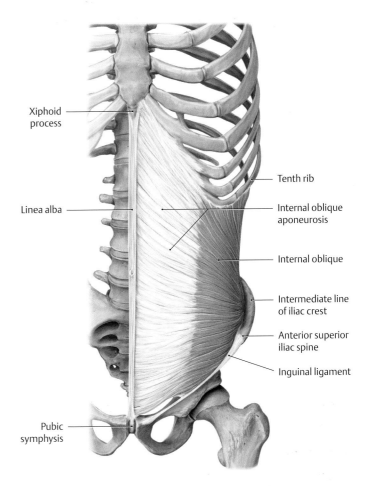

Xiphoid process
Linea alba
Pubic symphysis

Tenth rib
Internal oblique aponeurosis
Internal oblique
Intermediate line of iliac crest
Anterior superior iliac spine
Inguinal ligament

E Internal oblique
Left side, anterior view.

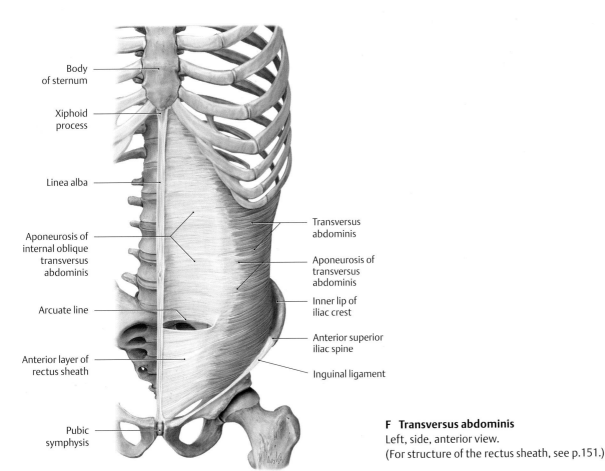

Body of sternum
Xiphoid process
Linea alba
Aponeurosis of internal oblique transversus abdominis
Arcuate line
Anterior layer of rectus sheath
Pubic symphysis

Transversus abdominis
Aponeurosis of transversus abdominis
Inner lip of iliac crest
Anterior superior iliac spine
Inguinal ligament

F Transversus abdominis
Left, side, anterior view.
(For structure of the rectus sheath, see p.151.)

2.6 The Muscles of the Abdominal Wall: Anterior and Posterior Muscles

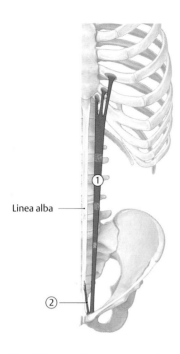

Linea alba

① Rectus abdominis

Origin:	Pubis (between the pubic tubercle and symphysis)
Insertion:	Cartilages of the fifth through seventh ribs, xiphoid process of the sternum
Action:	Flexes the lumbar spine, straightens the pelvis, active in expiration, maintenance of abdominal tone (abdominal press)
Innervation:	Intercostal nerves (T5–T12)

② Pyramidalis

Origin:	Pubis (anteriorly at the insertion of the rectus abdominis)
Insertion:	Linea alba (runs within the rectus sheath)
Action:	Tenses the linea alba
Innervation:	Subcostal nerve (twelfth intercostal nerve)

A Schematic of the anterior strap muscles of the abdominal wall: rectus abdominis and pyramidalis

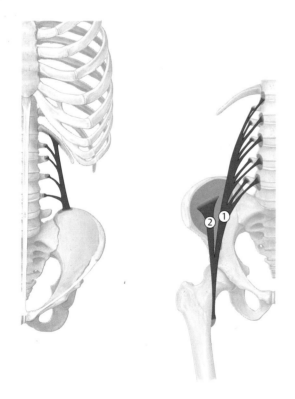

Quadratus lumborum

Origin:	Iliac crest
Insertion:	Twelfth rib, costal processes of the L1–L4 vertebrae
Action:	• Unilateral: bends the trunk to the same side
	• Bilateral: bearing down and expiration
Innervation:	Subcostal nerve (twelfth intercostal nerve)

Iliopsoas (① psoas major and ② iliacus)*

Origin:	• Psoas major (superficial layer): lateral surfaces of the T12 vertebral body, the L1–L4 vertebral bodies, and the associated intervertebral disks
	• Psoas major (deep layer): costal processes of the L1–L5 vertebrae
	• Iliacus: iliac fossa
Insertion:	Insert jointly as the iliopsoas muscle on the lesser trochanter of the femur
Action:	• Hip joint: flexion and external rotation
	• Lumbar spine: unilateral contraction (with the femur fixed) bends the trunk laterally, bilateral contraction raises the trunk from the supine position
Innervation:	Femoral nerve (T12–T14) and direct branches from the lumbar plexus

* Of these two muscles, only the psoas major belongs topographically to the posterior abdominal muscles. It is classified functionally as a hip muscle (see p. 422).

B Schematic of the deep posterior muscles of the abdominal wall: quadratus lumborum and psoas major

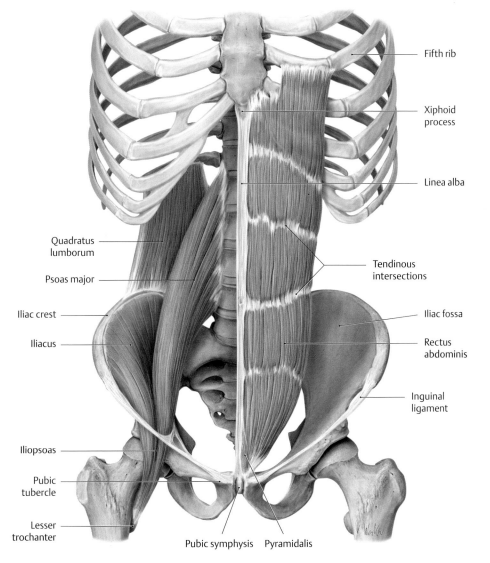

Fifth rib

Xiphoid process

Linea alba

Quadratus lumborum

Psoas major

Tendinous intersections

Iliac crest

Iliac fossa

Iliacus

Rectus abdominis

Inguinal ligament

Iliopsoas

Pubic tubercle

Lesser trochanter

Pubic symphysis   Pyramidalis

C Anterior (rectus abdominis and pyramidalis) and posterior muscles of the abdominal wall (quadratus lumborum and iliopsoas)
Anterior view. The anterior abdominal wall muscles are demonstrated on the left side and the posterior muscles on the right side.

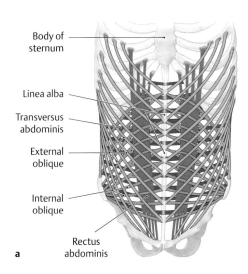

Body of sternum

Linea alba

Transversus abdominis

External oblique

Internal oblique

Rectus abdominis

a

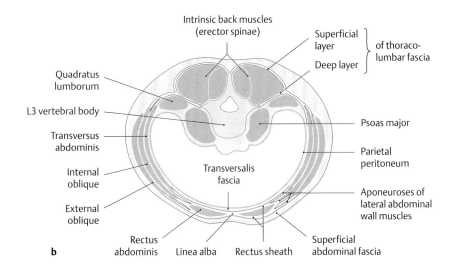

Intrinsic back muscles (erector spinae)

Superficial layer

Deep layer

of thoraco-lumbar fascia

Quadratus lumborum

L3 vertebral body

Transversus abdominis

Internal oblique

External oblique

Psoas major

Parietal peritoneum

Transversalis fascia

Aponeuroses of lateral abdominal wall muscles

Rectus abdominis   Linea alba   Rectus sheath

Superficial abdominal fascia

b

D Arrangement of the abdominal wall muscles and rectus sheath
a Anterior view, **b** transverse section at the level of L3.
The rectus abdominis and lateral oblique abdominal wall muscles and their aponeuroses comprise a functional unit. Fusion of the aponeuroses of the oblique muscles creates a sheath enclosing the rectus muscles which in turn meets the aponeurosis from the opposite side to form the linea alba in the abdominal midline. For the upper ¾ of the length of the rectus muscles, the aponeurosis of the internal oblique muscle splits, so portions pass both anterior and posterior to the rectus muscles. There-

fore, in the upper region of the rectus, the external oblique aponeurosis passes anterior, and the transverses abdominis aponeurosis passes posterior to the rectus muscles. Thus an anterior rectus sheath (external oblique and a portion of the internal oblique aponeuroses), and a posterior rectus sheath (the rest of the internal oblique and transverses aponeuroses) are formed. Over the lower ¼ of the rectus muscles, the aponeuroses of all three abdominal muscles pass anterior to the rectus muscles. No posterior sheath is present. The inferior edge of the posterior rectus sheath is called the arcuate line.

129

2.7 The Functions of the Abdominal Wall Muscles

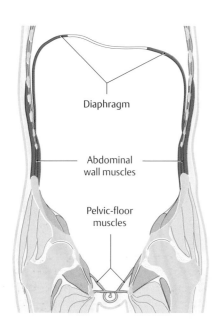

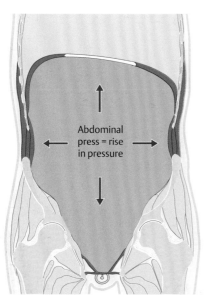

Functions of the Abdominal Wall Muscles

The different abdominal wall muscles perform numerous functions, which very often are carried out in concert with other muscle groups (e.g., the back and gluteal muscles and the diaphragm). The principal actions of the abdominal wall muscles are as follows:

- Maintenance of abdominal tone: tensing the abdominal wall and compressing the abdominal viscera (abdominal press)
- Stabilizing the vertebrae and reducing stresses on the spinal column
- Moving the trunk and pelvis
- Assisting in respiration

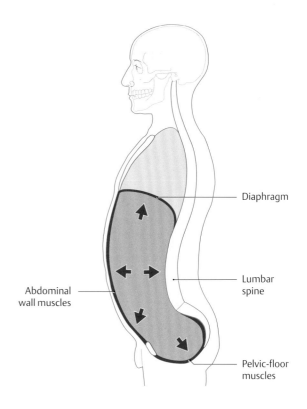

A Abdominal press = raising the intra-abdominal pressure by tensing the abdominal wall and pelvic floor muscles and the diaphragm

Schematic coronal section through the abdominal cavity, anterior view.

a The walls of the abdominal and pelvic cavity are formed by bony structures (spinal column, thoracic cage, pelvis) and also by muscles (diaphragm, muscles of the abdominal wall and pelvic floor).

b When the muscles about the abdomen contract (abdominal press), they reduce the volume of the abdominal cavity, thereby raising the intra-abdominal pressure and actively compressing the abdominal viscera. This action is important, for example, in expelling stool from the rectum (defecation), expelling urine from the bladder (micturition), and emptying the gastric contents (vomiting). The abdominal press is also an essential part of maternal pushing during the expulsive phase of labor.

B Abdominal press = stabilizing the spinal column by raising the intra-abdominal pressure

Schematic midsagittal section through the trunk, left lateral view. Simultaneous contraction of the diaphragm and the muscles of the abdominal wall and pelvic floor raises the pressure in the abdominal cavity (abdominal press). The hydrostatic effect of this maneuver stabilizes the trunk, reduces stresses on the spinal column (especially at the lumbar level), and stiffens the trunk wall like the wall of an inflated ball. This action is performed automatically during the lifting of heavy loads. The "inflatable space" of the trunk can be employed in this way to lighten the pressure load on the intervertebral disks by up to 50% in the upper lumbar spine and by approximately 30% in the lower lumbar spine. Meanwhile, the forces exerted by the intrinsic back muscles are reduced by more than 50%. This explains the importance of well-conditioned abdominal muscles in preventing and treating diseases of the spinal column.

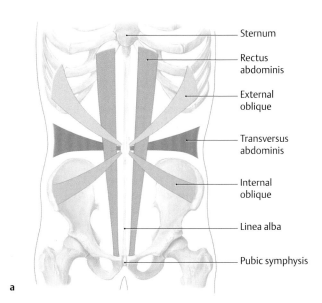

Sternum

Rectus abdominis

External oblique

Transversus abdominis

Internal oblique

Linea alba

Pubic symphysis

a

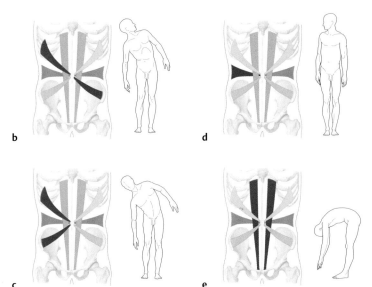

b

d

c

e

C Trunk movements aided by the straight and oblique muscles of the abdominal wall

a Course and arrangement of the straight and oblique abdominal wall muscles.

b Trunk flexion to the right with simultaneous rotation of the trunk to the left side by contraction of the external oblique muscle on the right side and the internal oblique muscle on the left side.

c Trunk flexion to the right by contraction of the right lateral abdominal muscles (aided by the right intrinsic back muscles).

d Rotating the trunk to the right side is effected by the right lateral abdominal muscles and the left intrinsic back muscles.

e Flexion of the trunk is effected by bilateral contraction of the rectus abdominis, lateral abdominal and psoas muscles.

.

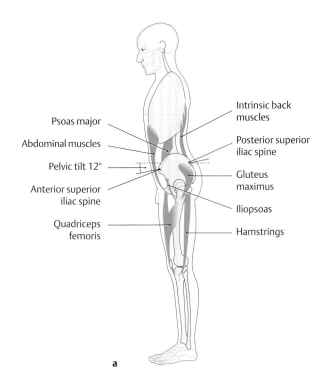

Psoas major

Abdominal muscles

Pelvic tilt 12°

Anterior superior iliac spine

Quadriceps femoris

Intrinsic back muscles

Posterior superior iliac spine

Gluteus maximus

Iliopsoas

Hamstrings

a

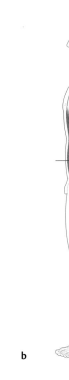

b

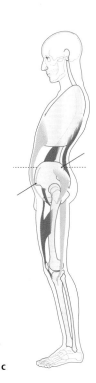

c

D Effect of the abdominal wall muscles on pelvic movements: active and passive posture

a Normal active posture, **b** active rigid posture, **c** passive slumped posture.

An imbalance between the intrinsic back muscles and abdominal muscles is particularly evident in the curvature of the lower spine and in the degree of pelvic tilt. In a normal active posture, the pelvis is tilted forward by approximately 12° (**a**). When a rigid posture is assumed ("stomach in, chest out"), the pelvis is held in a more upright position so that the anterior superior iliac spine and the posterior superior iliac spine are at the same level (**b**). The most active muscles are the abdominal wall muscles, the gluteal muscles, and the hamstrings. When the abdominal muscles are lax and are not well conditioned, the result is a passive slumped posture (**c**) with an excessive degree of anterior pelvic tilt. Also, the lordotic curvature of the lumbar spine is accentuated due to progressive shortening of the intrinsic back muscles. This posture is reinforced by the tendency of the iliopsoas muscles (psoas major and iliacus) to become shortened.

2.8 The Muscles of the Thoracic Cage (Intercostales, Subcostales, Scaleni, and Transversus thoracis)

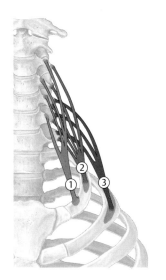

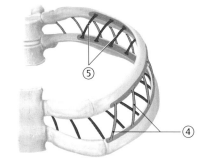

a

b

A Overview of the thoracic muscles
Anterior view.

a Scalene muscles.
b Intercostal muscles.

Scalene muscles

Origin:	① Anterior scalene: anterior tubercle of the transverse processes of the C3–C6 vertebrae
	② Middle scalene: posterior tubercle of the transverse processes of the C3–C7 vertebrae
	③ Posterior scalene: posterior tubercle of the transverse processes of the C5–C7 vertebrae
Insertion:	• Anterior scalene: scalene tubercle of first rib
	• Middle scalene: first rib (posterior to the groove for the subclavian artery)
	• Posterior scalene: outer surface of the second rib
Action:	• With the ribs mobile: raises the upper ribs (in inspiration)
	• With the ribs fixed: bends the cervical spine toward the same side (with unilateral contraction)
	• Flexes the neck (with bilateral contraction)
Innervation:	Direct branches from the cervical plexus and brachial plexus (C3–C6)

Intercostal muscles

Origin and insertion:	④ External intercostal muscles (costal tubercle to chondro-osseous junction): arise at the lower margin of a rib and insert on the upper margin of the next lower rib (course obliquely forward and downward)
	⑤ Internal intercostal muscles (costal angle to sternum): arise at the upper margin of a rib and insert on the lower margin of the next higher rib (course obliquely forward and upward)
	• Inntermost intercostal muscles: division of the internal intercostals (same course and action)
Action:	• External intercostals: raise the ribs (in inspiration), support the intercostal spaces, stabilize the chest wall
	• Internal intercostals: lower the ribs (in expiration), support the intercostal spaces, stabilize the chest wall
Innervation:	First through eleventh intercostal nerves

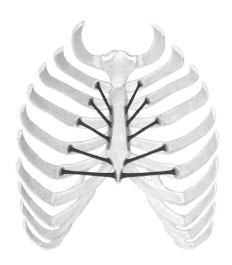

B Overview of the transversus thoracis
Posterior view.

Transversus thoracis

Origin:	Inner surface of the costal cartilage of the second through sixth ribs
Insertion:	Inner surface of the sternum and xiphoid process
Action:	Lowers the ribs (in expiration)
Innervation:	Second through seventh intercostal nerves

C Anterior, middle, and posterior scalene and the internal and external intercostal muscles

Anterior view with the thoracic cage partially removed. Topographically, the scaleni are included among the deep neck muscles but functionally they play an important role in thoracic breathing. Subcostal muscles have the same orientation as internal intercostals, but skip over one or two ribs to form continuous sheets, especially at the angle of the sixth through eleventh ribs.

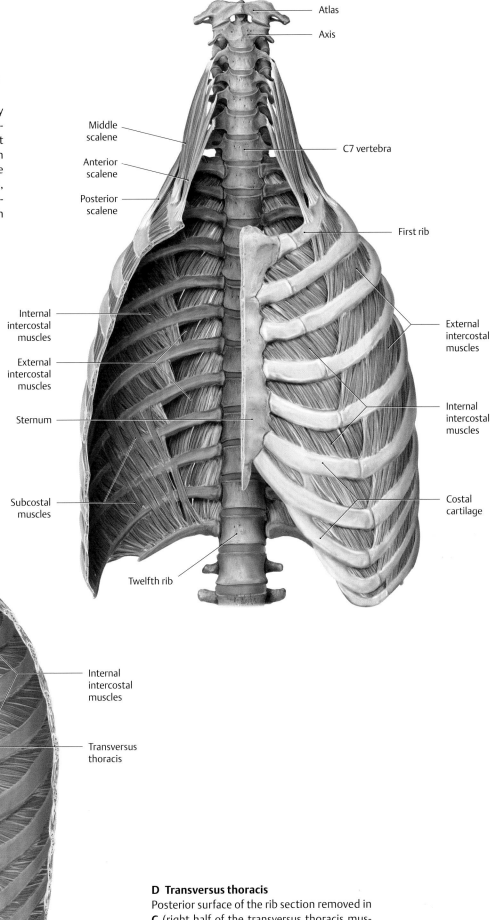

Atlas

Axis

Middle scalene

Anterior scalene

Posterior scalene

C7 vertebra

First rib

Internal intercostal muscles

External intercostal muscles

Sternum

External intercostal muscles

Internal intercostal muscles

Subcostal muscles

Costal cartilage

Twelfth rib

First rib

Manubrium sterni

Internal intercostal muscles

Body of sternum

Transversus thoracis

Xiphoid process

Costal cartilage

D Transversus thoracis
Posterior surface of the rib section removed in **C** (right half of the transversus thoracis muscle), posterior view.

133

2.9 The Muscles of the Thoracic Cage: The Diaphragm

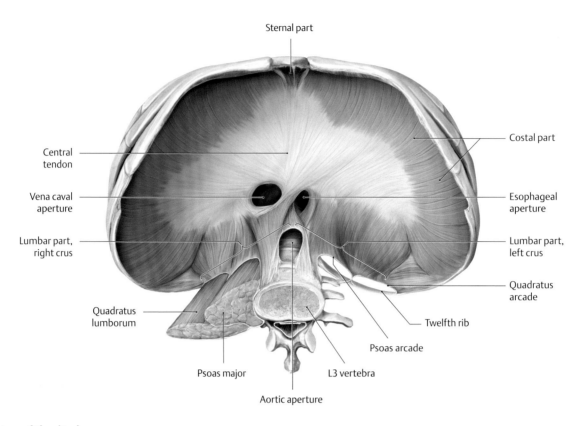

A Overview of the diaphragm

Origin:	• Costal part: lower margin of costal arch (inner surface of seventh through twelfth ribs)
	• Lumbar part (right and left crura):
	– Medial parts: L1–L3 vertebral bodies, second and third intervertebral disks, anterior longitudinal ligament
	– Lateral parts: first tendinous arch of the abdominal aorta (median arcuate ligament) at L1 associated with its anterior surface; second tendinous arch of the psoas arcade (medial arcuate ligament) from L2 vertebral body to associated costal process; third tendinous arch of the quadratus lumborum arcade (lateral arcuate ligament) from the costal process of L2 to the tip of rib 12
	• Sternal part: posterior surface of the xiphoid process
Insertion:	Central tendon
Action:	Principal muscle of respiration (diaphragmatic and thoracic breathing), aids in compressing the abdominal viscera (abdominal press)
Innervation:	Phrenic nerve from the cervical plexus (C3–C5)

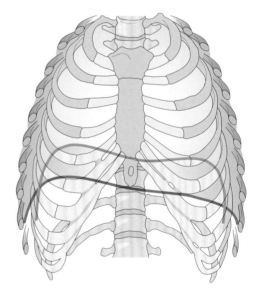

B Position of the diaphragm and ribs at full inspiration and expiration

Thoracic cage, anterior view.

Note the different positions of the diaphragm at full inspiration (red) and full expiration (blue). During a physical examination, the posterior lung boundaries can be identified by percussion (tapping the body surface). The respiratory movement of the diaphragm from end-expiration to end-inspiration should be determined; it is approximately 4–6 cm.

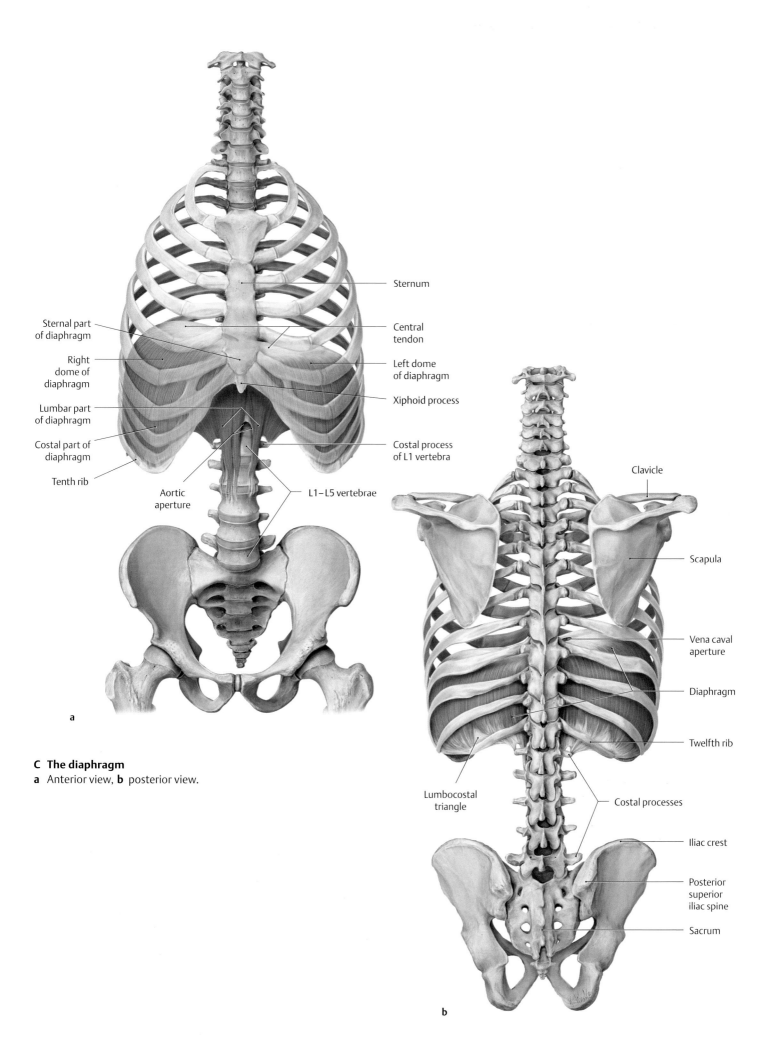

Sternum

Sternal part
of diaphragm

Central
tendon

Right
dome of
diaphragm

Left dome
of diaphragm

Lumbar part
of diaphragm

Xiphoid process

Costal part of
diaphragm

Costal process
of L1 vertebra

Tenth rib

Aortic
aperture

L1–L5 vertebrae

a

Clavicle

Scapula

Vena caval
aperture

Diaphragm

Twelfth rib

Lumbocostal
triangle

Costal processes

Iliac crest

Posterior
superior
iliac spine

Sacrum

b

C The diaphragm
a Anterior view, **b** posterior view.

2.10 The Muscles of the Pelvic Floor (Pelvic Diaphragm, Urogenital Diaphragm, Sphincter and Erectile Muscles)

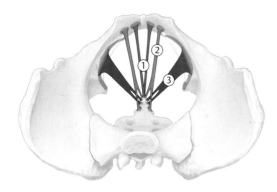

A Schematic of the pelvic diaphragm: the levator ani (puborectalis, pubococcygeus, and iliococcygeus) and coccygeus (not shown)
Inferior view.

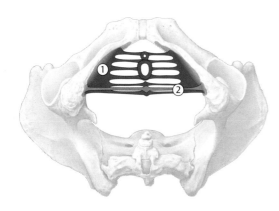

B Schematic of the urogenital diaphragm: deep and superficial transverse perineal
Inferior view.

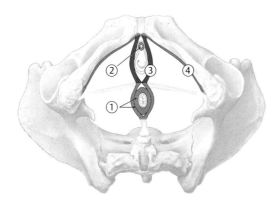

C Schematic of the sphincter and erectile muscles of the pelvic floor: external anal sphincter, external urethral sphincter, bulbospongiosus, and ischiocavernosus
Inferior view.

Levator ani

① **Puborectalis**

Origin:	Superior pubic ramus on both sides of the pubic symphysis
Insertion:	Anococcygeal ligament
Innervation:	Direct branches of the sacral plexus (S2–S4)

② **Pubococcygeus**

Origin:	Pubis (lateral at origin of the puborectalis)
Insertion:	Anococcygeal ligament, coccyx
Innervation:	Direct branches of the sacral plexus (S2–S4)

③ **Iliococcygeus**

Origin:	Tendinous arch of the internal obturator fascia (of the levator ani)
Insertion:	Anococcygeal ligament, coccyx
Function of the pelvic diaphragm:	Holds the pelvic organs in place
Innervation:	Direct branches of the sacral plexus (S2–S4)

① **Deep transverse perineal**

Origin:	Inferior pubic ramus, ischial ramus
Insertion:	Wall of vagina or prostate, central tendon of diaphragm
Innervation:	Pudendal nerve (S2–S4)

② **Superficial transverse perineal**

Origin:	Ischial ramus
Insertion:	Central tendon of diaphragm
Function of the urogenital diaphragm:	Holds the pelvic organs in place, closes the urethra
Innervation:	Pudendal nerve (S2–S4)

① **External anal sphincter**
The external anal sphincter runs posteriorly from the central tendon to the anococcygeal ligament (encircles the anus)

Action:	Closes the anus
Innervation:	Pudendal nerve (S2–S4)

② **External urethral sphincter**
Division of the deep transverse perineal (encircles the urethra)

Action:	Closes the urethra
Innervation:	Pudendal nerve (S2–S4)

③ **Bulbospongiosus**
Runs anteriorly from the central tendon to the clitoris in females, to the penile raphe in males

Action:	Narrows the vaginal introitus in females, surrounds the corpus spongiosum in males
Innervation:	Pudendal nerve (S2–S4)

④ **Ischiocavernosus**

Origin:	Ischial ramus
Insertion:	Crus of penis or clitoris
Action:	Squeezes blood into the corpus cavernosum of the penis or clitoris
Innervation:	Pudendal nerve (S2–S4)

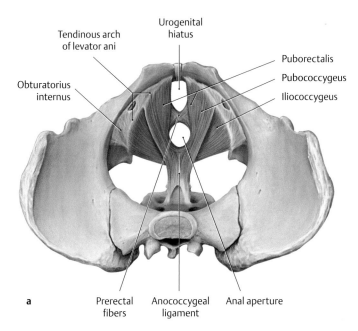

a

Urogenital hiatus — Tendinous arch of levator ani — Obturatorius internus — Puborectalis — Pubococcygeus — Iliococcygeus — Levator ani — Prerectal fibers — Anococcygeal ligament — Anal aperture

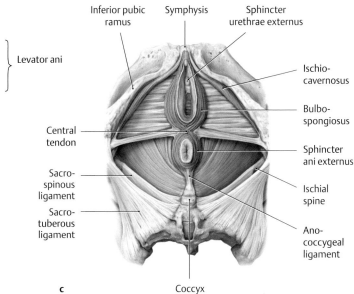

c

Inferior pubic ramus — Symphysis — Sphincter urethrae externus — Central tendon — Sacrospinous ligament — Sacrotuberous ligament — Ischiocavernosus — Bulbospongiosus — Sphincter ani externus — Ischial spine — Anococcygeal ligament — Coccyx

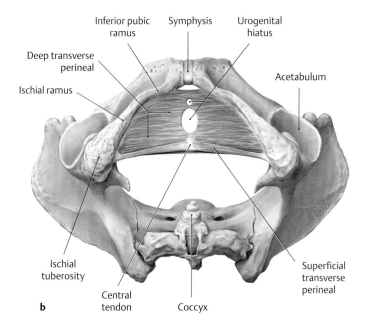

b

Inferior pubic ramus — Symphysis — Urogenital hiatus — Deep transverse perineal — Ischial ramus — Acetabulum — Ischial tuberosity — Central tendon — Coccyx — Superficial transverse perineal

D The muscles of the female pelvic floor
a Pelvic diaphragm, superior view.
b Urogenital diaphragm, inferior view.
c Sphincter and erectile muscles, inferior view.

The term "urogenital diaphragm" has been called into question due to controversy regarding the existence of the deep transverse perineal muscle in the female pelvis. This is because the deep transverse perineal becomes heavily permeated by connective tissue with aging and especially after vaginal deliveries. In older women, the deep perineal space (see p. 155) basically contains connective tissue that completely occupies the urogenital hiatus at the openings of the urethra and vagina (see also p. 160).

Important Functions of the Pelvic Floor Muscles
The pelvic floor performs a dual function:

- It supports the abdominal and pelvic organs by closing the abdominal and pelvic cavities inferiorly, bearing the bulk of the visceral load.
- It controls the openings of the rectum and urogenital passages (sphincter functions), which mechanically weaken the pelvic floor by piercing it.

To accomplish these inherently conflicting functions (sealing off the pelvic cavity while maintaining several apertures), the pelvic floor is lined by overlapping sheets of muscle and connective tissue. This complex structure, however, also makes the pelvic floor highly susceptible to damage, especially in women. Repetitive, extreme fluctuations in intra-abdominal pressure and other stresses, particularly at the end of pregnancy, can weaken the connective tissue apparatus and damage the pelvic floor muscles. Stretching and other injuries, as during labor and delivery (in multiparae), can eventually lead to pelvic floor insufficiency and its various clinical sequelae:

- Descent of the pelvic organs (e.g., *uterine descent*)
- In extreme cases, prolapse of the uterus with eversion of the vagina (*uterine prolapse*)

Visceral descent is generally associated with urinary or fecal incontinence in response to coughing or other acts (*stress incontinence*). Mild degrees of descent often respond well to regular pelvic floor exercises, but more serious cases may require surgical treatment with *pelvic floor repair* (surgical exposure and approximation of the two levator crura = puborectalis muscle).

137

3.1 The Back Muscles and Thoracolumbar Fascia

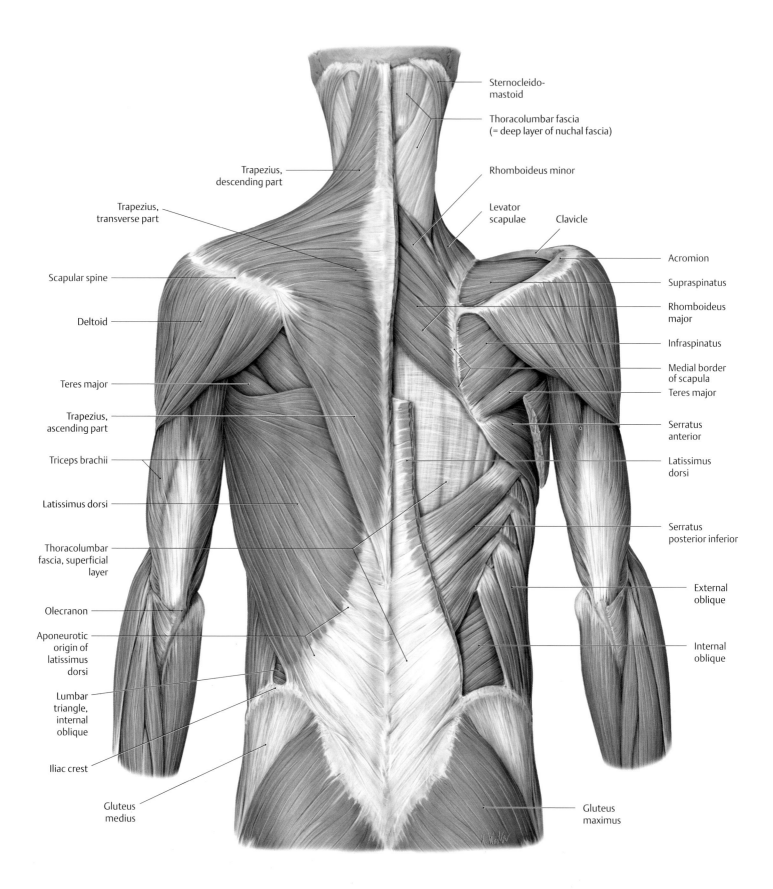

Sternocleido-
mastoid

Thoracolumbar fascia
(= deep layer of nuchal fascia)

Rhomboideus minor

Levator
scapulae   Clavicle

Acromion

Supraspinatus

Rhomboideus
major

Infraspinatus

Medial border
of scapula

Teres major

Serratus
anterior

Latissimus
dorsi

Serratus
posterior inferior

External
oblique

Internal
oblique

Gluteus
maximus

Trapezius,
descending part

Trapezius,
transverse part

Scapular spine

Deltoid

Teres major

Trapezius,
ascending part

Triceps brachii

Latissimus dorsi

Thoracolumbar
fascia, superficial
layer

Olecranon

Aponeurotic
origin of
latissimus
dorsi

Lumbar
triangle,
internal
oblique

Iliac crest

Gluteus
medius

A The thoracolumbar fascia as a "partition" between the intrinsic and nonintrinsic back muscles

The trapezius muscle has been completely removed on the right side of the drawing and the latissimus dorsi has been partially removed to demonstrate the thoracolumbar fascia. The superficial layer of the thoraco-lumbar fascia separates the intrinsic back muscles from the nonintrinsic muscles that have migrated to the back.

Note: The superficial layer of the thoracolumbar fascia is reinforced inferiorly by the aponeurotic origin of the latissimus dorsi.

138

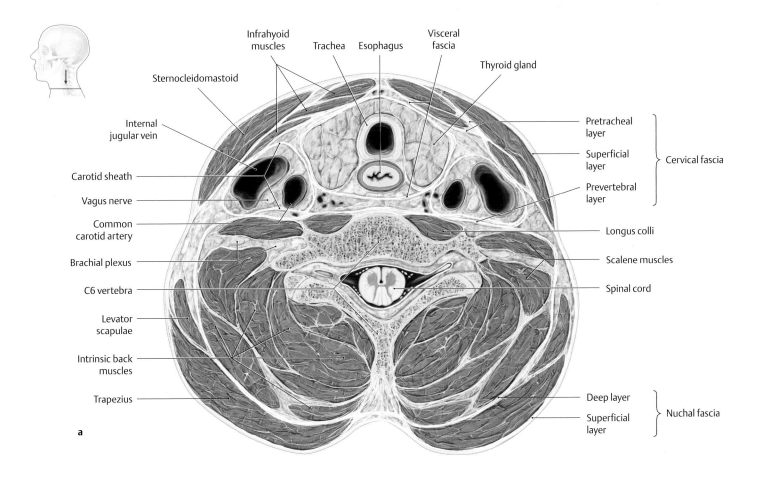

Infrahyoid muscles · Trachea · Esophagus · Visceral fascia · Thyroid gland · Sternocleidomastoid

Internal jugular vein · Pretracheal layer · Superficial layer · Cervical fascia · Prevertebral layer

Carotid sheath · Vagus nerve · Common carotid artery · Longus colli · Scalene muscles · Spinal cord

Brachial plexus · C6 vertebra · Levator scapulae · Intrinsic back muscles · Trapezius · Deep layer · Superficial layer · Nuchal fascia

a

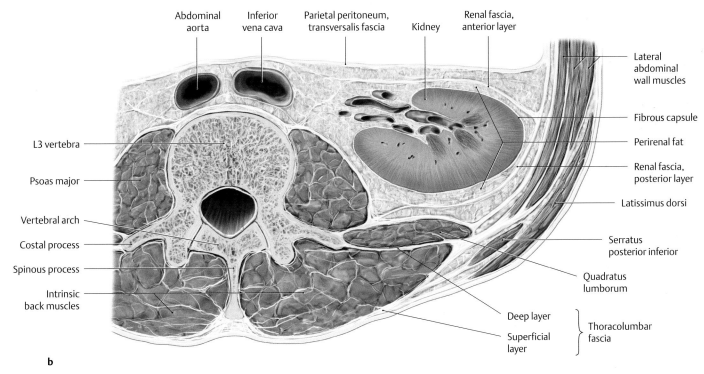

Abdominal aorta · Inferior vena cava · Parietal peritoneum, transversalis fascia · Kidney · Renal fascia, anterior layer

Lateral abdominal wall muscles · Fibrous capsule · Perirenal fat · Renal fascia, posterior layer · Latissimus dorsi

L3 vertebra · Psoas major · Vertebral arch · Costal process · Spinous process · Intrinsic back muscles · Serratus posterior inferior · Quadratus lumborum · Deep layer · Superficial layer · Thoracolumbar fascia

b

B Thoracolumbar fascia

a Transverse section through the neck at the level of the C6 vertebra, superior view.

b Transverse section through the posterior trunk wall at the level of the L3 vertebra (cauda equina removed), superior view.

The thoracolumbar fascia forms the lateral portion of an osseofibrous canal that encloses all of the *intrinsic back muscles*. Besides the thoracolumbar fascia, this canal is also formed by the vertebral arches and the spinous and costal processes of the associated vertebrae. The thoracolumbar fascia consists of a superficial and a deep layer, especially in the lumbar region; both layers unite at the lateral margin of the intrinsic back muscles. At the back of the neck, the superficial layer of the thoracolumbar fascia blends with the nuchal fascia (deep layer), becoming continuous with the prevertebral layer of the cervical fascia.

3.2 The Intrinsic Back Muscles: Lateral and Medial Tracts

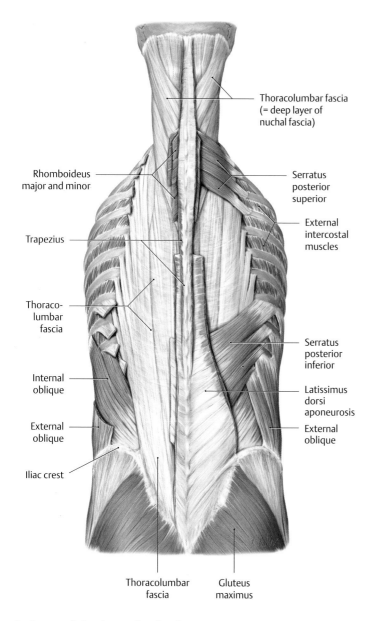

A Course of the thoracolumbar fascia
Posterior view. To demonstrate the thoracolumbar fascia, both shoulder girdles and the extrinsic back muscles have been removed (except for the serratus posterior superior and inferior and the aponeurotic origin of the latissimus dorsi on the right side).

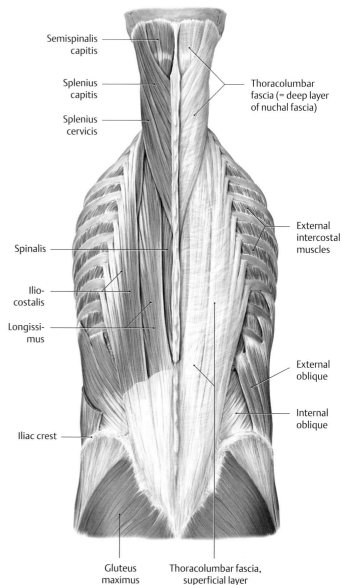

B Lateral tract of the intrinsic back muscles
Posterior view. Portions of the superficial layer of the thoracolumbar fascia have been removed on the left side of the back to expose the lateral tract muscles (iliocostalis, longissimus, splenii cervicis and capitis). The levator costarum and intertransversarii, also part of the lateral tract, are covered here by the iliocostal and longissimus muscles (see **C** and **D**).
Note that the thoracolumbar fascia on the back of the neck is continuous with the deep layer of the nuchal fascia.

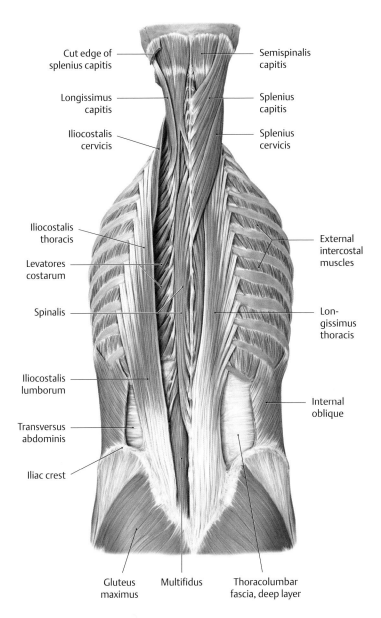

Cut edge of splenius capitis

Longissimus capitis

Iliocostalis cervicis

Iliocostalis thoracis

Levatores costarum

Spinalis

Iliocostalis lumborum

Transversus abdominis

Iliac crest

Semispinalis capitis

Splenius capitis

Splenius cervicis

External intercostal muscles

Longissimus thoracis

Internal oblique

Gluteus maximus

Multifidus

Thoracolumbar fascia, deep layer

C Medial tract of the intrinsic back muscles (portions of the lateral tract left in place)

Posterior view. The longissimus (except for longissimus capitis) and the splenii cervicis and capitis have been removed on the left side of the back, and the entire iliocostalis has been removed on the right side (see **C** for rotator muscles).

Note the deep layer of the thoracolumbar fascia, which gives origin to both the internal oblique and the transversus abdominis (see **D**).

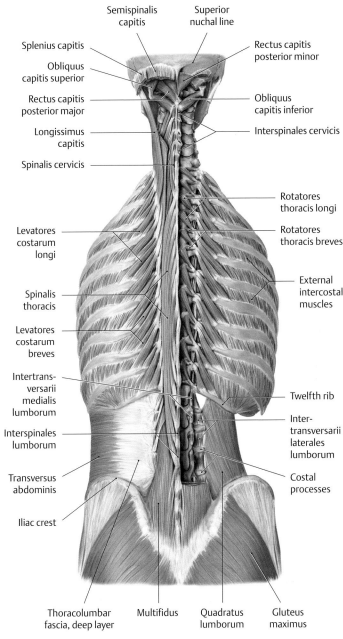

Semispinalis capitis

Splenius capitis

Obliquus capitis superior

Rectus capitis posterior major

Longissimus capitis

Spinalis cervicis

Levatores costarum longi

Spinalis thoracis

Levatores costarum breves

Intertransversarii medialis lumborum

Interspinales lumborum

Transversus abdominis

Iliac crest

Superior nuchal line

Rectus capitis posterior minor

Obliquus capitis inferior

Interspinales cervicis

Rotatores thoracis longi

Rotatores thoracis breves

External intercostal muscles

Twelfth rib

Intertransversarii laterales lumborum

Costal processes

Thoracolumbar fascia, deep layer

Multifidus

Quadratus lumborum

Gluteus maximus

D Medial tract of the intrinsic back muscles (with the entire lateral tract removed)

Posterior view. The entire lateral tract (except for the intertransversarii and levatores costarum) has been removed along with portions of the medial tract to demonstrate the various individual muscles of the medial tract.

Note the origin of the transversus abdominis from the deep layer of the thoracolumbar fascia in the lumbar region (left side).

On the right side, the deep fascial layer and multifidus muscle have been removed to display the intertransversarii (lateral tract) and the quadratus lumborum (posterior deep abdominal muscles).

141

3.3 The Intrinsic Back Muscles: Short Nuchal Muscles

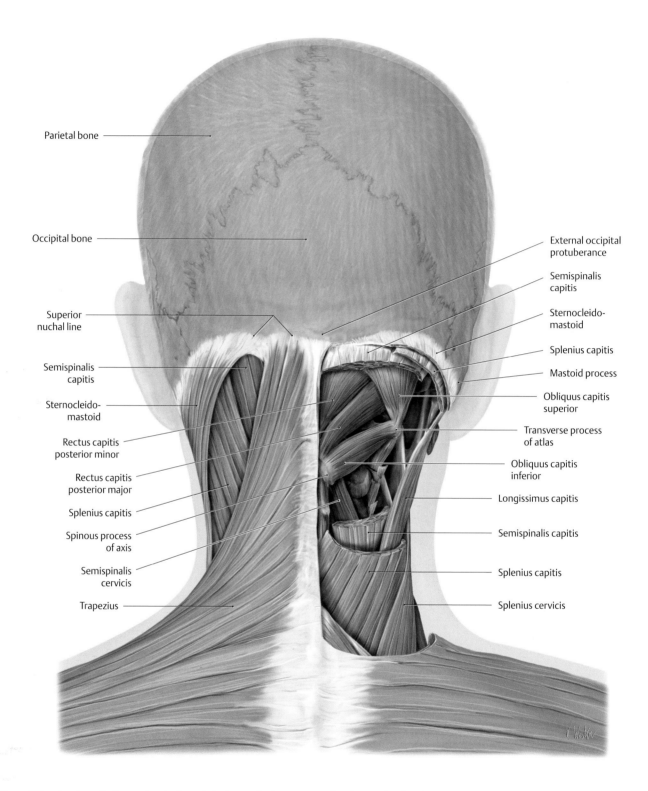

Parietal bone

Occipital bone

Superior nuchal line

Semispinalis capitis

Sternocleido-mastoid

Rectus capitis posterior minor

Rectus capitis posterior major

Splenius capitis

Spinous process of axis

Semispinalis cervicis

Trapezius

External occipital protuberance

Semispinalis capitis

Sternocleido-mastoid

Splenius capitis

Mastoid process

Obliquus capitis superior

Transverse process of atlas

Obliquus capitis inferior

Longissimus capitis

Semispinalis capitis

Splenius capitis

Splenius cervicis

A Location of the short nuchal muscles (suboccipital muscles)
Nuchal region, posterior view. The suboccipital muscles in the strict sense are the short or deep nuchal muscles that belong to the intrinsic back muscles (recti capitis posteriores major and minor and obliquii capitis superior and inferior). They meet the criterion of being innervated by a dorsal ramus—in this case the C1 dorsal ramus, the suboccipital nerve. Thus the recti capitis *anterior* and *lateralis* are *not* classified as intrinsic back muscles, despite their suboccipital location, because they are innervated by ventral rami. The short or deep nuchal muscles lie within the thoracolumbar fascia deep at the back of the neck and course between the occiput and the first two cervical vertebrae. They act mainly on the craniovertebral joints (see p. 96) and support differentiated head movements (e.g., for fine adjustments of head position). The following muscles have been partially removed to demonstrate their location in the right nuchal region: trapezius, sternocleidomastoid, splenius capitis, and semispinalis capitis. An important landmark in the deep nuchal region is the spinous process of the axis.

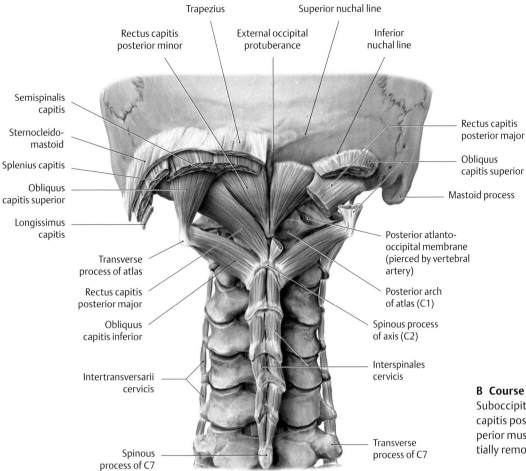

Trapezius

Superior nuchal line

Rectus capitis posterior minor

External occipital protuberance

Inferior nuchal line

Semispinalis capitis

Sternocleido-mastoid

Splenius capitis

Obliquus capitis superior

Longissimus capitis

Rectus capitis posterior major

Obliquus capitis superior

Mastoid process

Transverse process of atlas

Rectus capitis posterior major

Obliquus capitis inferior

Posterior atlanto-occipital membrane (pierced by vertebral artery)

Posterior arch of atlas (C1)

Spinous process of axis (C2)

Intertransversarii cervicis

Interspinales cervicis

Spinous process of C7

Transverse process of C7

B Course of the short nuchal muscles
Suboccipital region, posterior view. The rectus capitis posterior major and obliquus capitis superior muscles on the right side have been partially removed.

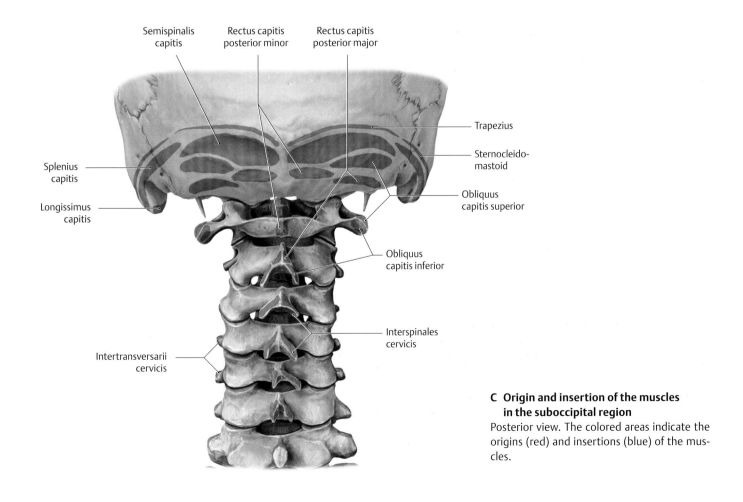

Semispinalis capitis

Rectus capitis posterior minor

Rectus capitis posterior major

Splenius capitis

Longissimus capitis

Trapezius

Sternocleido-mastoid

Obliquus capitis superior

Obliquus capitis inferior

Interspinales cervicis

Intertransversarii cervicis

C Origin and insertion of the muscles in the suboccipital region
Posterior view. The colored areas indicate the origins (red) and insertions (blue) of the muscles.

3.4 The Chest Wall Muscles and Endothoracic Fascia

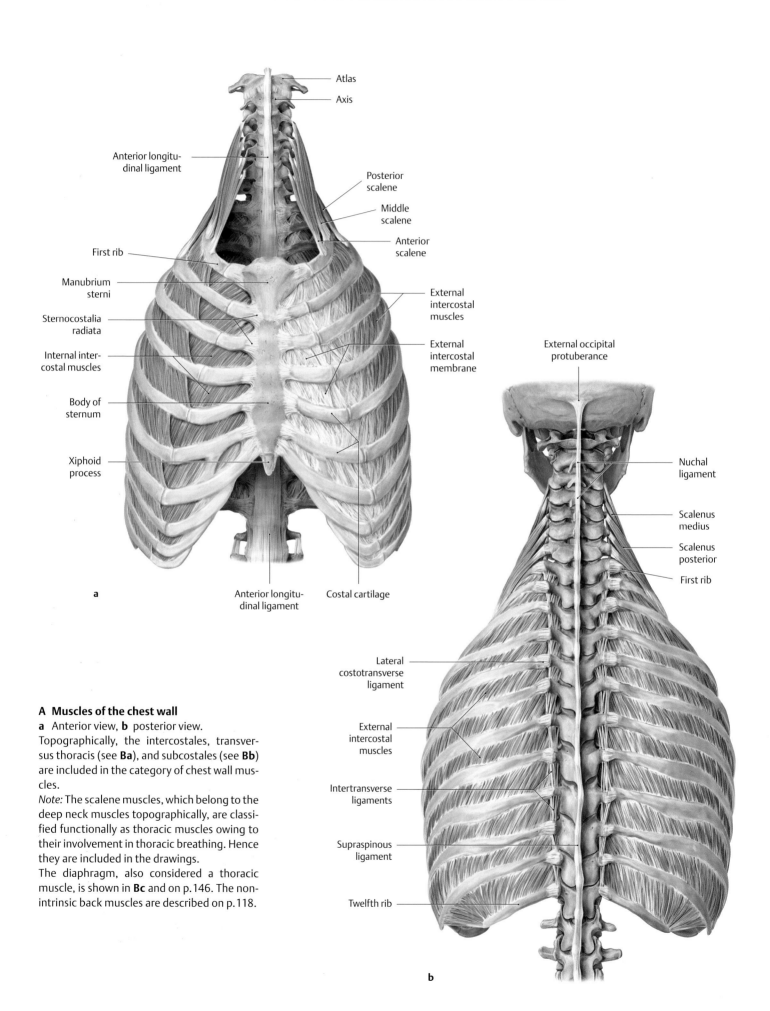

A Muscles of the chest wall
a Anterior view, **b** posterior view.
Topographically, the intercostales, transversus thoracis (see **Ba**), and subcostales (see **Bb**) are included in the category of chest wall muscles.
Note: The scalene muscles, which belong to the deep neck muscles topographically, are classified functionally as thoracic muscles owing to their involvement in thoracic breathing. Hence they are included in the drawings.
The diaphragm, also considered a thoracic muscle, is shown in **Bc** and on p. 146. The nonintrinsic back muscles are described on p. 118.

Labels for figure a:
- Atlas
- Axis
- Anterior longitudinal ligament
- Posterior scalene
- Middle scalene
- Anterior scalene
- First rib
- Manubrium sterni
- External intercostal muscles
- Sternocostalia radiata
- External intercostal membrane
- Internal intercostal muscles
- Body of sternum
- Xiphoid process
- Anterior longitudinal ligament
- Costal cartilage

Labels for figure b:
- External occipital protuberance
- Nuchal ligament
- Scalenus medius
- Scalenus posterior
- First rib
- Lateral costotransverse ligament
- External intercostal muscles
- Intertransverse ligaments
- Supraspinous ligament
- Twelfth rib

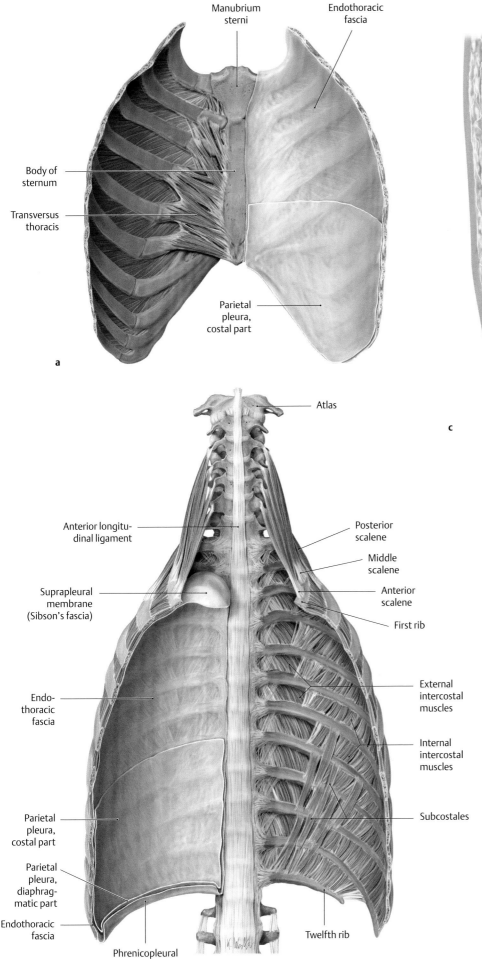

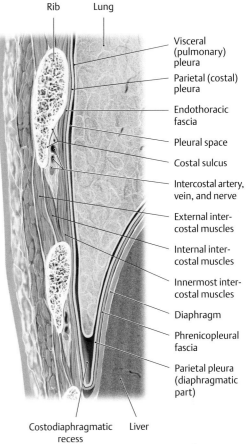

B Endothoracic fascia

a Posterior surface of the chest wall segment removed in **b**.
b Posterior chest wall, anterior view (endothoracic fascia removed on the left side).
c Coronal section through the lateral chest wall and costodiaphragmatic recess.

The thoracic cavity is lined by a fascialike layer of connective tissue, the *endothoracic fascia*. It lies between the deep muscles of the chest wall and the costal portion of the parietal pleura, to which it is firmly attached, and is analogous to the transversalis fascia of the abdominal cavity (**a**). The endothoracic fascia is thickened over the pleural apex to form the *suprapleural membrane (Sibson's fascia)*. The *phrenicopleural fascia* is the portion of the endothoracic fascia that connects the diaphragmatic part of the parietal pleura to the upper surface of the diaphragm (**b**). The costodiaphragmatic recess (**c**) between the chest wall and diaphragm is a potential space that enlarges on inspiration (lowering of the diaphragm) to accommodate the expanding lung. The pleural space is the potential space located between the parietal/costal pleura and the visceral pleura, which directly invests the lung tissue.

145

3.5 Thoracoabdominal Junction: The Diaphragm

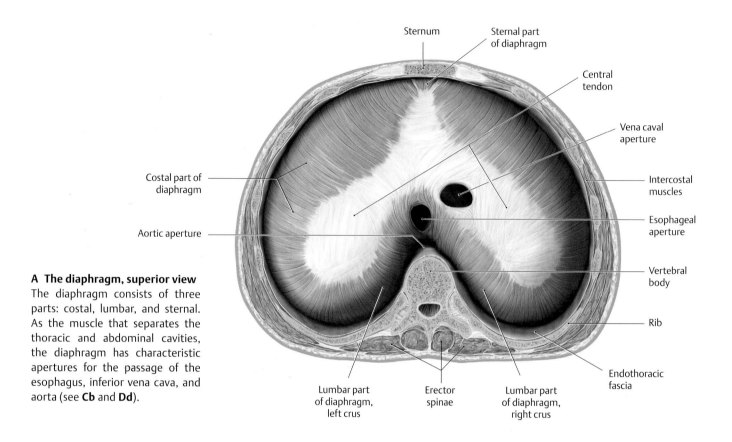

A The diaphragm, superior view
The diaphragm consists of three parts: costal, lumbar, and sternal. As the muscle that separates the thoracic and abdominal cavities, the diaphragm has characteristic apertures for the passage of the esophagus, inferior vena cava, and aorta (see **Cb** and **Dd**).

Labels for A:
Sternum
Sternal part of diaphragm
Central tendon
Vena caval aperture
Intercostal muscles
Esophageal aperture
Vertebral body
Rib
Endothoracic fascia
Costal part of diaphragm
Aortic aperture
Lumbar part of diaphragm, left crus
Erector spinae
Lumbar part of diaphragm, right crus

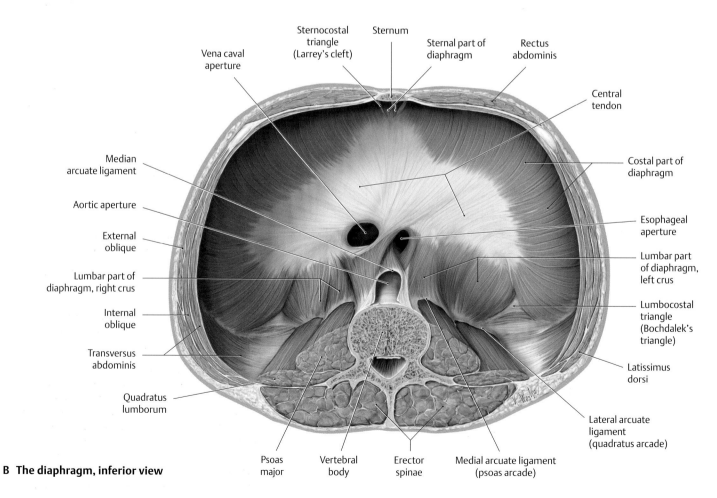

B The diaphragm, inferior view

Labels for B:
Sternocostal triangle (Larrey's cleft)
Sternum
Sternal part of diaphragm
Rectus abdominis
Vena caval aperture
Central tendon
Median arcuate ligament
Costal part of diaphragm
Aortic aperture
Esophageal aperture
External oblique
Lumbar part of diaphragm, left crus
Lumbar part of diaphragm, right crus
Lumbocostal triangle (Bochdalek's triangle)
Internal oblique
Transversus abdominis
Latissimus dorsi
Quadratus lumborum
Lateral arcuate ligament (quadratus arcade)
Psoas major
Vertebral body
Erector spinae
Medial arcuate ligament (psoas arcade)

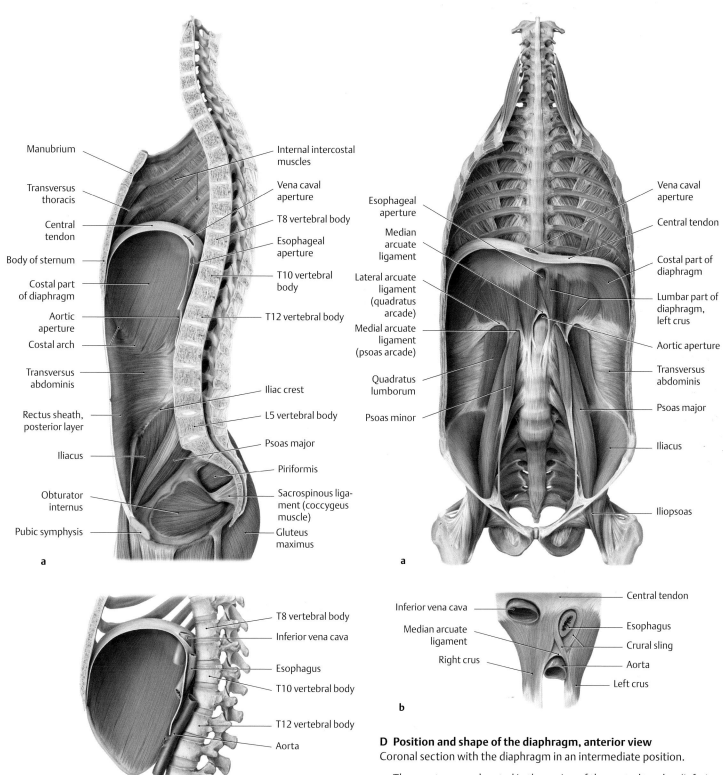

Manubrium

Transversus thoracis

Central tendon

Body of sternum

Costal part of diaphragm

Aortic aperture

Costal arch

Transversus abdominis

Rectus sheath, posterior layer

Iliacus

Obturator internus

Pubic symphysis

Internal intercostal muscles

Vena caval aperture

T8 vertebral body

Esophageal aperture

T10 vertebral body

T12 vertebral body

Iliac crest

L5 vertebral body

Psoas major

Piriformis

Sacrospinous ligament (coccygeus muscle)

Gluteus maximus

a

Esophageal aperture

Median arcuate ligament

Lateral arcuate ligament (quadratus arcade)

Medial arcuate ligament (psoas arcade)

Quadratus lumborum

Psoas minor

Vena caval aperture

Central tendon

Costal part of diaphragm

Lumbar part of diaphragm, left crus

Aortic aperture

Transversus abdominis

Psoas major

Iliacus

Iliopsoas

a

T8 vertebral body

Inferior vena cava

Esophagus

T10 vertebral body

T12 vertebral body

Aorta

b

Inferior vena cava

Median arcuate ligament

Right crus

Central tendon

Esophagus

Crural sling

Aorta

Left crus

b

C Position and shape of the diaphragm, viewed from the left side

Midsagittal section demonstrating the right half of the body. The diaphragm is in an intermediate position at end-expiration.

a The apertures in the diaphragm are depicted at vertical positions corresponding to the following landmarks in the lower thoracic spine: vena caval aperture = T 8 vertebral body, esophageal aperture = T 10 vertebral body, aortic aperture = T 12 vertebral body.

b The diaphragmatic apertures and the structures that they transmit.

D Position and shape of the diaphragm, anterior view

Coronal section with the diaphragm in an intermediate position.

a The apertures are located in the region of the central tendon (inferior vena cava) and in the lumbar part of the diaphragm (esophageal and aortic apertures).

b Enlarged view of the diaphragmatic apertures, with vessels transected. The vena caval aperture is located to the right of the midline, the esophageal and aortic apertures to the left.

In a *diaphragmatic hernia* (diaphragmatic rupture), abdominal viscera prolapse into the chest cavity through a congenital or acquired area of weakness in the diaphragm. By far the most common herniation site is the esophageal aperture, accounting for 90 % of cases. Typically the distal end of the esophagus and the gastric cardia (gastric inlet) "slide" upward through the esophageal aperture into the chest (axial hiatal hernia or sliding hernia; approximately 85 % of all hiatal hernias). Typical symptoms are acid reflux, heartburn, and a feeling of retrosternal pressure after meals. More severe cases may present with nausea, vomiting, and functional cardiac complaints.

3.6 The Lateral and Anterior Abdominal Wall Muscles*

* The posterior or deep abdominal wall muscles, most notably the psoas major, are actually hip muscles in a functional sense because they act predominantly on the hip joint. For this reason they are described in the chapters on the Lower Limb (see p. 420).

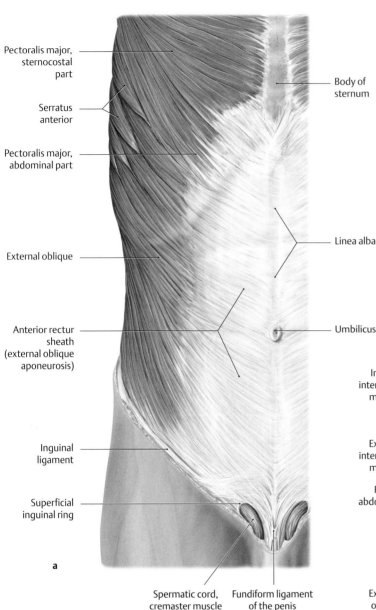

Pectoralis major, sternocostal part

Serratus anterior

Pectoralis major, abdominal part

External oblique

Anterior rectur sheath (external oblique aponeurosis)

Inguinal ligament

Superficial inguinal ring

Body of sternum

Linea alba

Umbilicus

Spermatic cord, cremaster muscle

Fundiform ligament of the penis

a

A Lateral (oblique) abdominal wall muscles in the male

Right side, anterior view. The oblique muscles of the abdominal wall consist of the external and internal oblique and the transversus abdominis.

a The external oblique aponeurosis borders the superficial inguinal ring, its inferior margin forming the inguinal ligament.

b The external oblique, pectoralis major, and serratus anterior muscles have been removed. The inferior border of the internal oblique forms the roof of the inguinal canal (see p. 182) and is continued onto the spermatic cord in the male as the cremaster muscle and fascia.

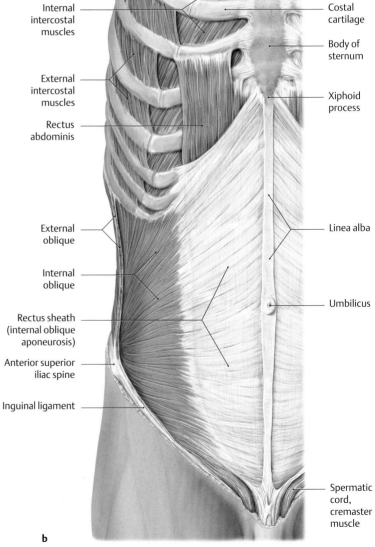

Internal intercostal muscles

External intercostal muscles

Rectus abdominis

External oblique

Internal oblique

Rectus sheath (internal oblique aponeurosis)

Anterior superior iliac spine

Inguinal ligament

Costal cartilage

Body of sternum

Xiphoid process

Linea alba

Umbilicus

Spermatic cord, cremaster muscle

b

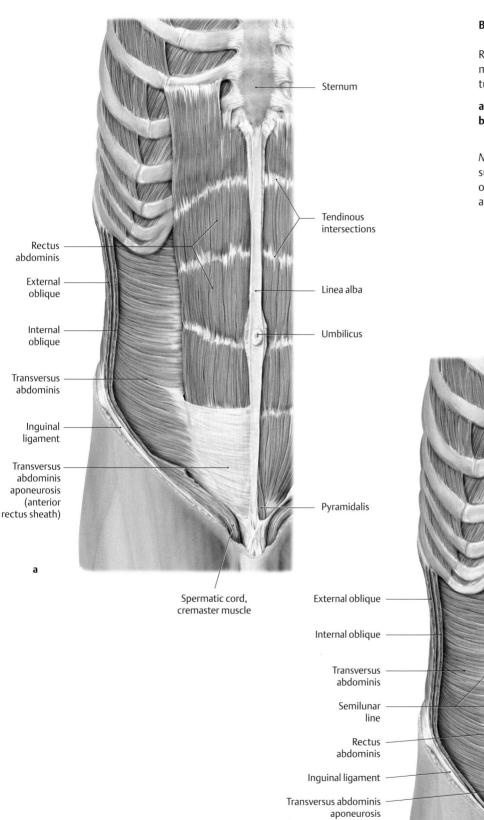

Sternum

Tendinous
intersections

Rectus
abdominis

External
oblique

Linea alba

Internal
oblique

Umbilicus

Transversus
abdominis

Inguinal
ligament

Transversus
abdominis
aponeurosis
(anterior
rectus sheath)

Pyramidalis

a

Spermatic cord,
cremaster muscle

B Anterior (straight) abdominal wall muscles in the male

Right side, anterior view. The straight or strap muscles of the abdominal wall include the rectus abdominis and pyramidalis.

a The internal oblique has been removed.
b The upper portion of the rectus abdominis has been removed.

Note: Below the arcuate line, the transversus abdominis aponeurosis and the internal oblique aponeurosis lie anterior to the rectus abdominis (see also p. 151).

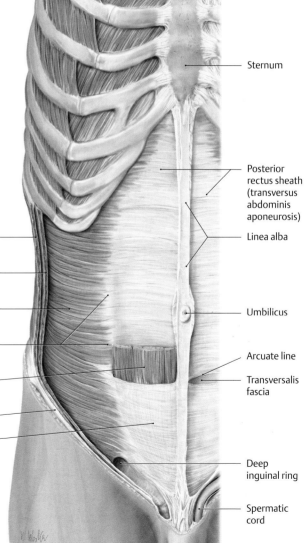

Sternum

Posterior
rectus sheath
(transversus
abdominis
aponeurosis)

Linea alba

External oblique

Internal oblique

Umbilicus

Transversus
abdominis

Arcuate line

Semilunar
line

Transversalis
fascia

Rectus
abdominis

Inguinal ligament

Deep
inguinal ring

Transversus abdominis
aponeurosis
(passes anterior to the
rectus abdominis
below the arcuate line)

Spermatic
cord

b

3.7 Structure of the Abdominal Wall and Rectus Sheath

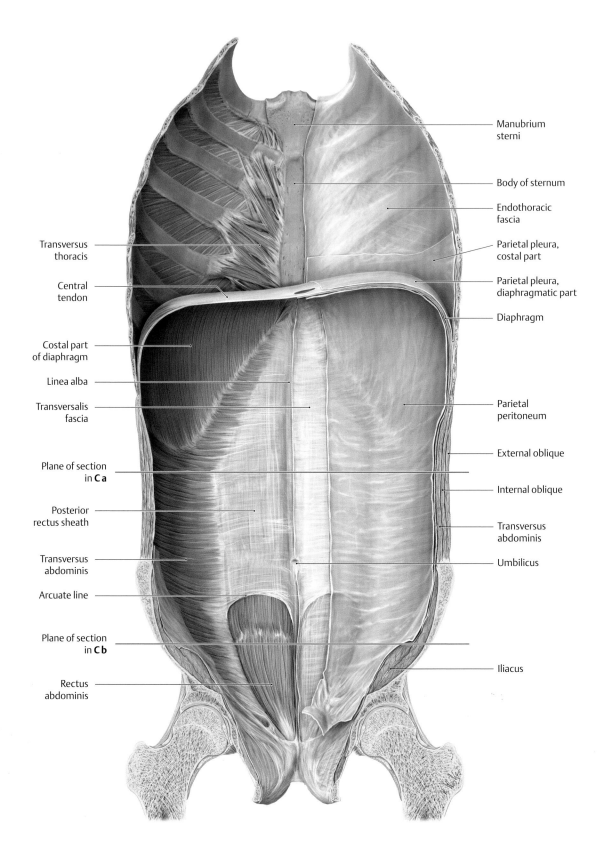

Manubrium sterni

Body of sternum

Endothoracic fascia

Parietal pleura, costal part

Parietal pleura, diaphragmatic part

Diaphragm

Parietal peritoneum

External oblique

Internal oblique

Transversus abdominis

Umbilicus

Iliacus

Transversus thoracis

Central tendon

Costal part of diaphragm

Linea alba

Transversalis fascia

Plane of section in **C a**

Posterior rectus sheath

Transversus abdominis

Arcuate line

Plane of section in **C b**

Rectus abdominis

A Overview of the abdominal wall and rectus sheath
Posterior view with the viscera removed. To show how the diaphragm separates the thoracic cavity from the abdominal cavity, the transversalis fascia and parietal peritoneum have been removed from the left *abdominal wall* while the endothoracic fascia and parietal pleura have been removed from the left *chest wall*. The *rectus sheath* (enclosing the rectus abdominis muscle) plays a special role in the abdominal wall, because its structure changes below the arcuate line to accommodate the increasing pressure of the viscera against the body wall (see **C**). The rectus sheath is formed by the aponeuroses of the lateral abdominal muscles (of which only the transversus is visible here; the others are hidden) and is divided into an anterior and a posterior layer.

B Structure of the abdominal wall

Cross section through the abdominal wall above the umbilicus, superior view. The following layers are distinguished in the lateral abdominal wall, from inside to outside:

- Parietal peritoneum
- Transversalis fascia
- Transversus abdominis muscle
- Internal oblique muscle
- External oblique muscle
- Superficial abdominal fascia
- Subcutaneous tissue
- Skin

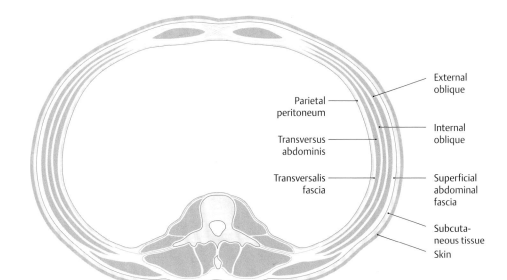

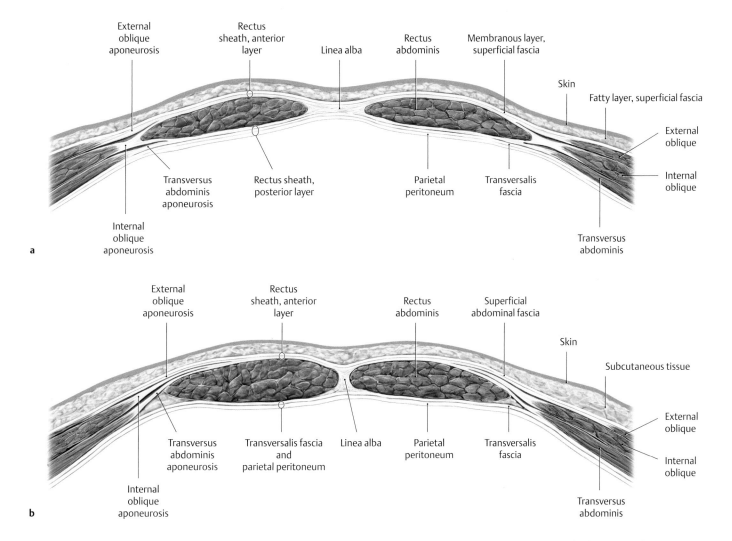

C Structure of the rectus sheath

Cross sections through the rectus sheath superior (**a**) and inferior (**b**) to the arcuate line, superior view. The aponeuroses of the lateral abdominal wall muscles ensheath the anterior strap muscles to form the rectus sheath. This creates a muscular compartment consisting of an anterior layer and a posterior layer. While the aponeuroses of the three lateral abdominal muscles contribute equally to the anterior and posterior layers of the sheath above the umbilicus, the two layers blend together approximately 3–5 cm below the umbilicus (at the level of the arcuate line) to form a single (and consequently more stable) sheet that passes in front of the rectus abdominis muscle. *Below the arcuate line*, the posterior layer of the rectus sheath is absent.

151

3.8 The Pelvic Floor Muscles: Overview of the Perineal Region and Superficial Fasciae

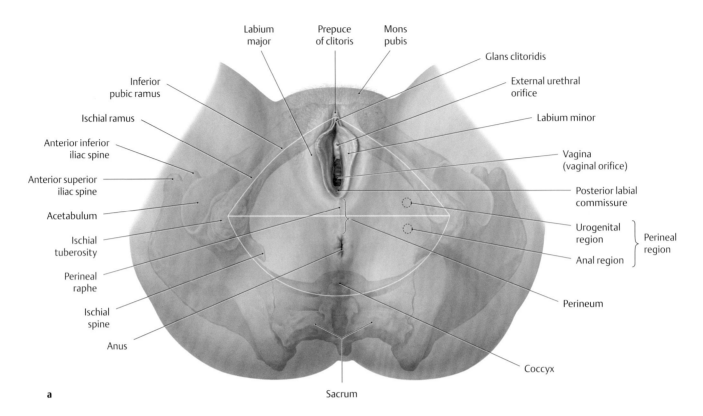

a

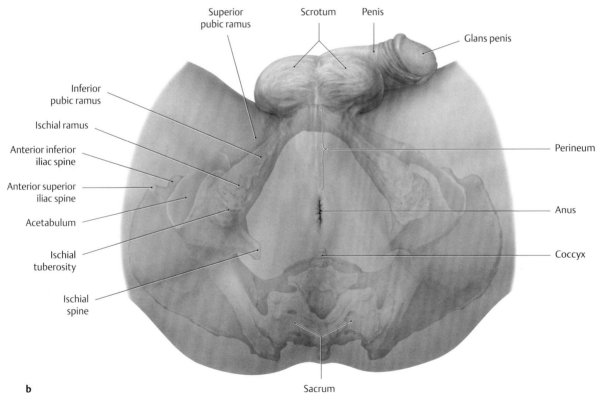

b

A Perineal region in the female (a) and male (b)
Lithotomy position, caudal (inferior) view. The perineal region in both sexes consists of the *urogenital region* anteriorly and the adjacent *anal region* posteriorly. The two regions are separated by a line that runs between the ischial tuberosities. The *perineum* denotes the soft-tissue area between the thighs and the buttocks. In the female, obstetricians refer to the perineum as the region from the anterior margin of the anus to the posterior commissure of the vagina. It is considerably longer in the male, extending from the anal margin to the root of the scrotum. The perineum is a region containing fibrous and fatty tissue, and *the perineal body* (see **Ba**), a fibromuscular mass also referred to as the *central tendon of the perineum*. A more detailed structural description of the perineum is given on p. 156.

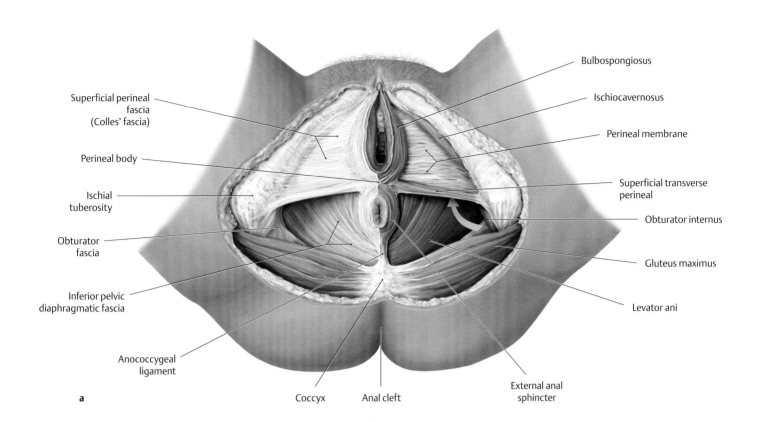

Superficial perineal fascia (Colles' fascia)

Perineal body

Ischial tuberosity

Obturator fascia

Inferior pelvic diaphragmatic fascia

Anococcygeal ligament

Coccyx

Anal cleft

Bulbospongiosus

Ischiocavernosus

Perineal membrane

Superficial transverse perineal

Obturator internus

Gluteus maximus

Levator ani

External anal sphincter

a

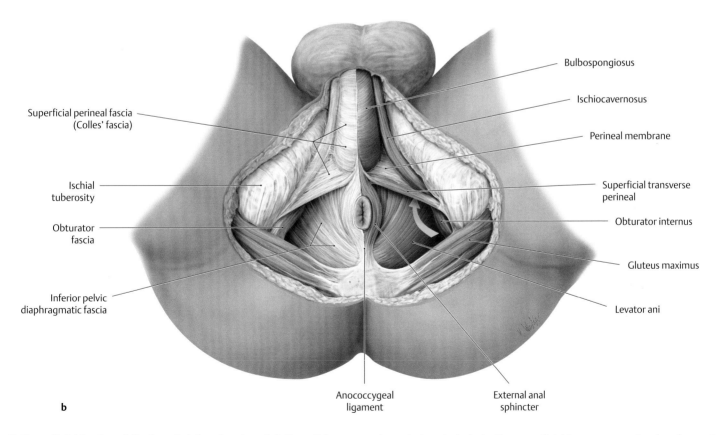

Superficial perineal fascia (Colles' fascia)

Ischial tuberosity

Obturator fascia

Inferior pelvic diaphragmatic fascia

Anococcygeal ligament

External anal sphincter

Bulbospongiosus

Ischiocavernosus

Perineal membrane

Superficial transverse perineal

Obturator internus

Gluteus maximus

Levator ani

b

B Superficial fasciae of the female (a) and male pelvic floor (b)
Lithotomy position, caudal view. The superficial perineal fascia (urogenital region) and the inferior pelvic diaphragmatic fascia (anal region) are intact on the right side but have been removed on the left side. In this way the superficial perineal space has been opened in the urogenital region on the left side of each dissection, and the levator ani muscle has been exposed in the anal region. The superficial perineal space is bounded posteriorly by the superficial transverse perineal and superiorly by the perineal membrane. The bulbospongiosus muscle is located in the medial part of this superficial perineal space, the ischiocavernosus is located laterally, and the superficial transverse perineal is located posteriorly. The green arrow in each figure points to the anterior recess of the left ischioanal fossa (see also p. 496).

153

3.9 Structure of the Pelvic Floor and Pelvic Spaces: Female versus Male

Plane of section in **A** and **B**

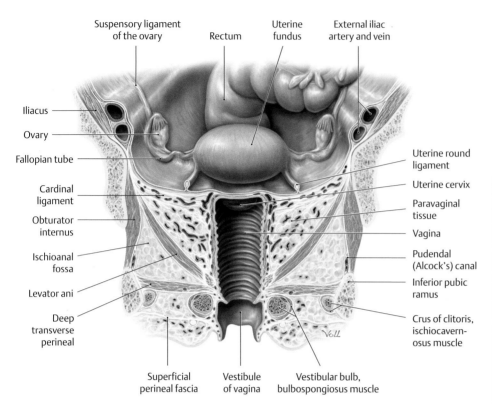

A Coronal section through the female pelvis
Anterior view.

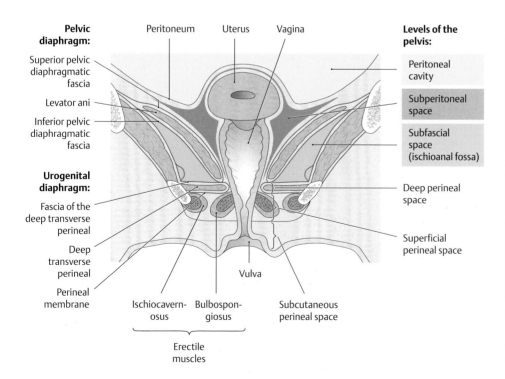

Levels of the pelvis:

Peritoneal cavity

Subperitoneal space

Subfascial space (ischioanal fossa)

Deep perineal space

Superficial perineal space

Subcutaneous perineal space

B Pelvic spaces, fasciae, and arrangement of the pelvic floor muscles in a female pelvis
Coronal section at the level of the vagina (see small diagram above for the exact location of the plane). The levels of the pelvis are shown in different colors.

C Subdivisions of the pelvis and structure of the pelvic floor (in both sexes)

Subdivisions of the pelvis

The pelvis is the portion of the abdominal cavity located in the lesser pelvis. It is surrounded by the skeleton of the lesser pelvis, which meets the greater pelvis at the *linea terminalis* (see p. 114). The pelvis is subdivided into upper, middle, and lower levels by the peritoneum and pelvic floor:

- **Upper level:** peritoneal cavity of the lesser pelvis
- **Middle level:** subperitoneal space
- **Lower level:** subfascial space (ischioanal fossa)

Subjacent to the pelvis are three more spaces that are considered to be separate from the pelvis itself: the *deep perineal space,* the *superficial perineal space,* and the *subcutaneous perineal space* (see **A**, **B**, and **F**).

Structure of the pelvic floor

The three muscular and connective-tissue sheets that contribute to the structure of the pelvic floor are also arranged in three levels:

- **Upper level:** pelvic diaphragm
- **Middle level:** deep urogenital muscles
- **Lower level:** sphincters and erectile muscles of the urogenital and intestinal tract

The funnel-shaped pelvic diaphragm is formed chiefly by the levator ani muscle and its superior and inferior fasciae (superficial and inferior pelvic diaphragmatic fasciae). The deep urogenital muscles (see p. 157) are a horizontal sheet of muscle and connective tissue that stretches between the ischial and pubic rami. It is formed mainly by the deep transverse perineal muscles and its inferior fasciae (perineal membrane). The sphincters and erectile muscles consist of the bulbospongiosus, ischiocavernosus, and the urethral and external anal sphincters with their associated muscular fasciae (see p. 136).

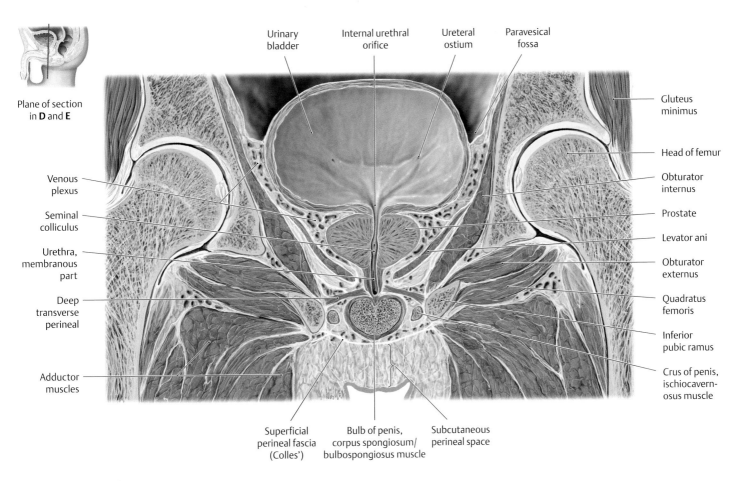

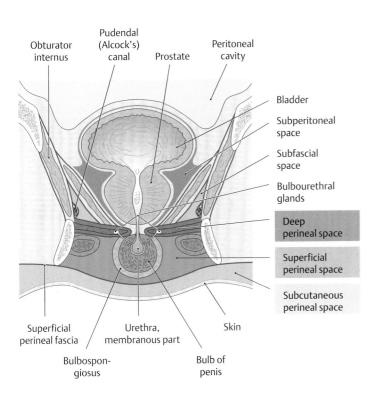

D Coronal section through the male pelvis
Anterior view.

E Pelvic spaces, fasciae, and arrangement of the pelvic floor muscles in a male pelvis
Coronal section at the level of the prostate (see small diagram above for the exact location of the plane). Different colors indicate the various levels of the pelvis and the perineal spaces.

F Boundaries and contents of the deep perineal space and superficial perineal space (Colles' space) in the male [and female]

Deep perineal space

- Boundaries:
  - Perineal membrane
  - Inferior pelvic diaphragmatic fascia
  - Superficial transverse perineal muscle
- Contents in the male [in the female]:
  - Deep transverse perineal muscle
  - Membranous part of the urethra
  - Bulbourethral glands
  - Terminal branches of the internal pudendal artery and vein
  - Terminal branches of the pudendal nerve

Superficial perineal space

- Boundaries:
  - Superficial perineal fascia (Colles')
  - Perineal membrane
  - Superficial transverse perineal muscle
- Contents in the male [in the female]:
  - Bulb of penis [vestibular bulb]
  - Crura of the corpus cavernosum [crura, shaft, and glans of the clitoris]
  - Bulbospongiosus muscles
  - Ischiocavernosus muscles
  - Terminal branches of the internal pudendal artery and vein
  - Terminal branches of the pudendal nerve

The **subcutaneous perineal space** is located between the superficial perineal fascia and skin and contains mostly fatty tissue.

3.10 The Muscles of the Female Pelvic Floor and Wall

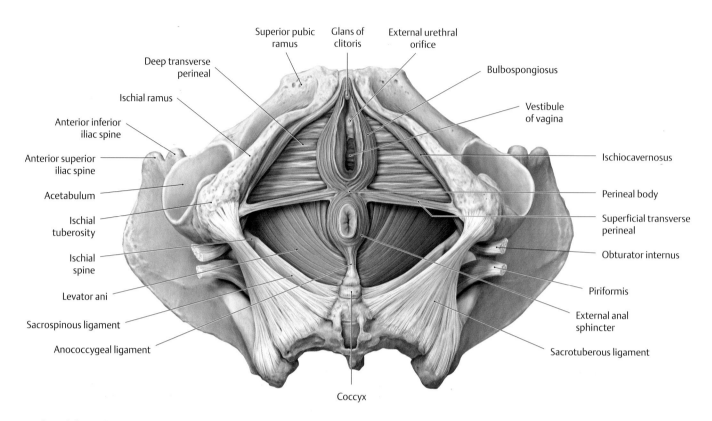

A Muscles of the pelvic floor after removal of the fasciae
Female pelvis, inferior view. The muscular layers are progressively removed from **B** through **D** to demonstrate the underlying muscles from a consistent perspective. The levator ani muscle is described more fully on subsequent pages.

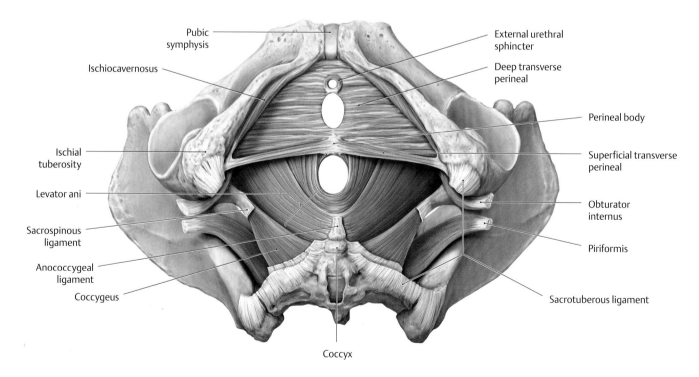

B Muscles of the pelvic floor with the sphincters removed
Female pelvis, inferior view. The sphincter muscles have been removed from the urogenital and intestinal tract (= bulbospongiosus and external anal sphincter), leaving the external urethral sphincter intact.

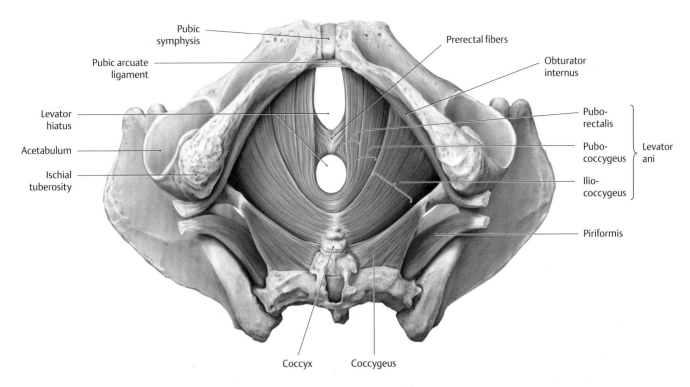

C Muscles of the pelvic floor with the urogenital muscles removed
Female pelvis, inferior view. The urogenital muscles (= superficial and deep transverse perineal and the ischiocavernosi) have been removed. *Note* the opening of the levator hiatus, which is bounded by the two crura of the puborectalis muscle (the "levator crura"). Note also the pre-rectal fibers that have split off from the puborectalis muscle. The pre-rectal fibers are interwoven with connective-tissue fibers and smooth muscle to form the fibromuscular framework of the perineum (see also p. 152).

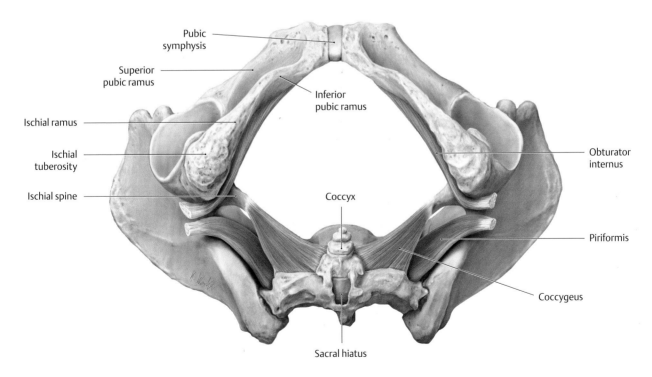

D Muscles of the pelvic wall (parietal muscles of the lesser pelvis)
Female pelvis, inferior view. All of the pelvic floor muscles have been removed, leaving the "parietal" pelvic muscles intact (obturator inter-nus, coccygeus, and piriformis). Along with the skeleton of the lesser pelvis, these muscles contribute structurally to the pelvic wall and assist in closing the posterior pelvic outlet. The obturator internus and its fas-cia provide a tendon of origin for the iliococcygeus, which is part of the levator ani complex (tendinous arch of the levator ani, see p. 159).

3.11 Pelvic Floor Muscles: The Levator ani

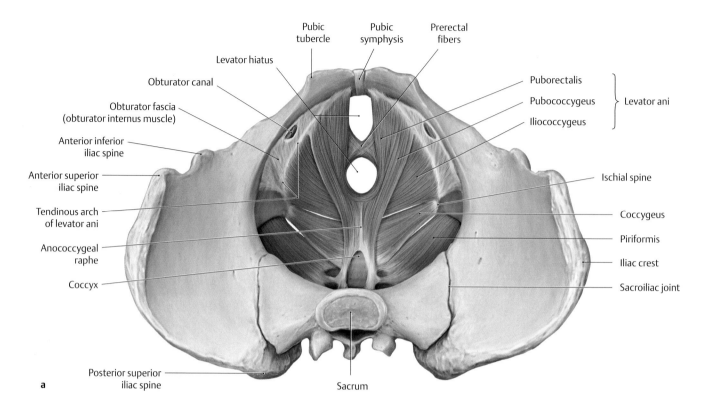

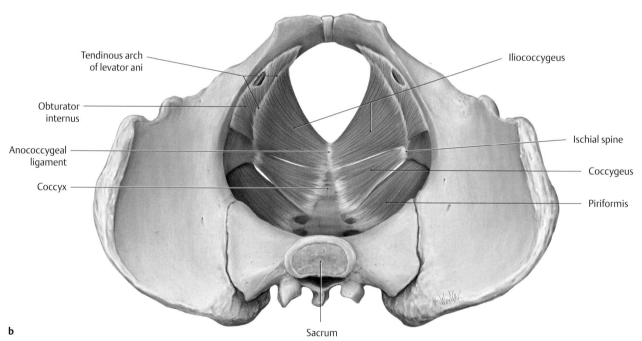

A Parts of the levator ani and the parietal muscles of the pelvic wall

Female pelvis, superior view.

a The levator ani muscle consists of three parts: the puborectalis, pubococcygeus, and iliococcygeus. It arises from the anterior and lateral pelvic wall on a line running from the center of the pubic symphysis to the ischial spine (= tendinous arch of the levator ani). As a contributor to continence, the *puborectalis* muscle assists the external anal sphincter (not visible here) in keeping the anus closed. It arises from the superior pubic ramus on both sides of the symphysis and extends posteriorly past the organs to unite at the midline behind the rectum (anococcygeal raphe). It has the shape of an arched gateway, its two crura (the levator crura) forming the boundaries of the levator hiatus. Contraction of the puborectalis draws the perineal flexure forward, as if through a sling.

b The puborectalis and pubococcygeus muscles have been removed. The coccygeus (muscle fibers on the sacrospinous ligament) and the piriformis complete the pelvic outlet posteriorly on both sides of the sacrum.

B Tendinous arch of the levator ani
Right hemipelvis, medial view. The tendinous arch of the levator ani is a thickening of the obturator internus fascia which serves as the origin of the iliococcygeus muscle.

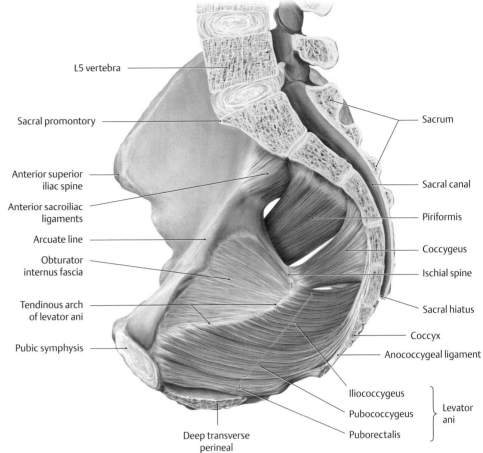

L5 vertebra

Sacral promontory

Anterior superior iliac spine

Anterior sacroiliac ligaments

Arcuate line

Obturator internus fascia

Tendinous arch of levator ani

Pubic symphysis

Sacrum

Sacral canal

Piriformis

Coccygeus

Ischial spine

Sacral hiatus

Coccyx

Anococcygeal ligament

Iliococcygeus

Pubococcygeus

Puborectalis

Levator ani

Deep transverse perineal

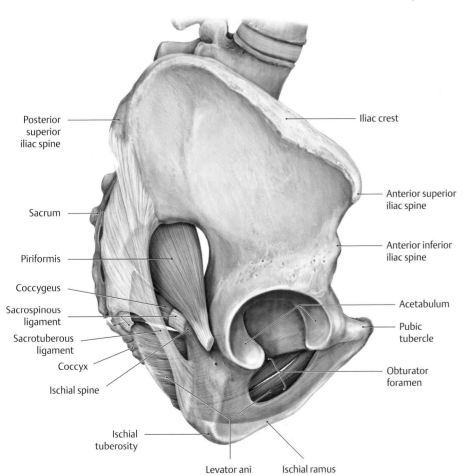

Posterior superior iliac spine

Sacrum

Piriformis

Coccygeus

Sacrospinous ligament

Sacrotuberous ligament

Coccyx

Ischial spine

Ischial tuberosity

Levator ani

Ischial ramus

Iliac crest

Anterior superior iliac spine

Anterior inferior iliac spine

Acetabulum

Pubic tubercle

Obturator foramen

C Funnel shape of the levator ani
Pelvis viewed from the right side. A portion of the ischium is shown transparent. Because the muscle is arranged in a cone or funnel-shape, contraction of the levator ani causes the anus to *descend* when there is a concomitant rise of the intra-abdominal pressure. Accordingly, *elevation* of the anus results from relaxation rather than contraction of the levator ani.

3.12 Pelvic Floor Muscles: Their Relation to Organs and Vessels in Males and Females

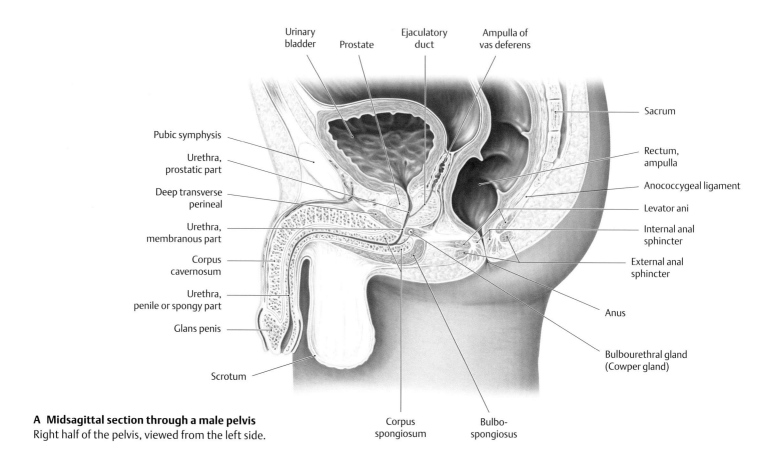

A Midsagittal section through a male pelvis
Right half of the pelvis, viewed from the left side.

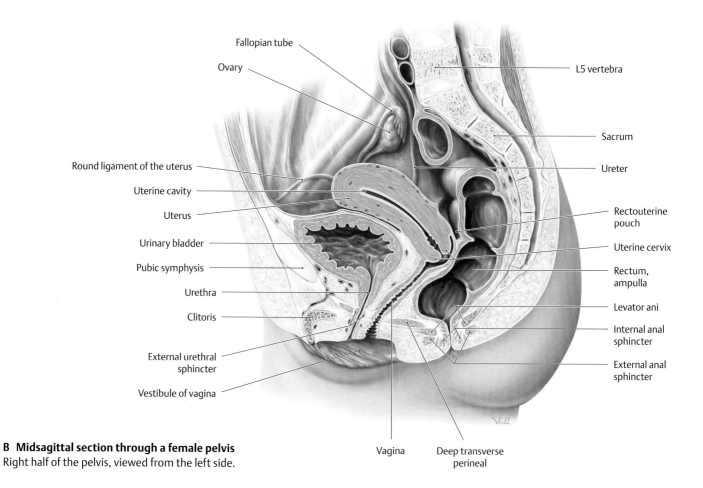

B Midsagittal section through a female pelvis
Right half of the pelvis, viewed from the left side.

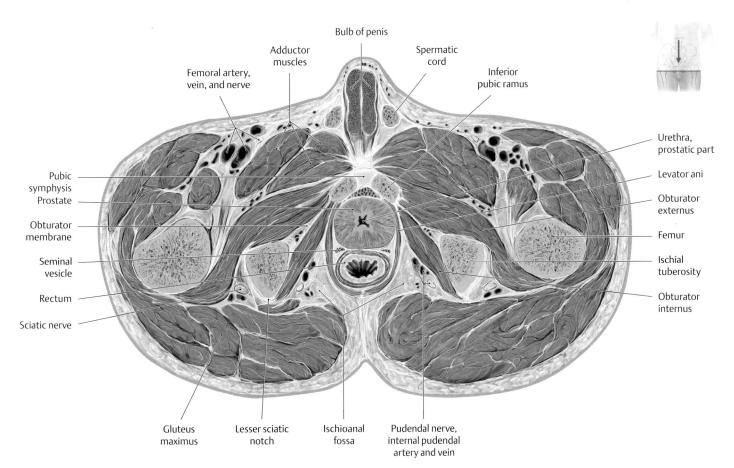

C Cross section through a male pelvis
Superior view.

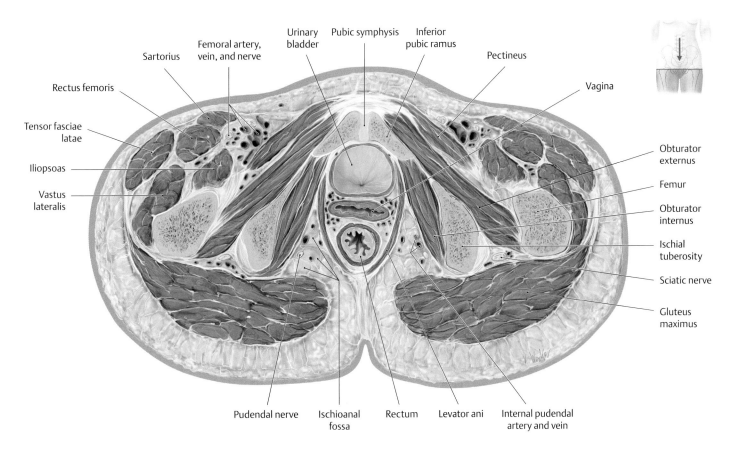

D Cross section through a female pelvis
Superior view.

161

4.1 The Arteries

A Overview of the arteries of the trunk wall

The arrangement of the neurovascular structures in the trunk reflects the segmental anatomy of the trunk wall, particularly in the thoracic region. Accordingly, each of the intercostal spaces is traversed by an intercostal artery, vein, and nerve.

The chest wall is supplied principally by the posterior intercostal arteries, which arise from the aorta, and by anterior intercostal branches arising from the internal thoracic artery:

- The first and second posterior intercostal arteries, which are given off by the superior intercostal artery (= branch of the costocervical trunk, see **D a**)
- The third through eleventh posterior intercostal arteries (each giving off a dorsal, a collateral, and a lateral cutaneous branch, see **D b**)
- The musculophrenic artery (one of the two terminal branches of the internal thoracic artery), which runs behind the costal arch, see **B**
- The subcostal artery (twelfth intercostal artery), see **B**
- The anterior intercostal arteries, which arise from the internal thoracic artery, see **B**

Many other "regional" arteries supply the anterior, lateral, and posterior trunk wall.

Anterior trunk wall

- The perforating branches (from the internal thoracic artery, e.g., the medial mammary branches that supply the breast), see **D b**
- The superior epigastric artery (continuation of the internal thoracic artery, see **B** and **C**)
- The inferior epigastric artery (from the external iliac artery, see **B** and **C**)
- The superficial epigastric artery, see **B**
- The superficial circumflex iliac artery, see **B**
- The deep circumflex iliac artery, see **B**

Posterior trunk wall

- Dorsal branches (from the posterior intercostal artery), each with a medial, a lateral cutaneous and a spinal branch, see **D c**
- The first through fourth lumbar arteries (each with a dorsal and spinal branch), see **B**
- The median sacral artery, see **B**

Lateral trunk wall

- The superior thoracic artery, see **B**
- The thoracoacromial artery, see **B**
- The lateral thoracic artery, see **B**
- The lateral cutaneous branches (from the intercostal artery), which distribute branches mainly to the breast (lateral mammary branches, see **D b**)
- The iliolumbar artery (from the internal iliac artery), which gives off an iliac, a lumbar, and a spinal branch, see **B**

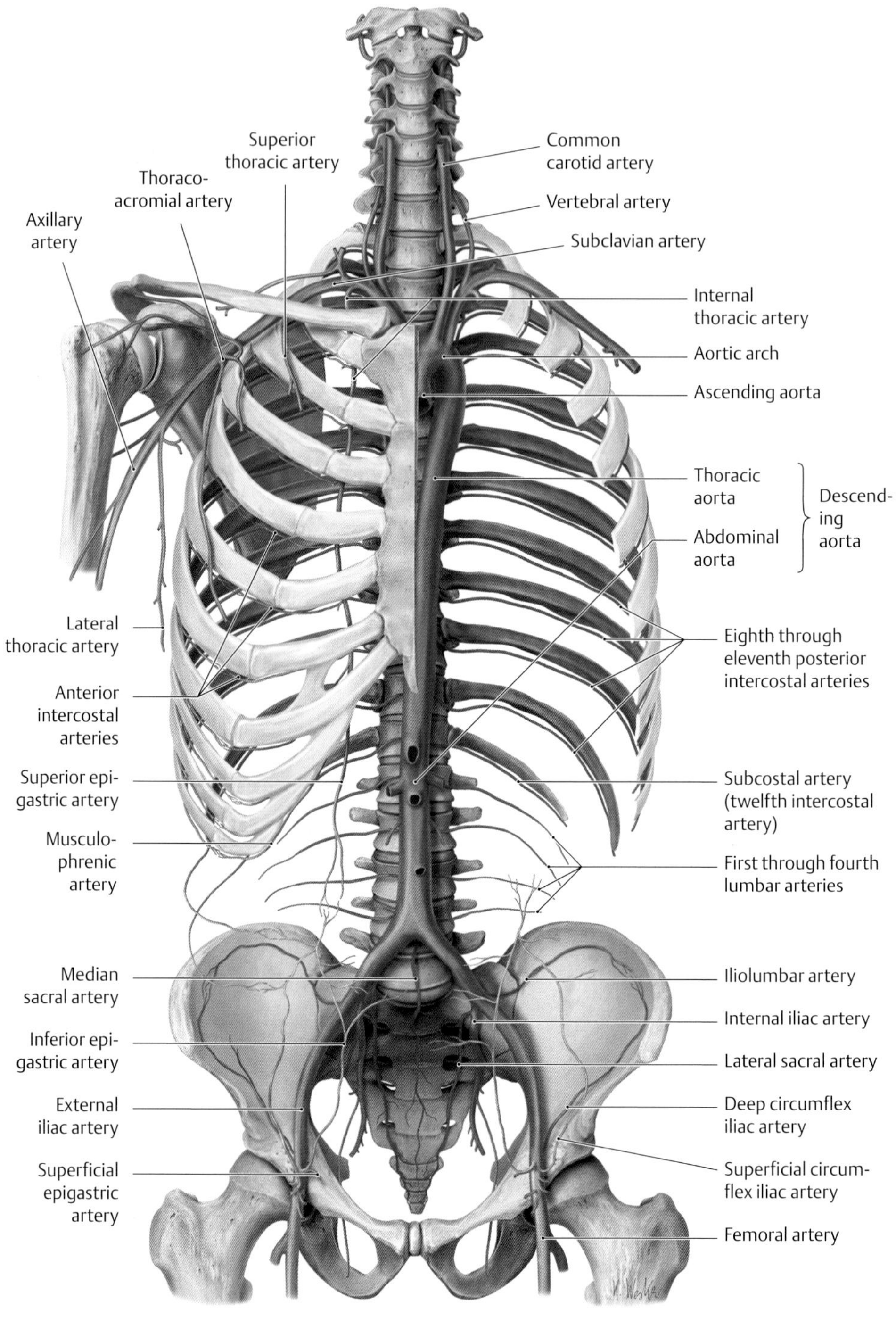
Superior thoracic artery
Thoraco-acromial artery
Axillary artery
Common carotid artery
Vertebral artery
Subclavian artery
Internal thoracic artery
Aortic arch
Ascending aorta
Thoracic aorta
Abdominal aorta
Descending aorta
Lateral thoracic artery
Anterior intercostal arteries
Eighth through eleventh posterior intercostal arteries
Superior epigastric artery
Subcostal artery (twelfth intercostal artery)
Musculophrenic artery
First through fourth lumbar arteries
Median sacral artery
Iliolumbar artery
Internal iliac artery
Inferior epigastric artery
Lateral sacral artery
External iliac artery
Deep circumflex iliac artery
Superficial epigastric artery
Superficial circumflex iliac artery
Femoral artery

B Arteries of the trunk wall
Anterior view. The anterior portions of the ribs have been removed on the left side.

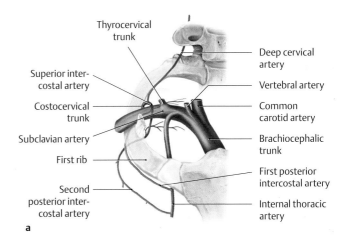

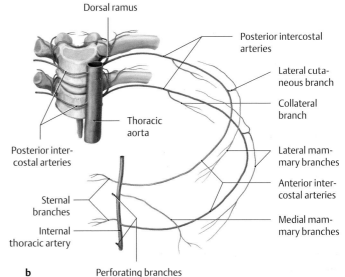

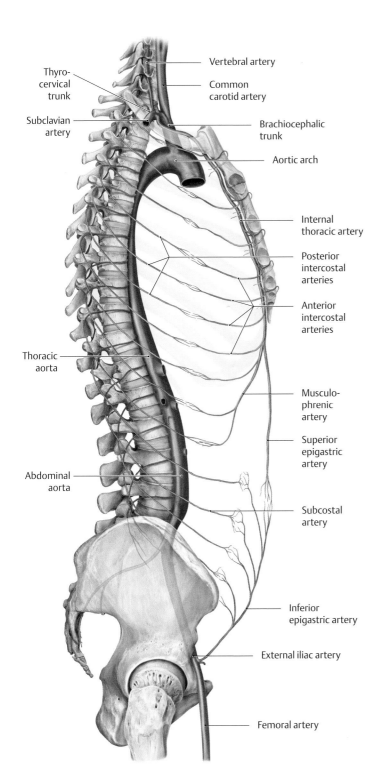

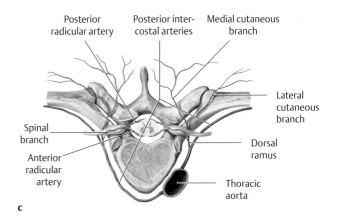

C Arteries of the trunk wall
Right lateral view.

D Course and branches of the intercostal arteries

a Anterior view of the superior intercostal artery, which gives off the first two intercostal arteries.
Note: The first and second posterior intercostal arteries are not branches of the thoracic aorta but arise from the superior intercostal artery (branch of the costocervical trunk), which are branches of the subclavian artery.

b Anterior view of the posterior intercostal arteries that are segmental branches of the thoracic aorta.
Note: The *anterior* intercostal arteries arise from the subclavian artery (via the internal thoracic artery), while the *posterior* intercostal arteries arise directly from the thoracic aorta.

c Branches of the posterior intercostal arteries, viewed from the superior view.

4.2 The Veins

A Overview of the veins of the trunk wall

The veins of the trunk wall drain into both the vena caval and azygos systems (see **B**). Within the vena caval system, we can distinguish between the tributary regions of the inferior vena cava and the superior vena cava. Connections between the superficial and inferior vena cavae are called *cavocaval anastomoses* (collateral channels).

Tributaries of the superior vena cava
- Superior intercostal vein (brachiocephalic vein) (see **B**)
- Anterior intercostal veins (internal thoracic vein, subclavian vein) (see **D**)
- Superior epigastric vein (internal thoracic vein, subclavian vein)
- Lateral thoracic vein (axillary vein) (see **C**)
- Thoracoepigastric vein (axillary vein) (see **C**)

Tributaries of the inferior vena cava (see **B**)
- Posterior intercostal veins ⎫
- Subcostal vein　　　　　　　⎬ Ascending lumbar vein
- First through fourth lumbar veins ⎭

- Iliolumbar vein ⎫
- Median sacral vein ⎬ Common iliac vein
- Lateral sacral vein ⎭

- Deep circumflex iliac vein ⎫
- Inferior epigastric vein 　⎬ External iliac vein
 ⎭

- Obturator vein (see p. 184) ⎫
- Internal pudendal vein (see p. 200) ⎬ Internal iliac vein

- External pudendal veins ⎫
- Superficial circumflex iliac vein ⎬ Femoral vein
- Superficial epigastric vein ⎭

Tributaries of the azygos vein (see **B**)
- Superior intercostal veins
- Posterior intercostal veins
- Hemiazygos vein
- Accessory hemiazygos vein
- Veins of the vertebral column, see **Ea**

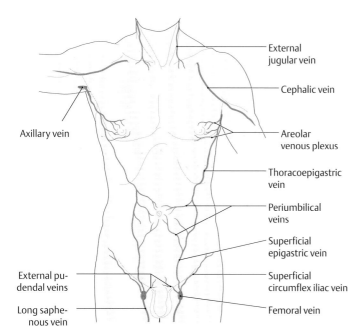

External jugular vein
Cephalic vein
Axillary vein
Areolar venous plexus
Thoracoepigastric vein
Periumbilical veins
Superficial epigastric vein
External pudendal veins
Superficial circumflex iliac vein
Long saphenous vein
Femoral vein

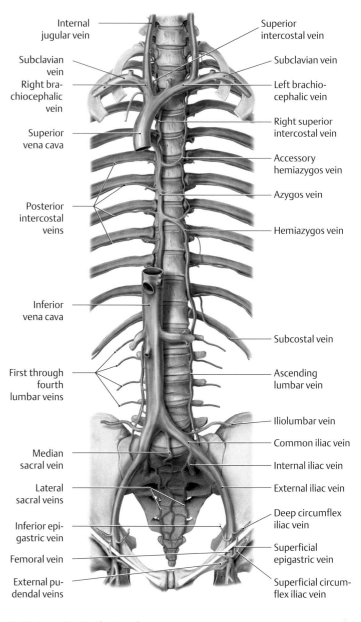

Internal jugular vein
Subclavian vein
Right brachiocephalic vein
Superior vena cava
Posterior intercostal veins
Inferior vena cava
First through fourth lumbar veins
Median sacral vein
Lateral sacral veins
Inferior epigastric vein
Femoral vein
External pudendal veins

Superior intercostal vein
Subclavian vein
Left brachiocephalic vein
Right superior intercostal vein
Accessory hemiazygos vein
Azygos vein
Hemiazygos vein
Subcostal vein
Ascending lumbar vein
Iliolumbar vein
Common iliac vein
Internal iliac vein
External iliac vein
Deep circumflex iliac vein
Superficial epigastric vein
Superficial circumflex iliac vein

B Major veins in the trunk
Anterior view.

C Superficial veins of the anterior trunk wall

Anterior view. Normally these veins are not palpable, but they are of key importance in the development of portocaval anastomoses, in which the former umbilical vein connects the portal vein of the liver to the superior and inferior vena cavae. In cases where portal hypertension develops as a result of liver disease (hepatic cirrhosis due to alcohol abuse), the portal venous blood must partially bypass the liver, flowing through the paraumbilical veins (see p. 184) to the superficial truncal veins in the umbilical region (periumbilical veins) and finally to the heart. Since the superficial veins must carry considerably more blood in this situation, they undergo varicose dilatation, becoming visible and palpable on the abdomen. This is also called a "Medusa's head" (*caput medusae*) because the serpentine, dilated veins around the umbilicus resemble the snake-haired head of the Gorgon.

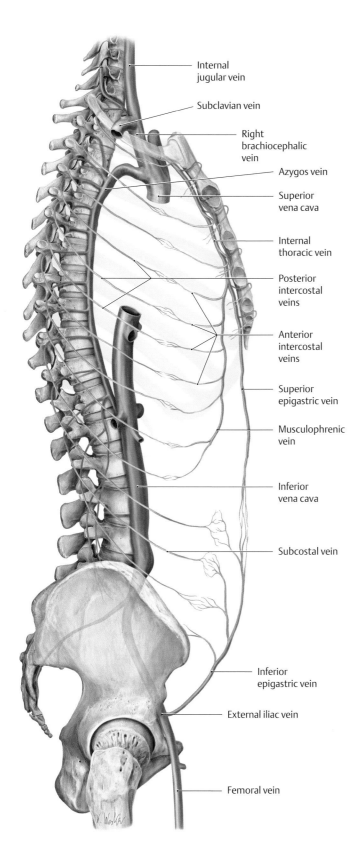

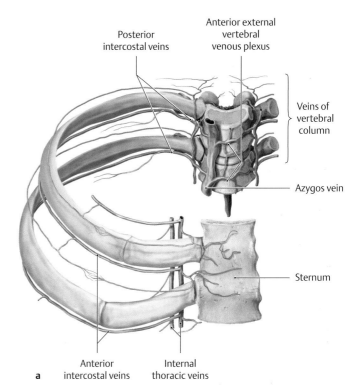

Internal jugular vein

Subclavian vein

Right brachiocephalic vein

Azygos vein

Superior vena cava

Internal thoracic vein

Posterior intercostal veins

Anterior intercostal veins

Superior epigastric vein

Musculophrenic vein

Inferior vena cava

Subcostal vein

Inferior epigastric vein

External iliac vein

Femoral vein

Posterior intercostal veins

Anterior external vertebral venous plexus

Veins of vertebral column

Azygos vein

Sternum

Anterior intercostal veins

Internal thoracic veins

a

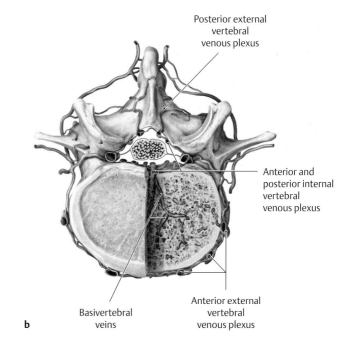

Posterior external vertebral venous plexus

Anterior and posterior internal vertebral venous plexus

Basivertebral veins

Anterior external vertebral venous plexus

b

E Intercostal veins and venous plexuses of the vertebral canal
a Vertebral column and rib segment, anterosuperior view.
b Lumbar vertebra, superior view.

D Veins of the trunk wall
Right lateral view.

4.3 The Lymphatic Vessels and Lymph Nodes

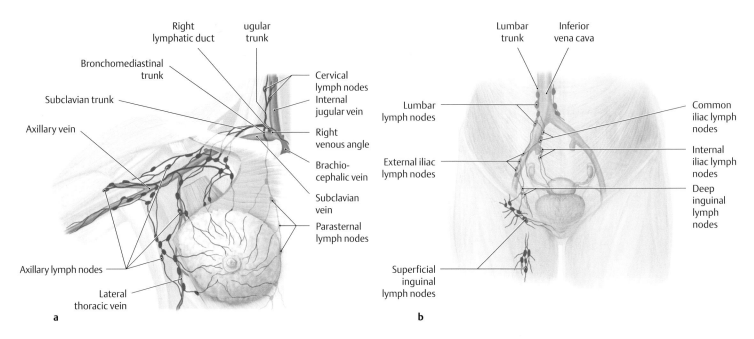

A Regional lymph nodes and their associated lymphatics
Anterior view.

a Axillary, parasternal, and cervical lymph nodes (right thoracic and axillary region with the arm abducted). The lymph node levels are described on p. 181.
b Lymph nodes of the inguinal region and lesser pelvis.

B Left and right venous angles
Anterior view. The approximately 1-cm-long *right lymphatic duct* collects lymph from the right upper quadrant of the body (see **Ca**) and empties into the **right venous angle** at the junction of the right internal jugular vein with the right subclavian vein. Its major tributaries are:

- the right jugular trunk (right half of the body and neck),
- the right subclavian trunk (right upper limb, right side of the chest and back wall), and
- the right bronchomediastinal trunk (organs of the right thoracic cavity).

The *thoracic duct* is approximately 40 cm long and transports lymph from the entire lower half of the body and left upper quadrant. It empties into the **left venous angle** between the left internal jugular vein and left subclavian vein. Its main tributaries are:

- the left jugular trunk (left half of the body and neck),
- the left subclavian trunk (left upper limb, left side of the chest and back wall),
- the left bronchomediastinal trunk (organs of the left thoracic cavity),
- the intestinal trunks (abdominal organs), and
- the right and left lumbar trunks (right and left lower limb; pelvic viscera; left pelvic, abdominal and back wall).

The intercostal lymphatic vessels transport lymph from the left and right intercostal spaces to the lymphatic duct.

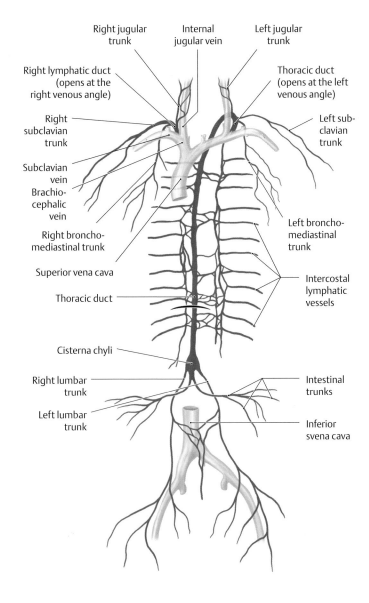

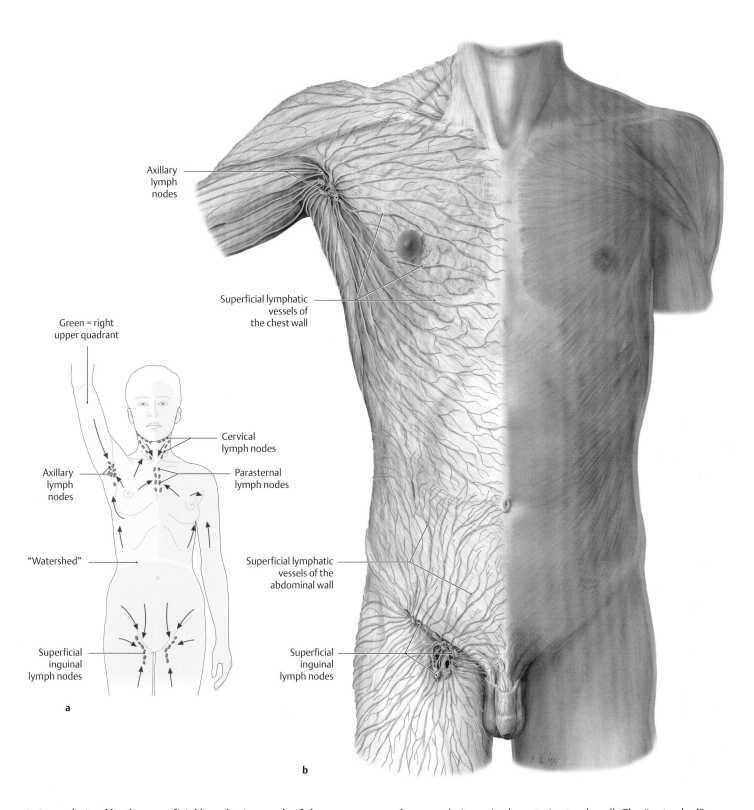

Axillary lymph nodes

Superficial lymphatic vessels of the chest wall

Green = right upper quadrant

Cervical lymph nodes

Axillary lymph nodes

Parasternal lymph nodes

"Watershed"

Superficial lymphatic vessels of the abdominal wall

Superficial inguinal lymph nodes

Superficial inguinal lymph nodes

a

b

C Areas drained by the superficial lymphatic vessels of the anterior trunk wall

Anterior view.

a Lymphatic pathways and regional lymph nodes of the anterior trunk wall (arrows indicate the direction of lymph flow).
b Superficial network of lymphatic vessels in the right anterior trunk wall.

Lymph from the skin of the trunk wall is collected mainly by the axillary and superficial inguinal lymph nodes, following the general pattern of venous drainage in the anterior trunk wall. The "watershed" zone between the two drainage regions is defined by a curved line above the umbilicus and below the costal arch. Lymph from the regional axillary and inguinal lymph nodes is finally collected by two lymphatic trunks, each of which drains into the jugulosubclavian venous junction on the corresponding side of the body (right or left venous angle, see **B**). Lymphatic fluid from the right upper quadrant (green) is returned to the venous system by the *right lymphatic duct*, while lymph from the other three body quadrants (violet) is returned to the veins by the *thoracic duct*.

167

4.4 The Nerves

A Anterior and posterior branches of the spinal nerves

The trunk wall receives most of its sensory nerve supply from the anterior and posterior branches of the T 1–T 12 spinal cord segments (intercostal nerves and dorsal rami of the spinal nerves) (see also p. 172).

Spinal cord segment	Anterior branches (ventral rami*)	Posterior branches (dorsal rami**)
C1		Suboccipital nerve
C2	Cervical plexus	Greater occipital nerve
C3		Third occipital nerve
C4		(see p. 172)
C5		
C6	Brachial plexus	
C7		
C8		
T1		
T2		
T3		
T4		
T5		
T6	Intercostal nerves	
T7		
T8		
T9		
T10		Dorsal rami ***
T11		
T12		
L1		
L2	Lumbar plexus	
L3		
L4		
L5		
S1		
S2	Sacral plexus	
S3		
S4		
S5		
Co1	Coccygeal plexus	
Co2	(see p. 482)	

*   Called also anterior rami
** Called also posterior rami
*** The dorsal rami of the L 1–L 3 spinal nerves are also known as the superior cluneal nerves, those from S 1–S 3 as the middle cluneal nerves (see **C**).
Note: The *inferior* cluneal nerves are anterior branches from the sacral plexus, see also p. 476.

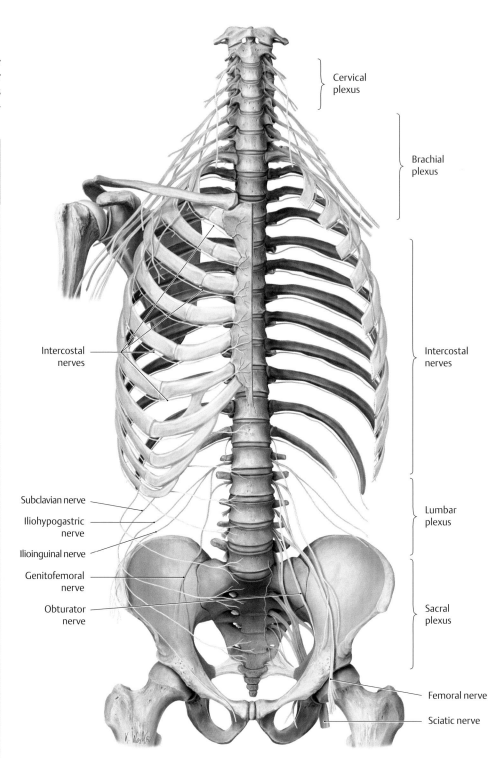

Cervical plexus

Brachial plexus

Intercostal nerves

Intercostal nerves

Subclavian nerve

Iliohypogastric nerve

Ilioinguinal nerve

Lumbar plexus

Genitofemoral nerve

Obturator nerve

Sacral plexus

Femoral nerve

Sciatic nerve

B Nerves of the trunk wall

Anterior view. The anterior part of the left half of the thoracic cage has been removed. The trunk wall receives most of its motor and sensory innervation from the twelve thoracic spinal nerves. Of all the spinal nerves, these twelve pairs most clearly reflect the original segmental (metameric) organization of the body.

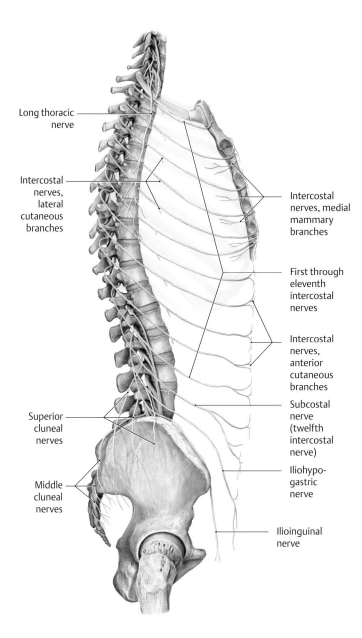

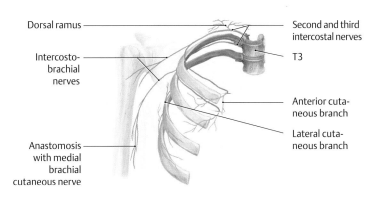

D Course of the intercostal nerves
Right side, anterior view.

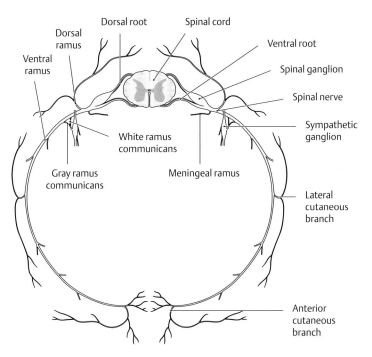

C Course of the nerves on the lateral trunk wall
Right lateral view.
Note the segmental arrangement of the intercostal nerves (compare with the segmental arrangement of the arteries and veins, pp. 162 and 164).

E Branches of a spinal nerve
Formed by the union of the dorsal (sensory) and ventral (motor) roots, the approximately 1-cm-long spinal nerve courses through the intervertebral foramen and divides into five branches after exiting the vertebral canal (see **F**).

F Spinal nerve branches and the territories they supply

Spinal nerve branch	Motor or visceromotor territory	Sensory territory
① Ventral ramus	All somatic muscles except for the intrinsic back muscles	Skin of the lateral and anterior trunk wall and of the upper and lower limbs
② Dorsal ramus	Intrinsic back muscles	Posterior skin of the head and neck, skin of the back and buttock
③ Meningeal ramus		Spinal meninges, ligaments of the spinal column, capsules of the facet joints
④ White ramus communicans	Carries preganglionic fibers from the spinal nerve to the sympathetic trunk ("white" because the preganglionic fibers are myelinated)	
⑤ Gray ramus communicans*	Carries postganglionic fibers from the sympathetic trunk back to the spinal nerve ("gray" because the fibers are unmyelinated)	

* Strictly speaking, the gray ramus communicans is not a spinal nerve branch but a branch passing from the sympathetic trunk to the spinal nerve.

169

5.1 Anterior Trunk Wall: Surface Anatomy and Superficial Nerves and Vessels

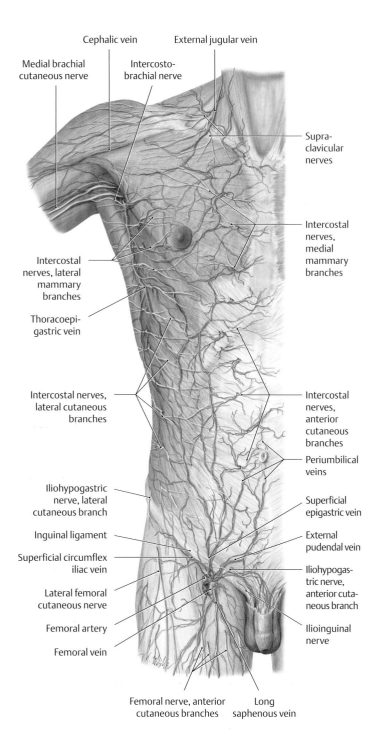

A Superficial cutaneous vessels and nerves of the anterior trunk wall
Anterior view.
Superficial vessels: Most of the *arterial supply* to the anterior trunk wall comes from two sources: the internal thoracic artery and the superficial epigastric artery. The superficial *veins* drain chiefly into the axillary vein (via the thoracoepigastric vein) and into the femoral vein (via the superficial epigastric and superficial circumflex iliac veins). The peri- and paraumbilical veins provide the main communication between the superficial veins of the trunk wall and the portal veins (portocaval anastomoses).
Superficial nerves: The *sensory supply* to the anterior trunk wall has a largely segmental arrangement (provided, for example, by lateral and anterior cutaneous branches from the intercostal nerves). The cervical plexus (supraclavicular nerves) is additionally involved in the thoracic region, as is the lumbar plexus (e.g., iliohypogastric and ilioinguinal nerves) in the lower abdominal region.

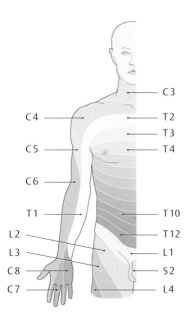

B Segmental (radicular) cutaneous innervation of the anterior trunk wall (dermatomes)
Right half of the trunk and adjacent upper limb, anterior view. Every sensory nerve root (dorsal root) innervates a specific skin area with its fibers. These "dermatomes" (see p. 66), then, correspond to associated spinal cord segments. The dermatomes are arranged in bandlike patterns that encircle the chest wall and upper abdomen. Below the umbilicus, the dermatomes become angled slightly downward toward the median plane. A "segmental gap" exists between the C 4 and T 2 dermatomes because the phylogenetic outgrowth of the human upper limb has removed the sensory fibers of C 5–C 8 and T 1 from the trunk wall (after Mumenthaler).

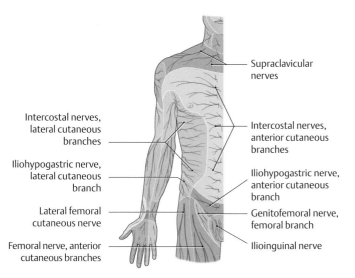

C Peripheral sensory cutaneous innervation of the anterior trunk wall
Right half of the trunk and adjacent upper limb, anterior view. The color-coded map of the peripheral cutaneous nerve territories follows the branching pattern of the cutaneous nerves in the subcutaneous connective tissue. Besides the cutaneous branches of the intercostal nerves (anterior and lateral cutaneous branches), it is chiefly the supraclavicular nerves and the iliohypogastric and ilioinguinal nerves that supply the skin of the anterior trunk wall (after Mumenthaler).

170

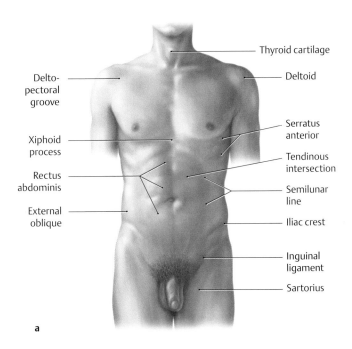

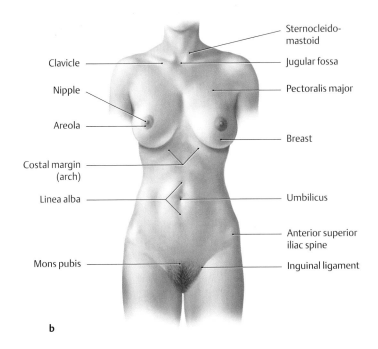

D Surface anatomy of the anterior trunk wall
a Male, **b** female.

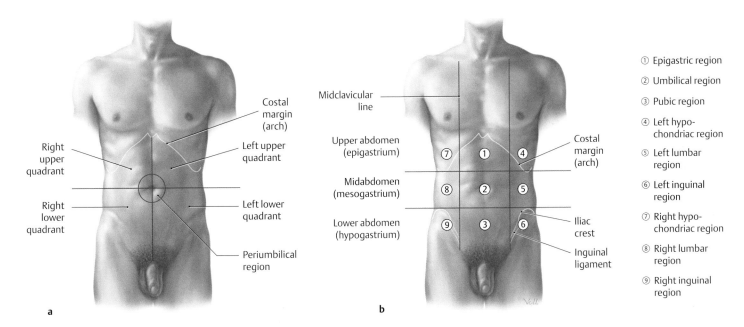

① Epigastric region

② Umbilical region

③ Pubic region

④ Left hypo-chondriac region

⑤ Left lumbar region

⑥ Left inguinal region

⑦ Right hypo-chondriac region

⑧ Right lumbar region

⑨ Right inguinal region

E Criteria for dividing the abdomen into regions
a The abdomen is divided into four quadrants by two perpendicular lines that intersect at the umbilicus.
b Coordinate system composed of two vertical and two horizontal lines. They divide the abdomen into nine regions, each located in either the upper, middle, or lower abdomen. The two vertical lines represent the left and right midclavicular lines. The two horizontal lines pass through the lowest point of the tenth ribs or the summit of the two iliac crests (see p. 31).

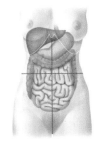
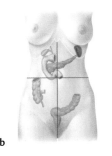
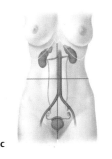

F Projection of the abdominal organs onto the four quadrants of the anterior abdominal wall
a Organs of the anterior layer, **b** organs of the middle layer,
c organs of the posterior layer.
The organs of the *anterior* layer abut the anterior abdominal wall. The organs of the *middle* layer are located in the posterior part of the abdominal cavity (some are partially retroperitoneal), and those of the *posterior* layer are located outside or behind the actual abdominal cavity (i.e., they are retroperitoneal).

5.2 Posterior Trunk Wall: Surface Anatomy and Superficial Nerves and Vessels

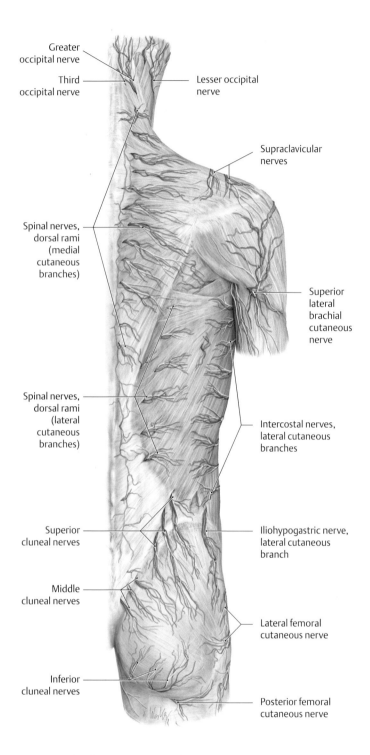

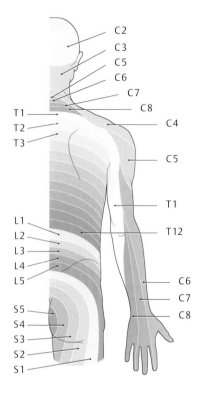

B Segmental (radicular) cutaneous innervation of the posterior trunk wall (dermatomes)
Right half of the trunk and adjacent upper limb, posterior view (after Mumenthaler).

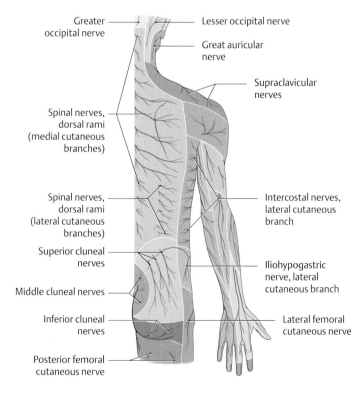

C Peripheral sensory cutaneous innervation of the posterior trunk wall
Right half of the trunk and adjacent upper limb, posterior view (after Mumenthaler).

A Superficial cutaneous vessels and nerves of the posterior trunk wall
Posterior view. Except for the lower buttocks and lateral portions of the trunk wall, the posterior trunk wall derives its sensory innervation from dorsal rami of the spinal nerves and from lateral cutaneous branches of the intercostal nerves. This is a predominantly segmental innervation pattern, analogous to that described in the anterior trunk wall. Both the medial and lateral cutaneous nerve branches pass with the cutaneous vessels through the intrinsic back muscles to the skin of the back. The skin of the buttocks is supplied by lateral branches from the three cranial lumbar and sacral nerves (superior and middle cluneal nerves).
Note: The lower part of the buttock is supplied by the inferior cluneal nerves, which are branches of the sacral plexus; thus they are derived from the *ventral* rami of the spinal nerves.

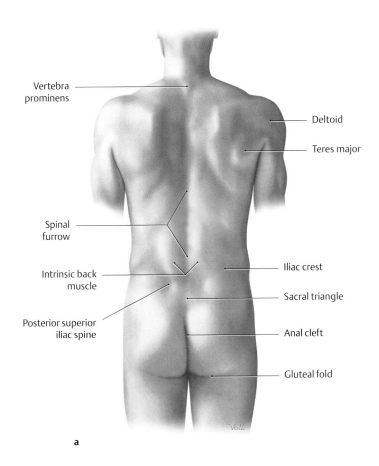

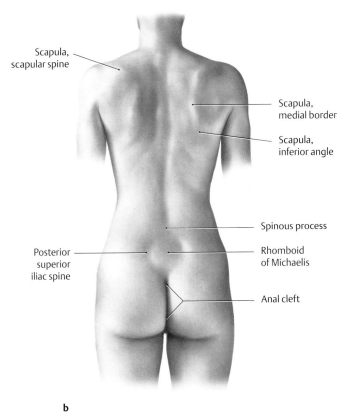

a Male, **b** female.

D Surface anatomy of the posterior trunk wall
a Male, **b** female.

In both sexes a *spinal furrow* runs vertically in the posterior midline of the trunk below the C7 spinous process. It is formed by the fixation of the subcutaneous tissue to the corresponding spinous processes. At the sacral level in males, the furrow widens to form the *sacral triangle* (bounded by the right and left posterior superior iliac spines and the upper part of the anal cleft. The corresponding diamond-shaped area in females is called the *rhomboid of Michaelis* (see **F**).

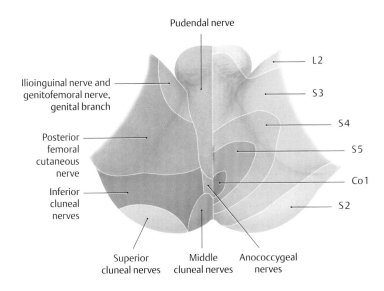

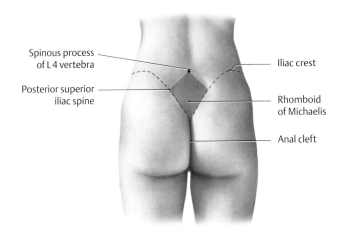

E Segmental and peripheral cutaneous innervation of the male perineal region
Lithotomy position. The segments or dermatomes have been mapped on the left side of the body, and the areas supplied by the peripheral cutaneous nerves are shown on the right side (after Mumenthaler).

F Anatomical boundaries of the Michaelis rhomboid
Female gluteal region, posterior view. In women the sacral triangle is expanded to form a diamond-shaped figure with the following boundaries: the left and right posterior superior iliac spines, the spinous process of the L4 vertebra, and the upper part of the anal cleft. With a normal female pelvis, the vertical and horizontal dimensions of the rhomboid are approximately equal. The shape of the Michaelis rhomboid (named for the German gynecologist G. A. Michaelis, 1798–1848) reflects the width of the female pelvis, providing an indirect indicator of the size of the birth canal.

173

5.3　Posterior Trunk Wall, Posterior View

A Neurovascular structures of the posterior trunk wall and nuchal region

Posterior view. The segmentally arranged neurovascular structures of the posterior trunk wall (dorsal rami of the spinal nerves and posterior branches of the posterior intercostal and lumbar vessels) are demonstrated on the left side of the trunk (all muscle fasciae have been removed except for the superficial layer of the thoracolumbar fascia). On the right side, the trapezius muscle has been detached from its origins and reflected laterally to show the course of the transverse cervical artery in the deep scapular region (compare with **B**).

Note: On the posterior trunk wall, only the lateral nuchal region (lesser occipital nerve, see **C**) and the lower gluteal region (inferior cluneal nerves) receive their sensory supply from ventral spinal nerve rami.

The latissimus dorsi muscle has been partially removed on the right side to demonstrate the upper costolumbar triangle (of Grynfeltt). The fibrous lumbar triangle (boundaries: twelfth rib, erector spinae, and internal oblique) is similar to the lower iliolumbar triangle (of Petit, bounded by the iliac crest, latissimus dorsi, and external oblique) in that it creates a site of predilection for rare, usually acquired lumbar hernias (Grynfeltt or Petit hernia, see also p. 189).

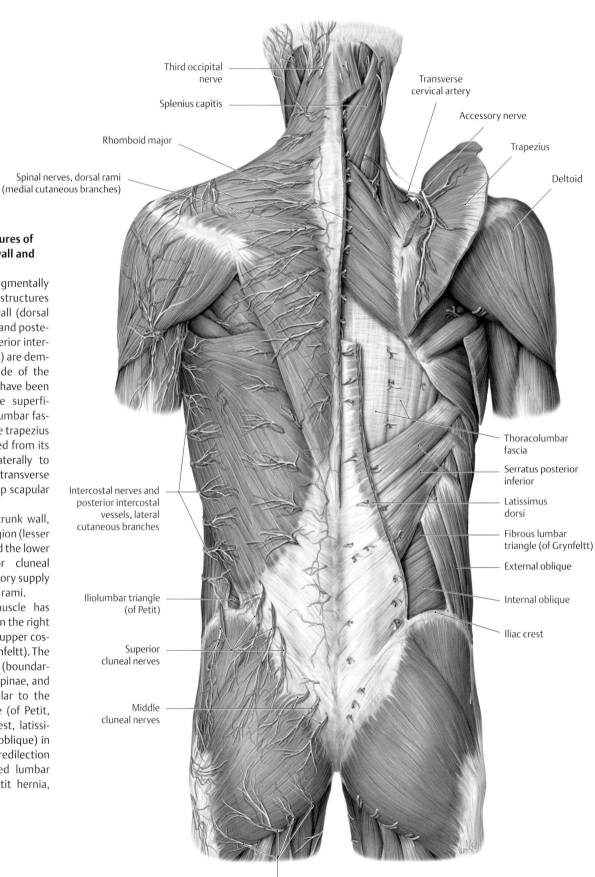

Third occipital nerve

Splenius capitis

Rhomboid major

Spinal nerves, dorsal rami (medial cutaneous branches)

Transverse cervical artery

Accessory nerve

Trapezius

Deltoid

Intercostal nerves and posterior intercostal vessels, lateral cutaneous branches

Iliolumbar triangle (of Petit)

Superior cluneal nerves

Middle cluneal nerves

Thoracolumbar fascia

Serratus posterior inferior

Latissimus dorsi

Fibrous lumbar triangle (of Grynfeltt)

External oblique

Internal oblique

Iliac crest

Inferior cluneal nerves

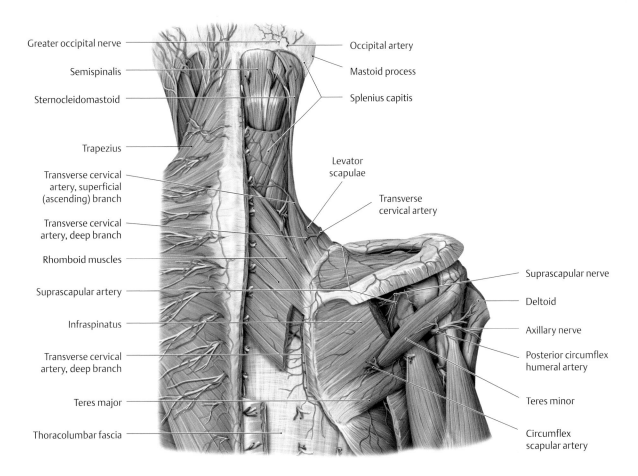

Greater occipital nerve

Semispinalis

Sternocleidomastoid

Trapezius

Transverse cervical artery, superficial (ascending) branch

Transverse cervical artery, deep branch

Rhomboid muscles

Suprascapular artery

Infraspinatus

Transverse cervical artery, deep branch

Teres major

Thoracolumbar fascia

Occipital artery

Mastoid process

Splenius capitis

Levator scapulae

Transverse cervical artery

Suprascapular nerve

Deltoid

Axillary nerve

Posterior circumflex humeral artery

Teres minor

Circumflex scapular artery

B Arteries of the deep scapular region

Right scapular region, posterior view. The trapezius, splenius capitis, deltoid, infraspinatus, and rhomboid major and minor muscles have been completely or partially removed on the right side. The deep scapular region is supplied by the transverse cervical artery, deep cervical artery (see C), suprascapular artery, circumflex scapular artery, and posterior circumflex humeral artery. All of these vessels arise directly or indirectly—via the thyrocervical trunk—from the subclavian artery (nei-

ther are visible here). The suprascapular, circumflex scapular and posterior circumflex humeral arteries form the *"scapular arcade"* (see p. 341). Medial to the mastoid process, the occipital artery appears below the tendon of insertion of the sternocleidomastoid muscle and runs upward with the sensory greater occipital nerve to the skin of the occiput. The greater occipital nerve pierces both the trapezius and semispinalis capitis muscles in the area of their firm tendinous attachments. It may become compressed at these sites, leading to *occipital neuralgia*.

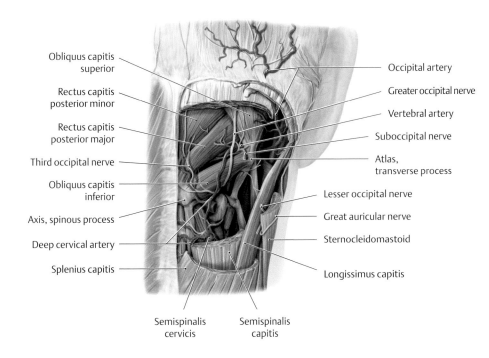

Obliquus capitis superior

Rectus capitis posterior minor

Rectus capitis posterior major

Third occipital nerve

Obliquus capitis inferior

Axis, spinous process

Deep cervical artery

Splenius capitis

Semispinalis cervicis

Semispinalis capitis

Occipital artery

Greater occipital nerve

Vertebral artery

Suboccipital nerve

Atlas, transverse process

Lesser occipital nerve

Great auricular nerve

Sternocleidomastoid

Longissimus capitis

C Suboccipital triangle (vertebral artery triangle)

Posterior view. The trapezius, sternocleidomastoid, splenius capitis, and semispinalis capitis muscles have been removed to display the suboccipital region on the right side. The suboccipital triangle is bounded by the suboccipital muscles (rectus capitis posterior major, and the obliquus capitis superior and inferior). In the deep portion of the triangle, the vertebral artery runs through its groove in the atlas. The suboccipital nerve (C 1), which is purely motor, emerges above the posterior arch of the atlas to supply the short muscles of the head. The greater occipital nerve (C 2) and, at a lower level, the third occipital nerve (C 3) wind posteriorly as they pass the lower margin of the obliquus capitis inferior. The deep cervical artery, a branch of the costocervical trunk, runs between the semispinalis capitis and cervicis muscles.

175

5.4　Posterior Trunk Wall, Anterior View

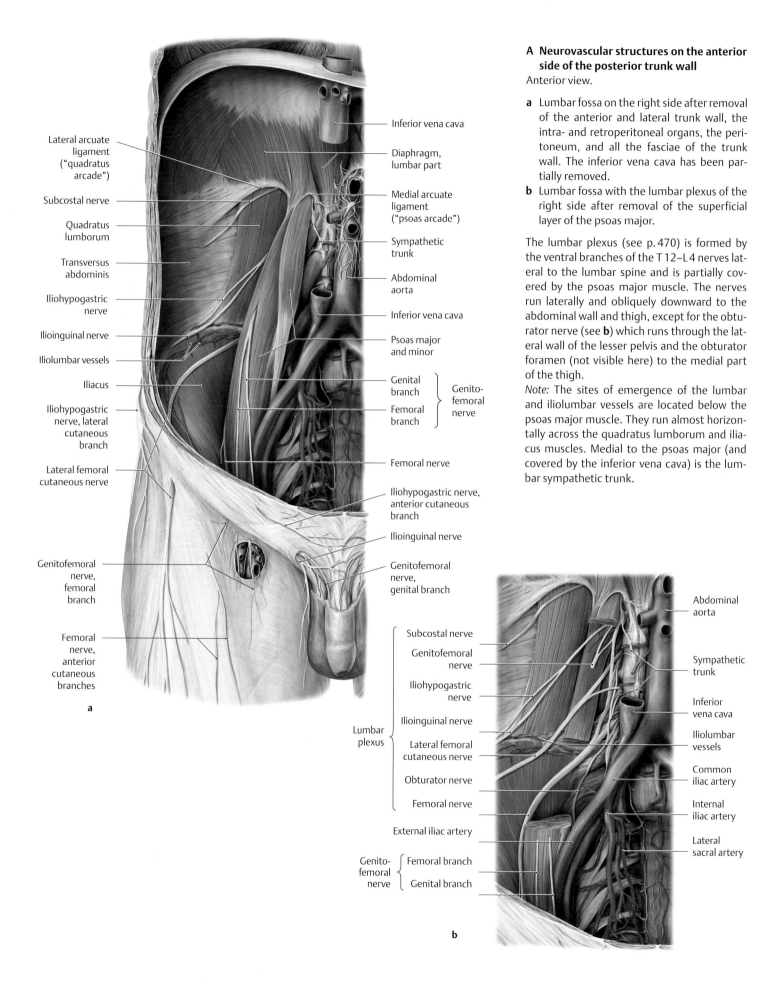

Lateral arcuate ligament ("quadratus arcade")

Subcostal nerve

Quadratus lumborum

Transversus abdominis

Iliohypogastric nerve

Ilioinguinal nerve

Iliolumbar vessels

Iliacus

Iliohypogastric nerve, lateral cutaneous branch

Lateral femoral cutaneous nerve

Genitofemoral nerve, femoral branch

Femoral nerve, anterior cutaneous branches

a

Inferior vena cava

Diaphragm, lumbar part

Medial arcuate ligament ("psoas arcade")

Sympathetic trunk

Abdominal aorta

Inferior vena cava

Psoas major and minor

Genital branch ⎫
　　　　　　 ⎬ Genito-
Femoral branch ⎭ femoral nerve

Femoral nerve

Iliohypogastric nerve, anterior cutaneous branch

Ilioinguinal nerve

Genitofemoral nerve, genital branch

Lumbar plexus {
Subcostal nerve

Genitofemoral nerve

Iliohypogastric nerve

Ilioinguinal nerve

Lateral femoral cutaneous nerve

Obturator nerve

Femoral nerve
}

External iliac artery

Genito-femoral nerve { Femoral branch / Genital branch }

Abdominal aorta

Sympathetic trunk

Inferior vena cava

Iliolumbar vessels

Common iliac artery

Internal iliac artery

Lateral sacral artery

b

A Neurovascular structures on the anterior side of the posterior trunk wall
Anterior view.

a Lumbar fossa on the right side after removal of the anterior and lateral trunk wall, the intra- and retroperitoneal organs, the peritoneum, and all the fasciae of the trunk wall. The inferior vena cava has been partially removed.

b Lumbar fossa with the lumbar plexus of the right side after removal of the superficial layer of the psoas major.

The lumbar plexus (see p. 470) is formed by the ventral branches of the T 12–L 4 nerves lateral to the lumbar spine and is partially covered by the psoas major muscle. The nerves run laterally and obliquely downward to the abdominal wall and thigh, except for the obturator nerve (see b) which runs through the lateral wall of the lesser pelvis and the obturator foramen (not visible here) to the medial part of the thigh.

Note: The sites of emergence of the lumbar and iliolumbar vessels are located below the psoas major muscle. They run almost horizontally across the quadratus lumborum and iliacus muscles. Medial to the psoas major (and covered by the inferior vena cava) is the lumbar sympathetic trunk.

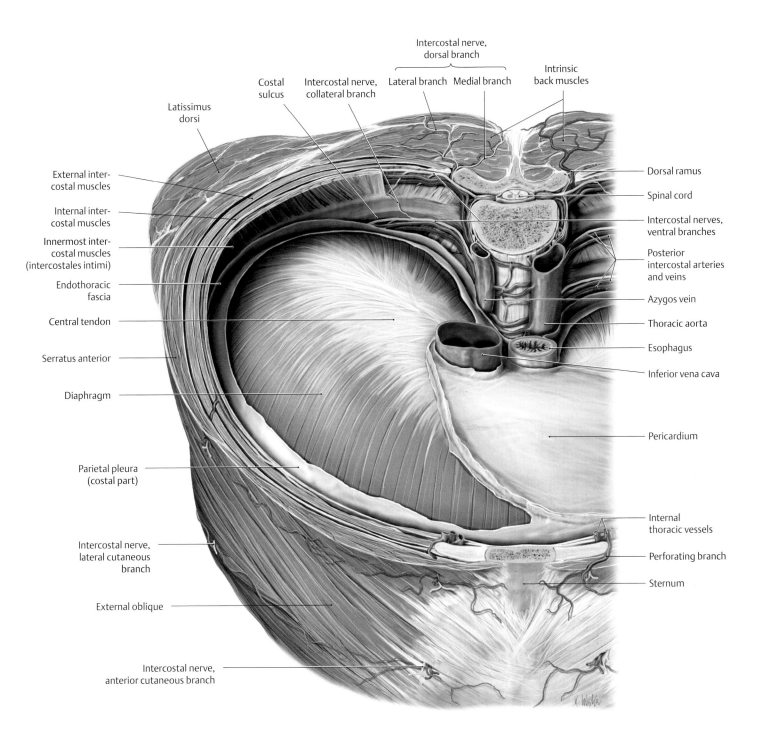

Intercostal nerve, dorsal branch

Costal sulcus

Intercostal nerve, collateral branch

Lateral branch   Medial branch

Intrinsic back muscles

Latissimus dorsi

External inter- costal muscles

Internal inter- costal muscles

Innermost inter- costal muscles (intercostales intimi)

Endothoracic fascia

Central tendon

Serratus anterior

Diaphragm

Parietal pleura (costal part)

Intercostal nerve, lateral cutaneous branch

External oblique

Intercostal nerve, anterior cutaneous branch

Dorsal ramus

Spinal cord

Intercostal nerves, ventral branches

Posterior intercostal arteries and veins

Azygos vein

Thoracic aorta

Esophagus

Inferior vena cava

Pericardium

Internal thoracic vessels

Perforating branch

Sternum

B Neurovascular structures of the posterior trunk wall at the thoracic level

Transverse section through the thorax after removal of the thoracic organs, parietal pleura, and part of the endothoracic fascia, anterosuperior view. The chest wall receives its arterial blood supply from the pos-terior intercostal arteries and is drained by the intercostal veins, which empty into the azygos system. The intercostal vessels run with the inter-costal nerves along the inferior border of the associated rib, lodged in the costal sulcus.

5.5 Anterior Trunk Wall: Overview and Location of Clinically Important Nerves and Vessels

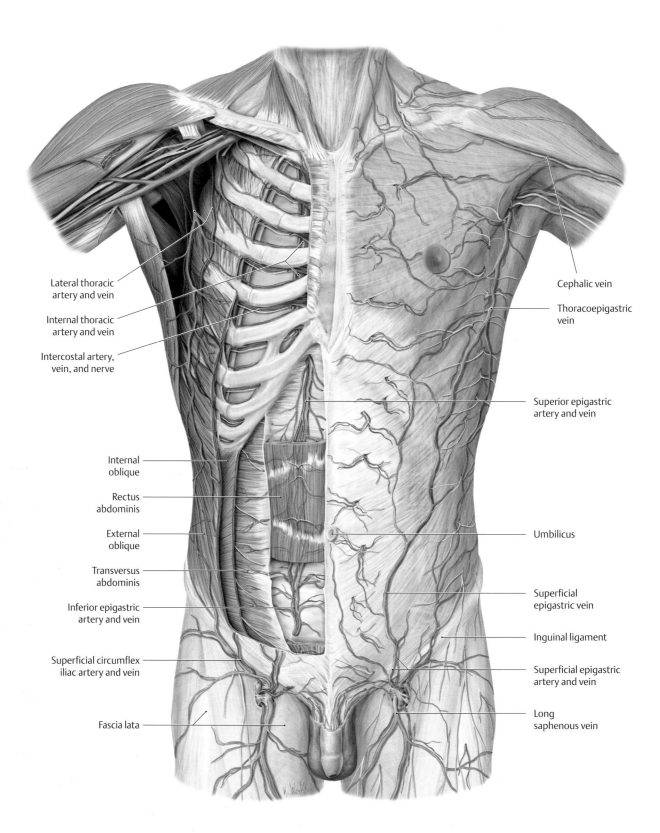

Lateral thoracic
artery and vein

Internal thoracic
artery and vein

Intercostal artery,
vein, and nerve

Internal
oblique

Rectus
abdominis

External
oblique

Transversus
abdominis

Inferior epigastric
artery and vein

Superficial circumflex
iliac artery and vein

Fascia lata

Cephalic vein

Thoracoepigastric
vein

Superior epigastric
artery and vein

Umbilicus

Superficial
epigastric vein

Inguinal ligament

Superficial epigastric
artery and vein

Long
saphenous vein

A Neurovascular structures on the anterior side of the anterior trunk wall

Anterior view. The superficial (subcutaneous) neurovascular structures are demonstrated on the left side of the trunk and the deep neurovascular structures on the right side. For this purpose the pectoralis major and minor muscles have been completely removed on the right side, and the external and internal oblique muscles have been partially removed. Portions of the right rectus abdominis muscle have been removed or rendered transparent to demonstrate the inferior epigastric vessels. Finally, the intercostal spaces have been exposed to display the course of the intercostal vessels and nerves.

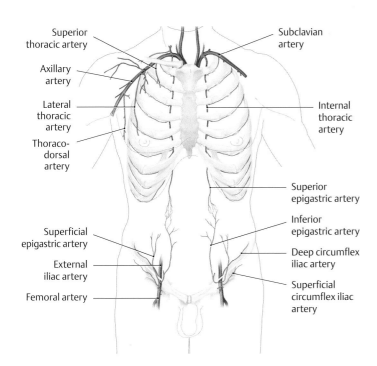

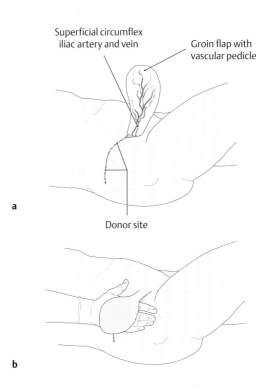

B The arterial supply of the anterior trunk wall

Anterior view. The anterior trunk wall receives its blood supply from two main sources: the internal thoracic artery, which arises from the subclavian artery, and the inferior epigastric artery, which arises from the external iliac artery. It is also supplied by smaller vessels arising from the axillary artery (superior thoracic artery, thoracodorsal artery, and lateral thoracic artery) and from the femoral artery (superficial epigastric artery and superficial circumflex iliac artery).

C Importance of the superficial circumflex iliac artery in harvesting skin flaps for plastic surgery

a Dissection of a skin flap based on the superficial circumflex iliac artery.

b The groin flap transferred to the dorsum of the right hand (after Weber).

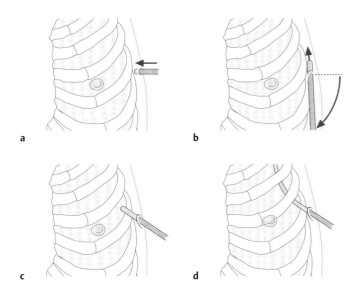

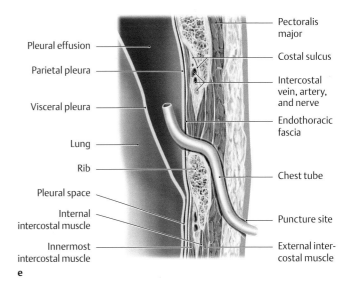

D Preserving the intercostal artery, vein, and nerve during the insertion of a chest tube

A chest tube may be inserted, for example, to drain an abnormal fluid collection from the pleural space, such as a pleural effusion due to bronchial carcinoma. The best site for placing the chest tube can be determined by percussion or ultrasound examination. Generally the optimum puncture site in the sitting patient is at the level of the seventh or eighth intercostal space on the posterior axillary line (see **e** and p. 30). The drain should always be introduced at the *upper margin of a rib* to avoid injuring the intercostal artery, vein, and nerve.

a–d Steps in the placement of a chest tube (anterior view; after Henne-Bruns, Dürig, and Kremer):

a A skin incision is made under local anesthesia, and the drainage tube is introduced perpendicular to the chest wall.

b On reaching the ribs, the tube is angled 90° and advanced cephalad in the subcutaneous plane, parallel to the chest wall.

c On reaching the next higher intercostal space, the tube is passed through the intercostal muscles above the rib.

d The tube is then advanced into the pleural cavity.

e Longitudinal section through the chest wall at the level of the posterior axillary line, after placement of the chest tube in the presence of pleural effusion.

5.6 Anterior Trunk Wall: Nerves, Blood Vessels, and Lymphatics in the Female Breast

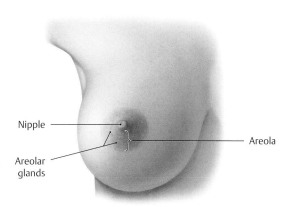

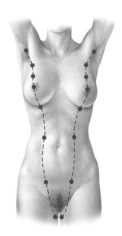

A Shape and appearance of the female breast
Right breast, anterior view. The female breast is shaped like a cone that is more rounded in its lower half than in the upper quadrants. It consists of the glandular tissue (mammary gland) and a fibrous stroma that contains fatty tissue. The excretory ducts of the glandular tissue open on the cone-shaped nipple, which lies at the center of the more heavily pigmented areola. Numerous small protuberances mark the openings of apocrine sweat glands and free sebaceous glands (areolar glands).

B The mammary ridges
The rudiments of the mammary glands form in both sexes along the mammary ridges, appearing as of an epidermal ridge extending from the axilla to the inguinal region on each side. Although rarely the mammary ridges may persist in humans to form accessory nipples (polythelia), normally all the rudiments disappear except for the thoracic pair. By the end of fetal development, lactiferous ducts have sprouted into the subcutaneous tissue from the two remaining epithelial buds. After menarche, breast development in females is marked by growth of the fibrous stroma and proliferation of the glandular tree in response to stimulation by sex hormones.

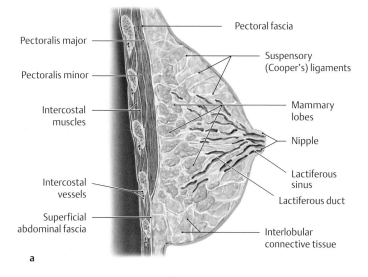

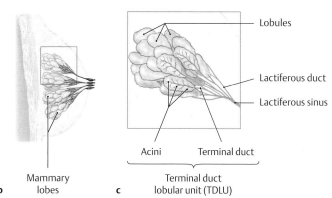

C Gross and microscopic anatomy of the breast

a The base of the adult female breast extends from the second to the sixth rib along the midclavicular line and directly overlies the pectoralis major, serratus anterior, and external oblique muscles. It is loosely attached to the pectoralis fascia and adjacent fascial planes (axillary and superficial abdominal fascia) by connective tissue. The breast is additionally supported, especially in its upper portion, by permeating bundles of connective tissue (the suspensory ligaments of the breast, or *Cooper's ligaments*). The glandular tissue is composed of 10–20 individual lobes, each of which has its lactiferous major duct that opens on the nipple by way of a dilated segment, the lactiferous sinus (structure of the lobe shown in **b**). The glands and lactiferous ducts are surrounded by firm, fibrofatty tissue that has a rich blood supply.

b Sagittal section of the duct system and portions of a lobe: A mammary lobe resembles a tree composed of branching lactiferous ducts, which terminate in smaller lobules (approximately 0.5 mm in diameter). In the *nonlactating breast* (as shown here), these lobules contain rudimentary acini that are arranged in clusters of small epithelial buds without a visible lumen.

c The terminal duct lobular unit (TDLU): One lobule and its terminal duct make up the basic secretory unit of the female breast. Each lobule is composed of acini that empty into a terminal ductule. The associated intralobular connective tissue (mantle tissue) contains stem cells that give rise to the tremendous cell growth (proliferation of the duct system and differentiation of the acini) that occurs during the transformation to the *lactating breast*. The TDLU is of key importance in pathohistology because it is the site where most malignant breast tumors originate (after Lüllmann).

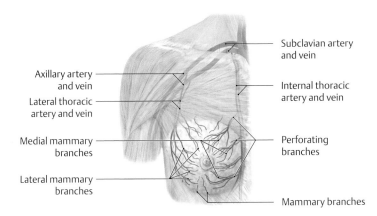

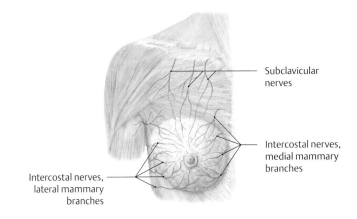

D Blood supply to the breast

The breast derives its blood supply from perforating branches of the internal thoracic artery (= medial mammary branches from the second through fourth intercostal spaces), branches of the lateral thoracic artery (lateral mammary branches), and direct branches from the second through fifth intercostal arteries (mammary branches). The breast is drained by the internal and lateral thoracic veins.

E Nerve supply to the breast

The sensory innervation of the breast has a segmental arrangement and is supplied by branches of the second through sixth intercostal nerves (lateral and medial mammary branches). Branches of the cervical plexus (supraclavicular nerves) also supply the upper portion of the breast.

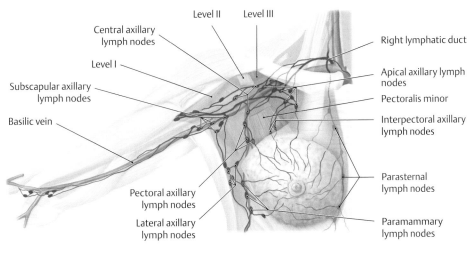

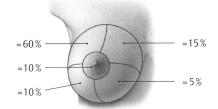

G Distribution of malignant tumors by quadrant in the female breast

The numbers indicate the average percentage location of malignant breast tumors.

F Lymphatic drainage of the breast

The lymphatic vessels of the breast can be divided into a superficial, subcutaneous, and deep system. The deep system begins with lymphatic capillaries at the acinar level (see **Cb** and **c**) and is particularly important as a route for tumor metastasis. The main regional filtering stations are the axillary and parasternal lymph nodes, the approximately 30–60 axillary lymph nodes receiving most of the lymphatic drainage. They are the first nodes to be affected by metastasis (see **G**) and therefore have major oncological significance. The axillary lymph nodes are subdivided into levels (see p. 312):

- **Level I: lower axillary group** (lateral to the pectoralis minor):
  – Pectoral axillary lymph nodes
  – Subscapular axillary lymph nodes
  – Lateral axillary lymph nodes
  – Paramammary lymph nodes
- **Level II: middle axillary group** (at the level of the pectoralis minor):
  – Interpectoral axillary lymph nodes
  – Central axillary lymph nodes
- **Level III: upper infraclavicular group** (medial to the pectoralis minor):
  – Apical axillary lymph nodes

The *parasternal lymph nodes* which are distributed along the thoracic vessels chiefly drain the medial portion of the breast. From there, tumor cells may spread across the midline to the opposite side. The survival rate in breast cancer patients correlates most strongly with the number of involved lymph nodes at the various *axillary* nodal levels. The parasternal lymph nodes are rarely important in this regard. According to Henne-Bruns, Dürig, and Kremer, the 5-year survival rate is approximately 65% with metastatic involvement of level I, 31% with involvement of level II, but approaches 0% in patients with level III involvement. This explains the key prognostic importance of a *sentinel lymphadenectomy* (removal of the sentinel lymph node). This technique is based on the assumption that every point in the integument drains via specific lymphatic pathways to a particular lymph node, rarely draining to more than one. Accordingly, the lymph node that is the first to receive lymph from the primary tumor will be the first node to contain tumor cells that have spread from the primary tumor by lymphogenous metastasis. The specific lymphatic drainage path, and thus the sentinel node, can be identified by scintigraphic mapping with radiolabeled colloids (^{99m}TC sulfur microcolloid), which has superseded the older technique of patent blue dye injection. The first lymph node to be visualized is the sentinel node. That node is selectively removed and histologically examined for the presence of tumor cells. If the sentinel node does not contain tumor cells, generally the rest of the axillary nodes will also be negative. This method is 98% accurate in predicting the level of axillary nodal involvement prior to surgery.

5.7 Anterior Trunk Wall: The Inguinal Canal

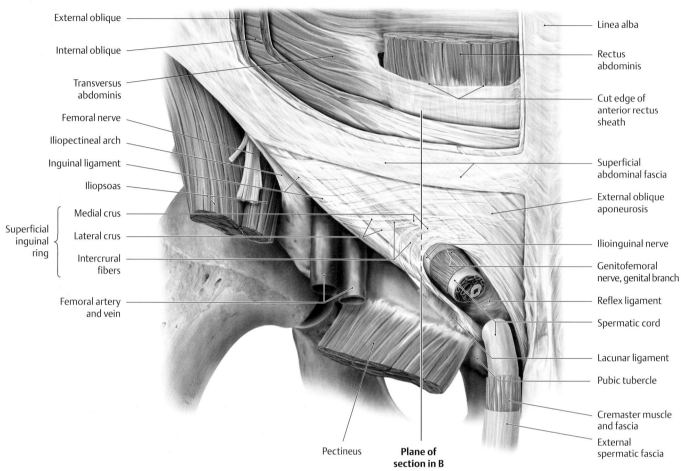

External oblique
Internal oblique
Transversus abdominis
Femoral nerve
Iliopectineal arch
Inguinal ligament
Iliopsoas
Superficial inguinal ring
— Medial crus
— Lateral crus
— Intercrural fibers
Femoral artery and vein

Linea alba
Rectus abdominis
Cut edge of anterior rectus sheath
Superficial abdominal fascia
External oblique aponeurosis
Ilioinguinal nerve
Genitofemoral nerve, genital branch
Reflex ligament
Spermatic cord
Lacunar ligament
Pubic tubercle
Cremaster muscle and fascia
External spermatic fascia

Pectineus
Plane of section in B

A Location of the inguinal canal in the male
Right inguinal region, anterior view. Approximately 4–6 cm long, the inguinal canal passes obliquely forward, downward, and medially above the inguinal ligament to pierce the anterior abdominal wall. It begins internally at the deep inguinal ring (**D** and **E**) in the lateral inguinal fossa (see p. 184) and opens externally at the superficial inguinal ring, lateral to the pubic tubercle. With the superficial abdominal fascia removed, this "external opening" of the canal can be identified as a slitlike orifice in the aponeurosis of the external oblique muscle (external oblique aponeurosis). It is bounded by the *medial crus* superomedially and by the *lateral crus* inferolaterally. Both crura are interconnected by the *intercrural fibers*. The superficial inguinal ring is completed internally by arched fibers from the inguinal ligament (reflex ligament), forming a deep groove. The inguinal canal in the male provides a pathway for the descent of the testis during fetal life (see p. 194). Its contents in the male (after testicular descent) include the spermatic cord, and its contents in the female include the round ligament of the ovary (ligamentum teres; see **C**).

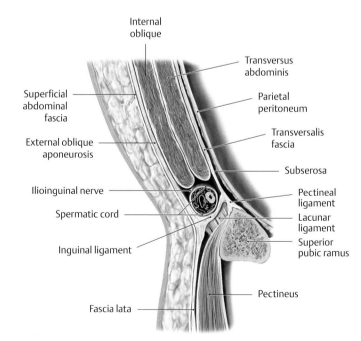

Internal oblique
Superficial abdominal fascia
External oblique aponeurosis
Ilioinguinal nerve
Spermatic cord
Inguinal ligament
Fascia lata

Transversus abdominis
Parietal peritoneum
Transversalis fascia
Subserosa
Pectineal ligament
Lacunar ligament
Superior pubic ramus
Pectineus

B Sagittal section through the inguinal canal in the male
Medial view. *Note* the structures that form the walls of the inguinal canal above and below the spermatic cord and on the anterior and posterior sides (compare with **C**). The openings and wall structures of the inguinal canal bear an important relationship to the pathophysiology of hernias (after Schumpelick).

C Openings and wall structures of the inguinal canal

The inguinal canal resembles a flattened tube with an internal and external opening (see below), a floor, a roof, and anterior and posterior walls. A lumen is present only after its contents have been removed (the spermatic cord in males, the uterine round ligament and its artery in females, the ilioinguinal nerve and lymphatic vessels in both sexes). The inguinal canal remains patent for life, especially in males, and thus forms a path for potential herniation through the abdominal wall (see p. 186).

Openings of the inguinal canal (see **A**)

Superficial inguinal ring	Opening in the external oblique aponeurosis bounded by the medial crus, lateral crus, intercrural fibers, and reflex ligament.
Deep inguinal ring	Opening between the interfoveolar ligament, inguinal ligament, and lateral umbilical fold; formed by an outpouching of the transversalis fascia (becomes the internal spermatic fascia) (see p. 185)

Wall structures of the inguinal canal (see **B**)

Floor	Inguinal ligament (densely interwoven fibers of the lower external oblique aponeurosis and adjacent fascia lata of the thigh)
Roof	Transversus abdominis and internal oblique muscles
Anterior wall	External oblique aponeurosis
Posterior wall	Transversalis fascia and peritoneum (partially thickened by the interfoveolar ligament)

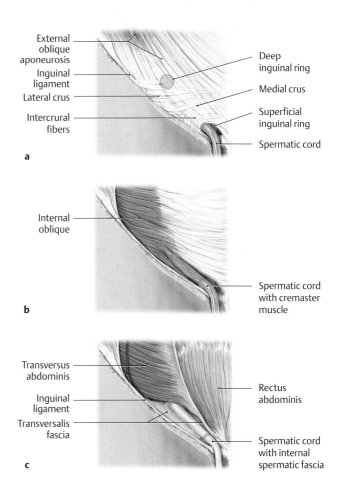

a

b

c

D Contribution of the oblique abdominal muscles to the structure of the male inguinal canal

Right inguinal region, anterior view.

a–c Progressive removal of the abdominal wall muscles.

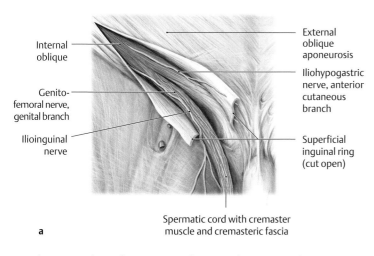

a

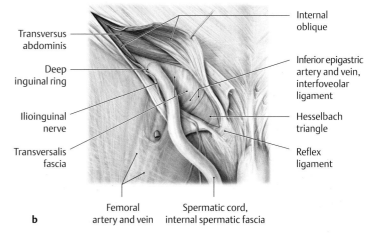

b

E The inguinal canal, progressively opened to expose the spermatic cord

a Division of the external oblique aponeurosis reveals the internal oblique muscle, some of whose fibers are continued onto the spermatic cord as the cremaster muscle. The genital branch of the genitofemoral nerve runs with it below the cremasteric fascia (see p. 472). The ilioinguinal nerve runs through the inguinal canal on the spermatic cord. Its sensory fibers pass through the superficial inguinal ring to the skin over the pubic symphysis and are distributed to the lateral portion of the scrotum or labia majora, and medial thigh.

b With the internal oblique muscle divided and the cremaster muscle split, the full course of the spermatic cord through the inguinal

canal can be displayed. The spermatic cord appears at the deep inguinal ring, where the transversalis fascia is invaginated into the inguinal canal (and encloses the spermatic cord on its way to the testis as the internal spermatic fascia). It runs below the transversus abdominis along the posterior wall of the inguinal canal (transversalis fascia and peritoneum). The wall at the midportion of the canal is formed by the interfoveolar ligament and is reinforced medially by the reflex ligament. Medial to the interfoveolar ligament, below which run the epigastric vessels, and above the inguinal ligament is the *Hesselbach triangle,* a weak spot in the abdominal wall which is a common site for direct inguinal hernias (after Schumpelick, see also p. 187).

5.8 Anterior Abdominal Wall: Anatomy and Weak Spots

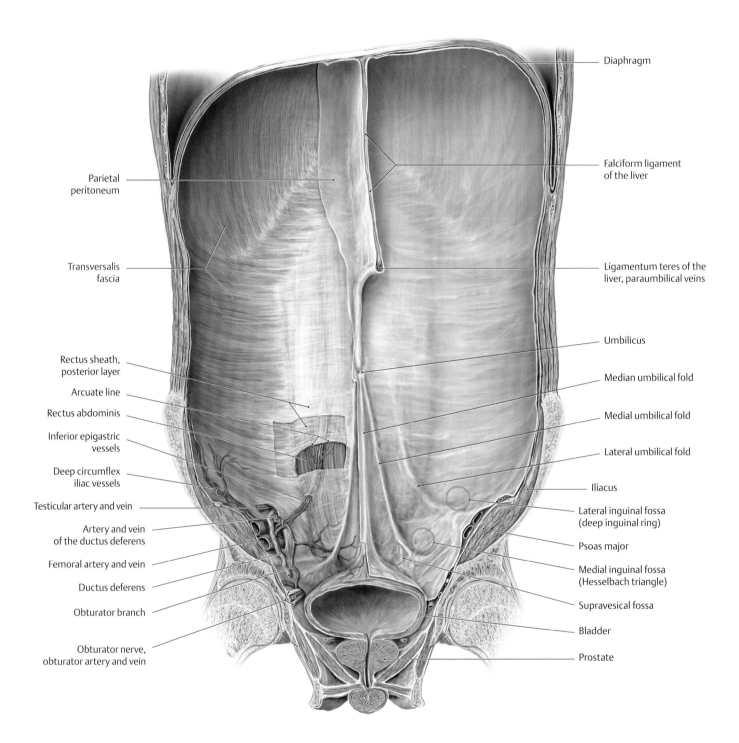

Parietal peritoneum

Transversalis fascia

Rectus sheath, posterior layer

Arcuate line

Rectus abdominis

Inferior epigastric vessels

Deep circumflex iliac vessels

Testicular artery and vein

Artery and vein of the ductus deferens

Femoral artery and vein

Ductus deferens

Obturator branch

Obturator nerve, obturator artery and vein

Diaphragm

Falciform ligament of the liver

Ligamentum teres of the liver, paraumbilical veins

Umbilicus

Median umbilical fold

Medial umbilical fold

Lateral umbilical fold

Iliacus

Lateral inguinal fossa (deep inguinal ring)

Psoas major

Medial inguinal fossa (Hesselbach triangle)

Supravesical fossa

Bladder

Prostate

A Internal surface anatomy of the anterior abdominal wall in the male

Coronal section through the abdominal and pelvic cavity at the level of the hip joints, posterior view. All of the abdominal and pelvic organs have been removed except for the urinary bladder and prostate. Portions of the peritoneum and transversalis fascia have also been removed on the left side. The internal surface anatomy of the lower abdominal wall is marked by five peritoneal folds, which extend toward the umbilicus:

- An unpaired *median umbilical fold* on the midline (contains the obliterated urachus)
- Paired left and right *medial umbilical folds* (contain the left and right obliterated umbilical artery)

- Paired left and right *lateral umbilical folds* (contain the left and right inferior epigastric vessels)

Located between the peritoneal folds on each side are three more or less distinct fossae, which are sites of potential herniation through the anterior abdominal wall:

- the *supravesical fossa,* located between the median and medial umbilical folds above the apex of the bladder;
- the *medial inguinal fossa* (Hesselbach triangle), located between the medial and lateral umbilical folds; and
- the *lateral inguinal fossa,* located lateral to the lateral umbilical fold (site of the deep inguinal ring).

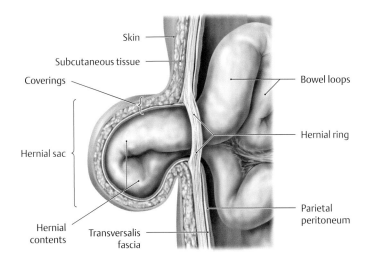

B Definition, occurrence, and structure of an abdominal hernia

Between the thorax and bony pelvis is an extended skeletal gap that is covered by multiple abdominal wall layers composed of broad muscles, fasciae, aponeuroses, and peritoneum. The muscular foundation is deficient at certain locations, and the abdominal wall at those sites is formed entirely by connective-tissue structures. These are the areas of greatest weakness (least resistance) in the abdominal wall. Occasionally these weak spots cannot withstand a rise of intra-abdominal pressure, and openings are created for the herniation of abdominal viscera. The term "hernia" (L. *hernia* = "rupture") refers to the protrusion of parietal peritoneum through an anatomical opening (e.g., inguinal or femoral hernia) or a secondary defect (e.g., umbilical hernia). An *external hernia* is one that protrudes from the abdominal cavity and is visible on the body surface, while an *internal hernia* protrudes into a peritoneal pouch that is contained within the abdomen. Hernias are also classified by the time of their occurrence as *congenital* (e.g., umbilical hernia, indirect inguinal hernia through a patent processus vaginalis) or *acquired* (e.g., direct inguinal hernia, femoral hernia). The following components of a hernia are important in terms of surgical treatment:

Hernial opening: the orifice or defect through which the viscus herniates.

Hernial sac: the pouch, generally lined by parietal peritoneum, that contains the herniated viscus. Its size is highly variable, depending on the extent of the hernia.

Hernial contents: may be almost any intra-abdominal viscus but usually consist of greater omentum or loops of small bowel.

Coverings: the tissue layers surrounding the hernial sac. The composition of the coverings depends on the location and mechanism of the hernia.

C Internal and external openings for abdominal hernias

Above the inguinal ligament, the median, medial, and lateral umbilical folds (see **A**) form three sites of weakness on each side of the abdominal wall where indirect and direct inguinal hernias and suprapubic hernias typically occur. Another weak spot is located *below the inguinal ligament* and medial to the femoral vein in the femoral ring. At that site the femoral ring is covered only by loose, compliant connective tissue, the femoral septum, which is permeated by numerous lymphatic vessels. The sharp-edged lacunar ligament forms the medial border of the femoral ring and can contribute to the incarceration of a femoral hernia (see p.187).

Internal opening	Hernia	External opening
Above the inguinal ligament:		
Supravesical fossa	Supravesical hernia	Superficial inguinal ring
Medial inguinal fossa (Hesselbach triangle)	Direct inguinal hernia	Superficial inguinal ring
Lateral inguinal fossa (deep inguinal ring)	Indirect inguinal hernia	Superficial inguinal ring
Below the inguinal ligament:		
Femoral ring	Femoral hernia	Saphenous hiatus

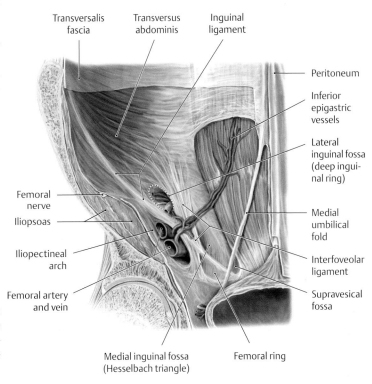

D Internal hernial openings in the male inguinal and femoral region

Detail from **A**, posterior view. The peritoneum and transversalis fascia have been partially removed to demonstrate the hernial openings more clearly. The internal openings (see **A** and **C**) for indirect and direct inguinal hernias, femoral hernias, and suprapubic (= supravesical) hernias are indicated by color shading.

5.9   Inguinal and Femoral Hernias

A Hernias of the groin region: inguinal and femoral hernias*

Hernia	Openings and course
• **Direct (medial) inguinal hernia** Always acquired	• *Internal opening:* Hesselbach triangle, i.e., above the inguinal ligament and medial to the inferior epigastric artery and vein • *Course:* sac is perpendicular to the abdominal wall • *External opening:* superficial inguinal ring
• **Indirect (lateral) inguinal hernia** Congenital (patent processus vaginalis) or acquired	• *Internal opening:* deep inguinal ring, i.e., above the inguinal ligament and lateral to the inferior epigastric artery and vein • *Course:* sac passes through the inguinal canal • *External opening:* superficial inguinal ring
• **Femoral hernia** Always acquired	• *Internal opening:* femoral ring and septum, i.e., below the inguinal ligament • *Course:* sac passes through the femoral canal below the fascia lata • *External opening:* saphenous hiatus

* 80 % of all hernias are inguinal hernias (90 % of which occur in males), and approximately 10 % are femoral hernias (more common in females) (see also p. 188). Inguinal hernias are among the most common structural defects in humans, accounting for some 20 % of all surgical operations.

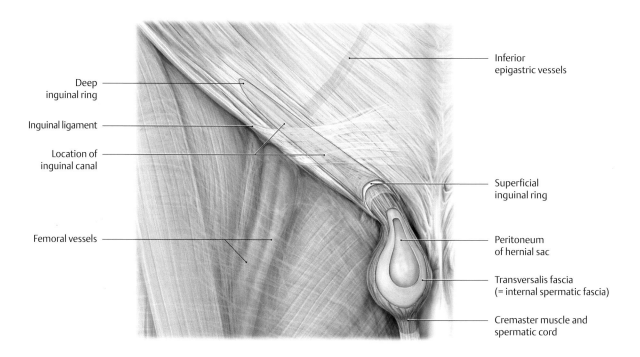

Deep inguinal ring

Inguinal ligament

Location of inguinal canal

Femoral vessels

Inferior epigastric vessels

Superficial inguinal ring

Peritoneum of hernial sac

Transversalis fascia (= internal spermatic fascia)

Cremaster muscle and spermatic cord

B Congenital or acquired indirect inguinal hernia
Right male inguinal region with the skin and superficial body fascia removed, anterior view. The fascia lata of the thigh is shown transparent, and the spermatic cord is windowed. Regardless of the location of the *internal* opening, both *indirect (lateral)* and *direct (medial)* inguinal hernias (see **C**) emerge from the superficial inguinal ring above the inguinal ligament. Indirect inguinal hernias may be congenital (due to a patent processus vaginalis) or acquired and follow a tract parallel to the abdominal wall. The hernial sac enters the expanded deep inguinal ring (internal opening), which is lateral to the epigastric vessels, and passes medially and obliquely along the inguinal canal. Invested by the fascia enclosing the spermatic cord, it finally emerges at the superficial inguinal ring and descends into the scrotum. The coverings of all indirect inguinal hernias include the peritoneum and the transversalis fascia (internal spermatic fascia).

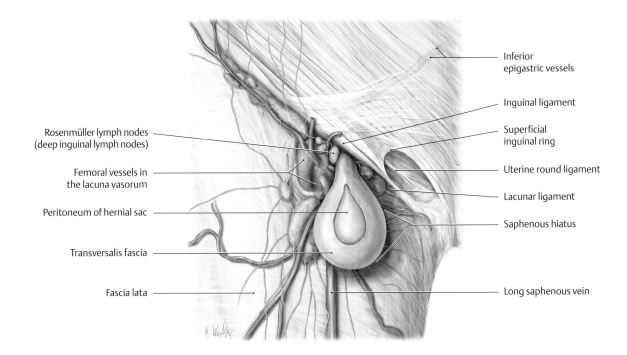

C Acquired direct inguinal hernia
Right inguinal region in the male with the skin and superficial body fascia removed, anterior view. The fascia lata of the thigh is lightly shaded. Direct inguinal hernias are always acquired and follow a tract that is perpendicular to the abdominal wall. The hernia will leave the abdominal cavity medial to the inferior epigastric vessels within Hesselbach's triangle (see p. 185). Such hernias may pass through the superficial inguinal ring, and in such instances the hernial sac is medial to the spermatic cord.

D Acquired femoral hernia
Right female inguinal region with the skin and superficial body fascia removed, anterior view. Femoral hernias are always acquired and are more common in women (broader pelvis and larger femoral ring). They always pass inferior to the inguinal ligament, and medial to the femoral vein, extending through the femoral ring to enter the femoral canal (not visible here). The funnel-shaped canal begins at the femoral ring (the internal opening of the hernia, not visible here) and ends approximately 2 cm inferiorly at the saphenous hiatus, and lies anterior to the pectineal fascia. The sharp-edged lacunar ligament forms the medial boundary of the femoral ring (risk of incarceration). Typically the femoral canal is occupied by loose fatty and connective tissue and deep inguinal lymph nodes. Femoral hernias may emerge at the saphenous hiatus (external opening), which is covered by the thin cribiform fascia, and thus become subcutaneous.

5.10   Rare External Hernias

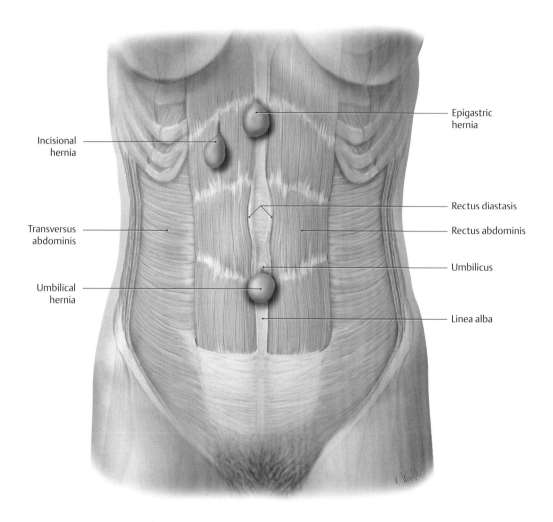

A Location of hernias in the anterior abdominal wall

B Hernias of the anterior abdominal wall *

Hernia	Location, occurrence, and typical features

• **Umbilical hernia**	• Umbilical region, passing through the umbilical ring:
	  – Congenital umbilical hernia: incomplete regression of the normal fetal umbilical hernia due to scarring of the umbilical papilla (hernial sac: amnion and peritoneum)
	  – Acquired umbilical hernia: common after multiple pregnancies, also in association with obesity, hepatic cirrhosis, or ascites (secondary widening of the umbilical ring)

• **Omphalocele**	• Congenital persistence (1 : 6000) of an abdominal wall defect with an incomplete reduction of abdominal viscera during fetal life; unlike an umbilical hernia, the omphalocele is not covered by epidermis but only by peritoneum, mucous connective tissue (Wharton jelly), and amniotic epithelium (so the contents are easily recognized)
• **Epigastric hernia**	• The hernial openings are gaps in the linea alba excluding the umbilicus (on a continuum with rectus diastasis, see below)
• **Rectus diastasis**	• The rectus muscles separate at the linea alba when the abdominal muscles are tightened, creating a site for potential for herniation (the hernia reduces on relaxation, and complaints are rare)
• **Incisional hernia**	• Occurs at a previous incision site (usually in the upper abdominal midline)

* Umbilical and epigastric hernias comprise approximately 10 % of all hernias.

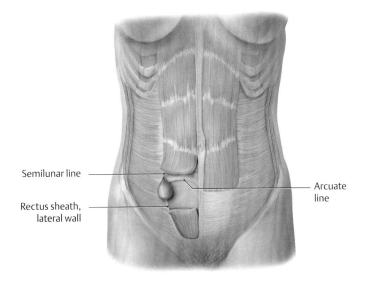

D Spigelian hernia

Semilunar line

Rectus sheath, lateral wall

Arcuate line

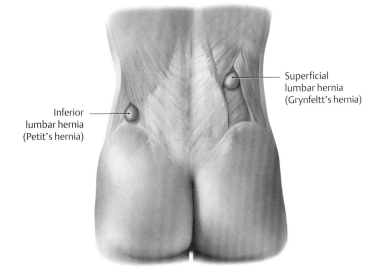

E Lumbar hernia

Superficial lumbar hernia (Grynfeltt's hernia)

Inferior lumbar hernia (Petit's hernia)

C Other rare hernias occurring elsewhere on the trunk*

Hernia	Location
• **Spigelian hernia**	• Anterior abdominal wall between the semilunar line and lateral rectus sheath, usually at the level of the arcuate line
• **Lumbar hernia**	• Between the twelfth rib and iliac crest: – Superior lumbar hernia (superior costolumbar triangle, Grynfeltt's triangle): between the twelfth rib and iliocostalis – Inferior lumbar hernia (inferior iliolumbar triangle, Petit's triangle): between the iliac crest, latissimus dorsi, and external oblique muscles
• **Obturator hernia**	• Through the obturator foramen and then between the pectineus, adductor longus, and external obturator muscles
• **Sciatic hernia**	• Through the greater sacrosciatic foramen: – Suprapiriform hernia (above the piriformis muscle) – Infrapiriform hernia (below the piriformis muscle) – Spinotuberous hernia (in front of the sacrotuberous ligament)
• **Perineal hernia**	• Through the pelvic floor: – Anterior perineal hernia (in front of the deep transverse perineal) – Posterior perineal hernia (behind the deep transverse perineal) – Ischiorectal hernia (through the levator ani into the ischioanal fossa)

* Less than 1% of all hernias, generally acquired (after Schumpelick)

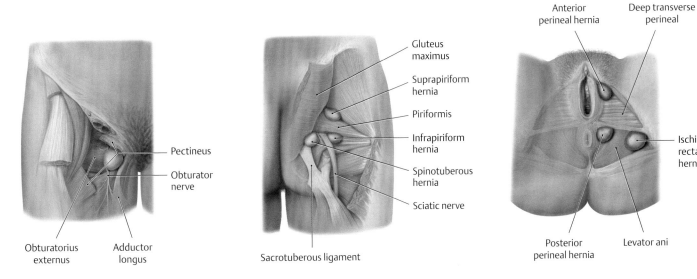

F Obturator hernia

Pectineus

Obturator nerve

Obturatorius externus

Adductor longus

G Sciatic hernia

Gluteus maximus

Suprapiriform hernia

Piriformis

Infrapiriform hernia

Spinotuberous hernia

Sciatic nerve

Sacrotuberous ligament

H Perineal hernia

Anterior perineal hernia

Deep transverse perineal

Ischio-rectal hernia

Posterior perineal hernia

Levator ani

5.11 Diagnosis and Treatment of Hernias

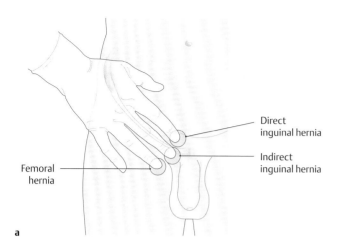

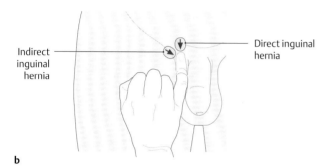

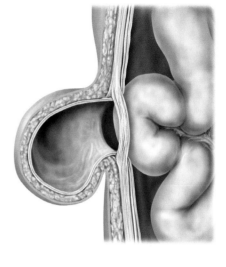

B Complete reduction of a hernia
When the herniated viscus can move freely within the hernial sac and at the hernial opening, generally the hernia can be reduced spontaneously (e.g., by lying down) or by manual manipulation. As a result, there is no risk of acute incarceration.

A Technique for the examination of inguinal and femoral hernias
Hernias of the groin region, like most hernias, are typically precipitated by a rise of intra-abdominal pressure (e.g., due to coughing, sneezing, or straining) and present as a palpable bulge or swelling in the inguinal region. Usually this swelling regresses spontaneously when the patient lies down. Spontaneous pain is generally absent with an uncomplicated hernia, and a foreign body sensation is more common. Persistent pain accompanied by a feeling of pressure at the hernia site, nausea, and vomiting are signs of incarceration (see **C**). In patients with a bulge in the inguinal region or a scrotal mass (see p. 197), the differential diagnosis should include hydrocele, varicocele, ectopic testis, lymphoma, and other tumors of the testis or epididymis. Since inguinal and femoral hernias are of the external type and are easily accessible to inspection and palpation, the diagnosis is generally made clinically.

a **Palpation from the iliac spine (the three-finger rule):** The "three-finger rule" makes it easier to appreciate the topographic anatomy of inguinal and femoral hernias and differentiate among direct and indirect inguinal hernias and femoral hernias. When the examiner places the thenar eminence on the anterior superior iliac spine, the index finger points to a direct hernia, the middle finger to an indirect hernia, and the ring finger to a femoral hernia. Thus when a hernia is felt below the index finger, for example, this means that the patient has a direct inguinal hernia.

b **Palpation from the scrotum:** This technique is particularly useful for palpating smaller inguinal hernias in the standing patient. By invaginating the scrotum and groin skin, the examiner palpates along the spermatic cord to the superficial inguinal ring and touches the posterior wall of the inguinal canal with the pad of the finger. When the patient coughs, an experienced examiner can distinguish an indirect hernia, which strikes the pad of the finger, from a direct hernia, which strikes the distal tip of the finger.

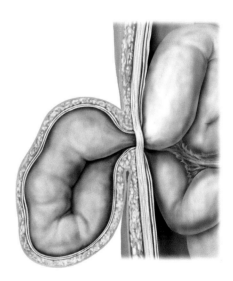

C Incarcerated hernia
Incarceration is the most serious complication of a hernia. Strangulation at the neck of the hernia restricts blood flow to the herniated bowel, with effects ranging from ischemia to necrosis. The patient may develop symptoms of a functional or mechanical bowel obstruction with a life-threatening interruption of intestinal transit due to narrowing or obstruction of the bowel lumen. Given the risk of bowel perforation and peritonitis in these cases, immediate surgery is indicated (see **D**).

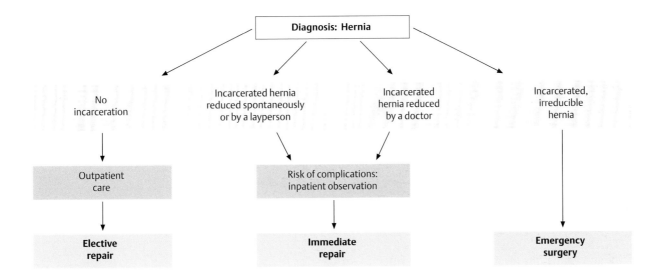

D Hernia symptoms and timing of the repair (after Henne-Bruns, Dürig, and Kremer)

As a rule, hernias do not respond definitively to conservative treatment (e.g., trusses or binders), and a permanent reduction is achieved only by surgical closure of the hernial opening (see **E**). The timing of the repair is based on the clinical presentation, i.e., the presence of a reducible, irreducible, or incarcerated hernia.

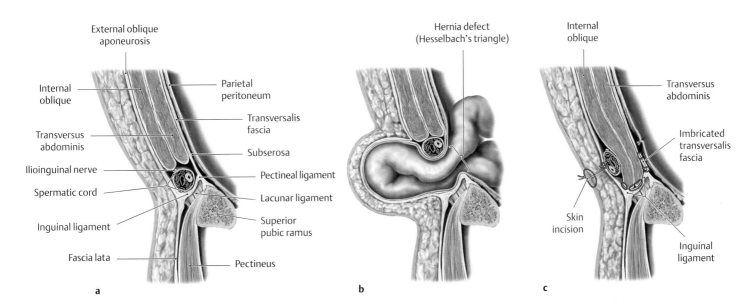

E Inguinal hernia repair: the Shouldice technique
Sagittal sections through the male groin region:

a Normal anatomy (see p.182).
b Acquired direct inguinal hernia.
c The Shouldice repair.

Various surgical methods are available for hernia repair. They differ mainly in the technique used to reinforce the posterior wall of the ingu-

inal canal. In all methods a skin incision is made approximately 2 cm above the inguinal ligament, the hernial sac is exposed and dissected free, the contents of the sac are returned to the abdominal cavity, and the defect is closed to restore the stability of the abdominal wall. In the *Shouldice repair* (the most successful and widely used operation), the posterior wall is reinforced by overlapping the transversalis fascia and suturing the internal oblique and transversus abdominis muscles to the inguinal ligament in two layers.

5.12 Development of the External Genitalia

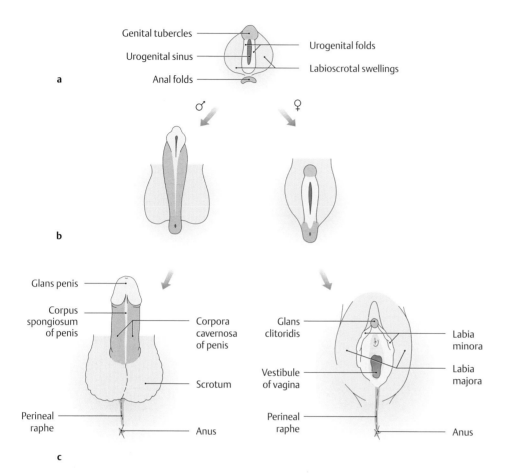

B Derivatives of the undifferentiated embryonic genital anlage during development of the external genital organs (after Starck)*

Undifferen-tiated anlage	Male	Female
Genital tubercles	Glans penis	Clitoris, glans clitoridis
Genital folds	Corpus spongiosum of the penis	Labia minora, vestibular bulb
Genital swellings	Scrotum	Labia majora
Urogenital sinus	Spongiose part of the urethra	Vestibule of the vagina
Anal folds	Perineal raphe	Perineal raphe

* Details on the development of the gonads and genital tracts can be found in text-books of embryology.

A Development of the external genitalia

a Rudimentary, undifferentiated external genitalia in a six-week-old embryo.
b Differentiation of the external genitalia along male or female lines in a 10-week-old fetus.
c Differentiated external genitalia in the newborn.

The external genital organs develop from an undifferentiated mesoder-mal primordium in the *cloaca* and, like the gonads, pass through an ini-tial **indifferent stage**. The anorectal area and urogenital sinus (cloaca) are not yet separated from each other and are closed externally by a common cloacal membrane. The following elevations develop around the cloacal membrane due to intensive mesodermal cell divisions:

• Anterior: the genital tubercles
• Lateral: the genital folds (urethral folds)
• Posterior: the anal folds
• Lateral to the genital folds: the genital swellings (labioscrotal swel-lings)

Later, between the sixth and seventh weeks of development, the urorec-tal septum divides the cloaca into an anterior part (urogenital sinus) and a posterior part (anus and rectum). The cloacal membrane disappears, and the urogenital ostium forms anteriorly. The early perineum forms at the level of the urorectal septum (by fusion of the paired anal folds to the perineal raphe). **Differentiation of the genital organs** begins approximately in the eighth to ninth week of fetal development. Sexual differentiation is clearly evident by the 13th week and is fully developed by the 16th week.

• In the *male fetus,* the genital tubercles enlarge *under the influence of testosterone* to form the phallus and future penis. The urogenital sinus closes completely by fusion of the genital folds and forms the spongy part of the urethra. The genital (scrotal) swellings unite to form the scrotum.
• In the *female fetus (absence of testosterone),* the genital tubercles give rise to the clitoris. The urogenital sinus persists as the vestibule of the vagina, and the two genital folds form the labia minora. The genital swellings enlarge to form the labia majora.

Male sex organs develop only in the presence of the factors listed below:

• A functionally competent *SRY (sex-determining region of the Y) gene* on the Y chromosome (otherwise, ovaries and a female phenotype will develop). The SRY gene ensures that anti-Müllerian hormone and Leydig cells are produced (see below).
• Among its other functions, the *anti-müllerian hormone* induces regression of the müllerian ducts. It is formed in the somatic cells of the testicular cords (future Sertoli cells) starting in the eighth week of fetal life.
• *Leydig cells* begin to form in the fetal testes by the ninth week and produce large amounts of androgens (testosterone) until birth. They stimulate differentiation of the *wolffian duct* into seminiferous tubu-les and the development of the male external genitalia.

Alteration or interruption of this process of differentiation at any stage can lead to incomplete midline fusion which leaves persistent clefts (hypospadias, epispadias, see **C**), or to more extensive external genital anomalies (see **E**) (after Starck).

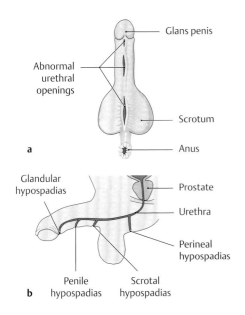

a

b Penile hypospadias   Scrotal hypospadias

C Hypospadias: a urethral anomaly in boys

a Cleft anomalies affecting the underside of the penis and scrotum.

b Possible sites of emergence of the urethra in hypospadias (penis viewed from the lateral view).

If the genital folds do not fuse completely during sexual differentiation (see **A**), the result is a cleft anomaly of the urethra, which may open on the underside of the penis *(hypospadias)* or on its dorsal surface *(epispadias)*. Hypospadias is much more common, with an incidence of 1:3000 compared with 1:100,000 for epispadias. It is most common to find an abnormal urethral orifice in the glans region of the penis (glandular hypospadias). Additionally, the shaft of the penis is usually shortened and angled downward by the presence of ventral fibrous bands. Surgical correction is generally performed between the sixth month and second year of life (after Sökeland, Schulze and Rübben).

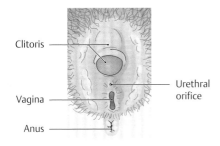

D External genitalia of a women with adrenogenital syndrome

Anterior view. The external genitalia show definite signs of masculinization. The clitoris is markedly enlarged. The labia majora and minora are partially fused, and the urogenital sinus forms an undersized vestibule (see **E**, female pseudohermaphroditism).

E Various forms of intersexuality*

Condition	Features
• True herma-phroditism**	• Very rare form of hermaphroditism (approximately 70% of cases have a female karyotype: 46,XX). The gonads contain both testicular and ovarian tissue *(ototestis)*, but with a preponderance of ovarian tissue. Hence the external genitalia tend to have a female appearance with a markedly enlarged clitoris. A uterus is frequently present. Most hermaphrodites are raised as girls.
• Pseudoherma-phroditism	• The pseudohermaphrodite has a definite chromosomal sex (female: 46,XX or male: 46,XY) but a phenotype of the *opposite* gender. The condition is termed male pseudohermaphroditism when a testis is present and female pseudohermaphroditism when an ovary is present.
– *Male pseudo-hermaphroditism* → Chromosomal sex: male (46,XY) → Phenotype: female	• **Etiology and pathogenesis** The female phenotype results from a lack of fetal androgen exposure: 1. Disturbance of testosterone synthesis 2. Disturbance of testosterone conversion 3. Androgen receptor defect 4. Testicular dysgenesis • **Example: testicular feminization** (1:20000 live births): – 46,XY chromosome complement – Individual has a female phenotype (estrogen synthesis present) but lacks pubic and axillary hair ("hairless woman"). The upper vagina and uterus are also absent. – *Cause:* androgen receptor defect or a disturbance of androgen metabolism (5α-reductase-2 defect) – *Result:* absence of spermatogenesis – *Treatment:* removal of the testes, which are usually in the inguinal region (risk of malignant transformation) and estrogen replacement for life.
– *Female pseudo-hermaphroditism* → Chromosomal sex: female (46,XX) → Phenotype: male	• **Etiology and pathogenesis** The male phenotype results from fetal androgen exposure: 1. Congenital enzyme defect 2. Diaplacental androgen exposure • **Example: congenital adrenogenital syndrome** (1:5000 live births): – 46,XX chromosome complement – Female internal genital organs with masculinized *external* genitalia (enlarged clitoris, partial fusion of the labia majora, small urogenital sinus, see **D**) – *Cause:* adrenocortical hyperplasia with impaired steroid synthesis based on a genetic enzyme defect (most commonly a 21-hydroxylase deficiency). The low hormone level causes increased ACTH secretion, leading to the overproduction of androgens. – *Treatment:* hydrocortisone therapy for life, which may be combined with a mineralocorticoid.

* Intersexuality refers to a condition marked by contradictions in the development of general external sex characteristics, the gonads, and the chromosomal sex.
** Named after *Hermaphroditos,* the androgynous son of Hermes and Aphrodite from Greek mythology.

5.13 Male External Genitalia: Testicular Descent and the Spermatic Cord

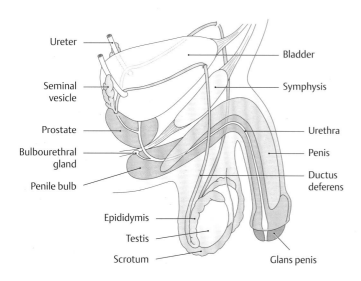

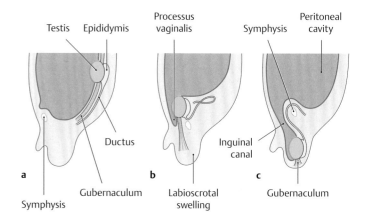

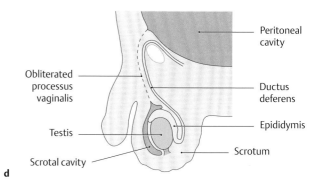

B Descent of the testis

Lateral view.

a Second month, **b** third month, **c** at birth, **d** after obliteration of the processus vaginalis of the peritoneum.

Near the end of the second month of development, the gonads and the rests of the mesonephros lie in a common peritoneal fold (urogenital fold), from which the "gonadal ligaments" are derived after regression of the mesonephros. The lower gonadal ligament, called the gubernaculum, is important for the descent of the testis. It passes below the genital ducts, pierces the abdominal wall in the area of the inguinal canal, and ends in the labioscrotal swelling, an outpouching of the ventral abdominal wall. Traction from this gonadal ligament (a consequence of body growth, which is more rapid than the growth of the genital organs) causes the testis and epididymis to slide downward along the dorsal trunk wall external to the peritoneum **(transabdominal descent)**. By the start of the third month, the testis has already reached the entrance of the future inguinal canal. The processus vaginalis, a funnel-shaped outpouching of peritoneum, forms ventral to the gubernaculum and is continued into the scrotal swelling with the other layers of the abdominal wall. It gives rise to the coverings of the spermatic cord and testis after the testis has completed its descent. A second phase, which is completed shortly before birth **(transinguinal descent)**, culminates in passage of the testis through the inguinal canal into the scrotum. After testicular descent is completed (by birth), the processus vaginalis is obliterated except for a small space that partially surrounds the testis as the scrotal cavity (tunica vaginalis of the testis with a visceral layer and a parietal layer, see p.196). Failure of this process of obliteration results in a persistent communication between the abdominal cavity and testicular cavity (congenital indirect inguinal hernia, see p.186) (after Starck).

A Overview of the male genital organs

The internal and external male genitalia are distinguished by their *origins:* The internal reproductive organs originate from the two urogenital ridges located above the pelvic floor (except for the prostate and Cowper glands, which develop from urethral epithelium and thus are derivatives of the urogenital sinus). By contrast, the external genital organs develop around the urogenital sinus from a genital anlage located below the pelvic floor (see p.192).

Male internal genital organs	Male external genital organs

• Testis
• Epididymis
• Ductus deferens (vas deferens)
• Accessory sex glands
  – Prostate
  – Seminal vesicles
  – Cowper glands (bulbourethral glands)
	• Penis
	• Scrotum
	• Coverings of the testis

Topographically, however, the testis, epididymis, and a portion of the ductus deferens are classified among the external genital organs because they migrate from the abdominal cavity into the scrotum during fetal development (testicular descent).

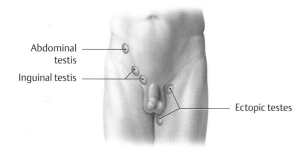

C Anomalous position of the testis

Abnormalities in the descent of the testis occur in approximately 3 % of all newborns. The testis may be retained in the abdominal cavity or in the inguinal canal (cryptorchidism or retained testis). A deficiency of androgen production is the presumed cause. An ectopic testis is one that strays from the normal tract and occupies an abnormal position. The principal results are infertility due to the higher ambient temperature and an increased risk of malignant transformation.

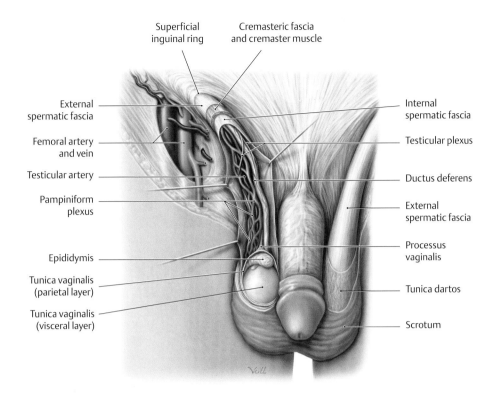

D The penis, scrotum, and spermatic cord
Anterior view. The skin has been partially removed from over the scrotum and spermatic cord. The tunica dartos and external spermatic fascia are exposed on the left side, and the spermatic cord on the right side has been opened in layers. The skin of the scrotum differs in many respects from the skin of the abdominal wall. It is more pigmented, markedly thinner, more mobile, and is devoid of subcutaneous fat. It also contains a network of myofibroblasts (tunica dartos), whose contraction causes a wrinkling of the skin. This reduces the surface area of the scrotum and, when accompanied by vasoconstriction of the cutaneous vessels, reduces heat loss from the testes. This mechanism regulates the temperature to optimize spermatogenesis.

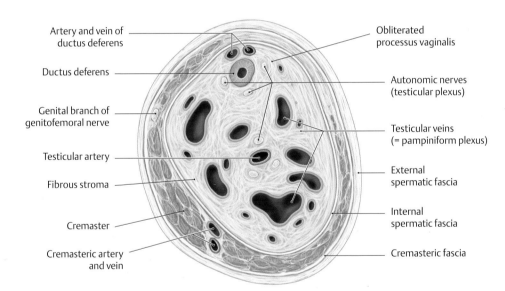

F Comparison of the abdominal wall layers and the corresponding coverings of the testis and spermatic cord
The coverings of the spermatic cord and testis are derived from the muscles and fasciae of the abdominal wall and from the peritoneum. They represent a continuation of the layers of the anterior abdominal wall and enclose the spermatic cord and testis in a pouch formed by the abdominal skin (testicular sac or scrotum).

Abdominal wall layers	Coverings of the spermatic cord and testis
• Abdominal skin	→ Scrotal skin with tunica dartos (myofibroblasts in the dermis)
• External abdominal oblique aponeurosis	→ External spermatic fascia
• Internal oblique muscle	→ Cremaster muscle with cremasteric fascia
• Transversalis fascia	
• Peritoneum	→ Internal spermatic fascia
	→ Tunica vaginalis with visceral layer (epiorchium) and parietal layer (periorchium)

E Contents of the spermatic cord
Cross section through a spermatic cord. The neurovascular structures that supply the testis converge at the level of the deep inguinal ring, forming a bundle the thickness of the small finger that is held together by loose connective tissue and by the coverings of the spermatic cord and testes. The coverings consist of the following structures:

- Cremasteric fascia with the cremaster muscle
- Genital branch of the genitofemoral nerve
- Cremasteric artery and vein
- Ductus deferens
- Artery and vein of the ductus deferens

- Testicular artery
- Testicular veins (pampiniform plexus)
- Autonomic nerve fibers (testicular plexus)
- Lymphatic vessels
- The obliterated processus vaginalis

Special features: The large veins of the pampiniform plexus are exceptionally thick-walled, with a three-layered media, and hence are easily mistaken for arteries. In life the ductus deferens, with its compact muscular wall, is palpable through the skin as a firm cord the thickness of a knitting needle. The ease of surgical access to this site is utilized in *vasectomy* or ligation of the ductus deferens to interrupt the transport of sperm (sterilization).

195

5.14 Male External Genitalia: The Testis and Epididymis

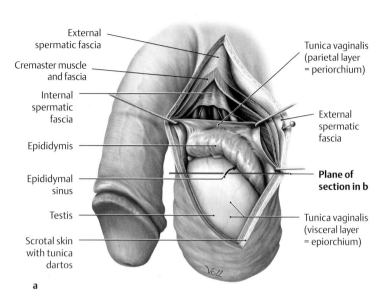

a

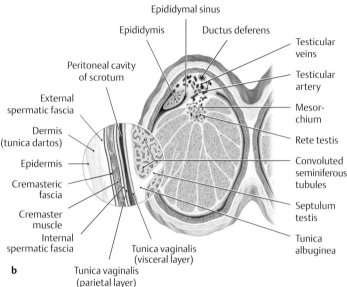

b

A Tunica vaginalis of the testis and peritoneal cavity of the scrotum (serous cavity of the testis)

a Opened tunica vaginalis of the left testis, lateral view.

b Cross section through the testis, epididymis, and scrotum, superior view.

The tunica vaginalis (unobliterated end of the processus vaginalis, see p.195) forms a serous coat surrounding the testis and epididymis. Its visceral layer is fused to the tunica albuginea of the testis. At the mediastinum testis, the *mesorchium* (suspensory ligament where nerves and

vessels enter and leave the testis), the tunica vaginalis is reflected to form the parietal layer, which is covered externally by the internal spermatic fascia. Between the two layers is a slitlike mesothelium-lined space (peritoneal cavity of the scrotum) that contains a scant amount of fluid and is partially continued between the testis and epididymis (epididymal sinus). An abnormal fluid collection in the serous cavity of the scrotum is called a *testicular hydrocele* (see **Fb**) (after Rauber and Kopsch).

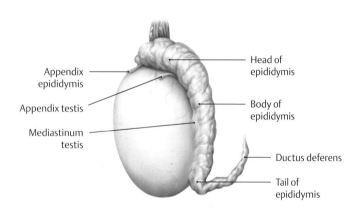

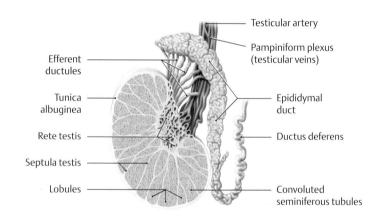

B Surface anatomy of the testis and epididymis

Left testis and epididymis, lateral view. The combined weight of the testis and epididymis at sexual maturity is approximately 20–30 g. The *testis* has an ovoid shape (approximately 5 cm long and 3 cm wide) and an average volume of approximately 18 mL (12–20 mL). The testicular tissue is enclosed in a tough fibrous capsule (tunica albuginea) and has a rubbery consistency. The *epididymis* consists of a head, which is attached to the upper pole of the testis, and a body and tail that curve down along the mediastinum on the posterior side of the testis. The tail of the epididymis becomes continuous with the ductus deferens at the lower pole of the testis.

C Structure of the testis and epididymis

Section through the testis (epididymis intact), lateral view. Fibrous septa (septula testis) extend radially from the tunica albuginea of the testis toward the mediastinum testis, subdividing the testicular tissue into approximately 370 wedge-shaped lobules. Each lobule contains one or more convoluted seminiferous tubules, in whose epithelium the spermatocytes are formed (spermatogenesis, see p. 4) and which open into the rete testis. From there, approximately 10–15 efferent ductules pass to the head of the epididymis, where the epididymal duct begins. This single duct is continuous distally with the ductus deferens, which passes through the inguinal canal in the spermatic cord to enter the abdominal cavity and opens into the prostatic part of the urethra via a short intervening segment, the ejaculatory duct (see p.199).

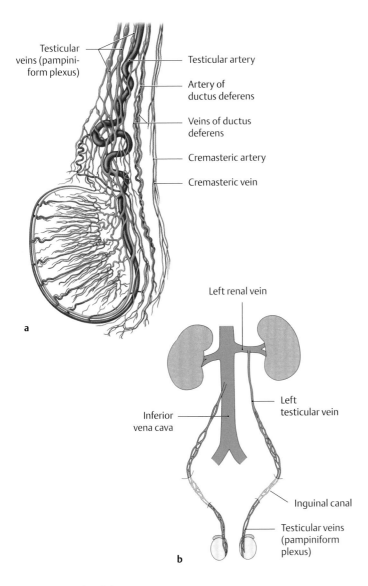

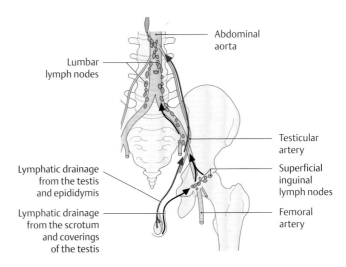

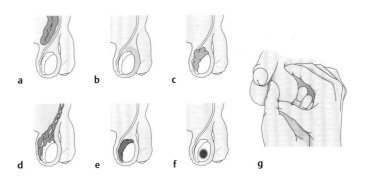

D Blood supply of the testis

a Arterial supply: The testis, epididymis, and their coverings are supplied by three different arteries, which anastomose with one another (after Hundeiker and Keller, quoted in Rauber and Kopsch):

- Testicular artery: arises directly from the aorta
- Artery of the ductus deferens: from the internal iliac artery
- Cremasteric artery: from the inferior epigastric artery

The vessels supplying the scrotum arise from the internal pudendal artery (see p. 496).

b Different venous drainage patterns of the right and left testes: Venous blood from the testis and epididymis flows into the testicular veins in the area of the mediastinum testis. These veins form an elongated venous network, especially distally, called the pampiniform plexus. It surrounds the branches of the testicular artery and ascends with it through the inguinal canal into the retroperitoneum. There the *right* testicular vein empties into the inferior vena cava, while the *left* testicular vein opens into the left renal vein. This asymmetry of venous drainage has major clinical relevance: The left testicular vein enters the left renal vein at a right angle. This creates a physiologically significant constriction that can obstruct venous outflow from the left testicular vein and thus from the pampiniform plexus (varicocele, see **Fd**). In this case the pampiniform plexus can no longer perform its "thermostat" function (cooling venous blood returning from the testicular artery), resulting in a local heat buildup that may compromise the fertility of the left testis.

E Lymphatic drainage and regional lymph nodes of the testis, the epididymis, the coverings of the testis, and the scrotum

The lymphatic vessels of the testis and epididymis drain to the lumbar lymph nodes, accompanied by the testicular vessels. The regional nodes that receive lymph from the scrotum and the coverings of the testis are the superficial inguinal nodes (see p. 468).

Note: Advanced testicular tumors tend to metastasize to retroperitoneal lymph nodes because they serve as the primary lymphatic conduit from the testis and epididymis.

F Abnormal findings on clinical examination of the external genitalia

a–f Diseases that may present with scrotal swelling: a inguinal hernia, **b** testicular hydrocele (serous fluid collection in the serous cavity), **c** spermatocele (retention cyst in the epididymis), **d** varicocele (painful, varicose dilatation of the pampiniform plexus), **e** epididymitis (painful bacterial inflammation of the epididymis), **f** testicular tumor (painless, usually unilateral induration of the testis).

g Bimanual examination of the testis and epididymis: Clinical examination of the external genitalia should include palpation of the testis and epididymis (bimanual examination). Based on the disease features noted above, the following questions should be addressed during the clinical examination:

- Is the mass confined to the scrotum?
- Is there transient enlargement of the mass when the patient coughs?
- Is the mass translucent when examined by *transillumination* (illumination with a flashlight)?
- Is the mass painless or tender to pressure?

Note: A painless induration of the testis, especially in young men, should always raise suspicion of a testicular tumor (after Sökeland, Schulze, and Rübben).

5.15 Male External Genitalia: The Fasciae and Erectile Tissues of the Penis

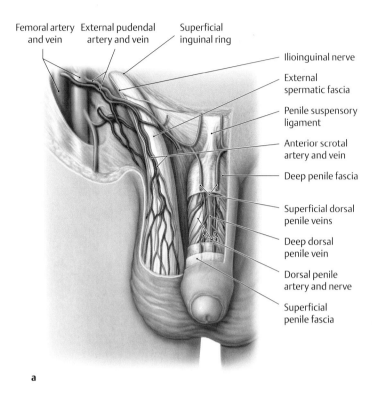

Femoral artery and vein
External pudendal artery and vein
Superficial inguinal ring

Ilioinguinal nerve

External spermatic fascia

Penile suspensory ligament

Anterior scrotal artery and vein

Deep penile fascia

Superficial dorsal penile veins

Deep dorsal penile vein

Dorsal penile artery and nerve

Superficial penile fascia

a

A Arrangement of the penile fasciae
a Anterior view of the penis (skin and fasciae partially removed).
b Right lateral view of the penis (skin and fasciae partially removed).
c Cross section through the shaft of the penis.

The penis is covered by thin, mobile skin that is devoid of fatty tissue. The skin over the glans penis is duplicated to form the prepuce (foreskin), which is attached to the undersurface of the glans by the median fold of the frenulum (see **b**). The erectile tissues of the penis are surrounded by a common, strong envelope of collagenous fibers, the *tunica albuginea.* The two layers of the penile fascia (superficial and deep) also surround the corpus spongiosum and corpora cavernosa. The erectile tissues, their fibrous sheaths, and the way in which the vessels are incorporated into these fibrous structures are of key interest in understanding the function of the penis (see p. 201).

Superficial penile fascia
Superficial dorsal penile vein
Dorsal penile artery and nerve, branch of the deep dorsal penile vein
Prepuce
Corona glandis
Glans penis
External urethral orifice
Frenulum
Penile skin
Deep penile fascia
Corpus cavernosum and corpus spongiosum with tunica albuginea

b

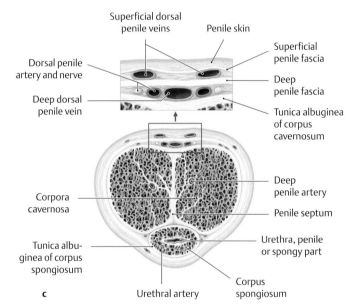

Superficial dorsal penile veins
Penile skin
Dorsal penile artery and nerve
Superficial penile fascia
Deep penile fascia
Deep dorsal penile vein
Tunica albuginea of corpus cavernosum
Corpora cavernosa
Deep penile artery
Penile septum
Tunica albuginea of corpus spongiosum
Urethra, penile or spongy part
Corpus spongiosum
Urethral artery

c

B Constriction of the prepuce (phimosis)
a Constriction of the prepuce in a 3-year-old boy.
b Appearance following circumcision.

The epithelium of the inner layer of the prepuce is adherent to the surface epithelium of the glans penis in newborns and infants. Because of this, the distal junction of the outer and inner layers of the prepuce is normally constricted, a condition characterized as **physiological phimosis**. During the first two years of life, the epithelial attachments become separated due to enlargement of the glans and the secretion of smegma (cellular debris sloughed from the stratified keratinized epithelium). If the pre-

puce still cannot slide over the glans by 3 years of age due to a functional stenosis (e.g., persistent epithelial attachments due to an absence of smegma secretion), the phimosis should be surgically corrected by circumcision. This procedure may be conservative or radical, resecting all the foreskin (as shown here), depending on the severity of the phimosis. Immediate surgical intervention (before 3 years of age) is necessary for **paraphimosis**—an emergency situation in which the glans is strangulated by the narrowed foreskin (painful, livid swelling of the glans due to decreased blood flow, with risk of necrosis) (after Sökeland, Schulze, and Rübben).

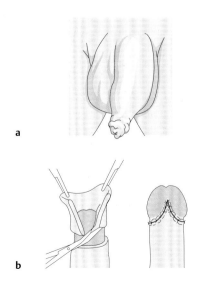

a

b

C The erectile tissues and erectile muscles of the penis

a Inferior view. The corpus spongiosum is partially mobilized, and the skin and fasciae have been removed. The ischiocavernosus and bulbospongiosus muscles have been removed on the left side along with the inferior fascia of the urogenital diaphragm.

b Cross section through the root of the penis. The root (radix) of the penis is firmly attached to the perineal membrane and pelvic skeleton. It is distinguished from the freely mobile shaft (body) of the penis, with its dorsal and urethral surfaces, and from the glans penis, which bears the external urethral orifice. The penis contains two types of erectile tissue:

• The paired corpora cavernosa
• The unpaired corpus spongiosum

At the root of the penis, each of the corpora cavernosa tapers to form a crus penis. Between the two crura lies the thickened end of the corpus spongiosum, the bulb of the penis. The glans penis forms the distal end of the corpus spongiosum. Its posterior margin is broadened to form the corona, which is turned over the ends of the corpora cavernosa. The erectile tissues receive their blood supply from branches of the internal pudendal artery, which branches in the deep perineal space (see pp. 155 and 200).

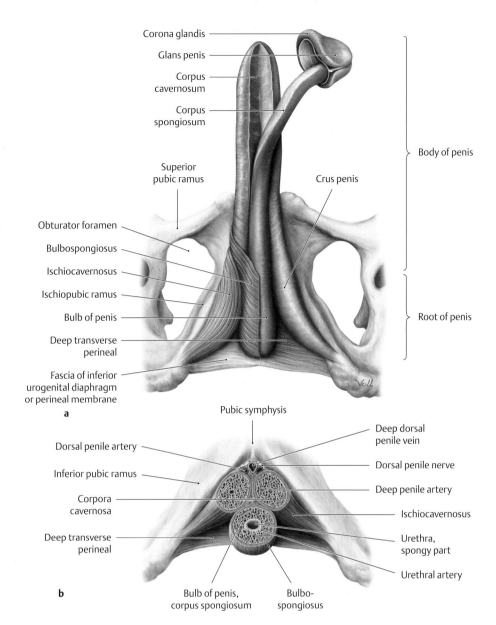

a

b

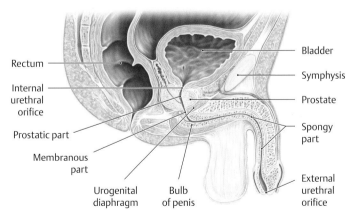

D Course of the male urethra
Midsagittal section through a male pelvis. The male urethra consists of a prostatic part, a membranous part, and a penile or spongy part named for different regions of the pelvis and external genitalia (see p. 193). The spongy part begins below the urogenital diaphragm at the bulb of the corpus spongiosum and terminates at the external urethral orifice.

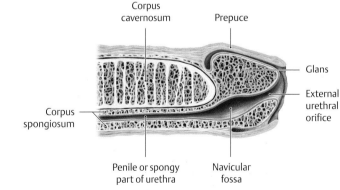

E Midsagittal section through the distal penis
The spongy part of the urethra undergoes an approximately 2-cm-long fusiform dilatation within the glans penis. In this area, the navicular fossa, the stratified columnar epithelium of the urethra gives way to stratified, nonkeratinized squamous epithelium. The upper cell layers of this epithelium are rich in glycogen, which—as in the vaginal milieu in females—provides a culture medium for the lactic acid bacteria that thrive there (acidic pH protects against pathogenic organisms).

199

5.16 Male External Genitalia: Nerves and Vessels of the Penis

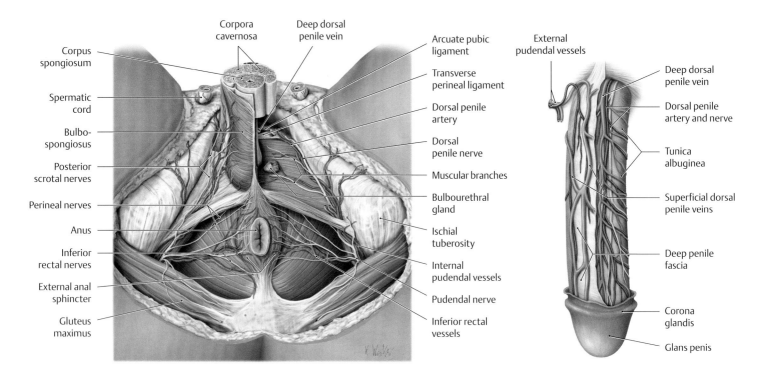

A Neurovascular structures of the male perineal region

Lithotomy position with the scrotum removed, inferior view. The superficial perineal space on the right side has been opened by removing the superficial perineal fascia. The erectile muscles and root of the penis have been removed on the left side, and the deep perineal space is partially exposed. The penis has been transected across the shaft, and the spermatic cords have been divided.

B Dorsal vessels and nerves of the penis

The prepuce, skin, and superficial fascia have been completely removed from the penile shaft. The deep penile fascia has also been removed from the left dorsum.

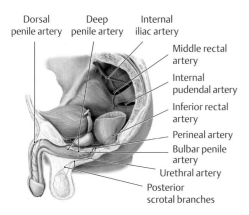

C Arterial supply to the penis and scrotum

Left lateral view. The penis and scrotum derive their arterial supply from the internal pudendal artery. This vessel enters the ischioanal fossa and, after giving off the inferior rectal artery to the anus, courses to the posterior border of the urogenital diaphragm. Then, after giving off the perineal artery, it passes through the deep perineal space into the superficial perineal space (see p.155) where it divides into its terminal branches: the dorsal penile artery, deep penile artery, bulbar penile artery, and urethral artery.

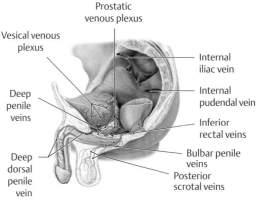

D Venous drainage of the penis and scrotum

Left lateral view. The veins of the penis (especially the deep dorsal penile vein and its tributaries the deep penile and bulbar penile veins) open initially into the internal pudendal vein and then into the prostatic venous plexus. Exceptions are the superficial dorsal penile veins (not seen here), which drain via the external pudendal veins into the long saphenous vein. On its way to the prostatic venous plexus, the deep dorsal penile vein passes through a narrow space just below the symphysis between the arcuate pubic ligament and the transverse perineal ligament (see ligaments in **A**).

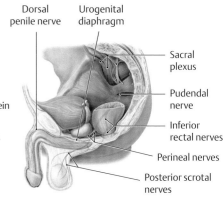

E Nerve supply to the penis and scrotum

Left lateral view. The pudendal nerve enters the ischioanal fossa and, after giving off the inferior rectal nerves, courses to the external anal sphincter and to the skin of the anus at the posterior border of the urogenital diaphragm. There it divides into its terminal branches, the perineal nerves. The superficial branches pass through the superficial perineal space to the skin of the perineum and posterior scrotum (posterior scrotal branches). The deep branches course in the deep perineal space. They innervate the erectile muscles (via muscular branches), the skin of the penis, and the erectile bodies (via the dorsal penile nerve). The course of the autonomic fibers is shown in **F**.

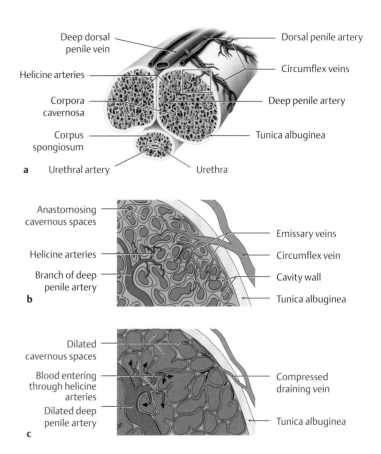

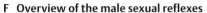

F Overview of the male sexual reflexes

The sexual reflexes in males are evoked by a variety of stimuli (e.g., tactile, visual, olfactory, acoustic, and psychogenic). Somatic and autonomic nerve pathways transmit the stimulus to the erection and ejaculation centers in the thoracolumbar and sacral spinal cord, from which it is relayed to higher centers (e.g., the hypothalamus and limbic system). For example, *tactile cutaneous stimuli* to the genitalia are transmitted to the sacral cord by *afferent somatic* fibers (dorsal penile nerve from the pudendal nerve, shown in green), and are relayed in the erection center (S2–S4) to *efferent parasympathetic* fibers (pelvic splanchnic nerves, shown in blue). These impulses, which stimulate vasodilation of the arteries supplying the erectile tissues (see **G**), are critically influenced by descending pathways from higher centers. Conversely, the excitatory impulses evoked by increasing mechanical stimulation of the glans penis ascend from the sacral cord to the ejaculation center located at the T12–L2 levels. There they are relayed to *efferent sympathetic* fibers (hypogastric nerves, shown in purple) and stimulate smooth muscle contractions in the epididymis, ductus deferens, prostate, and seminal vesicles. Simultaneous stimulation of the erectile muscles by efferent *somatic* nerve fibers (perineal nerves from the pudendal nerve, shown in red) produces rhythmic contractions that expel the ejaculate from the urethra (emission). Failure to achieve an erection, despite an active libido (psychological interest in sexual activity), is defined as erectile dysfunction. The recent development of successful medical treatment of *erectile dysfunction* with sildenafil (Viagra [Pfizer]) is based on its modulation of the second messenger cyclic guanosine monophosphate (cGMP). When the primary messenger nitrous oxide (NO) is released by neural stimulation, it activates the enzyme guanylate cyclase in penile erectile tissues. This enzyme generates cGMP as a second messenger, which in turn induces vasodilation and produces an erection. Sildenafil selectively inhibits cGMP breakdown by a specific phosphodiesterase (PDE5) that is prominent in erectile tissue. cGMP accumulates, vessels remain dilated, and penile erection is sustained. Sildenafil treatment thus effectively amplifies the initial neural stimuli, with the potential of prolonging normal erections and overcoming other, inhibitory physiological problems (after Klinke and Silbernagl).

G Mechanism of penile erection (after Lehnert)
a Penis in cross section, showing the blood vessels involved in erection (enlarged views in **b** and **c**).
b Corpus cavernosum in the flaccid state.
c Corpus cavernosum in the erect state.

Penile erection is based essentially on *maximum engorgement* and pressure elevation in the cavities (cavernous spaces) of the corpora cavernosa combined with a *constriction of venous outflow*. This mechanism raises the intracavernous blood pressure to approximately 10 times the normal systolic blood pressure (approximately 1200 mmHg in young men). Microscopically, the erectile tissue of the penis consists of an arborized trabecular meshwork of connective-tissue and smooth-muscle cells that is connected to the tunica albuginea. Among the trabeculae are interanastomosing cavities that are lined with endothelium. Branches of the deep penile artery, called the helicine arteries, open into these cavities. In the flaccid state, the helicine arteries are more or less occluded by "intimal pads." When an erection occurs, the afferent arteries dilate and the helicine arteries open under the influence of the autonomic nervous system. The result is that with each pulse wave, blood is forced into the cavernous spaces, increasing the volume of the erectile tissue, and raising the intracavitary pressure. The tunica albuginea, which has a limited capacity for distension, becomes taut and compresses the veins that pass through it. This mechanism, aided by the occlusion of emissary veins, causes a constriction of venous outflow, enabling the penis to remain stiff and hard. Meanwhile the dense venous plexuses in the corpus spongiosum and glans prevent excessive compression of the urethra. The flaccid phase begins with vasoconstriction of the afferent arteries. An undesired, prolonged, and painful erection is called *priapism* (from Priapus, the Greco-Roman god of procreation) and may occur, for example, in certain blood diseases or metabolic disorders. The initial treatment of this condition is medical; one option is the use of vasoconstrictors (etilefrine or norepinephrine). Surgical treatment involves making "punch anastomoses" to promote the outflow of blood.

5.17 Female External Genitalia: Overview and Episiotomy

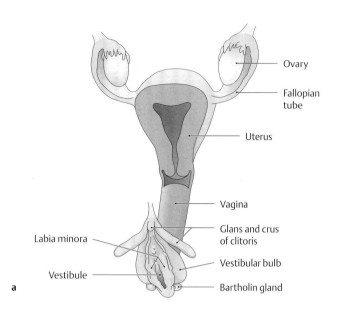

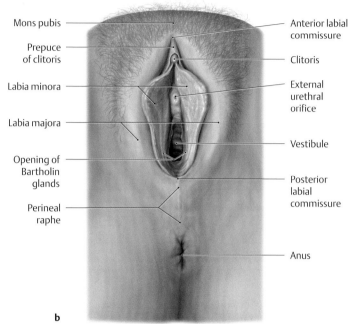

A Overview of the female genital organs
a Internal and some external genital organs.
b External genitalia, lithotomy position with the labia minora separated.

As in males, a distinction is drawn between the development and the topography of the female internal and external reproductive organs. The homology in the development of the male and female genital organs is reflected chiefly in the comparable histological features of the corresponding parts (see textbooks of histology). The female external genitalia (pudendum) is also known in clinical parlance as the *vulva*. It is separated from the internal genital organs by the *hymen* (not shown here). The outer boundaries of the vulva are formed by the mons pubis, a fatty-fleshy prominence over the pubic symphysis, and the labia majora, two pigmented ridges of skin that contain smooth muscle cells as well as sebaceous glands, sweat glands, and scent glands. The labia majora are interconnected anteriorly and posteriorly by a bridge of tissue called the anterior or posterior labial commissure. The area between the posterior commissure and anus is the perineal raphe. Specific structures are listed in the table at right.

Female internal genital organs	Female external genital organs (vulva)

• Ovary
 • Fallopian tube
 • Uterus
 • Vagina
	• Mons pubis
	 • Labia majora
	 • Labia minora
	 • Vestibule of vagina
	 • Vestibular bulb
	 • Clitoris
	 • Vestibular glands
	    – Greater vestibular glands (Bartholin glands)
	    – Lesser vestibular glands

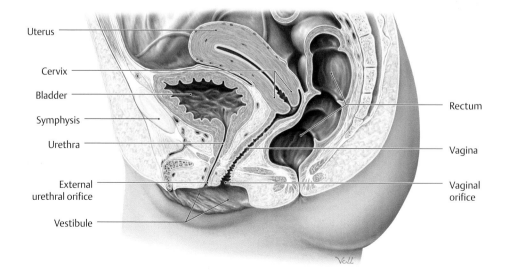

B Midsagittal section through a female pelvis
Left lateral view.
Note the close proximity of the external urethral orifice to the vaginal orifice, which opens into the vestibule.

Bulbospon-giosus

Lateral episiotomy

Midline episiotomy

Ischio-cavernosus

Deep transverse perineal

Superficial transverse perineal

Obturatorius internus

Levator ani

Perineum

Anus

Mediolateral episiotomy

b

Posterior commissure

External anal sphincter

Gluteus maximus

a

c

C Episiotomy: indications and technique
a Pelvic floor with crowning of the fetal head.
b Types of episiotomy: midline, mediolateral, lateral.
c Mediolateral episiotomy performed at the height of a contraction.

Episiotomy is a common obstetric procedure utilized to enlarge the birth canal during the expulsive stage of labor (see p. 482). When the fetal head crowns through the pelvic floor, the levator ani muscle in particular is passively stretched, forced downward, and rotated approximately 90°. The "levator plate" thus helps to form the wall of the distal birth canal along with the urogenital diaphragm and bulbospongiosus muscle. As such, it comes under considerable tension at the perineal body during the pushing stage of labor. To protect the perineal muscles from tearing, the obstetrician counteracts this tension by supporting the perineum with two fingers *(perineal protection)*. An *episiotomy* is often performed to prevent uncontrolled laceration of the perineum (maternal indication). There is an imminent danger of perineal laceration during the delivery when the perineal skin is stretched to the point that it turns white, indicating diminished blood flow. The primary purpose of an episiotomy, however, is to expedite the delivery of a baby

that is at risk for hypoxia during the expulsive stage. An *early episiotomy* is one that is made before the head crowns (the head is visible with contractions and pushing but recedes between contractions). A *timely episiotomy* is made after the head has crowned, when there is maximum tension on the perineal skin. Three types of episiotomy are available (see **D** for advantages and disadvantages):

- **Midline episiotomy:** straight down from the vagina toward the anus
- **Mediolateral episiotomy:** oblique incision from the posterior commissure
- **Lateral episiotomy:** lateral incision from the lower third of the vulva

After the placenta is delivered, the episiotomy is usually closed in at least three layers (vaginal suture, deep perineal suture, and cutaneous suture). Local anesthesia is generally required, especially when an early episiotomy has been done. If the episiotomy was made at the height of a contraction after crowning of the head, anesthesia is unnecessary. Local infiltration anesthesia and the pudendal block (PDB) are described on p. 482.

D Advantages and disadvantages of the different types of episiotomy (after Goerke)

Episiotomy	Divided muscles	Advantages	Disadvantages
• Midline	• None	• Easy to repair • Heals well	• May lengthen to a grade III perineal laceration
• Medio-lateral	• Bulbospongiosus • Superficial transverse perineal	• Gains more room • Low risk of laceration	• Heavier bleeding • More difficult to repair • More difficult healing
• Lateral*	• Bulbospongiosus • Superficial transverse perineal • Levator ani (puborectalis)	• Gains the most room	• Heaviest bleeding • Potential complications (e.g., anal incontinence) • Greatest postpartum complaints
* Very rarely used			

5.18 Female External Genitalia: Neurovascular Structures, Erectile Tissues, Erectile Muscles, and Vestibule

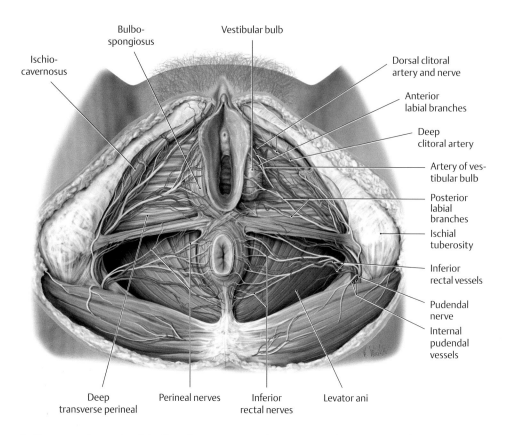

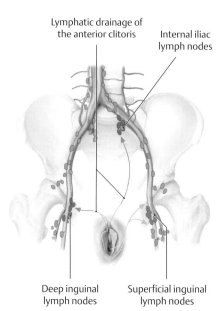

A Nerves and vessels of the female perineal region

Lithotomy position. The labia majora, skin, superficial perineal fascia, and fatty tissue in the ischioanal fossa have been removed to demonstrate the neurovascular structures. The bulbospongiosus and ischiocavernosus muscles and the inferior fascia of the urogenital diaphragm have also been dissected away on the left side.

B Lymphatic drainage of the female external genitalia

Female pelvis, anterior view. Lymph from the female external genitalia drains to the superficial inguinal lymph nodes. The only exceptions are the anterior portions of the clitoris (body and glans), which drain to the deep inguinal and internal iliac lymph nodes.

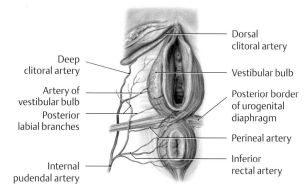

C Arterial supply to the female external genitalia

Perineal region, inferior view. The female external genitalia, like the penis and scrotum, are supplied by the internal pudendal artery, which enters the ischioanal fossa (not seen here). After giving off the inferior rectal artery to the anus, the internal pudendal artery passes to the posterior border of the urogenital diaphragm. Another branch, the perineal artery, supplies the perineal region, the erectile muscles, and the *posterior part* of the labia majora (posterior labial branches). In the superficial perineal space (not visible here, see p.155), the internal pudendal artery divides into its terminal branches, the artery of the vestibular bulb and the deep and dorsal clitoral arteries (which supply the corpus cavernosum of the clitoris). The *anterior part* of the labia majora is supplied by the external pudendal arteries (anterior labial branches), which arise from the femoral artery (not seen here).

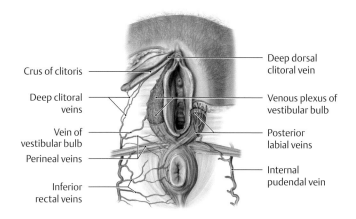

D Venous drainage of the female external genitalia

Venous drainage is handled by the following vessels:

- The deep clitoral veins, posterior labial veins, and vein of the vestibular bulb, which drain into the *internal pudendal vein*
- The superficial dorsal clitoral veins and anterior labial veins, which drain into the *external pudendal veins* (not seen here)
- The deep dorsal clitoral vein, which drains into the *vesical venous plexus*

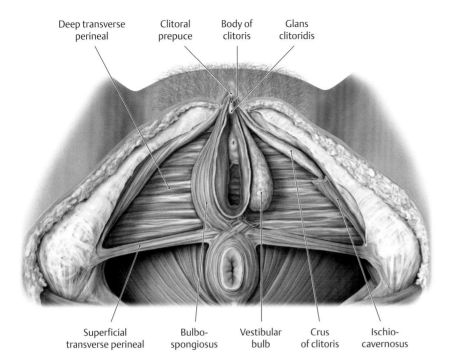

Deep transverse perineal — Clitoral prepuce — Body of clitoris — Glans clitoridis

Superficial transverse perineal — Bulbo-spongiosus — Vestibular bulb — Crus of clitoris — Ischio-cavernosus

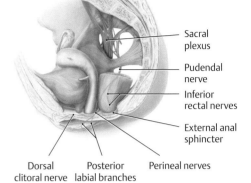

Sacral plexus — Pudendal nerve — Inferior rectal nerves — External anal sphincter

Dorsal clitoral nerve — Posterior labial branches — Perineal nerves

E Erectile tissues and erectile muscles in the female

Perineal region, lithotomy position. The labia majora and minora, skin, and superficial perineal fascia have been removed, as well as the erectile muscles on the left side.

Erectile tissues: The erectile tissues of the *clitoris* are distributed around both of its crura and its short shaft (body). They correspond to the erectile tissues in the male and are named accordingly: the right and left *corpora cavernosa of the clitoris,* homologous to the corpora cavernosa of the penis. The swelling at the end of the clitoral shaft is called the glans clitori-

dis, homologous to the glans penis. Its sensory innervation is like that of the penile glans, and it is mostly covered by a clitoral prepuce. The erectile tissue of the *labia minora* is located in the hairless, fat-free skin folds of the labia minora and is termed the *vestibular bulb,* which is the homologue of the corpus spongiosum in the male.

Erectile muscles: The two crura by which the clitoris arises from the inferior pubic ramus on each side are covered by the *ischiocavernosus* muscle, and the dense erectile venous plexus at the base of the labia is covered by the *bulbospongiosus.*

F Nerve supply to the female external genitalia

Lesser pelvis, left lateral view. The pudendal nerve enters the ischioanal fossa. After giving off the inferior rectal nerves to the external anal sphincter and anal skin, it courses to the posterior border of the urogenital diaphragm, where it divides into its terminal branches (perineal nerves). The *superficial branches* pass through the superficial perineal space (not seen here) to the skin of the perineum and the posterior portions of the labia majora (posterior labial branches). The *deep branches* course in the deep perineal space, distributing muscular branches to the erectile muscles and the dorsal clitoral nerve to the clitoris. The anterior portions of the labia majora are supplied by anterior labial branches from the ilioinguinal nerve (not seen here).

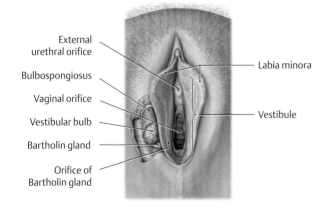

External urethral orifice — Bulbospongiosus — Vaginal orifice — Vestibular bulb — Bartholin gland — Orifice of Bartholin gland

Labia minora — Vestibule

G The vestibule and vestibular glands

Lithotomy position with the labia separated. The vestibule, bounded by the labia minora, contains the external openings of the urethra and vagina (external urethral orifice and vaginal orifice) and the vestibular glands. The *lesser vestibular glands* (not seen here) have numerous openings near the external urethral orifice, while the paired *greater vesti-*

bular glands (Bartholin glands) each open by a 1-cm-long duct at the posterior border of the vestibular bulb on the inner surface of the labia minora. The lesser vestibular glands are homologous to the urethral glands in the male, and the greater vestibular glands to the bulbourethral glands. The vestibular glands produce a mucous secretion that moistens the vestibule and reduces friction during coitus, preventing epithelial injury. Next to the external urethral orifice are two short, blind, rudimentary excretory ducts called paraurethral ducts (*Skene ducts,* not shown here). They correspond developmentally to the male prostate but have no known function in the female. Like the vestibular glands, however, they are susceptible to bacterial colonization. Bacterial colonization of the greater vestibular glands (Bartholin glands) can lead to *bartholinitis,* a painful inflammation with swelling and redness. An inflammation that occludes the excretory ducts of the glands can produce a painful *retention cyst,* which should be opened or removed.

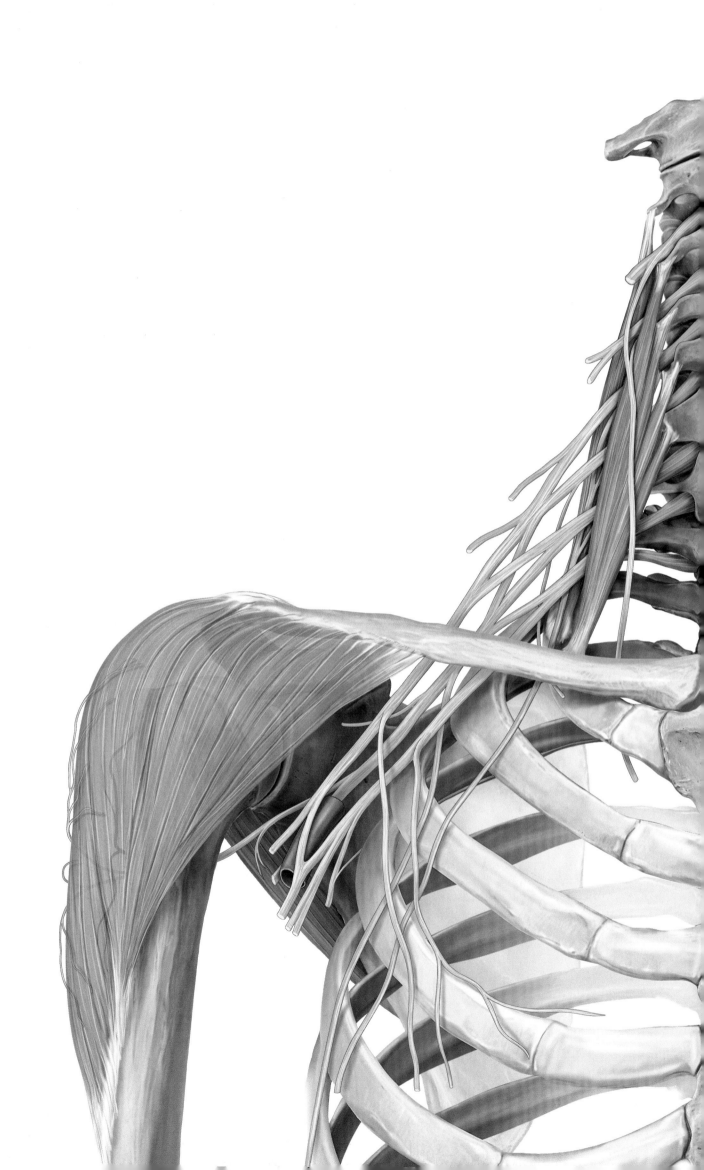

The Upper Limb

1.1 The Upper Limb as a Whole

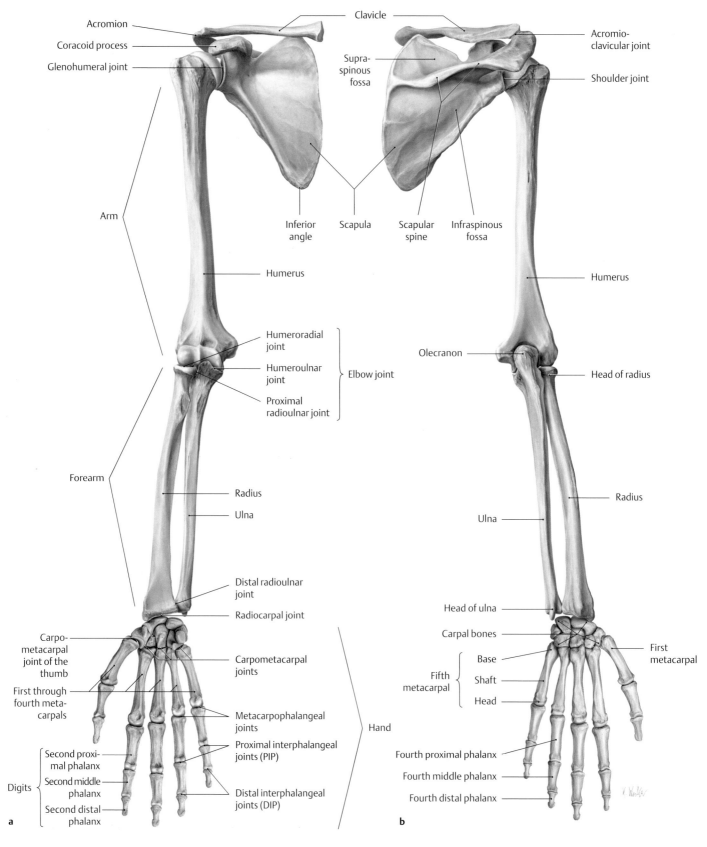

A Skeleton of the right upper limb

a Anterior view, **b** posterior view.

The skeleton of the upper limb consists of the shoulder girdle, arm, forearm, wrist and hand. The shoulder girdle (clavicle and scapula) is joined to the upper limb at the shoulder joint, and it joins the upper limb to

the thorax at the sternoclavicular joint (see p. 227). The limb itself consists of the:

- arm,
- forearm, and
- hand.

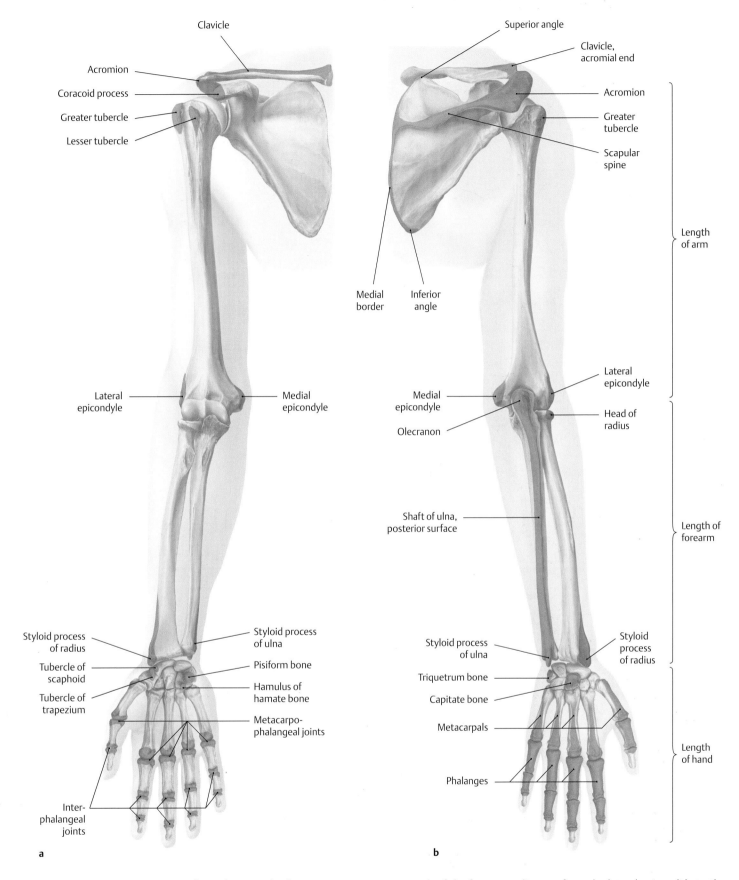

Clavicle

Acromion

Coracoid process

Greater tubercle

Lesser tubercle

Lateral epicondyle

Medial epicondyle

Styloid process of radius

Styloid process of ulna

Tubercle of scaphoid

Pisiform bone

Tubercle of trapezium

Hamulus of hamate bone

Metacarpo-phalangeal joints

Inter-phalangeal joints

a

Superior angle

Clavicle, acromial end

Acromion

Greater tubercle

Scapular spine

Medial border

Inferior angle

Length of arm

Lateral epicondyle

Medial epicondyle

Head of radius

Olecranon

Shaft of ulna, posterior surface

Length of forearm

Styloid process of ulna

Styloid process of radius

Triquetrum bone

Capitate bone

Metacarpals

Phalanges

Length of hand

b

B Palpable bony prominences on the right upper limb
a Anterior view, **b** posterior view.
Except for the lunate and trapezoid bones, all of the bones in the upper limb are palpable to some degree through the skin and soft tissues. By consensus, standard reference points have been defined for use in measuring the lengths of the segments of the dependent limb (with the palm turned forward):

- Length of the arm = distance from the acromion to the lateral epicondyle

- Length of the forearm = distance from the lateral epicondyle to the styloid process of the radius
- Length of the hand = distance from the styloid process of the radius to the tip of the third finger

The segment lengths of the limb may be measured, for example, to aid in the precise evaluation of isolated pediatric growth disturbances that are confined to a particular bone.

1.2 Integration of the Shoulder Girdle into the Skeleton of the Trunk

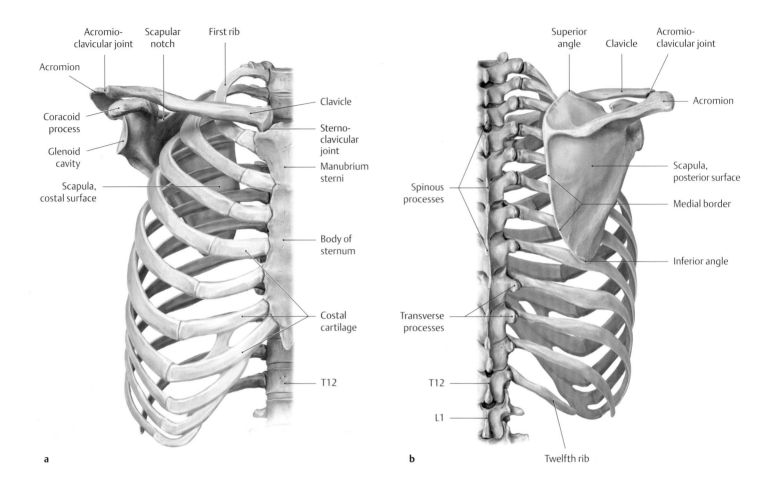

a

b

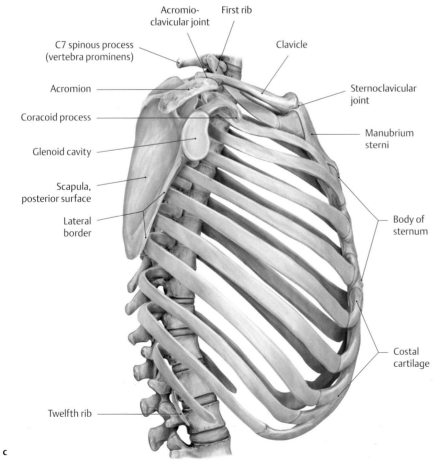

c

A Bones of the right shoulder girdle in their normal relation to the skeleton of the trunk

a Anterior view, **b** posterior view, **c** lateral view.

The two bones of the shoulder girdle (the clavicle and scapula) are connected at the acromioclavicular joint (see p. 227). In its normal anatomical position, the scapula extends from the second to the seventh rib. The inferior angle of the scapula is level with the spinous process of the seventh thoracic vertebra, and the scapular spine is level with the spinous process of the third thoracic vertebra. When the scapula occupies a normal position, its long axis is angled slightly laterally and its medial border forms a 3–5° angle with the midsagittal plane.

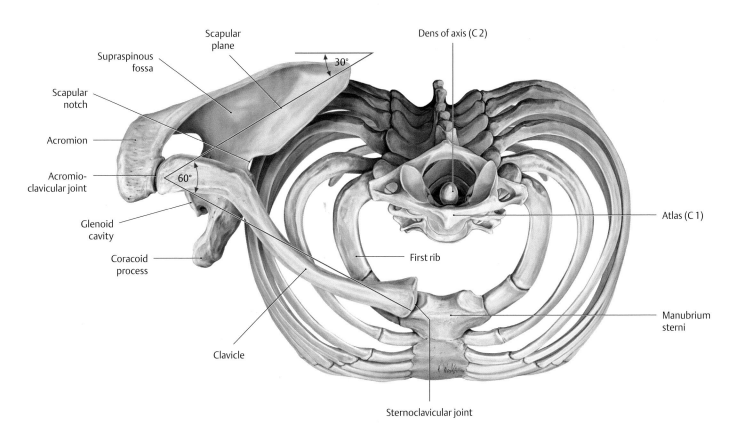

B Right shoulder girdle

Superior view. With the transition to a bipedal mode of locomotion, the human scapula moved from the more lateral placement in quadruped mammals to a more *posterior* position, and also a more frontal orientation, on the back of the thorax. Viewed from above, the scapula forms a 30° angle with the coronal plane. The scapula and clavicle subtend an angle of approximately 60°. Because of this arrangement, the two shoulder joints are angled slightly forward, shifting the range of arm movements forward into the field of vision and action. This reorientation in humans creates the opportunity for visual control of manual manipulations (hand–eye coordination).

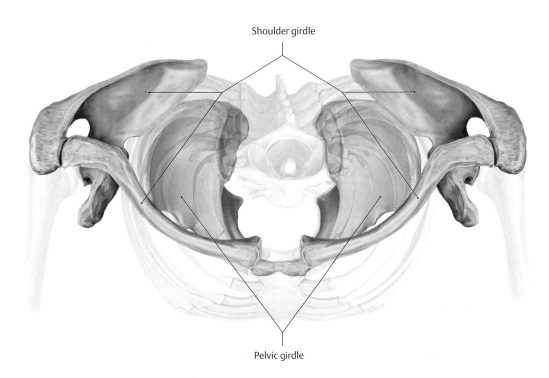

C Comparison of the shoulder girdle and pelvic girdle in their relation to the skeleton of the trunk

Superior view. Unlike the very mobile shoulder girdle, the pelvic girdle, consisting of the paired hip (innominate) bones, is firmly integrated into the axial skeleton. As the trunk assumes an upright position, the pelvis moves over the weight-bearing surface of the feet, making it necessary for the pelvis to support the total weight of the trunk. This basically limits the lower limbs to functions of locomotion and support while freeing the upper limbs from these tasks and making them a versatile organ of movement and expression that is particularly useful for touching and grasping.

211

1.3 The Bones of the Shoulder Girdle

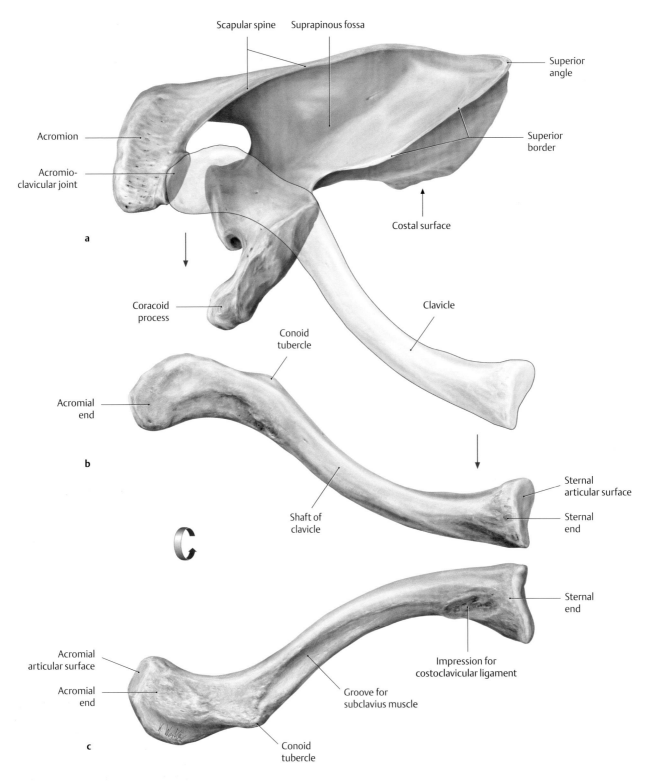

A Position and shape of the right clavicle
a Clavicle in its normal relation to the scapula, superior view.
b Isolated clavicle, superior view.
c Isolated clavicle, inferior view.

The clavicle is an S-shaped bone, approximately 12–15 cm long in adults, that is visible and palpable beneath the skin along its entire length. The medial or *sternal end* of the clavicle bears a saddle-shaped articular surface, while the lateral or *acromial end* has a flatter, more vertical articular surface. The clavicle is the *only* bone in the limbs that is not preformed in cartilage during embryonic development; instead, it ossifies directly from *connective tissue* (membranous ossi-

fication). A congenital failure or abnormality in the development of this connective tissue results in an anomaly called *cleidocranial dysostosis*. There may be associated ossification defects in the cranial vault, which are also formed by membranous ossification (*craniofacial dysostosis*). Besides fractures due to obstetric trauma (1–2% of all newborns), fractures of the middle third of the clavicle are one of the most common fractures that are sustained by children and adults (in children, some 50% of all clavicular fractures occur before six years of age).

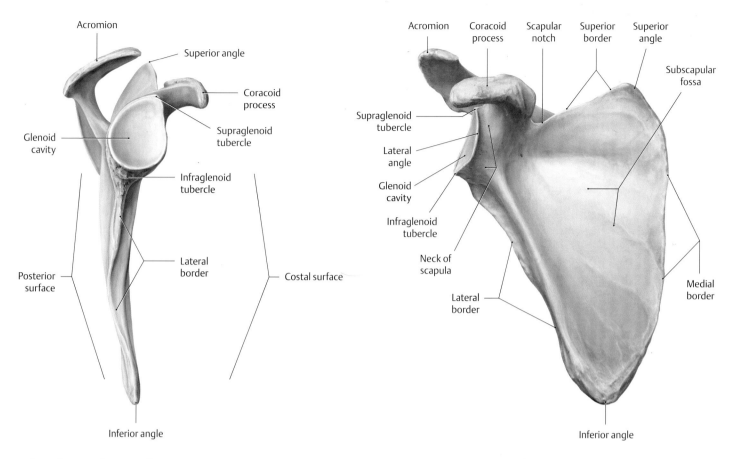

B The right scapula. Lateral view

C The right scapula. Anterior view

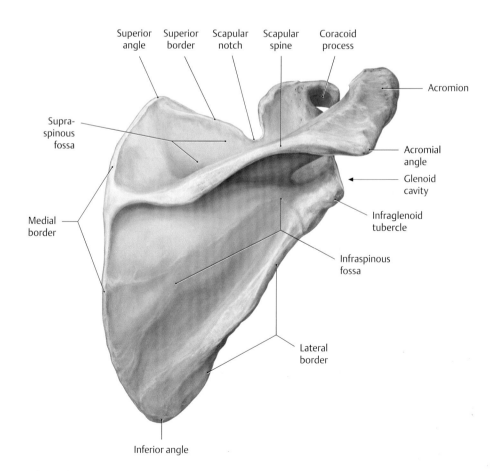

D The right scapula. Posterior view

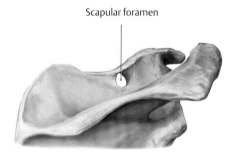

E The scapular foramen

The superior transverse ligament of the scapula (see p. 233) can become ossified, transforming the scapular notch into an anomalous bony canal referred to as a *scapular foramen*. This can lead to compression of the suprascapular nerve as it passes through this canal (see p. 340). Active rotational movements of the shoulder aggravate the nerve pressure, leading to significant symptoms (*scapular notch syndrome*). A common result is weakness and atrophy of the muscles—the supraspinatus and infraspinatus—that the suprascapular nerve innervates (see p. 263).

1.4 The Bones of the Upper Limb: The Humerus

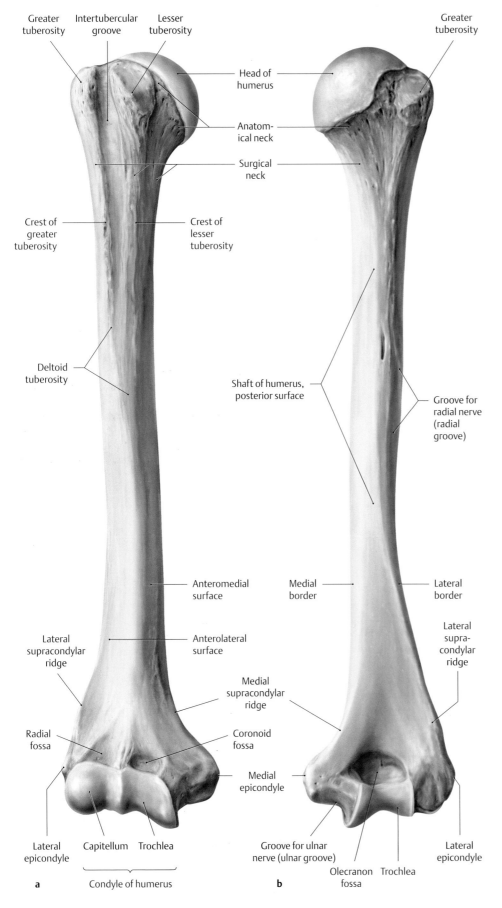

A The right humerus
a Anterior view, **b** posterior view.

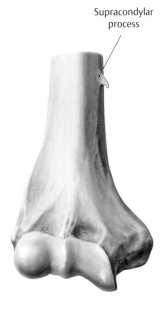

B Processus supracondylaris
An anomaly sometimes found on the distal humerus above the medial epicondyle is referred to as a supracondylar process. This bony outgrowth is a relatively rare atavistic feature in humans that corresponds to a normal structure in other vertebrates, in which it forms part of a supracondylar canal (see p. 345).

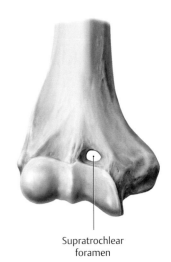

C The supratrochlear foramen
The presence of a supratrochlear foramen is another rare variant in which the two opposing olecranon and coronoid fossae communicate through an opening.

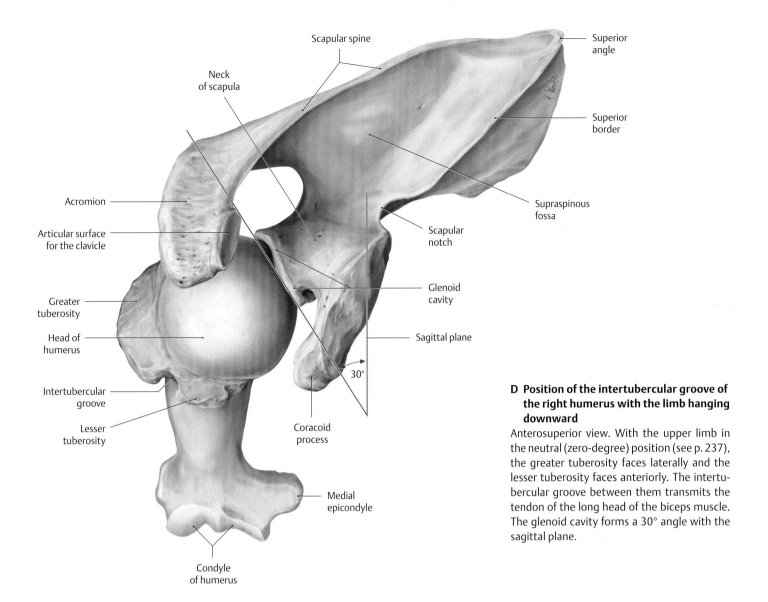

Scapular spine

Superior angle

Neck of scapula

Superior border

Acromion

Supraspinous fossa

Articular surface for the clavicle

Scapular notch

Greater tuberosity

Glenoid cavity

Head of humerus

Sagittal plane

Intertubercular groove

30°

Lesser tuberosity

Coracoid process

Medial epicondyle

Condyle of humerus

D Position of the intertubercular groove of the right humerus with the limb hanging downward

Anterosuperior view. With the upper limb in the neutral (zero-degree) position (see p. 237), the greater tuberosity faces laterally and the lesser tuberosity faces anteriorly. The intertubercular groove between them transmits the tendon of the long head of the biceps muscle. The glenoid cavity forms a 30° angle with the sagittal plane.

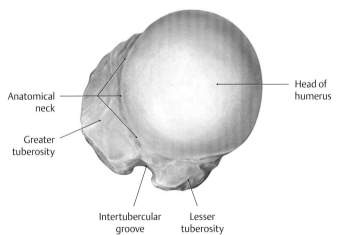

Anatomical neck

Head of humerus

Greater tuberosity

Intertubercular groove

Lesser tuberosity

Capitellum

Capitulotrochlear groove

Trochlea

Ulnar groove

Lateral epicondyle

Olecranon fossa

Medial epicondyle

E The proximal right humerus. Superior view

F The distal right humerus. Inferior view

1.5 The Bones of the Upper Limb: Torsion of the Humerus

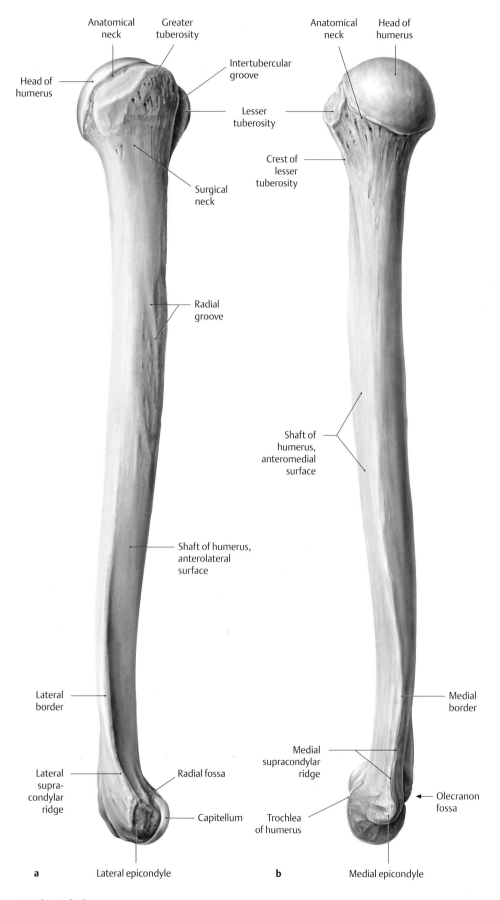

A The right humerus
a Lateral view, **b** medial view.

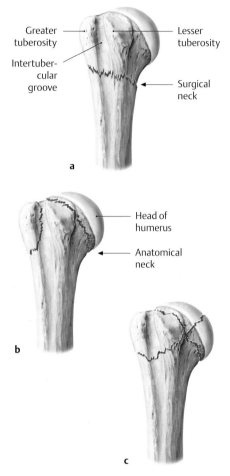

B Fractures of the proximal humerus
Anterior view. Fractures of the proximal humerus comprise approximately 4–5% of all fractures. They occur predominantly in older patients who sustain a fall onto the outstretched arm or directly onto the shoulder. Three main types are distinguished:

- Extra-articular fractures (**a**)
- Intra-articular fractures (**b**)
- Comminuted fractures (**c**)

Not infrequently, extra-articular fractures at the level of the *surgical neck* (site of predilection for extra-articular fractures of the proximal humerus) as well as intra-articular fractures at the level of the *anatomical neck* are accompanied by injuries of the blood vessels that supply the humeral head (anterior and posterior circumflex humeral arteries, see p. 309), with an associated risk of post-traumatic avascular necrosis. Besides proximal humeral fractures, other important injuries are fractures of the humeral shaft and fractures of the distal humerus (e.g., supracondylar fractures). Fractures of the humeral shaft are frequently associated with damage to the radial nerve in its groove (see p. 322 for neurological deficits following a radial nerve lesion).

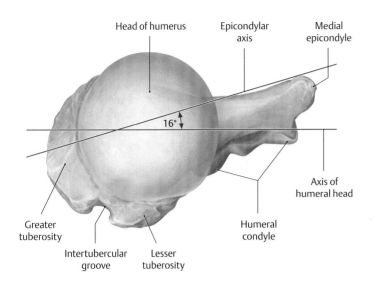

C Torsion of the humerus

Right humerus, superior view. The shaft of the adult humerus normally exhibits some degree of torsion, i.e., the proximal end of the humerus is rotated relative to its distal end. The degree of this torsion can be assessed by superimposing the axis of the humeral head (from the center of the greater tuberosity to the center of the humeral head) over the epicondylar axis of the elbow joint. This *torsion angle* equals approximately 16° in an adult, compared with about 60° in a newborn. The decrease in the torsion angle with body growth correlates with the change in the position of the scapulae. Thus, while the glenoid cavity in the newborn still faces anteriorly, it is directed much more laterally in the adult (see p. 211). As the position of the scapula changes, there is a compensatory decrease in the torsion angle to ensure that hand movements will remain within the visual field of the adult.

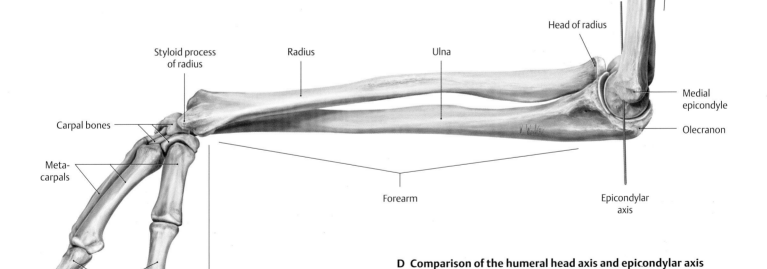

D Comparison of the humeral head axis and epicondylar axis

Skeleton of the right arm, viewed from the medial view with the forearm pronated.

1.6 The Bones of the Upper Limb: The Radius and Ulna

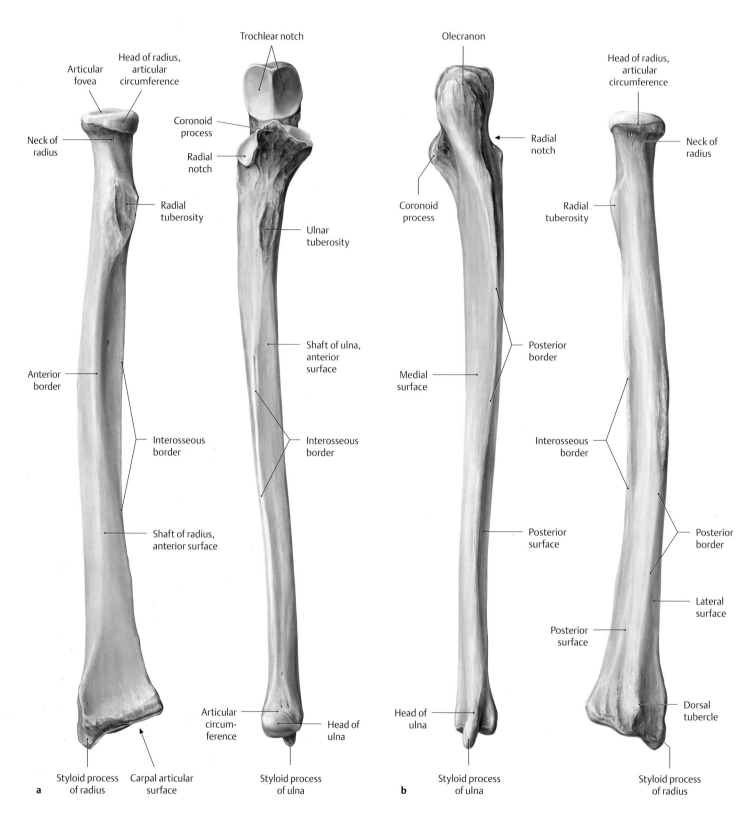

A The radius and ulna of the right forearm
a Anterior view, **b** posterior view.
The radius and ulna are not shown in their normal relationship; they have been separated to demonstrate the articular surfaces of the proximal and distal radioulnar joints.

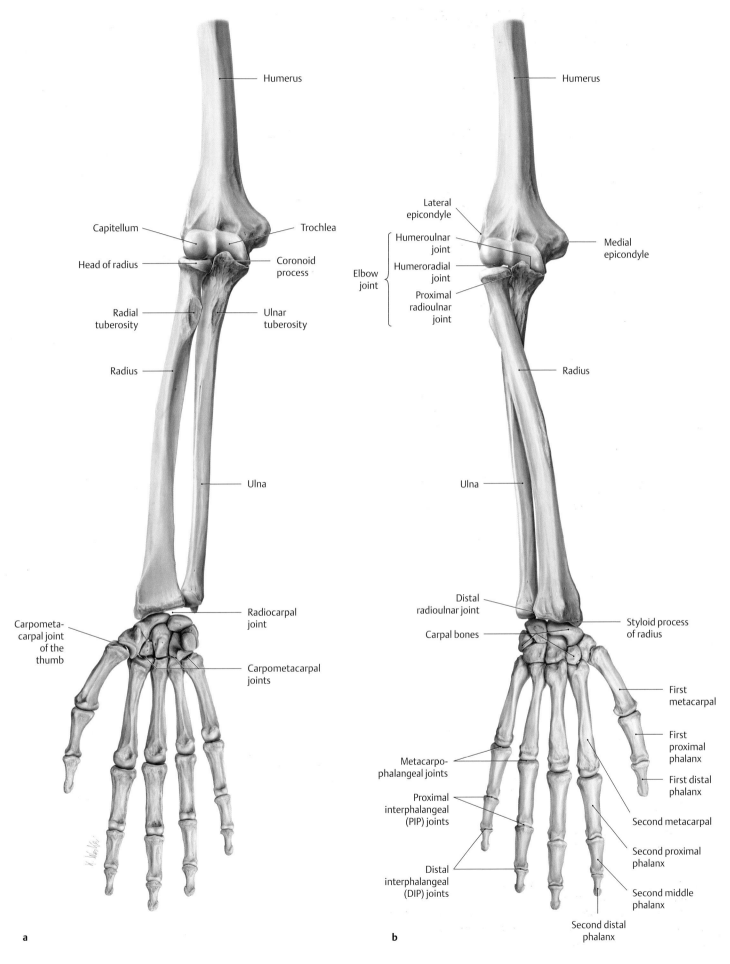

Humerus

Capitellum

Head of radius

Radial tuberosity

Radius

Ulna

Carpometa-carpal joint of the thumb

Trochlea

Coronoid process

Ulnar tuberosity

Radiocarpal joint

Carpometacarpal joints

a

Lateral epicondyle

Humeroulnar joint

Humeroradial joint

Proximal radioulnar joint

Elbow joint

Humerus

Medial epicondyle

Radius

Ulna

Distal radioulnar joint

Carpal bones

Metacarpo-phalangeal joints

Proximal interphalangeal (PIP) joints

Distal interphalangeal (DIP) joints

Second distal phalanx

Styloid process of radius

First metacarpal

First proximal phalanx

First distal phalanx

Second metacarpal

Second proximal phalanx

Second middle phalanx

b

B The radius and ulna of the right arm in supination (a) and pronation (b)

The radius and ulna are parallel to each other in supination, whereas in pronation the radius crosses over the ulna. The movement of turning the palm upward or downward (supination/pronation) takes place at the proximal and distal radioulnar joints (see p. 242).

1.7 The Bones of the Upper Limb: The Articular Surfaces of the Radius and Ulna

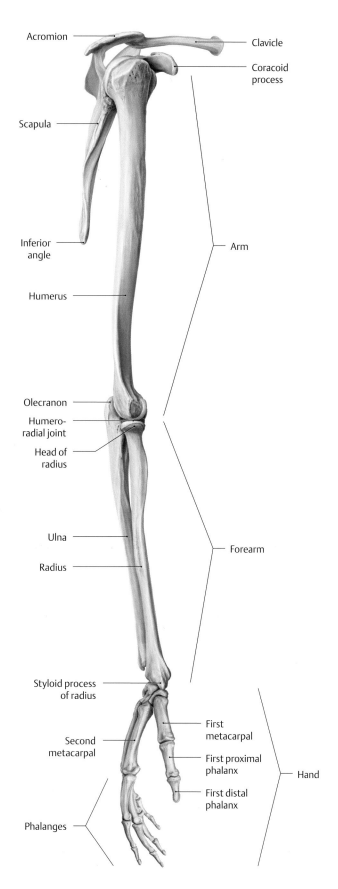

A The right upper limb
Lateral view. The forearm is supinated (the radius and ulna are parallel).

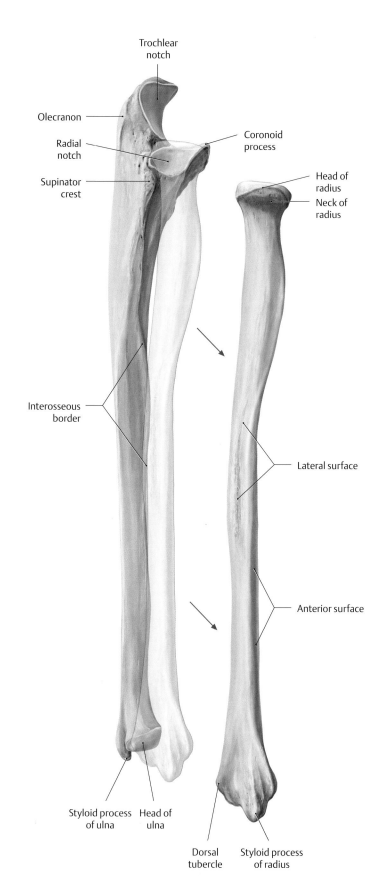

B Right forearm
Lateral view. The radius and ulna are shown in a disarticulated position to demonstrate the articular surfaces of the ulna for the proximal and distal radioulnar joints (see **C**).

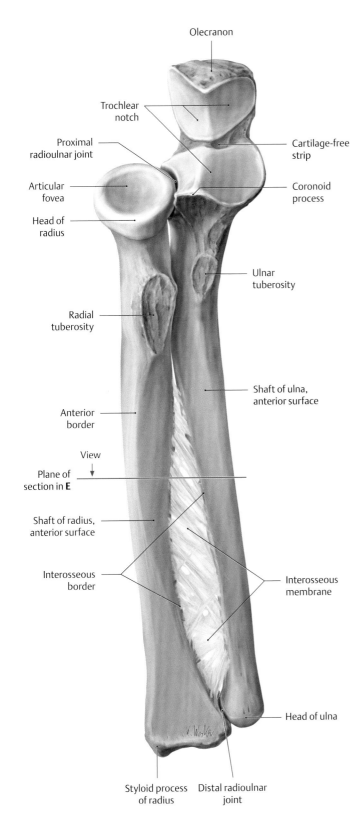

Olecranon

Trochlear notch

Proximal radioulnar joint

Articular fovea

Head of radius

Cartilage-free strip

Coronoid process

Ulnar tuberosity

Radial tuberosity

Shaft of ulna, anterior surface

Anterior border

View

Plane of section in **E**

Shaft of radius, anterior surface

Interosseous border

Interosseous membrane

Head of ulna

Styloid process of radius

Distal radioulnar joint

C The radius and ulna of the right forearm

Anterosuperior view. The proximal and distal radioulnar joints are functionally interlinked by the interosseous membrane between the radius and ulna. As a result, motion in one joint is invariably combined with motion in the other (see p. 244).

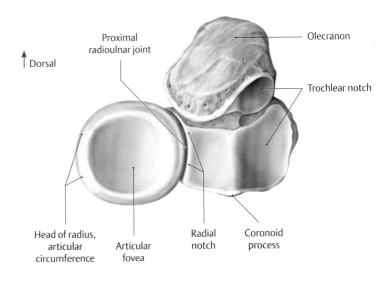

Proximal radioulnar joint

↑ Dorsal

Olecranon

Trochlear notch

Head of radius, articular circumference

Articular fovea

Radial notch

Coronoid process

D The proximal articular surfaces of the radius and ulna of the right forearm. Proximal view

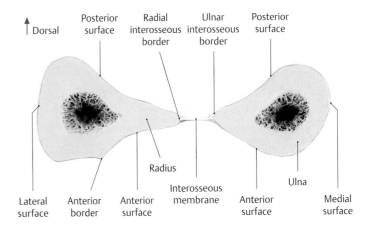

↑ Dorsal

Posterior surface

Radial interosseous border

Ulnar interosseous border

Posterior surface

Lateral surface

Anterior border

Anterior surface

Interosseous membrane

Radius

Anterior surface

Ulna

Medial surface

E Cross section through the right radius and ulna. Proximal view.

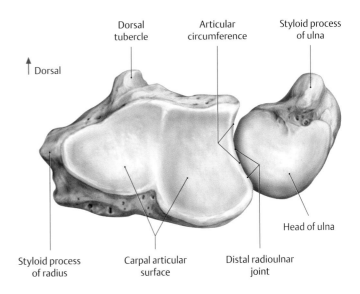

Dorsal tubercle

Articular circumference

Styloid process of ulna

↑ Dorsal

Styloid process of radius

Carpal articular surface

Head of ulna

Distal radioulnar joint

F The distal articular surfaces of the radius and ulna of the right forearm. Distal view

221

1.8 The Bones of the Upper Limb: The Hand

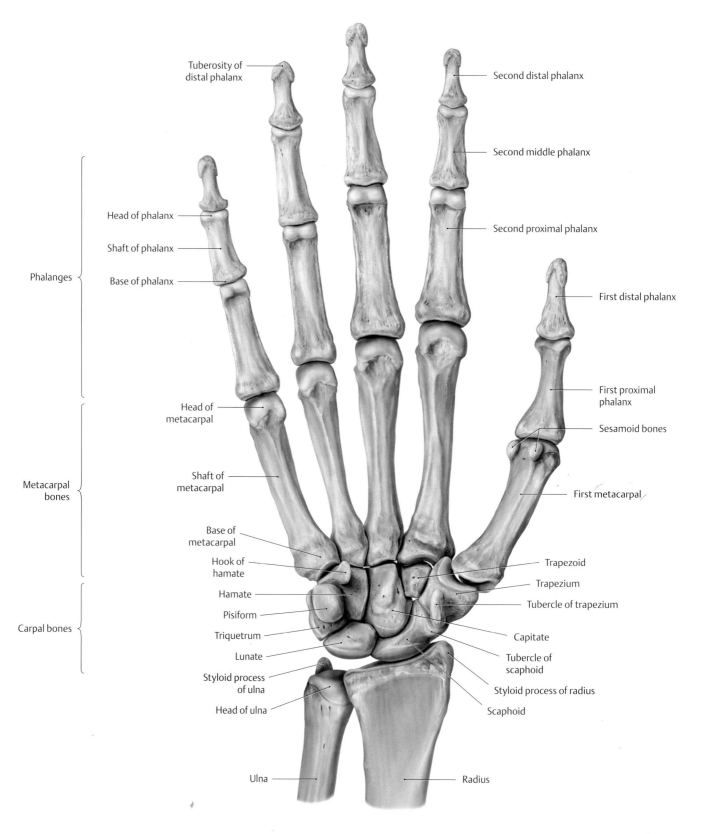

Tuberosity of distal phalanx

Second distal phalanx

Second middle phalanx

Head of phalanx

Shaft of phalanx

Second proximal phalanx

Base of phalanx

Phalanges

First distal phalanx

Head of metacarpal

First proximal phalanx

Sesamoid bones

Shaft of metacarpal

Metacarpal bones

First metacarpal

Base of metacarpal

Hook of hamate

Trapezoid

Trapezium

Hamate

Tubercle of trapezium

Pisiform

Carpal bones

Triquetrum

Capitate

Lunate

Tubercle of scaphoid

Styloid process of ulna

Styloid process of radius

Head of ulna

Scaphoid

Ulna

Radius

A The bones of the right hand. Palmar view
The skeleton of the hand consists of:

- the carpal bones
- the metacarpal bones
- the phalanges.

The palm refers to the anterior (flexor) surface of the hand, the dorsum to the posterior (extensor) surface. The terms of anatomical orientation in the hand are palmar or volar (toward the anterior surface), dorsal (toward the posterior surface), ulnar (toward the ulna or small finger), and radial (toward the radius or thumb).

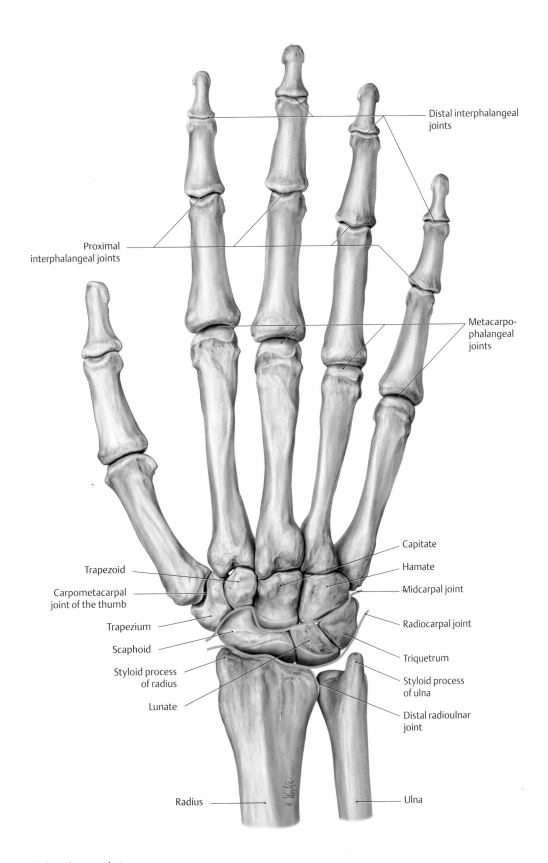

B The bones of the right hand. Dorsal view
The radiocarpal and midcarpal joints are indicated by blue lines.

1.9 The Bones of the Upper Limb: The Carpal Bones

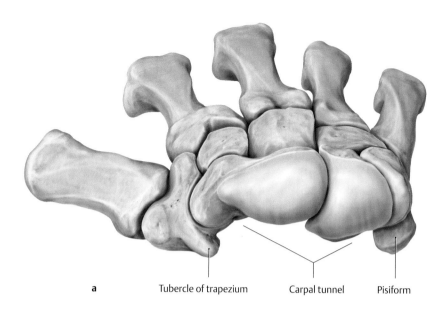

a — Tubercle of trapezium — Carpal tunnel — Pisiform

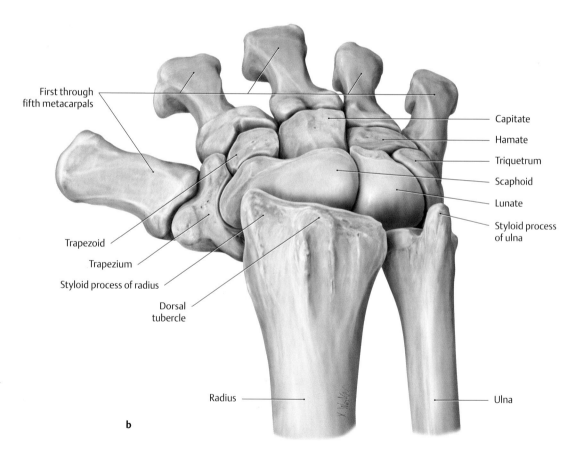

First through fifth metacarpals

Capitate

Hamate

Triquetrum

Scaphoid

Lunate

Styloid process of ulna

Trapezoid

Trapezium

Styloid process of radius

Dorsal tubercle

Radius

Ulna

b

A Carpal bones of the right hand, proximal view
a After removal of the radius and ulna, **b** with the wrist in flexion.
The carpal bones are arranged in two rows of four bones each—one proximal row and one distal row (see also **B**). From a biomechanical and clinical standpoint, the carpal bones do not form two transverse rows but are arranged in three longitudinal columns: a radial scaphoid column (consisting of the scaphoid, trapezium, and trapezoid bones), a central lunate column (consisting of the lunate and capitate), and an ulnar triquetral column (consisting of the triquetrum and hamate). In this functional classification, the pisiform is regarded as a sesamoid bone embedded in the tendon of the flexor carpi ulnaris muscle (see p. 356). The bones in each row are interconnected by tight joints, their surfaces exhibiting a palmar concavity and a dorsal convexity. This creates the carpal tunnel on the palmar surface (see p. 248), which is bounded by a bony eminence on the radial and ulnar sides.

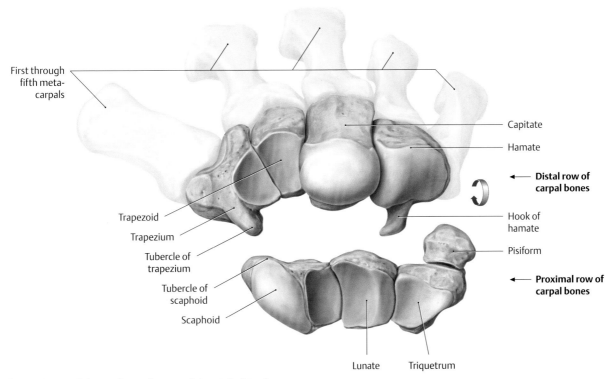

First through fifth meta-carpals

Capitate

Hamate

← **Distal row of carpal bones**

Hook of hamate

Pisiform

← **Proximal row of carpal bones**

Trapezoid

Trapezium

Tubercle of trapezium

Tubercle of scaphoid

Scaphoid

Lunate   Triquetrum

B Articular surfaces of the midcarpal joint of the right hand
The *distal* row of carpal bones is shown from the *proximal* view. The *proximal* row is shown from the *distal* view.

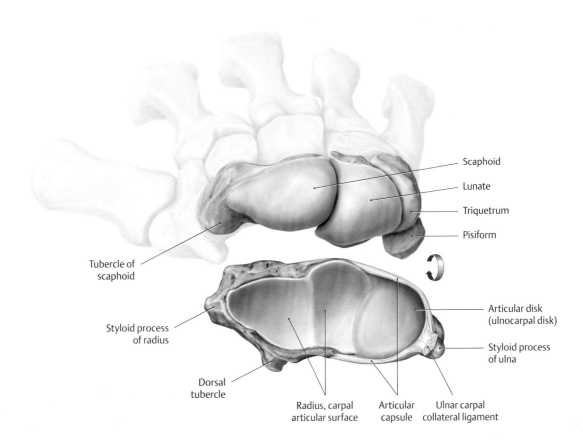

Scaphoid

Lunate

Triquetrum

Pisiform

Tubercle of scaphoid

Articular disk (ulnocarpal disk)

Styloid process of radius

Styloid process of ulna

Dorsal tubercle

Radius, carpal articular surface   Articular capsule   Ulnar carpal collateral ligament

C Articular surfaces of the radiocarpal joint of the right hand
The proximal row of carpal bones is shown from the proximal view. The articular surfaces of the radius and ulna and the articular disk (ulnocarpal disk) are shown from the distal view.
Clinically, the radiocarpal joint is subdivided into a radial compartment and an ulnar compartment. This takes into account the presence of the interposed ulnocarpal disk, which creates a second, ulnar half of the radiocarpal joint in addition to the radial half. Accordingly, the radius articulates with the proximal row of carpal bones in the radial compartment while the head of the ulna and ulnocarpal disk articulate with the proximal row of carpal bones in the ulnar compartment.

1.10 The Joints of the Shoulder: Overview, Clavicular Joints

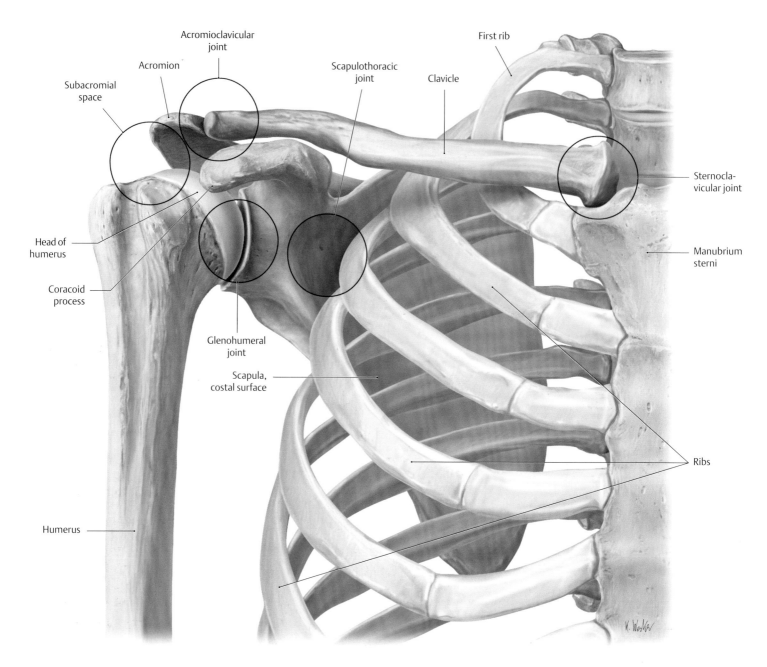

A The five joints of the shoulder

Right shoulder, anterior view. A total of five joints contribute to the wide range of arm motions at the shoulder joint. There are three true shoulder joints and two functional articulations:

- **True joints:**
  1. Sternoclavicular joint
  2. Acromioclavicular joint
  3. Glenohumeral joint
- **Functional articulations:**
  4. Subacromial space: a space lined with bursae (subacromial and subdeltoid bursae) that allows gliding between the acromion and the rotator cuff (= muscular cuff of the glenohumeral joint, consisting of the supraspinatus, infraspinatus, subscapularis, and teres minor muscles, which press the head of the humerus into the glenoid cavity; see p. 263).
  5. Scapulothoracic joint: loose connective tissue between the subscapularis and serratus anterior muscles that allows gliding of the scapula on the chest wall.

Besides the true joints and functional articulations, the two ligamentous attachments between the clavicle and first rib (costoclavicular ligament) and between the clavicle and coracoid process (coracoclavicular ligament) contribute to the mobility of the upper limb. All of these structures together comprise a functional unit, and free mobility in all the joints is necessary to achieve a full range of motion. This expansive mobility is gained at the cost of stability, however. Since the shoulder has a loose capsule and weak reinforcing ligaments, it must rely on the stabilizing effect of the rotator cuff tendons. As the upper limb changed in mammalian evolution from an organ of support to one of manipulation, the soft tissues and their pathology assumed increasing importance. As a result, a large percentage of shoulder disorders involve the soft tissues.

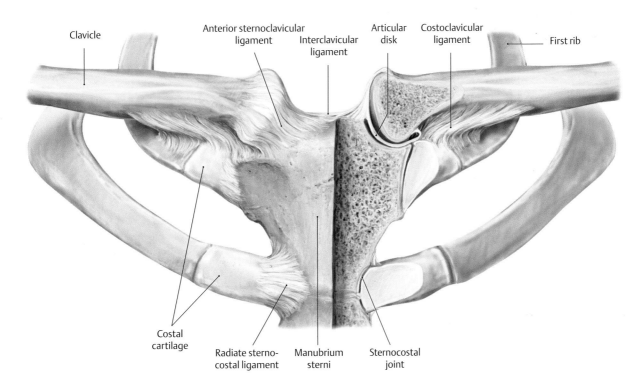

B The sternoclavicular joint and its ligaments

Anterior view. The sternoclavicular joint (called also the *medial* clavicular joint) and the acromioclavicular joint (the *lateral* clavicular joint, see below) together make up the true joints within the shoulder girdle itself. In the figure, a coronal section has been made through the sternum and adjacent clavicle to demonstrate the inside of the left sternoclavicular joint. A fibrocartilaginous articular disk compensates for the mismatch of surfaces between the two saddle-shaped articular faces of the clavicle and manubrium sterni.

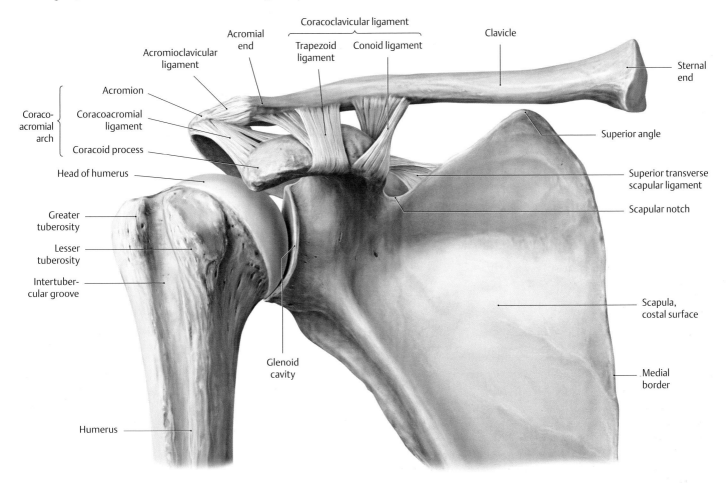

C The acromioclavicular joint and its ligaments

Anterior view. The acromioclavicular joint (the *lateral* clavicular joint) has the form of a *plane joint*. Because the articulating surfaces are flat, they must be held in place by strong ligaments (acromioclavicular, coraco-acromial and coracoclavicular ligaments). This greatly limits the mobility of the acromioclavicular joint. In some individuals the acromioclavicular joint has a variably shaped articular disk which gives the joint greater mobility.

227

1.11 The Joints of the Shoulder: Ligaments of the Clavicular and Scapulothoracic Joints

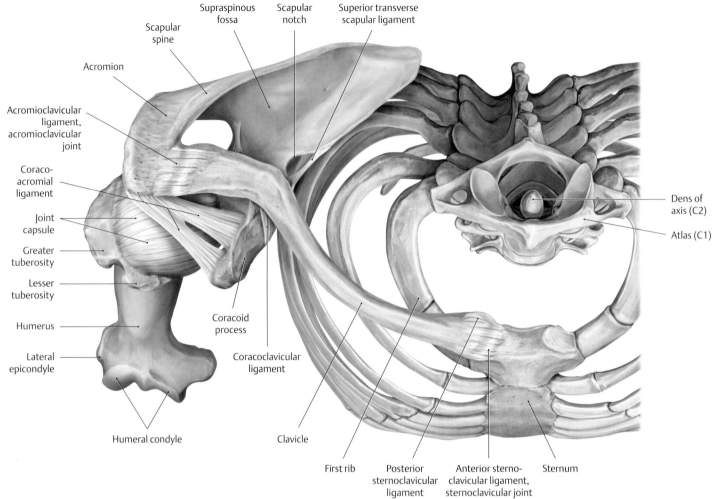

A Ligaments of the sternoclavicular and acromioclavicular joints
Right side, superior view.

B Injuries of the acromioclavicular joint
A fall onto the shoulder or outstretched arm frequently causes dislocation of the acromioclavicular joint and damage to the coracoclavicular ligaments. Ligament injury allows the lateral end of the clavicle to move independently of the scapula, causing it to appear upwardly displaced. The clavicle can be pushed down (with significant pain), but will spring back up when pressure is released ("piano-key sign"). Three grades of acromioclavicular separation can be distinguished clinically based on the degree of ligament damage (Tossy classification).

Tossy I The acromioclavicular and coracoclavicular ligaments are stretched but still intact.
Tossy II The acromioclavicular ligament is ruptured, with subluxation of the joint.
Tossy III Ligaments are all disrupted, with complete dislocation of the acromioclavicular joint.

Radiographs in different planes will show widening of the space in the acromioclavicular joint. Comparative-stress radiographs with the patient holding approximately 10-kg weights in each hand will reveal the extent of upward displacement of the lateral end of the clavicle on the affected side.

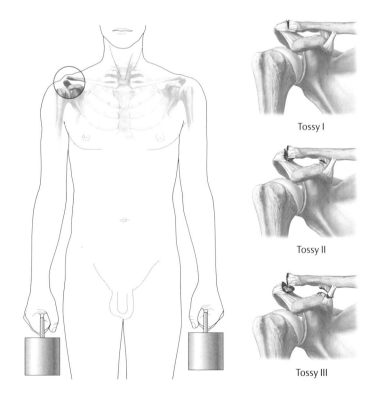

Tossy I

Tossy II

Tossy III

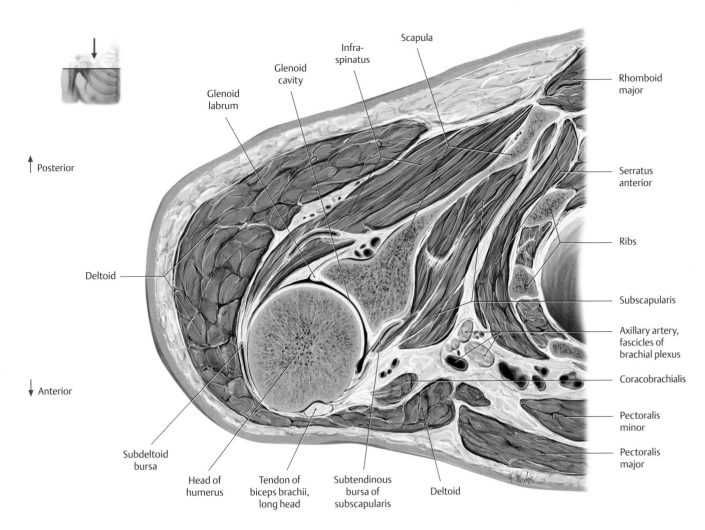

↑ Posterior

↓ Anterior

Glenoid labrum

Glenoid cavity

Infra-spinatus

Scapula

Rhomboid major

Serratus anterior

Ribs

Deltoid

Subscapularis

Axillary artery, fascicles of brachial plexus

Coracobrachialis

Pectoralis minor

Pectoralis major

Subdeltoid bursa

Head of humerus

Tendon of biceps brachii, long head

Subtendinous bursa of subscapularis

Deltoid

C Transverse section through the right shoulder joint
Superior view. In all movements of the shoulder girdle, the scapula glides on a curved surface of loose connective tissue between the serratus anterior and subscapularis muscles (see **D**). This surface can be considered a "scapulothoracic" joint that allows the scapula not only to change the position of the shoulder (translational motion), but also to pivot, with the glenohumeral joint maintained in relatively stable position on the thorax (rotational motion) (see p. 236). (drawing based on a specimen from the Anatomical Collection at the University of Kiel).

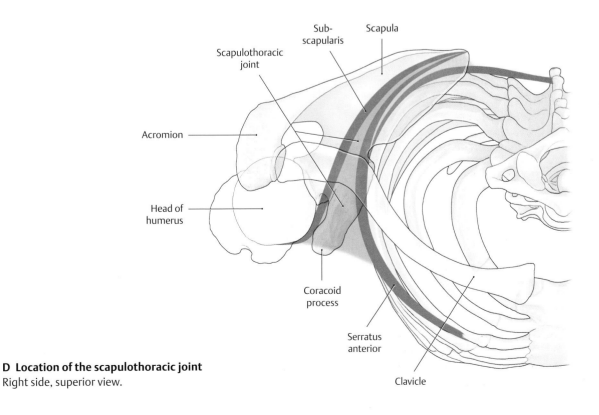

Scapulothoracic joint

Sub-scapularis

Scapula

Acromion

Head of humerus

Coracoid process

Serratus anterior

Clavicle

D Location of the scapulothoracic joint
Right side, superior view.

1.12 The Joints of the Shoulder: The Capsule and Ligaments of the Glenohumeral Joint

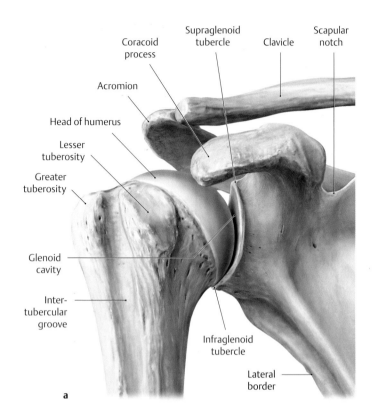

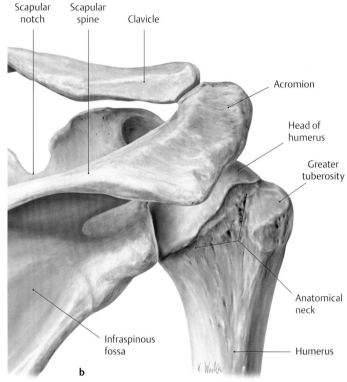

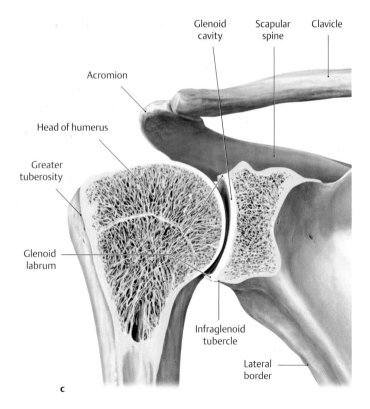

A Articulating bony elements of the right shoulder joint (glenohumeral joint)

a Anterior view.

b Posterior view.

c Coronal section through the shoulder joint, anterior view.

In the shoulder joint—the most mobile joint in the human body but also the most susceptible to injury—the head of the humerus articulates with the glenoid cavity of the scapula to form a spheroidal type of joint. The articular surface of the humeral head is three to four times larger than the articular surface of the scapula. To help correct for this disparity, the glenoid cavity is slightly deepened and enlarged by a rim of fibrocartilage, the glenoid labrum (see **c**). While this size discrepancy of the articulating surfaces serves to increase the range of shoulder motion, it compromises the stability of the joint. Since the joint capsule and ligaments are weak, the rotator cuff tendons are the primary stabilizers of the glenohumeral joint (see p. 264).

Dislocations of the shoulder joint are notoriously common. Approximately 45 % of all dislocations involve the shoulder joint. In typical cases the head of the humerus dislocates anteriorly or anteroinferiorly in response to forcible external rotation of the raised arm. Whereas considerable trauma is generally needed to cause the initial dislocation, certain movements of the shoulder (e.g., excessive arm rotation during sleep) may be sufficient to redislocate the humeral head from the glenoid cavity (recurrent shoulder dislocation).

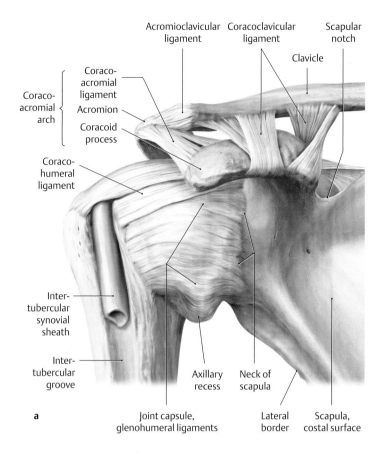

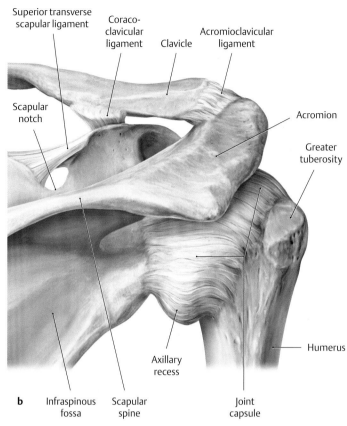

a

Coraco-acromial arch
- Coraco-acromial ligament
- Acromion
- Coracoid process

Acromioclavicular ligament

Coracoclavicular ligament

Scapular notch

Clavicle

Coraco-humeral ligament

Inter-tubercular synovial sheath

Inter-tubercular groove

Axillary recess

Joint capsule, glenohumeral ligaments

Neck of scapula

Lateral border

Scapula, costal surface

b

Superior transverse scapular ligament

Coraco-clavicular ligament

Clavicle

Acromioclavicular ligament

Scapular notch

Acromion

Greater tuberosity

Humerus

Axillary recess

Infraspinous fossa

Scapular spine

Joint capsule

c

Acromioclavicular ligament

Coracoclavicular ligament

Superior transverse scapular ligament

Coracoacromial ligament

Coracoid process

Clavicle

Acromion

Subcoracoid bursa

Transverse ligament of humerus

Tendon of biceps brachii, long head

Intertubercular groove

Axillary recess

Intertuber-cular synovial sheath

Subtendinous bursa of subscapularis

B Capsule, ligaments, and joint cavity of the right shoulder

a Anterior view.
b Posterior view.
c Joint cavity from the anterior view.

The capsule of the shoulder joint is broad and is very thin posteriorly, where it is not reinforced by ligaments. But it is strengthened anteriorly by three ligamentous structures (the superior, medial, and inferior glenohumeral ligaments) and superiorly by the coracohumeral ligament. The coracoacromial ligament, acromion, and coracoid process together form the "coracoacromial arch," which helps stabilize the humeral head in the glenoid cavity but also limits upward movement of the humerus. When the arm is hanging at the side, the lower part of the joint capsule, which is not reinforced by muscle, sags to form the axillary recess. This redundant fold provides a reserve capacity that is particularly useful during abduction movements of the arm. With prolonged disuse of the arm, the axillary recess may become atrophic or obliterated by adhesions, causing significant limitation of arm motion.

The cavity of the shoulder joint is connected to the adjacent bursae. The subtendinous bursa of the subscapularis muscle and the subcoracoid bursa consistently communicate with the joint cavity. The long biceps tendon sheath also communicates with the joint cavity in its passage through the intertubercular groove.

231

1.13 The Joints of the Shoulder: The Subacromial Space

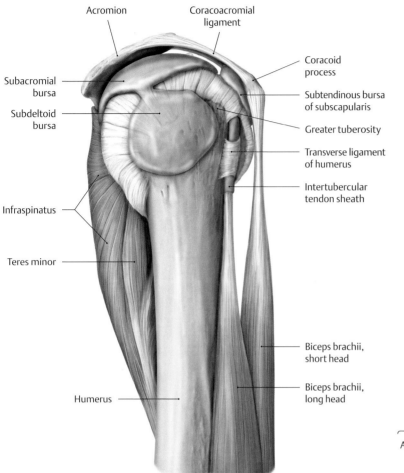

Labels (clockwise):
Acromion · Coracoacromial ligament · Coracoid process · Subtendinous bursa of subscapularis · Greater tuberosity · Transverse ligament of humerus · Intertubercular tendon sheath · Biceps brachii, short head · Biceps brachii, long head · Humerus · Teres minor · Infraspinatus · Subdeltoid bursa · Subacromial bursa

A Subacromial space, right shoulder

Lateral view. The deltoid muscle has been removed to demonstrate the following structures:

- The attachments of the rotator cuff muscles (supraspinatus, infraspinatus, teres minor, and subscapularis) to the proximal humerus (see also **B**)
- The tendons of origin of the biceps brachii muscle
- The subacromial space with the subacromial bursa, which consistently communicates with the subdeltoid bursa

The two bursae allow frictionless gliding between the humeral head and the rotator cuff tendons (especially the supraspinatus and the upper part of the infraspinatus) beneath the coracoacromial arch during abduction and elevation of the arm (see p. 237).

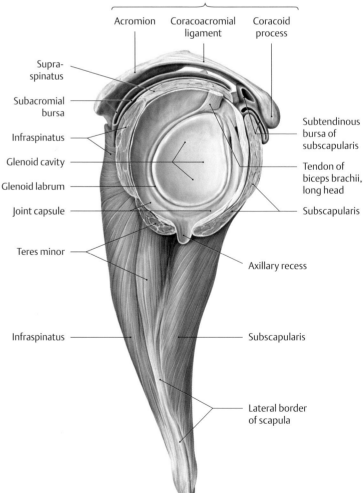

Labels: Coracoacromial arch (Acromion · Coracoacromial ligament · Coracoid process) · Supraspinatus · Subacromial bursa · Infraspinatus · Glenoid cavity · Glenoid labrum · Joint capsule · Teres minor · Infraspinatus · Subtendinous bursa of subscapularis · Tendon of biceps brachii, long head · Subscapularis · Axillary recess · Subscapularis · Lateral border of scapula

B Subacromial bursa and glenoid cavity of the right shoulder joint

Lateral view. The humeral head has been removed and the rotator cuff tendons of insertion have been divided to demonstrate the glenoid cavity of the shoulder joint. The *glenoid labrum* enlarges and deepens the glenoid only very slightly. Just before inserting into the humeral head, the muscles of the rotator cuff send tendinous expansions to the joint capsule that help to press the humeral head into the glenoid cavity. The subacromial bursa is located between the coracoacromial arch and the tendons that insert on the humeral head (see **D**).

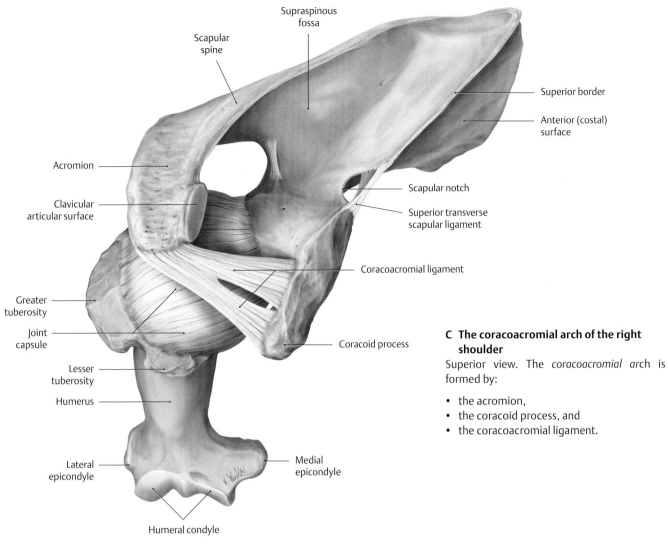

C The coracoacromial arch of the right shoulder
Superior view. The *coracoacromial arch* is formed by:

- the acromion,
- the coracoid process, and
- the coracoacromial ligament.

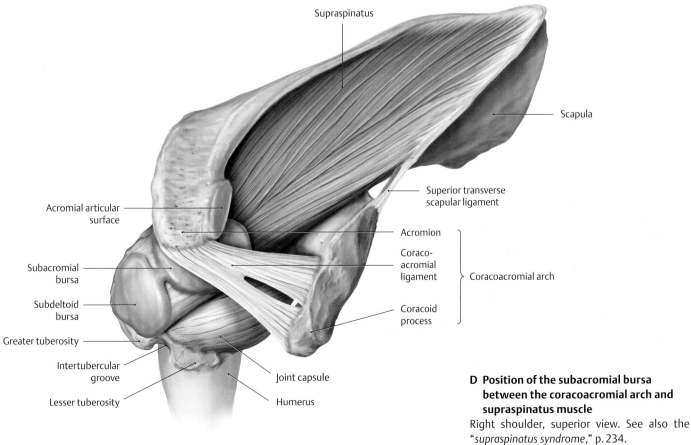

D Position of the subacromial bursa between the coracoacromial arch and supraspinatus muscle
Right shoulder, superior view. See also the "*supraspinatus syndrome*," p. 234.

233

1.14 The Subacromial Bursa and Subdeltoid Bursa

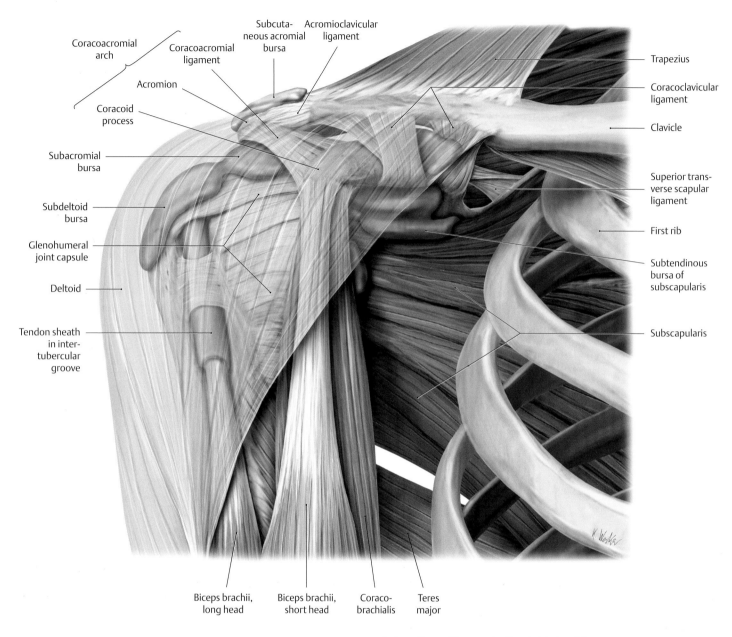

A Location of bursae in the right shoulder
Anterior view. The pectoralis major and minor and serratus anterior muscles have been removed. The location of the bursae can be seen through the deltoid muscle, which is lightly shaded.
Note in particular the coracoacromial arch and the underlying subacromial bursa.

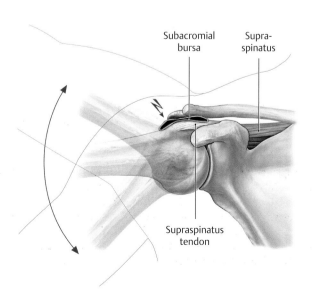

B Supraspinatus (impingement) syndrome
A supraspinatus tendon that has been thickened by calcification or other degenerative changes can be caught underneath the acromion, impinging upon the subacromial bursa, when the arm is abducted. Pain from this *supraspinatus* or *impingement syndrome* occurs in an arc of motion between 60° and 120° of abduction.

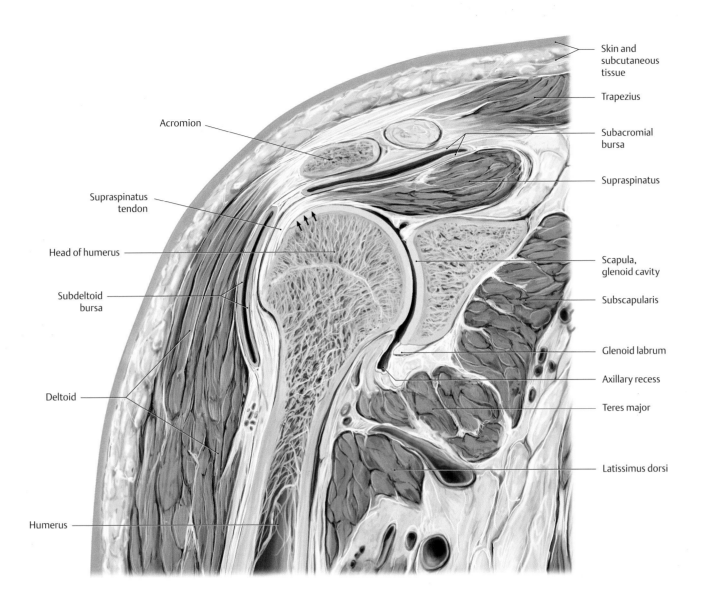

C Coronal section through the right shoulder joint

Anterior view. The tendon of insertion of the supraspinatus muscle differs structurally from ordinary traction tendons. Its distal course gives it the function of a gliding tendon, which passes over the fulcrum of the humeral head (arrows). In that area, located approximately 1–2 cm proximal to its insertion on the greater tuberosity, the tendon tissue in contact with the humeral head is composed of fibrocartilage. This fibrocartilage zone is avascular, representing an adaptation of the tendon to the pressure loads imposed by the bony fulcrum (drawing based on a specimen from the Anatomical Collection at the University of Kiel).

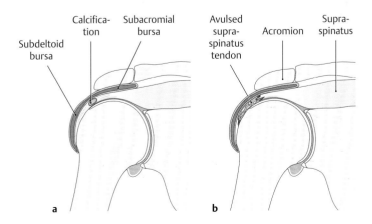

D Damage to the supraspinatus tendon

a Calcification (calcifying tendinitis) and related degenerative changes.

b Rotator cuff tear (supraspinatus tendon avulsion).

The supraspinatus tendon is the most frequently damaged component of the rotator cuff. When it is ruptured, the subacromial and subdeltoid bursae are no longer isolated from the joint cavity, becoming one continuous space. When the function of the supraspinatus muscle is lost after rupture of its tendon, the initial phase of arm abduction is specifically impaired. The supraspinatus normally contributes significantly to the first 10° of abduction ("starter function"; see p. 262).

1.15 Movements of the Shoulder Girdle and Shoulder Joint

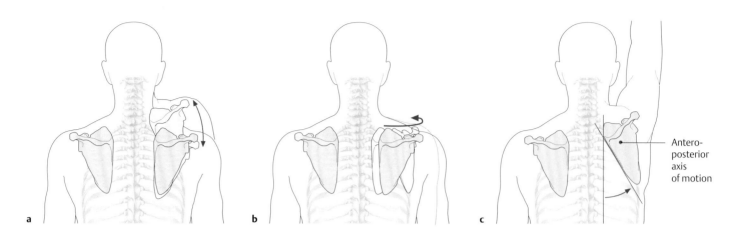

a   **b**   **c**

Antero-
posterior
axis
of motion

A Movements of the scapula

The sternoclavicular and acromioclavicular joints are mechanically linked in such a way that all movements of the clavicle are accompanied by movements of the scapula. The scapula moves by gliding on the chest wall in the scapulothoracic joint. Both its movement and its fixation are effected by muscular slings. The following types of scapular movement are distinguished:

a Elevation and depression (during elevation and depression of the shoulder girdle): translation of the scapula in the craniocaudal direction.

b Abduction and adduction (during protraction and retraction of the shoulder girdle): horizontal translation of the scapula in the posteromedial-to-anterolateral direction.

c Lateral rotation of the inferior angle (during abduction or elevation of the arm): rotation of the scapula about an anteroposterior axis through the center of the scapula. With an approximately 60° range of rotation, the inferior angle of the scapula moves about 10 cm laterally while the superior angle moves about 2–3 cm inferomedially.

40°

Axis of
motion

0°

10°

a

Axis of
motion

30°

0°

b

25°

B Movements (and range of motion) in the sternoclavicular joint

a Elevation and depression of the shoulder about a para-sagittal axis.

b Protraction and retraction of the shoulder about a longitudinal (vertical) axis.

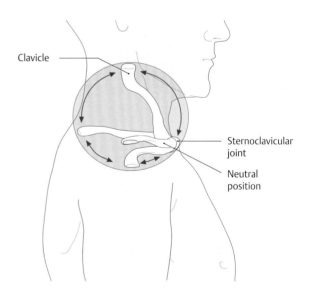

Clavicle

Sternoclavicular
joint

Neutral
position

C Range of motion of the clavicle

Lateral view of the right clavicle. Viewing the range of motion of the clavicle in the sternoclavicular joint from the lateral view, we find that the clavicle moves roughly within a conical shell whose apex is directed toward the sternum, and with a slightly oval base approximately 10–13 cm in diameter. The clavicle also rotates about its own axis, particularly during elevation of the shoulder girdle, where its S shape significantly increases the range of shoulder elevation. The range of this rotation is approximately 45° and creates a third degree of freedom which gives the sternoclavicular joint the *function* of a spheroidal joint.

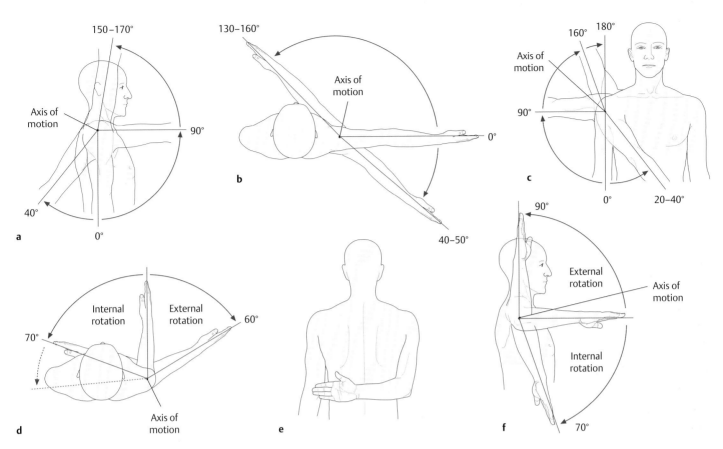

D Movements in the shoulder joint

As a typical spheroidal joint, the shoulder joint has three mutually perpendicular cardinal axes with three degrees of freedom and a total of six main directions of movement. In a very basic sense, all movements in the shoulder girdle can be classified as vertical, horizontal, or rotational. In *vertical movements*, the arm is elevated in various directions from a neutral adducted position. In *horizontal movements*, the arm is moved forward or backward while in 90° of abduction. *Rotational movements* can be performed with the arm in any position. The maximum *range* of these various movements can be achieved only by concomitant movement of the shoulder girdle, however.

a Anteversion and retroversion (flexion and extension) occur about a horizontal axis.

b Anteversion and retroversion of the arm raised to 90° abduction are also described as horizontal movements.

c Abduction and adduction occur about a sagittal axis, with movements past 90° often referred to as elevation. In clinical parlance, however, the term "elevation" is generally applied to all vertical movements. Past 80–90° of abduction, an automatic external rotation occurs which keeps the greater tuberosity from impinging on the coracoacromial arch. When the arm is abducted while internally rotated, the range of abduction is decreased to approximately 60°.

d–f Internal and external rotation of the arm occur about the longitudinal (shaft) axis of the humerus. When the arm is flexed at the elbow during these movements, the forearm can be used as a pointer. When the arm is hanging at the side, the maximum range of internal rotation is limited by the trunk. Placing the arm behind the back is equivalent to 95° of internal rotation (**e**). When the arm is abducted 90°, the range of external rotation is increased while the maximum range of internal rotation is slightly reduced (**f**).

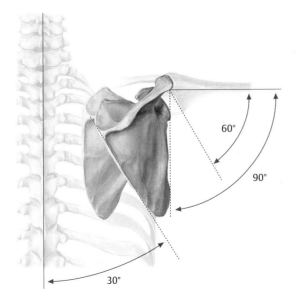

E Humeroscapular rhythm

The arm and scapula move in a 2:1 ratio during abduction. This means that when the arm is abducted 90°, for example, 60° of that movement occurs in the glenohumeral joint while 30° is accomplished by concomitant movement of the shoulder girdle. This "humeroscapular rhythm" is dependent upon freedom of movement of the scapula during abduction. Diseases of the shoulder joint can alter this rhythm, often causing the scapula to begin its rotation considerably earlier. This is best illustrated by cases involving ankylosis or arthrodesis of the glenohumeral joint (pathological or intentional operative stiffening or fixation), in which movements in the shoulder girdle alone still permit the arm to be abducted 40–60° and still allow for one-third the normal range of flexion/extension.

237

1.16 The Elbow Joint as a Whole

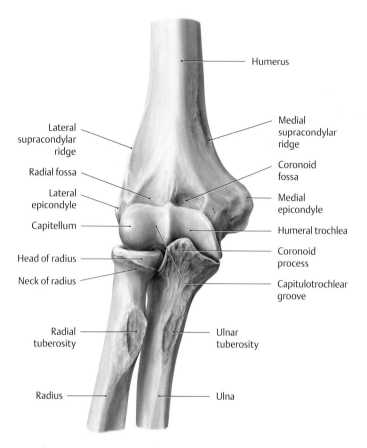

a Anterior view

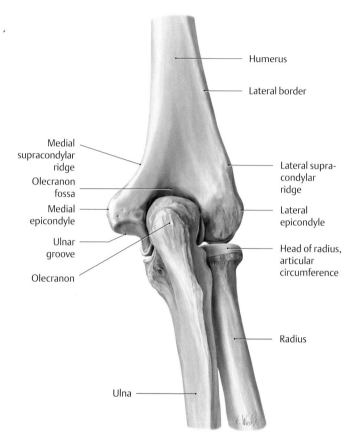

b Posterior view

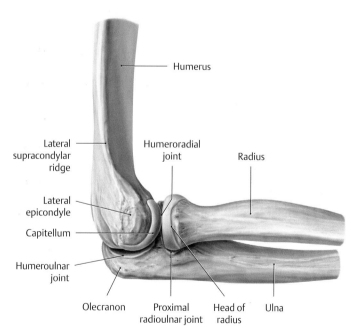

c Lateral view

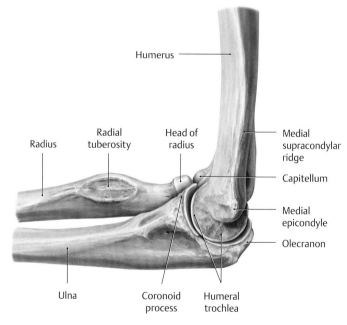

d Medial view

A The articulating skeletal elements of the right elbow joint
The *humerus, radius,* and *ulna* articulate with one another at the elbow (cubital) joint. The elbow consists of three articulations:

- The humeroulnar joint between the humerus and ulna
- The humeroradial joint between the humerus and radius
- The proximal radioulnar joint between the proximal ends of the ulna and radius

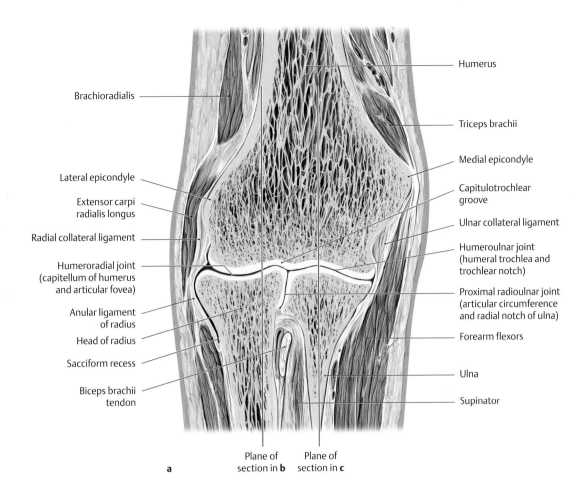

Brachioradialis

Humerus

Triceps brachii

Lateral epicondyle

Medial epicondyle

Extensor carpi radialis longus

Capitulotrochlear groove

Radial collateral ligament

Ulnar collateral ligament

Humeroradial joint (capitellum of humerus and articular fovea)

Humeroulnar joint (humeral trochlea and trochlear notch)

Anular ligament of radius

Proximal radioulnar joint (articular circumference and radial notch of ulna)

Head of radius

Forearm flexors

Sacciform recess

Ulna

Biceps brachii tendon

Supinator

Plane of section in **b**   Plane of section in **c**

a

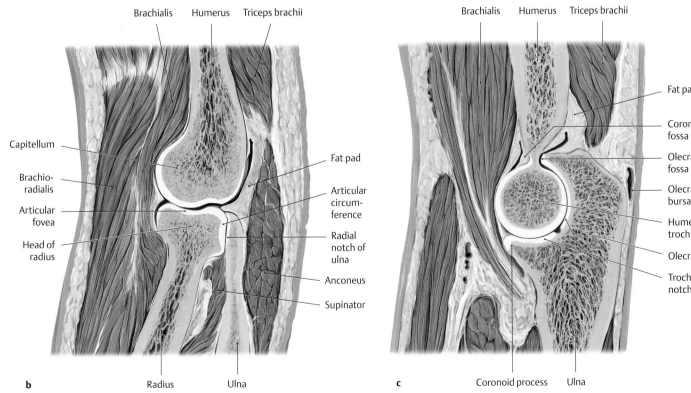

Brachialis   Humerus   Triceps brachii

Brachialis   Humerus   Triceps brachii

Capitellum

Fat pad

Fat pad

Brachio-radialis

Coronoid fossa

Articular circum-ference

Olecranon fossa

Articular fovea

Radial notch of ulna

Olecranon bursa

Head of radius

Anconeus

Humeral trochlea

Supinator

Olecranon

Trochlear notch

b   Radius   Ulna

c   Coronoid process   Ulna

B Skeletal and soft-tissue elements of the right elbow joint

a Coronal section viewed from the front (*note* the planes of section shown in **b** and **c**).

b Sagittal section through the humeroradial joint and proximal radioulnar joint, medial view.

c Sagittal section through the humeroulnar joint, medial view.

(Drawings based on specimens from the Anatomical Collection at the University of Kiel).

1.17 The Elbow Joint: Capsule and Ligaments

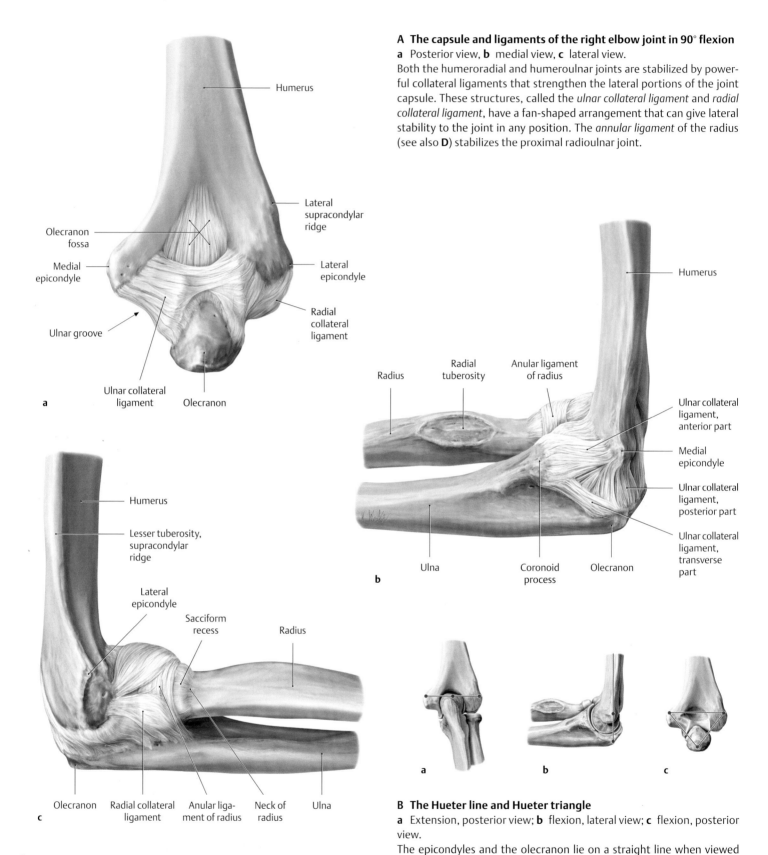

A The capsule and ligaments of the right elbow joint in 90° flexion
a Posterior view, **b** medial view, **c** lateral view.

Both the humeroradial and humeroulnar joints are stabilized by powerful collateral ligaments that strengthen the lateral portions of the joint capsule. These structures, called the *ulnar collateral ligament* and *radial collateral ligament*, have a fan-shaped arrangement that can give lateral stability to the joint in any position. The *annular ligament* of the radius (see also **D**) stabilizes the proximal radioulnar joint.

Humerus

Olecranon fossa

Medial epicondyle

Ulnar groove

Ulnar collateral ligament

Olecranon

Lateral supracondylar ridge

Lateral epicondyle

Radial collateral ligament

a

Humerus

Lesser tuberosity, supracondylar ridge

Lateral epicondyle

Sacciform recess

Radius

Olecranon

Radial collateral ligament

Anular ligament of radius

Neck of radius

Ulna

c

Radius

Radial tuberosity

Anular ligament of radius

Humerus

Ulnar collateral ligament, anterior part

Medial epicondyle

Ulnar collateral ligament, posterior part

Ulnar collateral ligament, transverse part

Ulna

Coronoid process

Olecranon

b

a **b** **c**

B The Hueter line and Hueter triangle
a Extension, posterior view; **b** flexion, lateral view; **c** flexion, posterior view.

The epicondyles and the olecranon lie on a straight line when viewed from the posterior view in the extended elbow. They also lie on a straight line when viewed from the lateral view in the flexed elbow. But when the flexed elbow is viewed from behind, the two epicondyles and the tip of the olecranon form an equilateral triangle. Fractures and dislocations alter the shape of the triangle.

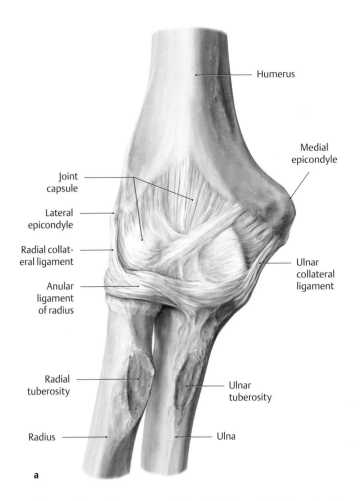

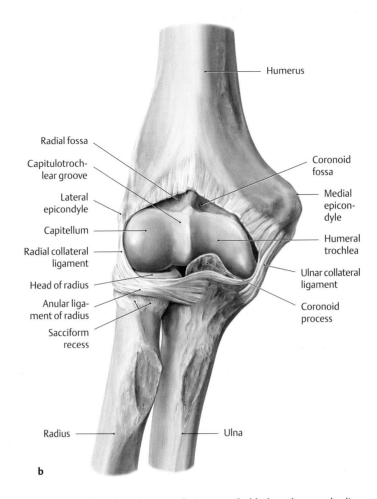

a

b

C The capsule and ligaments of the right elbow joint in extension

a Anterior view, **b** Anterior view with the ventral portions of the capsule removed.

The joint capsule of the elbow encloses all three articulations in the elbow joint complex. While the capsule is very thin in front and behind, it is reinforced on each side by the collateral ligaments (see **A**). Over the end of the radius, the joint capsule is expanded below the annular ligament to form the sacciform recess—a redundant tissue fold that provides a reserve capacity during pronation and supination of the forearm. During flexion and extension, the brachialis and anconeus muscles tighten the joint capsule to prevent entrapment of the capsule between the articular surfaces (see p. 272).

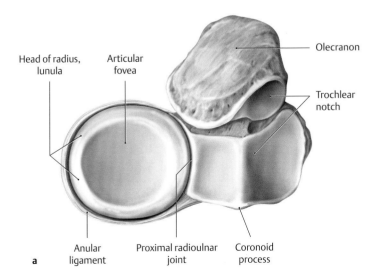

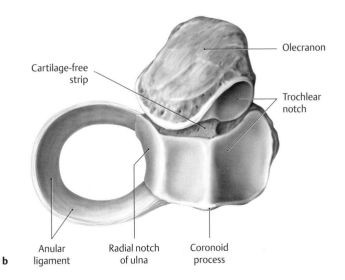

a

b

D Course of the anular ligament in the right proximal radioulnar joint

a View of the proximal articular surfaces of the radius and ulna after removal of the humerus. **b** Same view as in **a** with the radius also removed.

The anular ligament is of key importance in stabilizing the proximal radioulnar joint. It runs from the anterior to the posterior border of the radial notch of the ulna (= cartilage-covered articular surface on the ulna), wrapping around the radial head and pressing it into the ulnar articular surface. Histologically, the inner surface of the anular ligament has the fibrocartilaginous structure of a gliding tendon, enabling it to withstand the compressive loads that are transmitted to the ligament.

1.18 The Forearm: Proximal and Distal Radioulnar Joints

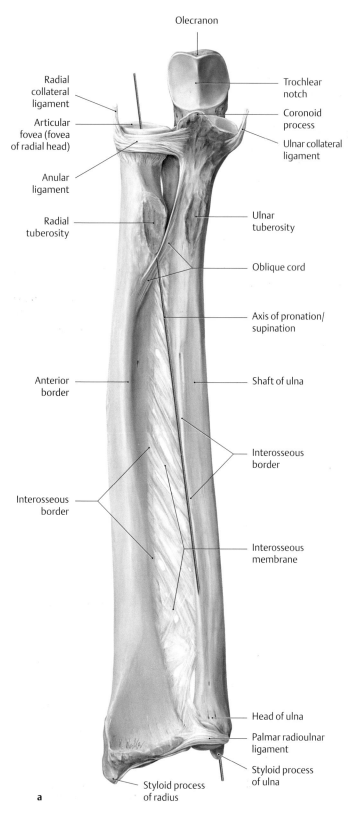

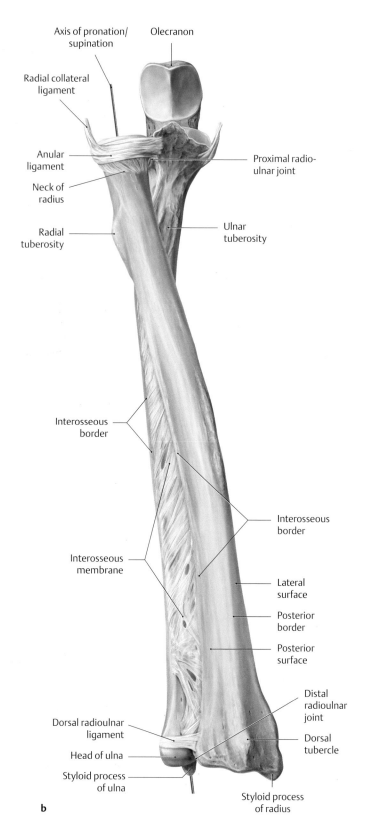

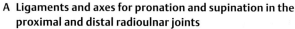

A Ligaments and axes for pronation and supination in the proximal and distal radioulnar joints

Right forearm, anterior view.

a Supination (the radius and ulna are parallel to each other).
b Pronation (the radius crosses over the ulna).

The proximal radioulnar joint functions together with the distal radioulnar joint to enable pronation and supination movements of the hand.

The movements of both joints are functionally interlinked by the interosseous membrane, so that the movement of one is necessarily associated with movement of the other. The axis for pronation and supination runs obliquely from the center of the humeral capitellum (not shown) through the center of the radial articular fovea down to the styloid process of the ulna.

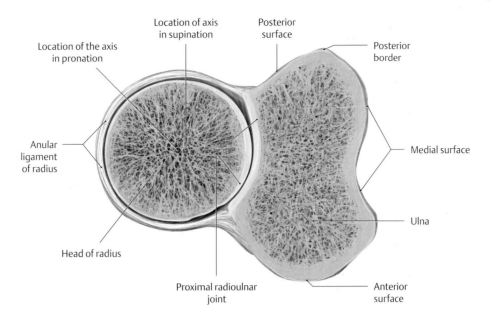

B Cross section through the right proximal radioulnar joint in pronation

Distal view. Owing to the slightly oval shape of the radial head, the pronation/supination axis that runs through the radial head moves approximately 2 mm radially during pronation (the long diameter of the radial head is transverse when pronation is reached). This ensures that when the hand is pronated, there will be sufficient space for the radial tuber-

osity within the interosseous space (= the space between the radial tuberosity and oblique cord; see **Aa**, for example).

Note the thicker articular cartilage of the radial articular circumference on the pronation side. This thickening occurs as an adaptation to the greater articular pressure in the proximal radioulnar joint in the pronated position.

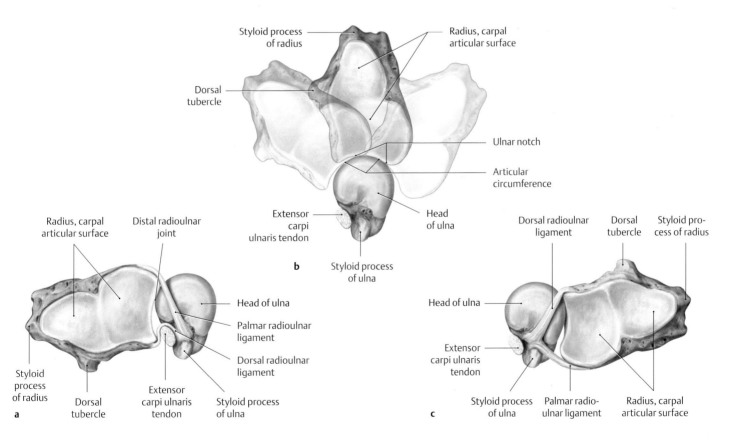

C Rotation of the radius and ulna during pronation and supination

View of the distal articular surfaces of the radius and ulna of the right forearm. For clarity, the ulnocarpal disk is not shown.

a Supination
b Semipronation
c Pronation

The dorsal and palmar radioulnar ligaments are part of the "ulnocarpal complex", which serves to stabilize the distal radioulnar joint. The mode of contact between the two distal articular surfaces varies with the position of the radius and ulna. They are in close apposition only in an intermediate (semipronated or neutral) position (after Schmidt and Lanz).

1.19 Movements of the Elbow and Radioulnar Joints

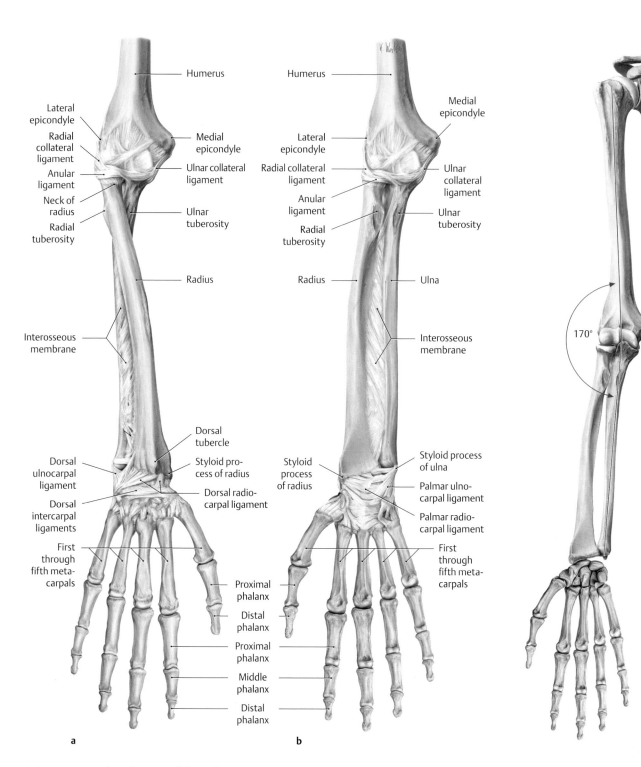

a

b

A Pronation and supination of the right hand

Anterior view.

a Pronation, **b** supination.

Pronation/supination of the hand makes it possible to raise an object to the mouth for eating and to touch any area of the body for protection or cleaning. Pronation and supina-

tion are also essential for the working hand in actions such as turning a screwdriver, screwing in a light bulb, emptying a bucket, unlocking a door, etc. The range of hand movements can be further increased by adding movements of the shoulder girdle and trunk. This may be done, for example, to enable a full 360° twisting movement of the hand.

B Normal valgus of the elbow joint

Skeleton of the right upper limb with the forearm supinated. Anterior view.

The shape of the humeral trochlea (see p. 238) results in a normal valgus angulation between the humeral shaft and ulna (*cubitus valgus*) [valgus = bend or twist outward, away from the body axis]). This applies particularly during extension and supination. This "cubital angle" equals approximately 170°.

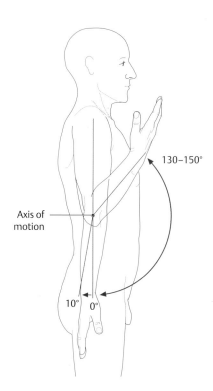

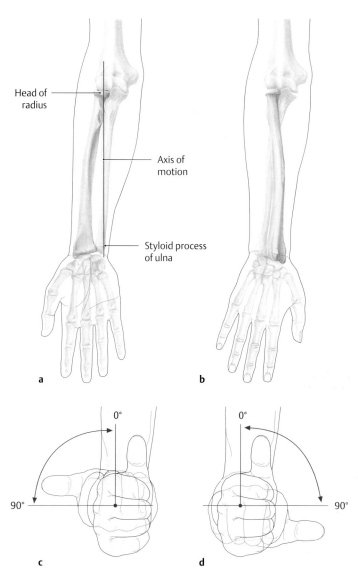

C Range of motion in the humeroradial and humeroulnar joints of the elbow

The flexion/extension axis of the forearm runs below the epicondyles through the capitellum and trochlea of the humerus. Starting from the neutral (zero-degree) position, both joints have a maximum range of 150° in flexion and approximately 10° in extension. Both movements are constrained either by soft tissues (muscles, fat, etc. = soft-tissue restraint) or by bone (olecranon = bony restraint).

D Range and axis of pronation/supination of the right hand

The neutral (zero-degree) position of the hand and forearm is also called semipronation. The axis of pronation/supination extends through the head of the radius and the styloid process of the ulna.

a Supination (the radius and ulna are parallel to each other).
b Pronation (the radius crosses over the ulna).
c Supination of the hand with the elbow flexed, viewed from the front (the palmar surface of the hand is up).
d Pronation of the hand with the elbow flexed, viewed from the front (the palmar surface of the hand is down).

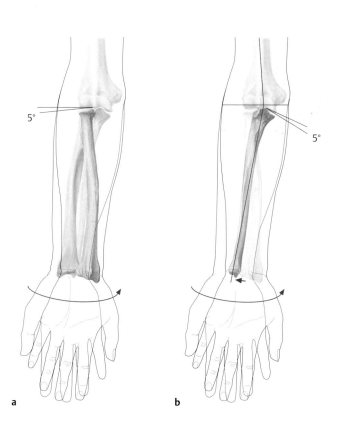

E Displacement and angulation of the radius and ulna during pronation

a Due to the crossed position of the radius and ulna in pronation, the articular fovea of the radius is angled approximately 5° distally.
b Because the distal part of the ulna moves laterally during pronation, the ulna is also angled approximately 5° distally in that position.

245

1.20   The Ligaments of the Hand

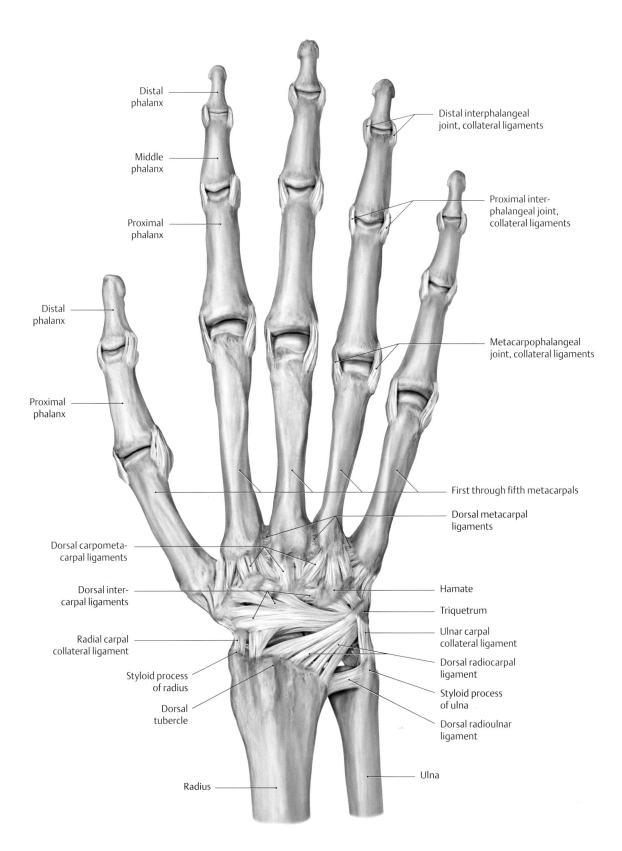

Distal
phalanx

Distal interphalangeal
joint, collateral ligaments

Middle
phalanx

Proximal inter-
phalangeal joint,
collateral ligaments

Proximal
phalanx

Distal
phalanx

Proximal
phalanx

Metacarpophalangeal
joint, collateral ligaments

First through fifth metacarpals

Dorsal metacarpal
ligaments

Dorsal carpometa-
carpal ligaments

Dorsal inter-
carpal ligaments

Hamate

Triquetrum

Radial carpal
collateral ligament

Ulnar carpal
collateral ligament

Dorsal radiocarpal
ligament

Styloid process
of radius

Styloid process
of ulna

Dorsal
tubercle

Dorsal radioulnar
ligament

Ulna

Radius

A The ligaments of the right hand. Posterior view.
The various ligaments in the carpal region form a dense network that strengthens the joint capsule of the wrist. *Four groups* of ligaments can be distinguished based on their location and arrangement (see also the palmar view in **B**):

1. The ligaments between the forearm and carpal bones (radiocarpal and ulnocarpal ligaments, collateral ligaments)
2. The ligaments between individual carpal bones (intercarpal ligaments)
3. The ligaments between the carpal and metacarpal bones (carpometacarpal ligaments)
4. The ligaments between the bases of the metacarpals (metacarpal ligaments)

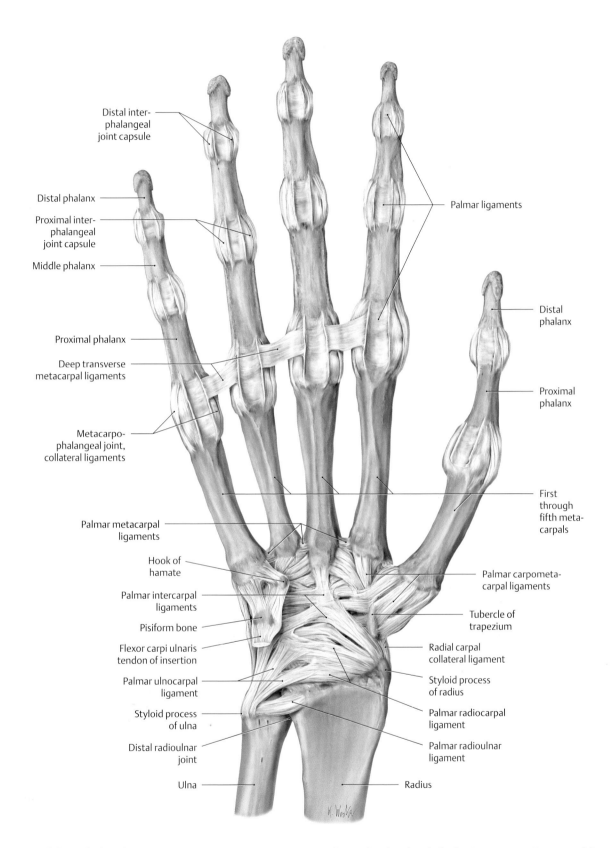

Distal inter-
phalangeal
joint capsule

Distal phalanx

Proximal inter-
phalangeal
joint capsule

Middle phalanx

Proximal phalanx

Deep transverse
metacarpal ligaments

Metacarpo-
phalangeal joint,
collateral ligaments

Palmar metacarpal
ligaments

Hook of
hamate

Palmar intercarpal
ligaments

Pisiform bone

Flexor carpi ulnaris
tendon of insertion

Palmar ulnocarpal
ligament

Styloid process
of ulna

Distal radioulnar
joint

Ulna

Palmar ligaments

Distal
phalanx

Proximal
phalanx

First
through
fifth meta-
carpals

Palmar carpometa-
carpal ligaments

Tubercle of
trapezium

Radial carpal
collateral ligament

Styloid process
of radius

Palmar radiocarpal
ligament

Palmar radioulnar
ligament

Radius

B The ligaments of the right hand. Anterior view.
Among the ligaments that bind the carpal bones together (intercarpal
ligaments), a distinction is made between *internal ligaments* and *surface
ligaments*. The internal ligaments interconnect the individual bones at
a deeper level and include the interosseous intercarpal ligaments (not
shown here). The surface ligaments consist of the dorsal (see **A**) and
palmar intercarpal ligaments.

1.21 The Carpal Tunnel

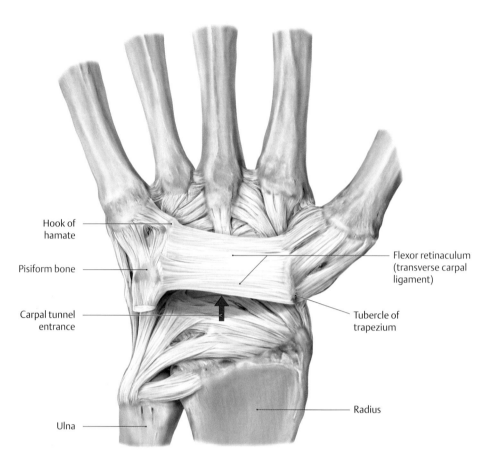

A Flexor retinaculum (transverse carpal ligament) and carpal tunnel, right hand

Anterior view. The bony elements of the wrist form a concave groove on the palmar side (see also **C**), which is closed by the flexor retinaculum (referred to clinically as the transverse carpal ligament) to form a fibroosseous tunnel called the carpal tunnel or carpal canal. The narrowest part of this canal is located approximately 1 cm beyond the midline of the distal row of carpal bones (see **D**). The cross-sectional area of the tunnel at that site measures only about 1.6 cm². The carpal tunnel is traversed by a total of *ten flexor tendons* (enclosed in tendon sheaths and embedded in connective tissue) and by the *median nerve* (see p. 326).

The tight fit of sensitive neurovascular structures with closely apposed, frequently moving tendons in this narrow space often causes problems when any of the structures swell or degenerate, leading to *carpal tunnel syndrome*. Narrowing of the tunnel can entrap or compress the median nerve, altering its function both by direct mechanical action and by restricting the blood flow within the nerve sheath. With chronic compression, the median nerve itself begins to degenerate beyond the site of entrapment, causing progressive pain and paresthesia, and, ultimately, denervation and wasting of the muscles it serves, particularly the abductor pollicis brevis (see p. 326).

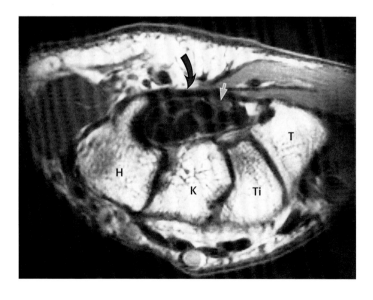

B Axial magnetic resonance image (T1-weighted) of the right hand at the level of the carpal tunnel

Proximal view. The flexor retinaculum (transverse carpal ligament) can be recognized as a band of low signal intensity (red arrow). Just below it toward the radial side is the median nerve (small arrow), whose water and lipid contents cause it to display a higher signal intensity than the superficial and deep flexor tendons. The primary diagnosis of carpal tunnel syndrome is based on clinical signs and electrophysiological measurements such as nerve conduction velocity. While conventional radiographs and CT scans can detect bony causes of the syndrome, magnetic resonance imaging can also demonstrate soft-tissue causes (e.g., edema or swelling of the median nerve, fibrosis, neuroma, etc.).

H = Hamate bone with hook
K = Capitate bone
T = Trapezium
Ti = Trapezoid

(from Vahlensieck and Reiser: MRT des Bewegungsapparates, 2. ed. Thieme, Stuttgart 2001).

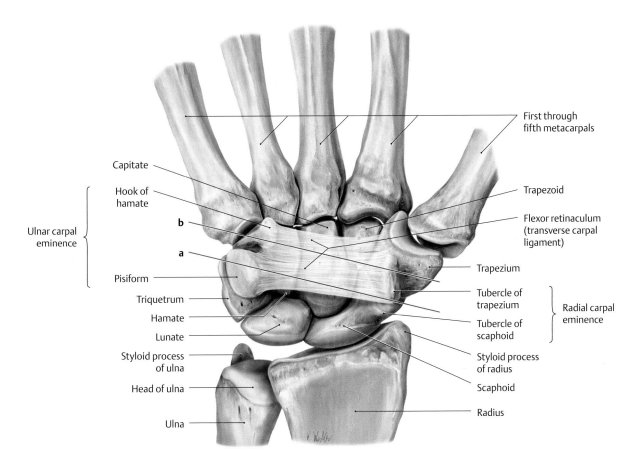

First through
fifth metacarpals

Capitate

Hook of
hamate

Ulnar carpal
eminence

Pisiform

Triquetrum

Hamate

Lunate

Styloid process
of ulna

Head of ulna

Ulna

Trapezoid

Flexor retinaculum
(transverse carpal
ligament)

Trapezium

Tubercle of
trapezium

Tubercle of
scaphoid

Radial carpal
eminence

Styloid process
of radius

Scaphoid

Radius

C Bony boundaries of the carpal tunnel of the right hand
Anterior view. The carpal bones form a convex arch on the dorsal side of the wrist and a concave arch on the palmar side. This creates a *carpal tunnel* on the palmar side, which is bounded by bony elevations on the radial and ulnar sides (the radial and ulnar carpal eminences). The tubercle of the trapezium forms the palpable eminence on the radial side, while the hook of the hamate and the pisiform bone form the eminence on the ulnar side. Stretched between them is the flexor retinaculum (transverse carpal ligament), which closes the carpal tunnel on the palmar side (the planes of section marked **a** and **b** correspond to the cross sections in Fig. **D**).

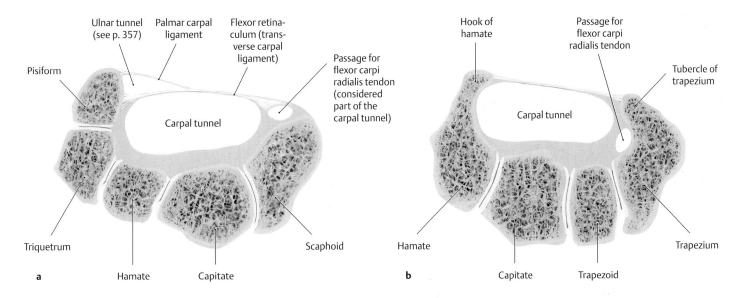

Ulnar tunnel
(see p. 357)

Palmar carpal
ligament

Flexor retina-
culum (trans-
verse carpal
ligament)

Passage for
flexor carpi
radialis tendon
(considered
part of the
carpal tunnel)

Pisiform

Carpal tunnel

Triquetrum

Hamate   Capitate

Scaphoid

a

Hook of
hamate

Passage for
flexor carpi
radialis tendon

Tubercle of
trapezium

Carpal tunnel

Hamate

Capitate   Trapezoid

Trapezium

b

D Cross sections through the carpal tunnel
a Cross section through the proximal part of the carpal tunnel (plane **a** in **C**).
b Cross section through the distal part of the carpal tunnel (plane **b** in **C**).

Note: The carpal tunnel is narrowest over the center of the distal row of carpal bones (**b**) (after Schmidt and Lanz).

249

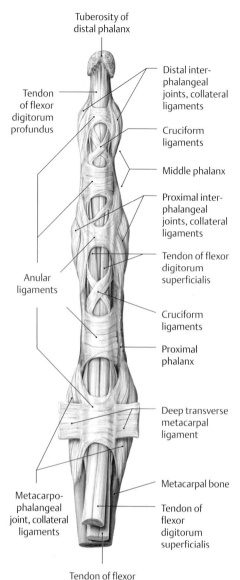

Tuberosity of distal phalanx

Tendon of flexor digitorum profundus

Distal interphalangeal joints, collateral ligaments

Cruciform ligaments

Middle phalanx

Proximal interphalangeal joints, collateral ligaments

Anular ligaments

Tendon of flexor digitorum superficialis

Cruciform ligaments

Proximal phalanx

Deep transverse metacarpal ligament

Metacarpophalangeal joint, collateral ligaments

Metacarpal bone

Tendon of flexor digitorum superficialis

b Tendon of flexor digitorum profundus

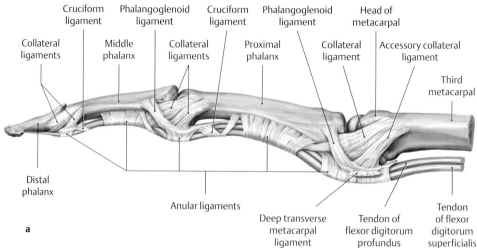

Collateral ligaments

Cruciform ligament

Phalangoglenoid ligament

Middle phalanx

Collateral ligaments

Cruciform ligament

Phalangoglenoid ligament

Proximal phalanx

Collateral ligament

Head of metacarpal

Accessory collateral ligament

Third metacarpal

Distal phalanx

Anular ligaments

Deep transverse metacarpal ligament

Tendon of flexor digitorum profundus

Tendon of flexor digitorum superficialis

a

A The joint capsules, ligaments, and digital tendon sheath of the right middle finger

a Lateral view, **b** Anterior view.

The long flexor tendons (flexor digitorum superficialis and profundus) run in a strong, common synovial tendon sheath (not shown here) on the palmar side of the fingers. The *tendon sheaths* are guide mechanisms that allow for frictionless gliding of the long flexor tendons. The outer fibrous layer of the tendon sheaths, the stratum fibrosum, is strengthened by *anular ligaments* and *cruciform ligaments* (see **B**), which also bind the sheaths to the palmar surface of the phalanx and prevent palmar deviation of the sheaths during flexion. The gaps between the anular and cruciform ligaments are necessary to allow flexion of the fingers (see also p. 298, Musculature: Topographical Anatomy).

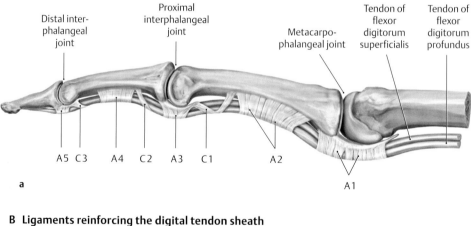

Distal interphalangeal joint

Proximal interphalangeal joint

Metacarpophalangeal joint

Tendon of flexor digitorum superficialis

Tendon of flexor digitorum profundus

A5 C3 A4 C2 A3 C1 A2

A1

a

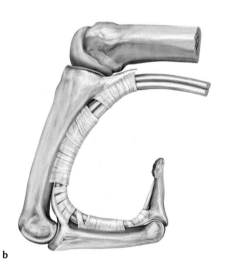

b

B Ligaments reinforcing the digital tendon sheath

a Lateral view in extension, **b** lateral view in flexion.

A 1–5 = anular ligaments, C 1–3 = cruciform ligaments.

- First anular ligament (A1): at the level of the metacarpophalangeal joint
- Second anular ligament (A2): on the shaft of the proximal phalanx
- Third anular ligament (A3): at the level of the proximal interphalangeal joint
- Fourth anular ligament (A4): on the shaft of the middle phalanx
- Fifth anular ligament (A5): at the level of the distal interphalangeal joint

The cruciform ligaments are highly variable in their course.

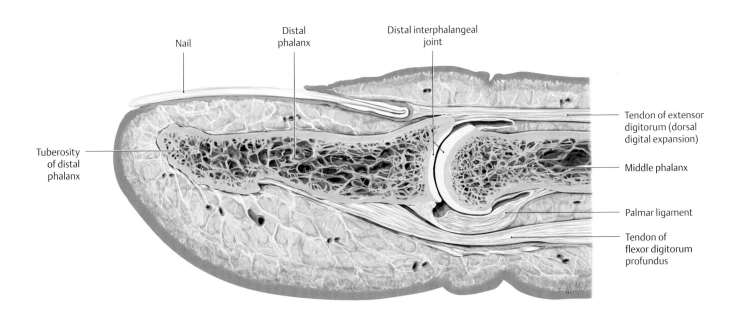

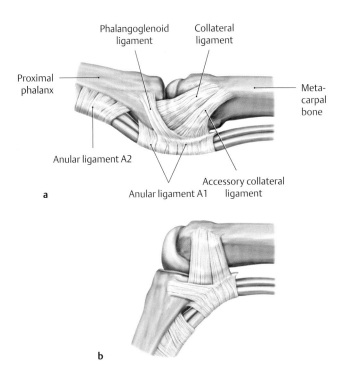

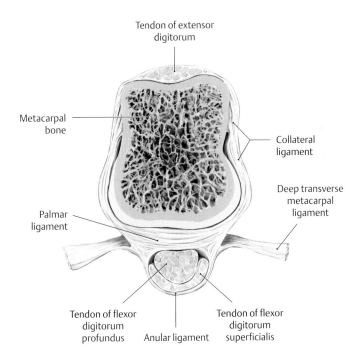

C Longitudinal section through the distal part of a finger

In the metacarpophalangeal joint as well as the proximal and distal interphalangeal joints, the palmar articular surfaces of the phalanges are enlarged proximally by a fibrocartilaginous plate called the palmar ligament (volar plate). The palmar ligaments also form the floor of the digital tendon sheaths at these locations (after Schmidt and Lanz).

D The capsule and ligaments of the metacarpophalangeal joint

a Extension, b flexion. Lateral view.

Note: The collateral ligament is *lax* in extension and *taut* in flexion. For this reason, the finger joints should always be placed in a "functional position" (e.g., with the metacarpophalangeal joints flexed approximately 50–60°, see p. 255) if the hand is to be immobilized (e.g., in a cast) for a long period of time. If this is not done and the finger joints remain extended for a prolonged period, the collateral ligaments will shorten and create an extension deformity after the cast is removed. The accessory collateral ligament and phalangoglenoid ligament are taut in both flexion and extension and act mainly as restraints to limit extension.

E Cross section through the head of the third metacarpal of the right hand

Proximal view. At the level of the second through fifth metacarpal heads, the volar fibrocartilage plates (palmar ligaments) are interconnected by transverse bands, the deep transverse metacarpal ligaments. By binding the palmar ligaments to the A 1 anular ligaments (see **B**) of the flexor tendon sheaths, they also strengthen the distal metacarpus and stabilize the transverse metacarpal arch (after Schmidt and Lanz).

1.23 The Carpometacarpal Joint of the Thumb

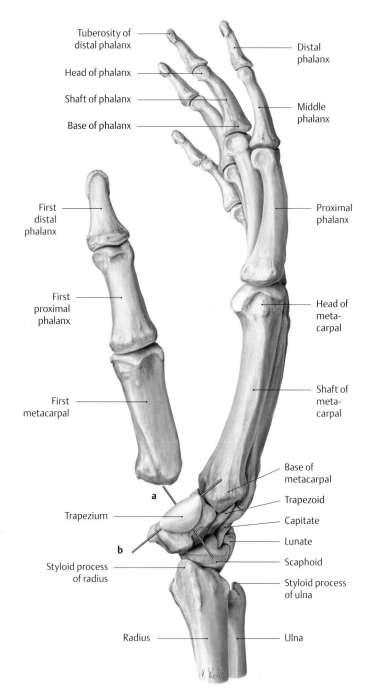

Tuberosity of distal phalanx

Head of phalanx

Shaft of phalanx

Base of phalanx

Distal phalanx

Middle phalanx

First distal phalanx

Proximal phalanx

First proximal phalanx

Head of metacarpal

First metacarpal

Shaft of metacarpal

Base of metacarpal

Trapezoid

Trapezium

Capitate

Lunate

Scaphoid

Styloid process of radius

Styloid process of ulna

Radius

Ulna

A Axes of motion of the carpometacarpal joint of the thumb
Skeleton of the right hand, radial view. The first metacarpal bone has been moved slightly distally to facilitate orientation. The saddle-shaped articular surfaces of the trapezium and first metacarpal allow movements about two cardinal axes:

• An abduction/adduction axis (**a**)
• A flexion/extension axis (**b**)

While the axis for abduction/adduction runs approximately on a dorsopalmar line, the axis for flexion/extension runs transversely through the sellar limb of the trapezium. When the thumb is moved toward the small finger (opposition), a rotary movement takes place about a longitudinal axis through the first metacarpal bone (third degree of freedom). This oppositional movement of the thumb—essential for precision grasping movements of the hand—is made possible by the natural mismatch of the articular surfaces (see **F**).

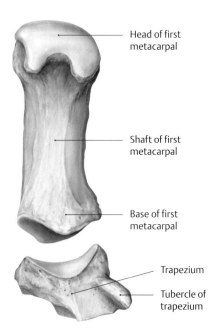

Head of first metacarpal

Shaft of first metacarpal

Base of first metacarpal

Trapezium

Tubercle of trapezium

B Articulating surfaces of the carpometacarpal joint of the thumb
Palmar-ulnar view. The articular surface of the trapezium is convex in the dorsopalmar direction and concave in the radioulnar direction. This is opposite to the curvatures found in the corresponding articular surface of the first metacarpal bone.

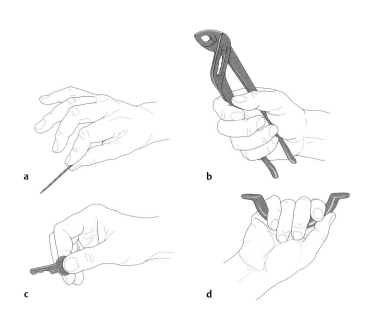

a   b

c   d

C Types of grip
Normal hand actions can be reduced to four primary types of grip:
a Pinch or precision grip, **b** power grip, **c** key grip, **d** hook grip.
The clinical examination should include function testing of the hand, giving particular attention to disturbances of fine motor skills and gross strength. It is important, for example, to evaluate the pinch grip and key grip, the pinch grip between the thumb and index finger having fundamental importance for the function of the hand. This is why, in issues pertaining to workers' compensation, loss of the thumb or index finger is considered to have a more serious impact on occupational capacity than the loss of the other long fingers.

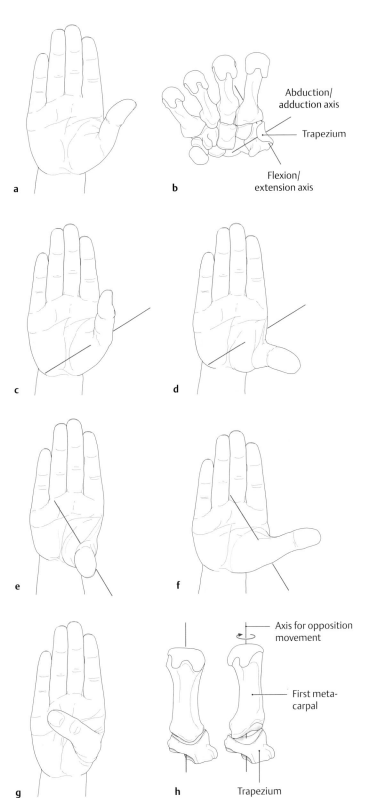

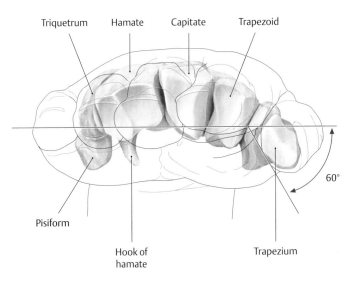

E Relationship of the thumb to the fingers in the neutral (zero-degree) position
Right hand, distal view. Owing to the concave arch of the carpal bones, the scaphoid and trapezium have a markedly radiopalmar orientation. As a result, the metacarpus of the thumb is not placed in line with the other fingers but is rotated approximately 60° toward the palm.

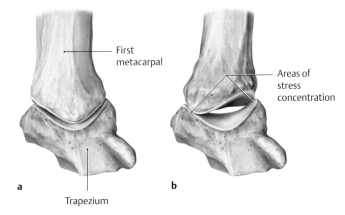

F Rotation-induced incongruity of the carpometacarpal joint during opposition of the thumb
a Neutral (zero-degree) position, **b** the thumb in opposition.
As a sellar (saddle-shaped) joint, the carpometacarpal joint of the thumb is subjected to functional stresses that may promote osteoarthritis (after Koebke). The potentially harmful stresses are created by rotation of the first metacarpal bone during opposition of the thumb. When the thumb is maximally opposed, this rotation greatly reduces the surface area available for stress transfer across the joint (contrast this with the large area available in **a**). This concentration of stresses in a localized area predisposes to degenerative changes in the ascending sellar limb of the first metacarpal bone as well as the articular surface of the trapezium (first carpometacarpal osteoarthritis).

D Movements in the carpometacarpal joint of the thumb
Right hand. Palmar view.

a The neutral (zero-degree) position.
b Axes of motion in the carpometacarpal joint of the thumb.
c Adduction.
d Abduction.
e Flexion.
f Extension.
g Opposition.
h Axis for opposition of the thumb. As the first metacarpal rotates, its area of contact with the articular surface of the trapezium is greatly diminished (see **F**).

1.24 Movements of the Hand and Finger Joints

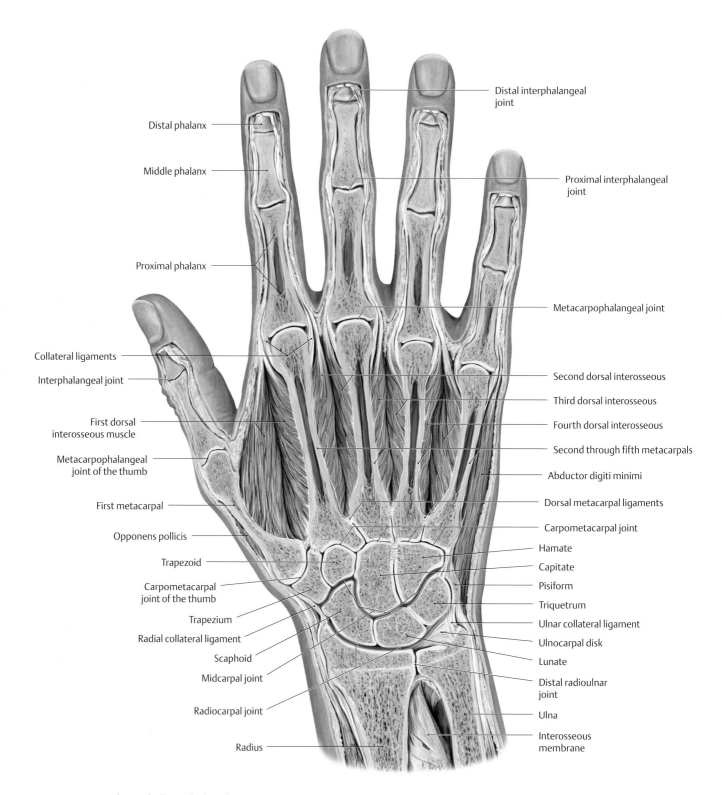

A Transverse section through the right hand
Posterior view. The hand and forearm are connected at the **radiocarpal and midcarpal joints** (both indicated by blue lines in the drawing). Morphologically, the *radiocarpal joint* is an ovoid or ellipsoidal joint, while the *midcarpal joint* is an interdigitating hinge joint (with an approximately S-shaped joint space between the proximal and distal rows of carpal bones). Except for the carpometacarpal joint of the thumb, the joints between the distal row of carpal bones and the bases of the metacarpals (the carpometacarpal joints) are *amphiarthroses* (joined by fibrocartilage) that permit very little motion.

The **finger joints** are classified as follows:

- *Metacarpophalangeal joints* between the metacarpal bones and the proximal phalanges (MCP joints, spheroidal type)
- *Proximal interphalangeal joints* between the proximal and middle phalanges (PIP joints, hinge type)
- *Distal interphalangeal joints* between the middle and distal phalanges (DIP joints, hinge type)

Since the *thumb* lacks a middle phalanx, it has but two joints: a metacarpophalangeal joint and an interphalangeal joint (drawing based on a specimen from the Anatomical Collection at the University of Kiel).

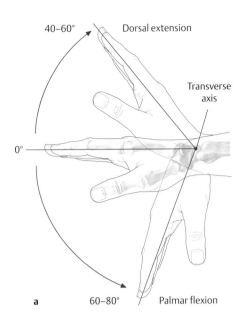

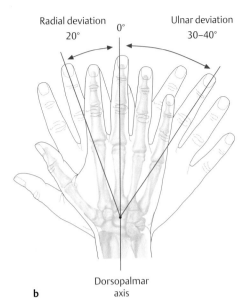

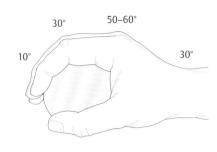

B Movements of the radiocarpal and midcarpal joints

Starting from the "neutral (zero-degree) position," palmar *flexion* and dorsal *extension* are performed about a transverse axis (**a**), while radial and ulnar deviation occur about a dorsopalmar axis (**b**). The *transverse* axis runs through the lunate bone for the radiocarpal joint and through the capitate bone for the midcarpal joint. The *dorsopalmar* axis runs through the capitate bone. Thus, while palmar flexion and dorsal extension can occur in both the radiocarpal and midcarpal joints, radial and ulnar deviation can occur only in the radiocarpal joint.

C Functional position of the hand

For postoperative immobilization of the hand, the desired position of the wrist and fingers should be considered when the cast, splint, or other device is applied. Otherwise the ligaments may shorten and the hand can no longer assume a normal resting position.

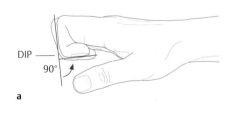

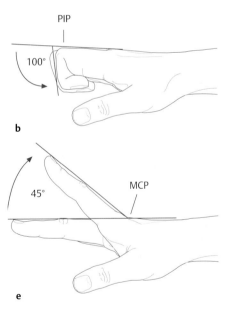

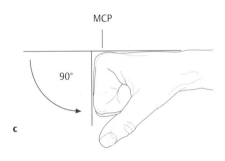

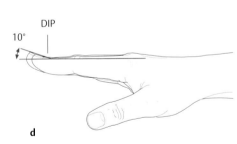

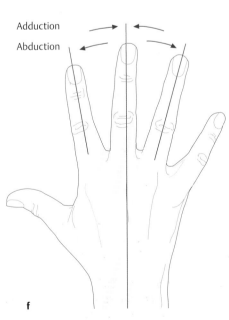

D Range of motion of the finger joints

The proximal interphalangeal (PIP) and distal interphalangeal (DIP) joints are pure hinge joints with only one degree of freedom (flexion/extension). The metacarpophalangeal (MCP) joints of the second through fifth fingers are shaped like spheroidal joints with three theoretical degrees of freedom, but rotation is so limited by the collateral ligaments that only two degrees of freedom exist: flexion/extension and abduction/adduction. The following specific movements of the finger joints are distinguished:

a Flexion in the distal interphalangeal joint (DIP).

b Flexion in the proximal interphalangeal joint (PIP).

c Flexion in the metacarpophalangeal joint (MCP).

d Extension in the distal interphalangeal joint (DIP).

e Extension in the metacarpophalangeal joint (MCP).

f Abduction and adduction in the metacarpophalangeal joints (spreading the fingers apart and bringing them together about a dorsopalmar axis through the heads of the metacarpals).

Abduction/adduction movements are described in relation to the middle finger: all movements away from the middle finger are classified as abduction, all movements toward the middle finger as adduction.

2.1 Functional Muscle Groups

A Principles used in the classification of muscles
The muscles of the upper limb can be classified according to various criteria. An optimum system for classification should be logical and clear. The following criteria are suitable for classifying muscles:

- Origin
- Topography
- Function
- Innervation

While function and topography in the upper limb are often interrelated (muscles with the same action on a joint are often located close together), muscles that have similar actions in the shoulder region (e.g., muscles of the shoulder joint and shoulder girdle) vary considerably in their location. The following classification (**B**), then, is a compromise between topographical and functional considerations. In section **C**, a different muscle classification system, based on innervation, is presented.
The grouping of muscles by the pattern of their innervation reveals features of their embryological and phylogenetic origin, and provides clinical insights into the clusters of consequences from damage to particular nerves.

B Functional-topographical classification of the muscles of the upper limb

Muscles of the shoulder girdle

Shoulder girdle muscles that have migrated from the head
- Trapezius
- Sternocleidomastoid
- Omohyoid

Posterior muscles of the trunk and shoulder girdle
- Rhomboid major
- Rhomboid minor
- Levator scapulae

Anterior muscles of the trunk and shoulder girdle
- Subclavius
- Pectoralis minor
- Serratus anterior

Muscles of the shoulder joint

Posterior muscle group
- Supraspinatus
- Infraspinatus
- Teres minor
- Subscapularis
- Deltoid
- Latissimus dorsi
- Teres major

Anterior muscle group
- Pectoralis major
- Coracobrachialis

Muscles of the arm

Posterior muscle group
- Triceps brachii
- Anconeus

Anterior muscle group
- Brachialis
- Biceps brachii

Muscles of the forearm

Posterior forearm muscles
- Superficial extensors
  - Extensor digitorum
  - Extensor digiti minimi
  - Extensor carpi ulnaris

- Deep extensors
  - Supinator
  - Abductor pollicis longus
  - Extensor pollicis brevis
  - Extensor pollicis longus
  - Extensor indicis

Anterior forearm muscles
- Superficial flexors
  - Pronator teres
  - Flexor digitorum superficialis
  - Flexor carpi radialis
  - Flexor carpi ulnaris
  - Palmaris longus

- Deep flexors
  - Flexor digitorum profundus
  - Flexor pollicis longus
  - Pronator quadratus

Radial forearm muscles
- Radialis group
  - Brachioradialis
  - Extensor carpi radialis longus
  - Extensor carpi radialis brevis

Muscles of the hand

Metacarpal muscles
- First through fourth lumbricals
- First through fourth dorsal interossei
- First through third palmar interossei

Thenar muscles
- Abductor pollicis brevis
- Adductor pollicis
- Flexor pollicis brevis
- Opponens pollicis

Hypothenar muscles
- Abductor digiti minimi
- Flexor digiti minimi
- Opponens digiti minimi
- Palmaris brevis

C Classification of the muscles of the upper limb by their innervation

Almost all the muscles of the upper limb are innervated by the brachial plexus arising from spinal cord segments C 5–T 1. Exceptions are the trapezius, sternocleidomastoid, and omohyoid; originating in vertebrate evolution as muscles of the head, they are supplied by cranial nerve XI (accessory nerve) and the cervical plexus (ansa cervicalis).

Nerve	Innervated muscles
Accessory nerve	Trapezius Sternocleidomastoid
Ansa cervicalis	Omohyoid
Dorsal scapular nerve	Levator scapulae Rhomboid major Rhomboid minor
Suprascapular nerve	Supraspinatus Infraspinatus
Long thoracic nerve	Serratus anterior
Nerve to the subclavius	Subclavius
Subscapular nerve	Subscapularis Teres major
Thoracodorsal nerve	Latissimus dorsi
Medial and lateral pectoral nerves	Pectoralis major Pectoralis minor
Musculocutaneous nerve	Coracobrachialis Biceps brachii Brachialis
Axillary nerve	Deltoid Teres minor
Radial nerve	Triceps brachii Anconeus Supinator Brachioradialis Extensor carpi radialis longus Extensor carpi radialis brevis Extensor digitorum Extensor digiti minimi Extensor carpi ulnaris Extensor pollicis longus Extensor pollicis brevis Extensor indicis Abductor pollicis longus
Median nerve	Pronator teres Pronator quadratus Palmaris longus Flexor carpi radialis Flexor pollicis longus Flexor digitorum profundus (½) Flexor digitorum superficialis Abductor pollicis brevis Opponens pollicis Flexor pollicis brevis (superficial head) First and second lumbricals
Ulnar nerve	Flexor carpi ulnaris Flexor digitorum profundus (½) Palmaris brevis Flexor digiti minimi Abductor digiti minimi Opponens digiti minimi Adductor pollicis Flexor pollicis brevis (deep head) Palmar and dorsal interossei Third and fourth lumbricals

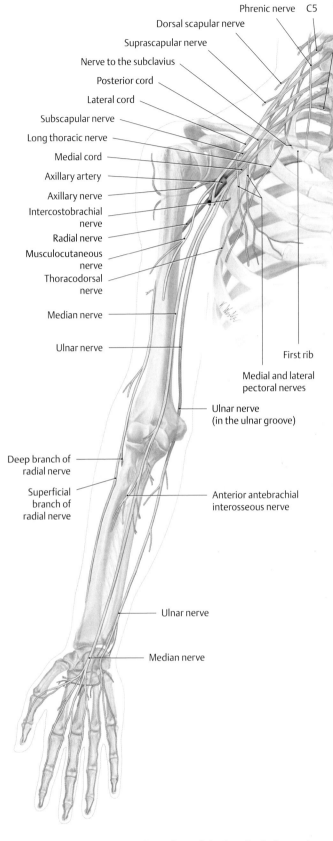

D Overview of the motor branches of the brachial plexus that supply the muscles of the upper limb

With the outgrowth of the limb buds from the trunk during embryonic development, the branches of the brachial plexus follow the genetically determined *posterior* extensor muscles and *anterior* flexor muscles. The nerves for the *extensors* (radial and axillary nerves) arise from the three *posterior* divisions of the brachial plexus, while the nerves for the *flexors* (musculocutaneous nerve, ulnar nerve, median nerve) arise from the three *anterior* divisions of the plexus (see p. 346, Neurovascular Systems: Topographical Anatomy).

2.2 The Muscles of the Shoulder Girdle: Trapezius, Sternocleidomastoid, and Omohyoid

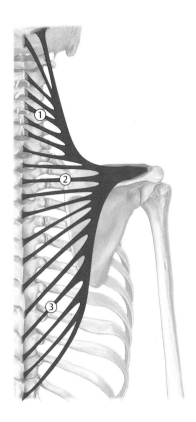

Origin:	① Descending part1[1]:
	• Occipital bone (superior nuchal line and external occipital protuberance)
	• The spinous processes of all cervical vertebrae via the nuchal ligament
	② Transverse part:
	Broad aponeurosis at the level of the T 1–T 4 spinous processes
	③ Ascending part:
	Spinous processes of T 5–T 12
Insertion:	• Lateral third of the clavicle (descending part)
	• Acromion (transverse part)
	• Scapular spine (ascending part)
Actions:	• Descending part:
	– Draws the scapula obliquely upward and rotates the glenoid cavity inferiorly (acting with the inferior part of the serratus anterior)
	– Tilts the head to the same side and rotates it to the opposite side (with the shoulder girdle fixed)
	• Transverse part: draws the scapula medially
	• Ascending part: draws the scapula medially downward (supports the rotating action of the descending part)
	• Entire muscle: steadies the scapula on the thorax
Innervation:	Cranial nerve XI (accessory nerve) and cervical plexus (C 2–C 4)

A Schematic of the trapezius

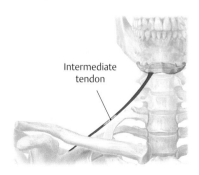

Sternal head

Clavicular head

Origin:	• Sternal head: manubrium sterni
	• Clavicular head: medial third of the clavicle
Insertion:	Mastoid process and superior nuchal line
Actions:	• Unilateral: – Tilts the head to the same side
	– Rotates the head to the opposite side
	• Bilateral: – Extends the head
	– Assists in respiration when the head is fixed
Innervation:	Accessory nerve (cranial nerve XI) and direct branches from the cervical plexus (C 1–C 2)

B Schematic of the sternocleidomastoid

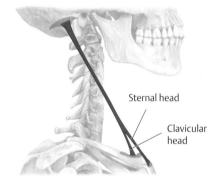

Intermediate tendon

Origin:	Superior border of the scapula
Insertion:	Body of the hyoid bone
Actions:	• Depresses (fixes) the hyoid bone
	• Moves the larynx and hyoid bone downward (for phonation and the final phase of swallowing)
	• Tenses the cervical fascia with its intermediate tendon and maintains patency of the internal jugular vein
Innervation:	Ansa cervicalis of the cervical plexus (C1–C4)

C Schematic of the omohyoid

1 The structures listed in the tables are not all illustrated in the drawings at right because they are not necessarily visible in those views. The tables and associated diagrams are intended to give a systematic overview of the named muscles and their actions, while the drawings at right are intended to display the muscles as they would appear in a dissection.

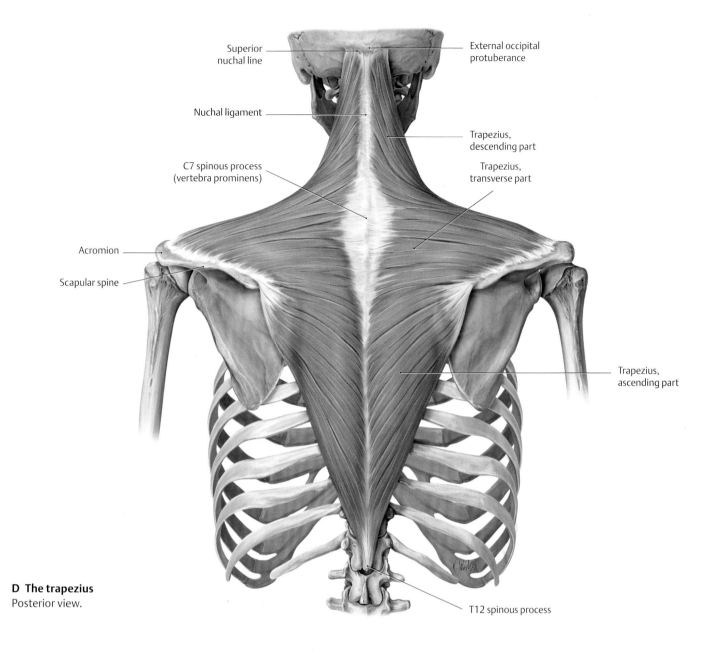

Superior nuchal line

External occipital protuberance

Nuchal ligament

Trapezius, descending part

C7 spinous process (vertebra prominens)

Trapezius, transverse part

Acromion

Scapular spine

Trapezius, ascending part

T12 spinous process

D The trapezius
Posterior view.

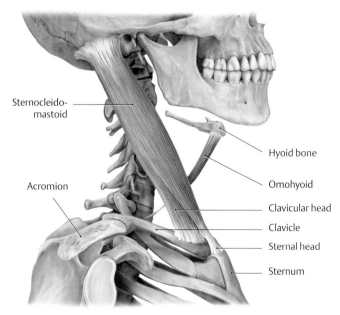

Sternocleido-mastoid

Hyoid bone

Omohyoid

Clavicular head

Acromion

Clavicle

Sternal head

Sternum

E The sternocleidomastoid and omohyoid
Right side, lateral view.

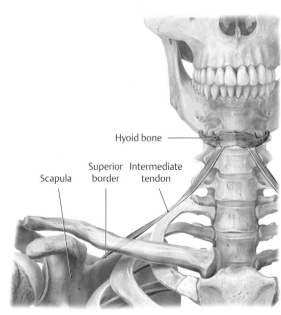

Hyoid bone

Scapula

Superior border

Intermediate tendon

F The omohyoid
Right side, anterior view.

2.3 The Muscles of the Shoulder Girdle: Serratus anterior, Subclavius, Pectoralis minor, Levator scapulae, and Rhomboid major and minor

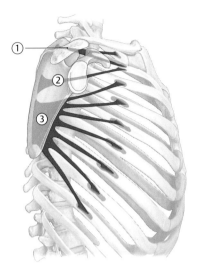

Origin:	First through ninth ribs
Insertion:	Scapula: ① Superior part (superior angle)
	② Intermediate part (medial border)
	③ Inferior part (inferior angle and medial border)
Actions:	• Entire muscle: draws the scapula laterally forward, elevates the ribs when the shoulder girdle is fixed (assists in respiration)
	• Inferior part: rotates the scapula and draws its inferior angle laterally forward, (rotates glenoid cavity superiorly)
	• Superior part: lowers the raised arm (antagonist to the inferior part)
Innervation:	Long thoracic nerve (C 5–C 7)

A Schematic of the serratus anterior

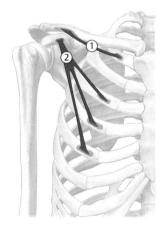

① Subclavius

Origin:	First rib (chondro-osseous junction)
Insertion:	Inferior surface of the clavicle (lateral third)
Action:	Steadies the clavicle in the sternoclavicular joint
Innervation:	Nerve to the subclavius (C 5, C 6)

② Pectoralis minor

Origin:	Third through fifth ribs
Insertion:	Coracoid process of the scapula
Actions:	• Draws the scapula downward, causing its inferior angle to move posteromedially (lowers the raised arm), rotates glenoid inferiorly
	• Assists in respiration
Innervation:	Medial and lateral pectoral nerves (C6–T1)

B Schematic of the subclavius and pectoralis minor

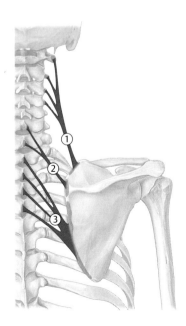

① Levator scapulae

Origin:	Transverse processes of the C 1–C 4 vertebrae
Insertion:	Superior angle of the scapula
Actions:	• Draws the scapula medially upward while moving the inferior angle medially (returns the raised arm to the neutral [zero-degree] position)
	• Inclines the neck toward the same side (when the scapula is fixed)
Innervation:	Dorsal scapular nerve (C4–C5)

② Rhomboid minor

Origin:	Spinous processes of the C 6 and C 7 vertebrae
Insertion:	Medial border of the scapula (above the scapular spine)
Actions:	• Steadies the scapula
	• Draws the scapula medially upward (returns the raised arm to the neutral [zero-degree] position)
Innervation:	Dorsal scapular nerve (C4–C5)

③ Rhomboid major

Origin:	Spinous processes of the T 1–T 4 vertebrae
Insertion:	Medial border of the scapula (below the scapular spine)
Actions:	• Steadies the scapula
	• Draws the scapula medially upward (returns the raised arm to the neutral [zero-degree] position)
Innervation:	Dorsal scapular nerve (C 4–C 5)

C Schematic of the levator scapulae and rhomboideus minor and major

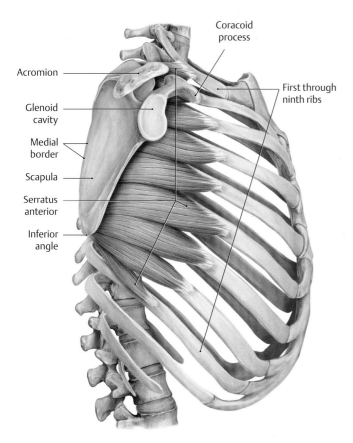

Coracoid process

Acromion

Glenoid cavity

Medial border

Scapula

Serratus anterior

Inferior angle

First through ninth ribs

D The serratus anterior
Right side, lateral view.

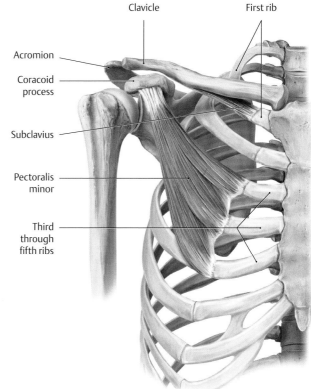

Clavicle

First rib

Acromion

Coracoid process

Subclavius

Pectoralis minor

Third through fifth ribs

E The pectoralis minor and subclavius
Right side, anterior view.

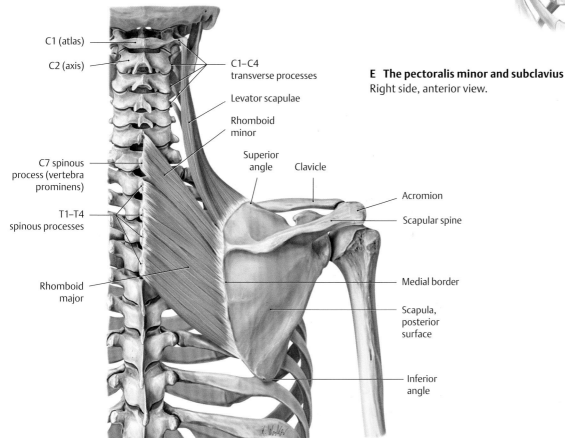

C1 (atlas)

C2 (axis)

C1–C4 transverse processes

Levator scapulae

Rhomboid minor

Superior angle

Clavicle

C7 spinous process (vertebra prominens)

T1–T4 spinous processes

Rhomboid major

Acromion

Scapular spine

Medial border

Scapula, posterior surface

Inferior angle

F The levator scapulae, rhomboideus major, and rhomboideus minor
Right side, posterior view.

2.4   The Muscles of the Shoulder Girdle: The Rotator Cuff

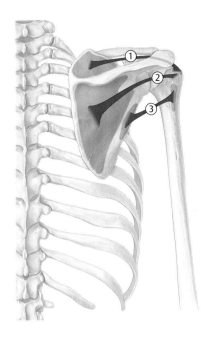

① **Supraspinatus**

Origin:	Supraspinous fossa of the scapula
Insertion:	Greater tuberosity of the humerus
Action:	Abduction
Innervation:	Suprascapular nerve (C 4–C 6)

② **Infraspinatus**

Origin:	Infraspinous fossa of the scapula
Insertion:	Greater tuberosity of the humerus
Action:	External rotation
Innervation:	Suprascapular nerve (C 4–C 6)

③ **Teres minor**

Origin:	Lateral border of the scapula
Insertion:	Greater tuberosity of the humerus
Action:	External rotation, weak adduction
Innervation:	Axillary nerve (C 5, C 6)

A Schematic of the supraspinatus, infraspinatus, and teres minor

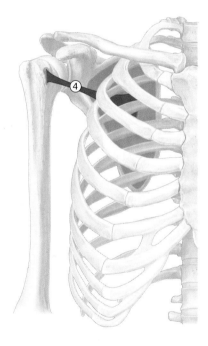

④ **Subscapularis**

Origin:	Subscapular fossa of the scapula
Insertion:	Lesser tuberosity of the humerus
Action:	Internal rotation
Innervation:	Subscapular nerve (C 5, C 6)

B Schematic of the subscapularis

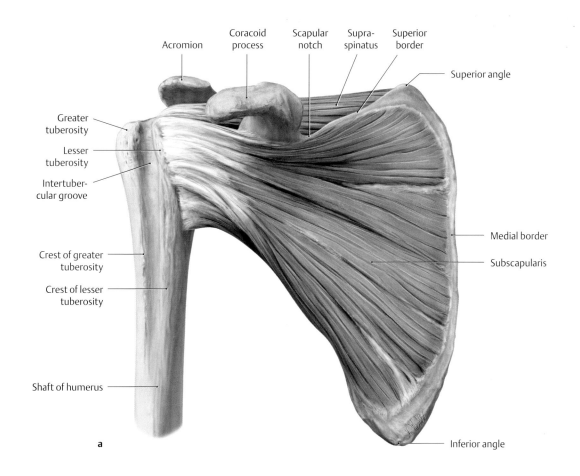

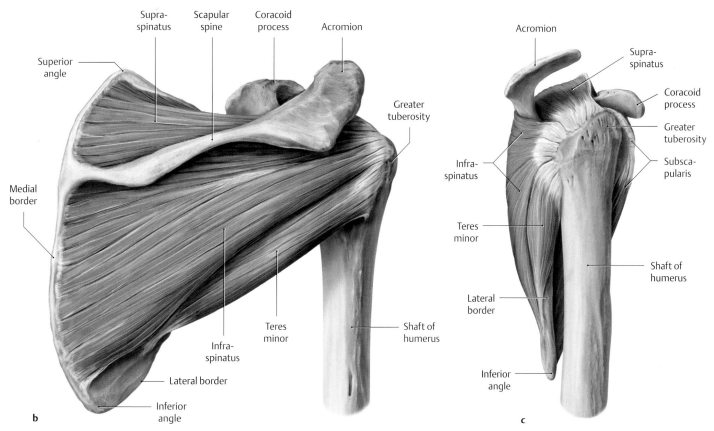

C Muscles of the rotator cuff: supraspinatus, infraspinatus, teres minor, and subscapularis
Right shoulder joint.

a Anterior view.
b Posterior view.
c Lateral view.

263

2.5 The Muscles of the Shoulder Girdle: The Deltoid

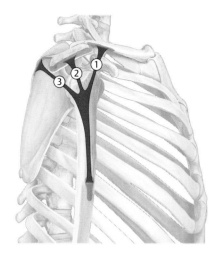

Origin: ① Clavicular part: lateral third of the clavicle
             ② Acromial part: acromion
             ③ Spinal part: scapular spine
Insertion: Deltoid tuberosity on the humerus
Actions: • Clavicular part: anteversion (moves the arm and shoulder forward), internal rotation, adduction
             • Acromial part: abduction
             • Spinal part: retroversion (moves the arm and shoulder backward), external rotation, adduction

Between 60° and 90° of abduction, the clavicular and spinal parts of the deltoid assist the acromial part of the muscle with abduction.
Innervation: Axillary nerve (C 5, C 6)

A Schematic of the deltoid

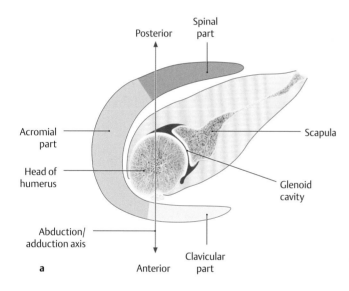

a

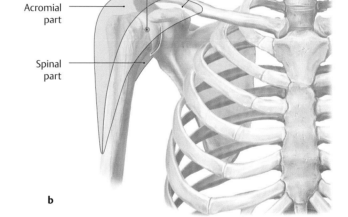

b

B The variable actions of the deltoid components
a Cross section through the right shoulder joint.
b Right shoulder joint in the neutral (zero-degree) position, anterior view.
c Right shoulder joint in 60° of abduction, anterior view.

The actions of the three parts of the deltoid muscle (clavicular, acromial, and spinal) depend on their relationship to the position of the humerus and its axis of motion. As a result, the parts of the deltoid can act antagonistically as well as synergistically. At *less than 60°* abduction, the clavicular and spinal parts of the deltoid act as antagonists to the acromial part, but at *more than 60°* abduction the acromial part assists in the abduction. Starting from the neutral (zero-degree) position, the acromial part of the deltoid abducts the arm and steadies it in any position it assumes. When the arm is abducted past approximately 60°, the clavicular and spinal parts also become active as they move past the sagittal motion axis (abduction/adduction axis, **c**). This alters the action of these parts: they act as adductors below 60°, but when the arm passes 60° they become abductors.

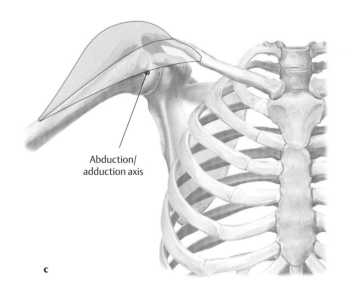

c

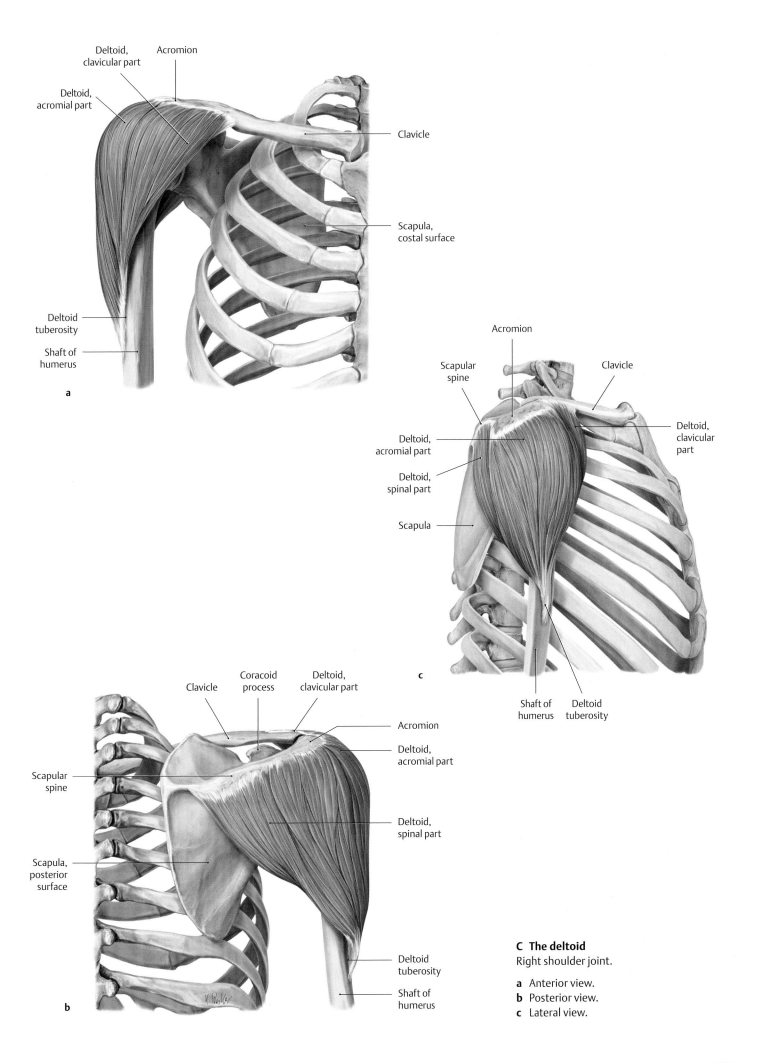

Deltoid, clavicular part

Acromion

Deltoid, acromial part

Clavicle

Scapula, costal surface

Deltoid tuberosity

Shaft of humerus

a

Acromion

Scapular spine

Clavicle

Deltoid, acromial part

Deltoid, clavicular part

Deltoid, spinal part

Scapula

Shaft of humerus

Deltoid tuberosity

c

Clavicle

Coracoid process

Deltoid, clavicular part

Acromion

Deltoid, acromial part

Scapular spine

Deltoid, spinal part

Scapula, posterior surface

Deltoid tuberosity

Shaft of humerus

b

C The deltoid
Right shoulder joint.

a Anterior view.
b Posterior view.
c Lateral view.

265

2.6 The Muscles of the Shoulder Girdle: Latissimus dorsi and Teres major

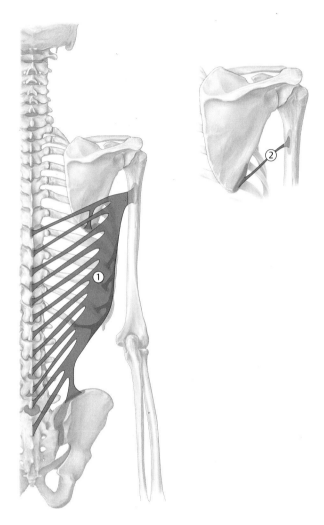

A Schematic of the latissimus dorsi and teres major

① **Latissimus dorsi**

Origin:	• Vertebral part:
	  – Spinous processes of the T 7–T 12 vertebrae
	  – Thoracolumbar fascia of the spinous processes of all lumbar vertebrae and the sacrum
	• Iliac part: posterior third of the iliac crest
	• Costal part: 9th through 12th ribs
	• Scapular part: inferior angle of the scapula

Insertion:	Crest of the lesser tuberosity (anterior view) of the humerus
Actions:	Internal rotation, adduction, retroversion (moves the arm backward), respiration (expiration, "cough muscle")
Innervation:	Thoracodorsal nerve (C 6–C 8)

② **Teres major**

Origin:	Inferior angle of the scapula
Insertion:	Crest of the lesser tuberosity of the humerus
Action:	Internal rotation, adduction, retroversion
Innervation:	Thoracodorsal nerve (C 6–C 8)

B Course of the tendon of insertion of latissimus dorsi in the neutral position and in elevation

Posterior view. The latissimus dorsi muscle is most active in the abducted or elevated arm. Raising the arm untwists the muscle fibers in the area of insertion, increasing the muscle's stretch and maximizing the force it can exert. When the position of the arm is fixed, the latissimus dorsi can pull the body upwards as in the act of climbing or can depress the arm against a resistance. This makes the latissimus dorsi an important muscle for paraplegics, for example, who can use that muscle to raise themselves from wheelchairs.

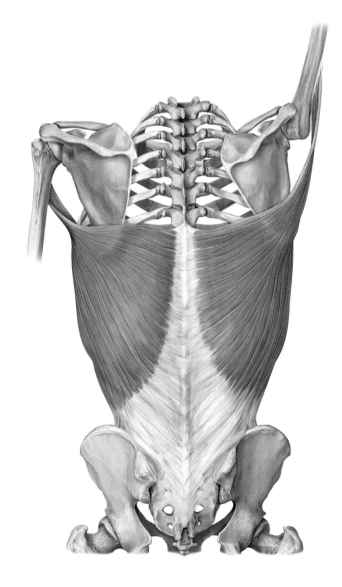

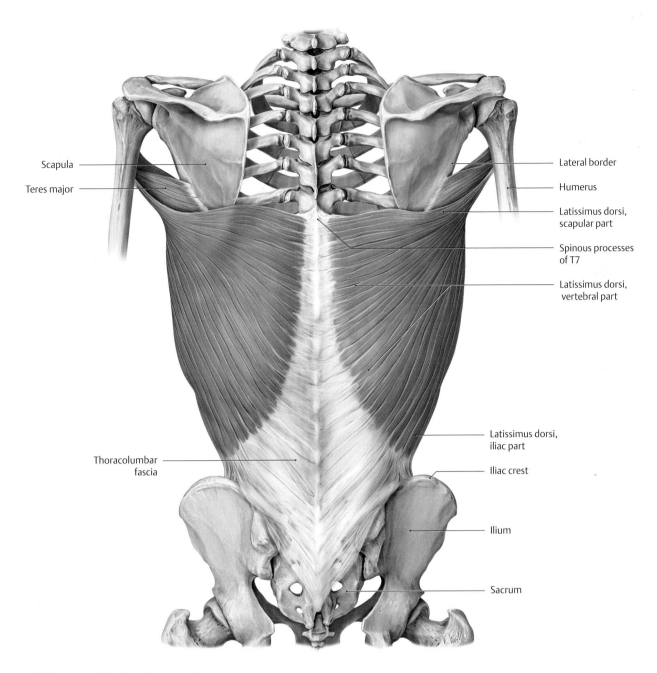

Scapula

Teres major

Lateral border

Humerus

Latissimus dorsi, scapular part

Spinous processes of T7

Latissimus dorsi, vertebral part

Latissimus dorsi, iliac part

Thoracolumbar fascia

Iliac crest

Ilium

Sacrum

C The latissimus dorsi and teres major
Posterior view.

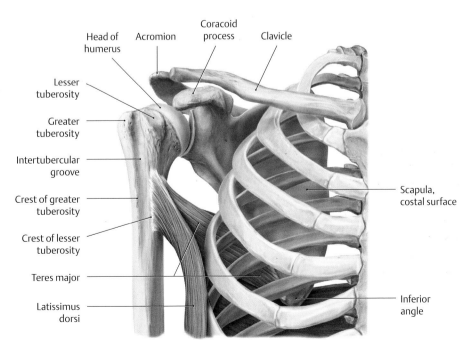

Head of humerus

Acromion

Coracoid process

Clavicle

Lesser tuberosity

Greater tuberosity

Intertubercular groove

Crest of greater tuberosity

Crest of lesser tuberosity

Teres major

Latissimus dorsi

Scapula, costal surface

Inferior angle

D Common insertion of the latissimus dorsi and teres major on the crest of the lesser tuberosity
Anterior view.

2.7 The Muscles of the Shoulder Girdle: Pectoralis major and Coracobrachialis

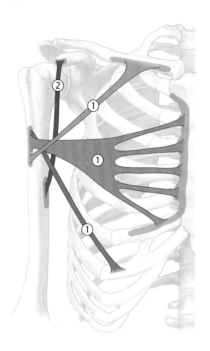

① **Pectoralis major**

Origin:	• Clavicular part: medial half of the clavicle
	• Sternocostal part: sternum and the second through sixth costal cartilages
	• Abdominal part: anterior layer of the rectus sheath
Insertion:	Crest of the greater tuberosity of the humerus
Actions:	• Adduction and internal rotation (entire muscle)
	• Anteversion (clavicular part and sternocostal part)
	• Assists respiration when the shoulder girdle is fixed
Innervation:	Medial and lateral pectoral nerves (C 5–T 1)

② **Coracobrachialis**

Origin:	Coracoid process of the scapula
Insertion:	Humerus (in line with the crest of the lesser tuberosity)
Actions:	Anteversion, adduction, internal rotation
Innervation:	Musculocutaneous nerve (C 6, C 7)

A Schematic of the pectoralis major and coracobrachialis

B Twisting of the tendon of insertion of pectoralis major

Anterior view. The three parts of the pectoralis major (clavicular, sternocostal, and abdominal) converge laterally and insert on the crest of the greater tuberosity by a broad tendon that has a horseshoe-shaped cross section. The tendon fiber bundles are twisted on themselves in such a way that the clavicular part inserts lower on the humerus than the sternocostal part, which inserts lower than the abdominal part. As with the latissimus dorsi, the muscle fibers of the pectoralis major become untwisted and stretched with increasing elevation of the arm, increasing the force that the muscle can exert.

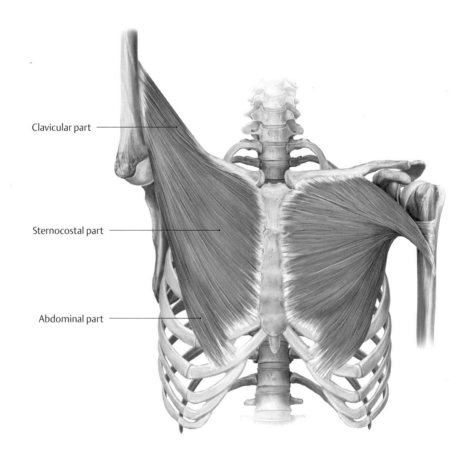

Clavicular part

Sternocostal part

Abdominal part

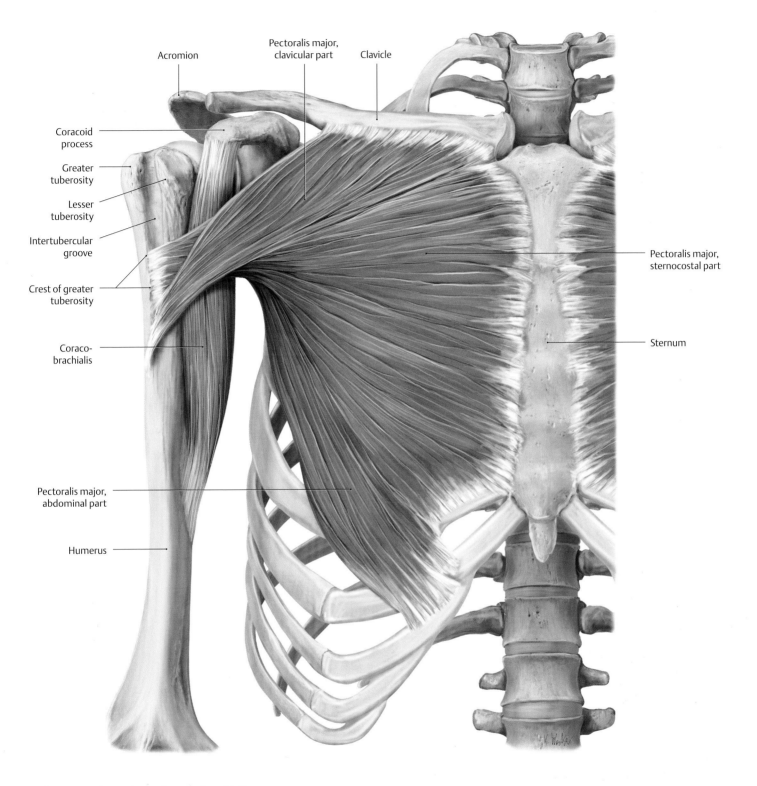

Acromion

Pectoralis major, clavicular part

Clavicle

Coracoid process

Greater tuberosity

Lesser tuberosity

Intertubercular groove

Crest of greater tuberosity

Coraco-brachialis

Pectoralis major, abdominal part

Humerus

Pectoralis major, sternocostal part

Sternum

C The pectoralis major and coracobrachialis
Right side, anterior view.

2.8 The Muscles of the Arm: Biceps brachii and Brachialis

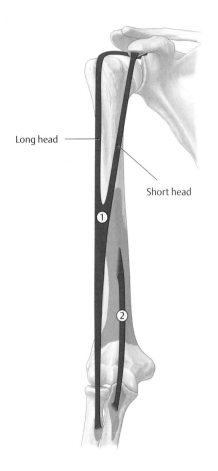

Long head

Short head

① **Biceps brachii**

Origin:
- Long head: supraglenoid tubercle of the scapula
- Short head: coracoid process of the scapula

Insertion: Radial tuberosity

Actions:
- Elbow joint:
  - Flexion, supination (with the elbow flexed)
- Shoulder joint:
  - Flexion (forward motion of humerus)
  - Stabilization of humeral head during deltoid contraction
  - Abduction and internal (medial) rotation of the humerus

Innervation: Musculocutaneous nerve (C 5–C 6)

② **Brachialis**

Origin: Distal half of the anterior surface of the humerus, also the medial and lateral intermuscular septa

Insertion: Ulnar tuberosity

Action: Flexion at the elbow joint

Innervation: Musculocutaneous nerve (C 5–C 6) and radial nerve (C 7)

A Schematic of the biceps brachii and brachialis

B Supinating action of the biceps brachii with the elbow flexed

a The forearm is pronated with the elbow flexed (right arm, medial view).

b Cross section at the level of the radial tuberosity with the forearm pronated (proximal view).

c The forearm is supinated with the elbow flexed (right arm, medial view).

d Cross section at the level of the radial tuberosity with the forearm supinated (proximal view).

When the elbow is flexed, the biceps brachii acts as a powerful supinator in addition to its role as a flexor, because the lever arm in that position is almost perpendicular to the axis of pronation/supination (see p. 242). This is why *supination movements* are particularly effective when the elbow is flexed. When the forearm is *pronated* (**a**), the tendon of insertion of biceps brachii is wrapped around the radius. When the muscle then contracts to flex the elbow, the tendon unwraps like a rope coiled around a crank (**b**).

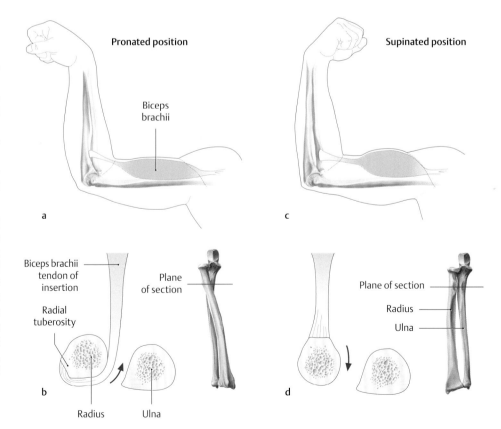

Pronated position

Biceps brachii

a

Biceps brachii tendon of insertion

Radial tuberosity

Plane of section

b

Radius   Ulna

Supinated position

c

Plane of section

Radius

Ulna

d

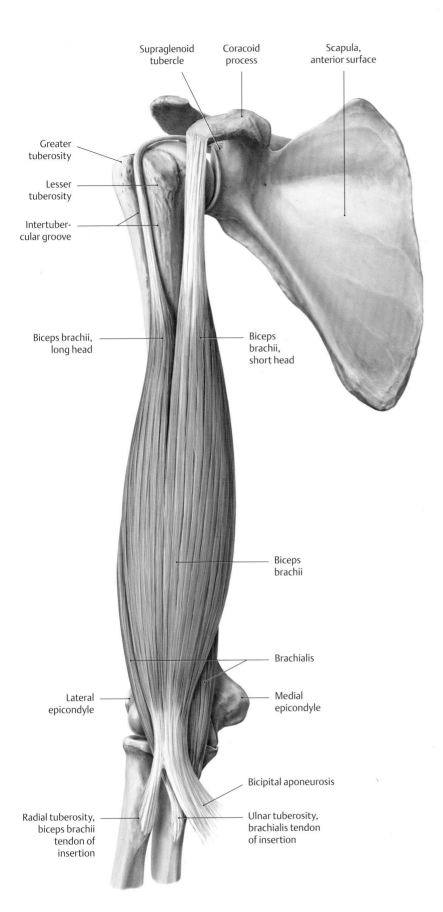

Supraglenoid tubercle

Coracoid process

Scapula, anterior surface

Greater tuberosity

Lesser tuberosity

Intertuber- cular groove

Biceps brachii, long head

Biceps brachii, short head

Biceps brachii

Brachialis

Lateral epicondyle

Medial epicondyle

Bicipital aponeurosis

Radial tuberosity, biceps brachii tendon of insertion

Ulnar tuberosity, brachialis tendon of insertion

C The biceps brachii and brachialis
Right arm, anterior (ventral) view.

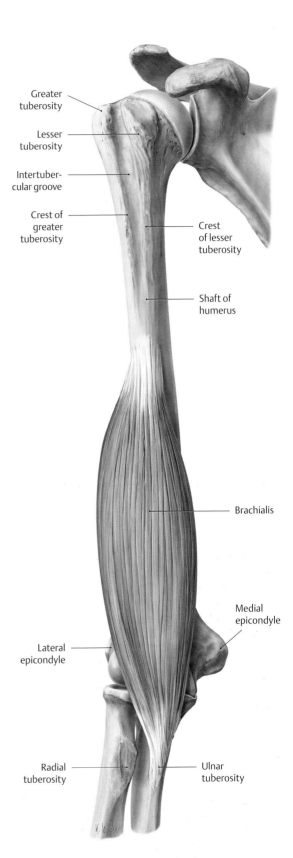

Greater tuberosity

Lesser tuberosity

Intertuber- cular groove

Crest of greater tuberosity

Crest of lesser tuberosity

Shaft of humerus

Brachialis

Lateral epicondyle

Medial epicondyle

Radial tuberosity

Ulnar tuberosity

D The brachialis
Right arm, anterior (ventral) view.

271

2.9 The Muscles of the Arm: Triceps brachii and Anconeus

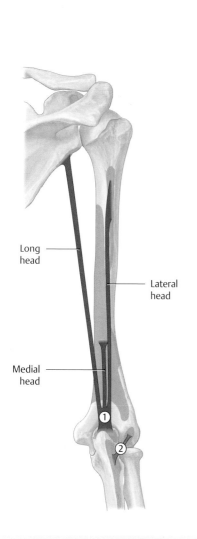

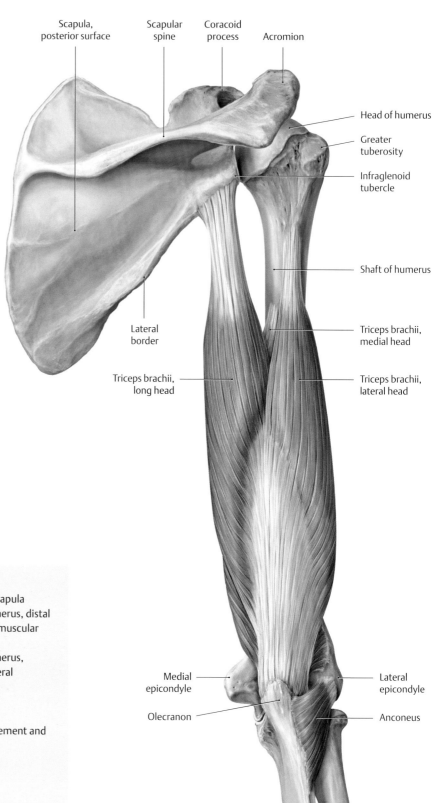

① **Triceps brachii**

Origin:
- Long head: infraglenoid tubercle of the scapula
- Medial head: posterior surface of the humerus, distal to the radial groove, and the medial intermuscular septum
- Lateral head: posterior surface of the humerus, proximal to the radial groove, and the lateral intermuscular septum

Insertion: Olecranon of the ulna

Actions:
- Elbow joint: extension
- Shoulder joint: long head: backward movement and adduction of the arm

Innervation: Radial nerve (C 6–C 8)

② **Anconeus**

Origin: Lateral epicondyle of the humerus (and the posterior joint capsule in some cases)

Insertion: Olecranon of the ulna (radial surface)

Actions: Extends the elbow and tightens its joint capsule

Innervation: Radial nerve (C 6–C 8)

A Schematic of the triceps brachii and anconeus

B The triceps brachii and anconeus
Right upper arm, posterior (dorsal) view.

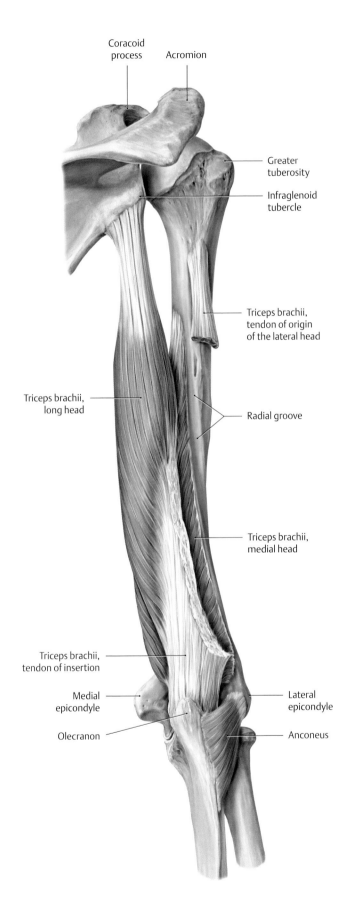

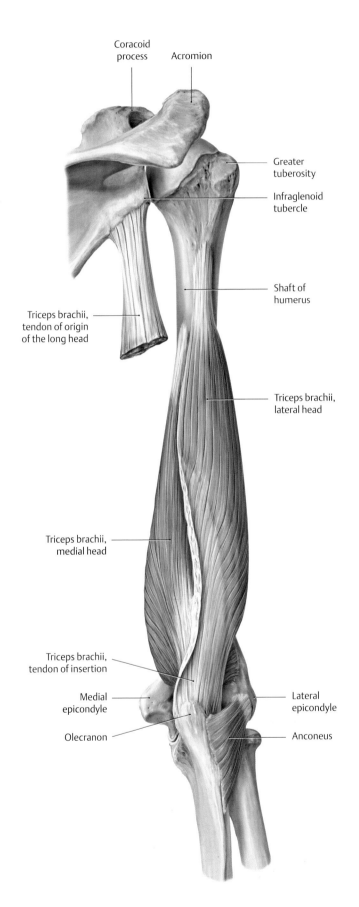

C The triceps brachii and anconeus
Right upper arm, posterior (dorsal) view. The lateral head of triceps brachii has been partially removed.

D The triceps brachii and anconeus
Right upper arm, posterior (dorsal) view. The long head of triceps brachii has been partially removed.

273

2.10 The Muscles of the Forearm: The Superficial and Deep Flexors

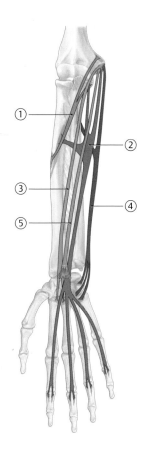

A Schematic of the superficial flexors

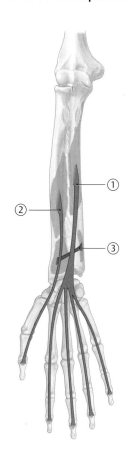

B Schematic of the deep flexors

① **Pronator teres**

Origin:	• Humeral head: medial epicondyle of the humerus
	• Ulnar head: coronoid process of the ulna
Insertion:	Lateral surface of the radius (distal to the supinator insertion)
Actions:	• Elbow joint: weak flexor
	• Forearm joints: pronation
Innervation:	Median nerve (C 6, C 7)

② **Flexor digitorum superficialis**

Origin:	• Humeral head: medial epicondyle of the humerus
	• Ulnar head: coronoid process of the ulna
	• Radial head: distal to the radial tuberosity
Insertion:	The sides of the middle phalanges of the second through fifth digits
Actions:	• Elbow joint: weak flexor
	• Wrist joints and the MCP and PIP joints of the second through fifth digits: flexion
Innervation:	Median nerve (C 8, T 1)

③ **Flexor carpi radialis**

Origin:	Medial epicondyle of the humerus
Insertion:	Base of the second metacarpal (and sometimes of the third metacarpal)
Actions:	Wrist joints: flexion and abduction (radial deviation) of the hand
Innervation:	Median nerve (C 6, C 7)

④ **Flexor carpi ulnaris**

Origin:	• Head of humerus: medial epicondyle
	• Head of ulna: olecranon
Insertion:	Pisiform hook of the hamate, base of the fifth metacarpal
Actions:	Wrist joints: flexion and adduction (ulnar deviation) of the hand
Innervation:	Ulnar nerve (C 7–T 1)

⑤ **Palmaris longus**

Origin:	Medial epicondyle of the humerus
Insertion:	Palmar aponeurosis
Actions:	• Elbow joint: weak flexor
	• Wrist joints: palmar flexion, tightens the palmar aponeurosis for gripping
Innervation:	Median nerve (C 7, C 8)

① **Flexor digitorum profundus**

Origin:	Proximal two-thirds of the flexor surface of the ulna and the adjacent interosseous membrane
Insertion:	Palmar surface of the distal phalanges of the second through fifth digits
Actions:	Wrist joints and the MCP, PIP, and DIP joints of the second through fifth digits: flexion
Innervation:	• Median nerve (radial part, second and third digits), C 8, T 1
	• Ulnar nerve (ulnar part, fourth and fifth digits), C 7–T 1

② **Flexor pollicis longus**

Origin:	Mid-anterior surface of the radius and the adjacent interosseous membrane
Insertion:	Palmar surface of the distal phalanx of the thumb
Actions:	• Wrist joints: flexion and radial abduction of the hand
	• Carpometacarpal joint of the thumb: opposition
	• Metacarpophalangeal and interphalangeal joints of the thumb: flexion
Innervation:	Median nerve (C 7, C 8)

③ **Pronator quadratus**

Origin:	Distal one-fourth of the anterior surface of the ulna
Insertion:	Distal one-fourth of the anterior surface of the radius
Actions:	Pronates the hand, stabilizes the distal radioulnar joint
Innervation:	Median nerve (C 7, C 8)

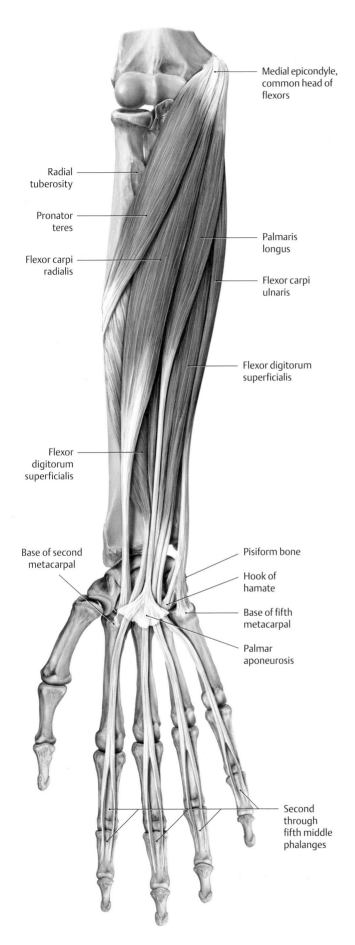

Medial epicondyle, common head of flexors

Radial tuberosity

Pronator teres

Flexor carpi radialis

Palmaris longus

Flexor carpi ulnaris

Flexor digitorum superficialis

Flexor digitorum superficialis

Base of second metacarpal

Pisiform bone

Hook of hamate

Base of fifth metacarpal

Palmar aponeurosis

Second through fifth middle phalanges

C The superficial flexors (pronator teres, flexor digitorum superficialis, flexor carpi radialis, flexor carpi ulnaris, and palmaris longus)
Right forearm, anterior (ventral) view.

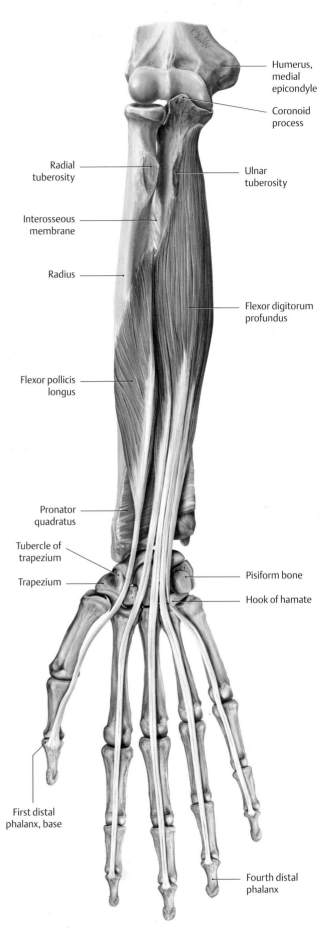

Humerus, medial epicondyle

Coronoid process

Radial tuberosity

Ulnar tuberosity

Interosseous membrane

Radius

Flexor digitorum profundus

Flexor pollicis longus

Pronator quadratus

Tubercle of trapezium

Trapezium

Pisiform bone

Hook of hamate

First distal phalanx, base

Fourth distal phalanx

D The deep flexors (flexor digitorum profundus, flexor pollicis longus, and pronator quadratus)
Right forearm, anterior (ventral) view.

275

2.11 The Muscles of the Forearm: The Radialis Muscles

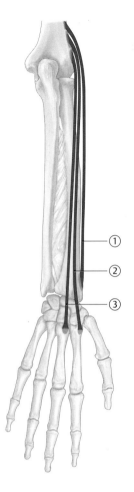

① **Brachioradialis**

Origin: Lateral surface of the distal humerus, lateral intermuscular septum
Insertion: Styloid process of the radius
Actions: • Elbow joint: flexion
• Forearm joints: semipronation
Innervation: Radial nerve (C5, C6)

② **Extensor carpi radialis longus**

Origin: Lateral surface of the distal humerus (lateral supracondylar ridge), lateral intermuscular septum
Insertion: Dorsal base of the second metacarpal
Actions: • Elbow joint: weak flexor
• Wrist joints: dorsal extension (assists in fist closure), abduction (radial deviation) of the hand
Innervation: Radial nerve (C6, C7)

③ **Extensor carpi radialis brevis**

Origin: Lateral epicondyle of the humerus
Insertion: Dorsal base of the third metacarpal
Actions: • Elbow joint: weak flexor
• Wrist joints: dorsal extension (assists in fist closure), abduction (radial deviation) of the hand
Innervation: Radial nerve (C7, C8)

A Schematic of the radialis muscles

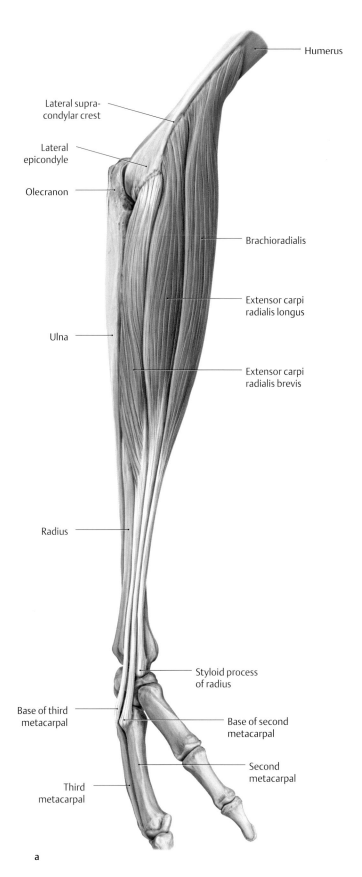

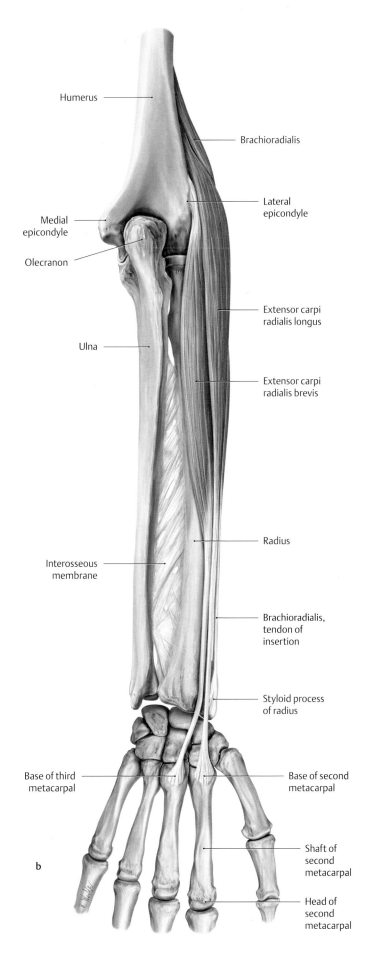

B The radialis muscles (brachioradialis, extensor carpi radialis longus, and extensor carpi radialis brevis)
Right forearm.

a Lateral (radial) view.
b Posterior (dorsal) view.

2.12 The Muscles of the Forearm: The Superficial and Deep Extensors

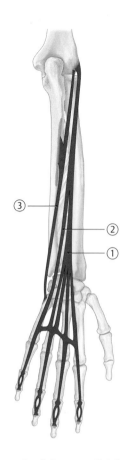

A Schematic of the superficial extensors

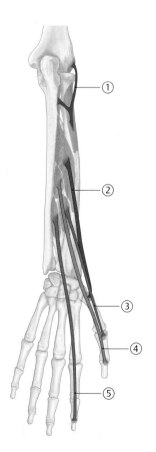

B Schematic of the deep extensors

① **Extensor digitorum**

Origin:	Common head (lateral epicondyle of the humerus)
Insertion:	Dorsal digital expansion of the second through fifth digits
Actions:	• Wrist joints: extension
	• MCP, PIP, and DIP joints of the second through fifth digits: extension and abduction of the fingers
Innervation:	Radial nerve (C 7, C 8)

② **Extensor digiti minimi**

Origin:	Common head (lateral epicondyle of the humerus)
Insertion:	Dorsal digital expansion of the fifth digit
Actions:	• Wrist joints: extension, ulnar abduction of the hand
	• MCP, PIP, and DIP joints of the fifth digit: extension and abduction of the fifth digit
Innervation:	Radial nerve (C 7, C 8)

③ **Extensor carpi ulnaris**

Origin:	Common head (lateral epicondyle of the humerus), ulnar head (dorsal surface of the ulna)
Insertion:	Base of the fifth metacarpal
Actions:	Wrist joints: extension, adduction (ulnar deviation) of the hand
Innervation:	Radial nerve (C 7, C 8)

① **Supinator**

Origin:	Olecranon of the ulna, lateral epicondyle of the humerus, radial collateral ligament, annular ligament of the radius
Insertion:	Radius (between the radial tuberosity and the insertion of pronator teres)
Action:	Supinates the forearm joints
Innervation:	Radial nerve (C 6, C 7)

② **Abductor pollicis longus**

Origin:	Dorsal surfaces of the radius and ulna, also the interosseous membrane
Insertion:	Base of the first metacarpal
Actions:	• Radiocarpal joint: abduction (radial deviation) of the hand
	• Carpometacarpal joint of the thumb: abduction
Innervation:	Radial nerve (C 7, C 8)

③ **Extensor pollicis brevis**

Origin:	Posterior surface of the radius and the interosseous membrane (distal to abductor pollicis longus)
Insertion:	Base of the proximal phalanx of the thumb
Actions:	• Radiocarpal joint: abduction (radial deviation) of the hand
	• Carpometacarpal and MCP joints of the thumb: extension
Innervation:	Radial nerve (C 7, C 8)

④ **Extensor pollicis longus**

Origin:	Posterior surface of the ulna and the interosseous membrane
Insertion:	Base of the distal phalanx of the thumb
Actions:	• Wrist joints: extension and abduction (radial deviation) of the hand
	• Carpometacarpal joint of the thumb: adduction
	• MCP and interphalangeal joints of the thumb: extension
Innervation:	Radial nerve (C 7, C 8)

⑤ **Extensor indicis**

Origin:	Posterior surface of the ulna, the interosseous membrane
Insertion:	Posterior digital expansion of the second digit
Actions:	• Wrist joint: extension
	• MCP, PIP, and DIP joints of the second digit: extension
Innervation:	Radial nerve (C 7, C 8)

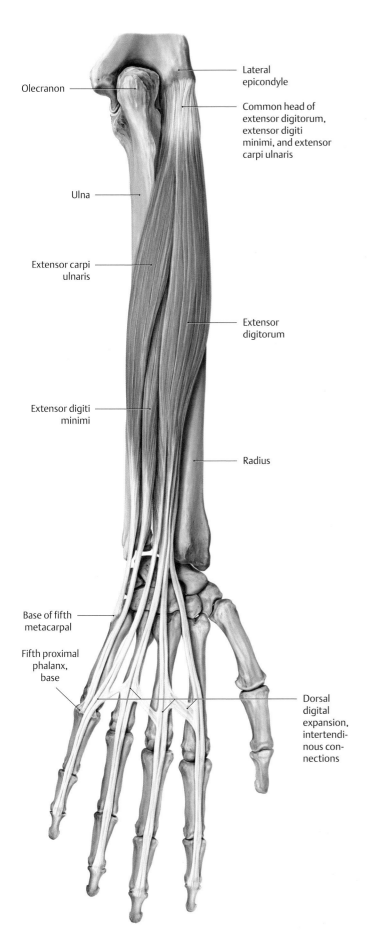

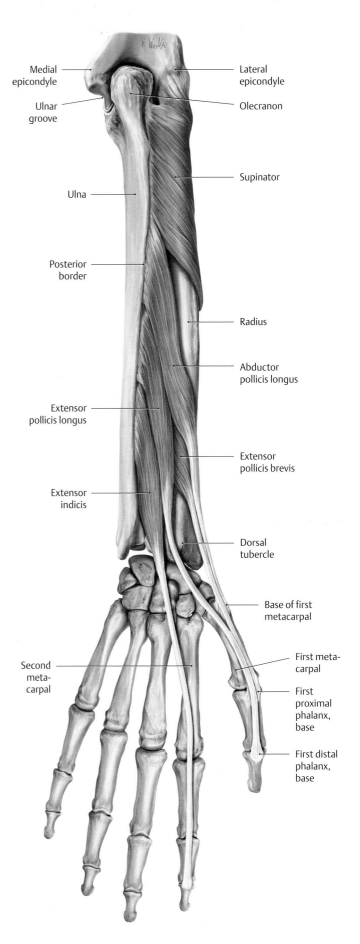

C The superficial extensors (extensor digitorum, extensor digiti minimi, and extensor carpi ulnaris)
Right forearm, posterior (dorsal) view.

D The deep extensors (supinator, abductor pollicis longus, extensor pollicis brevis, extensor pollicis longus, and extensor indicis)
Right forearm, posterior (dorsal) view.

2.13 The Intrinsic Muscles of the Hand: The Thenar and Hypothenar Muscles

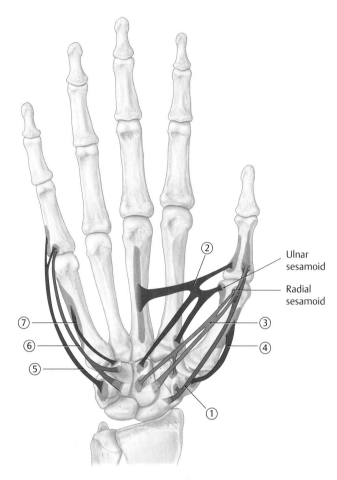

A Schematic of the thenar (①–④) and hypothenar muscles (⑤–⑦)

Labels on figure: Ulnar sesamoid, Radial sesamoid

① **Abductor pollicis brevis**

Origin:	Scaphoid bone and trapezium, flexor retinaculum
Insertion:	Base of the proximal phalanx of the thumb (via the radial sesamoid)
Actions	Abduction of the thumb
Innervation:	Median nerve (C 8, T 1)

② **Adductor pollicis**

Origin:	• Transverse head: palmar surface of the third metacarpal • Oblique head: capitate bone, base of second metacarpal
Insertion:	Base of the proximal phalanx of the thumb (via the ulnar sesamoid)
Actions:	• Carpometacarpal joint of the thumb: opposition • Metacarpophalangeal joint of the thumb: flexion
Innervation:	Ulnar nerve (C 8, T 1)

③ **Flexor pollicis brevis**

Origin:	• Superficial head: flexor retinaculum • Deep head: capitate bone, trapezium
Insertion:	Base of the proximal phalanx of the thumb (via the radial sesamoid)
Actions:	• Carpometacarpal joint of the thumb: flexion, opposition • Metacarpophalangeal joint of the thumb: flexion
Innervation:	• Median nerve, C 8, T 1 (superficial head) • Ulnar nerve, C 8, T 1 (deep head)

④ **Opponens pollicis**

Origin:	Trapezium
Insertion:	Radial border of the first metacarpal
Action:	Carpometacarpal joint of the thumb: opposition
Innervation:	Median nerve (C 8, T 1)

⑤ **Abductor digiti minimi**

Origin:	Pisiform bone
Insertion:	Ulnar base of the proximal phalanx and the dorsal digital expansion of the fifth digit
Actions:	• Metacarpophalangeal joint of the little finger: flexion and abduction of the little finger • PIP and DIP joints of the little finger: extension
Innervation:	Ulnar nerve (C 8, T 1)

⑥ **Flexor digiti minimi**

Origin:	Hook of the hamate, the flexor retinaculum
Insertion:	Base of the proximal phalanx of the fifth digit
Action:	MCP joint of the little finger: flexion
Innervation:	Ulnar nerve (C 8, T 1)

⑦ **Opponens digiti minimi**

Origin:	Hook of the hamate
Insertion:	Ulnar border of the fifth metacarpal
Action:	Draws the metacarpal in the palmar direction (opposition)
Innervation:	Ulnar nerve (C 8, T 1)

Palmaris brevis (not shown)

Origin:	Ulnar border of the palmar aponeurosis
Insertion:	Skin of the hypothenar eminence
Action:	Tightens the palmar aponeurosis (protective function)
Innervation:	Ulnar nerve (C 8, T 1)

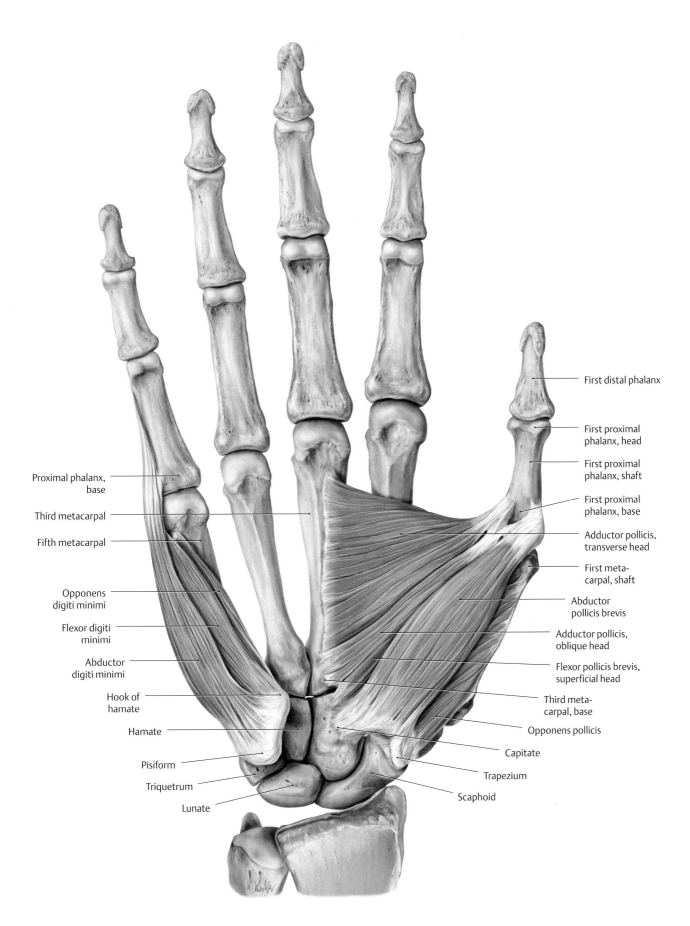

First distal phalanx

First proximal phalanx, head

First proximal phalanx, shaft

First proximal phalanx, base

Adductor pollicis, transverse head

First meta-carpal, shaft

Abductor pollicis brevis

Adductor pollicis, oblique head

Flexor pollicis brevis, superficial head

Third meta-carpal, base

Opponens pollicis

Capitate

Trapezium

Scaphoid

Proximal phalanx, base

Third metacarpal

Fifth metacarpal

Opponens digiti minimi

Flexor digiti minimi

Abductor digiti minimi

Hook of hamate

Hamate

Pisiform

Triquetrum

Lunate

B The thenar muscles (abductor pollicis brevis, adductor pollicis, flexor pollicis brevis, and opponens pollicis) and the hypothenar muscles (abductor digiti minimi, flexor digiti minimi, and opponens digiti minimi)
Right hand, anterior view

The Intrinsic Muscles of the Hand: Lumbricals and Interossei (Metacarpal Muscles)

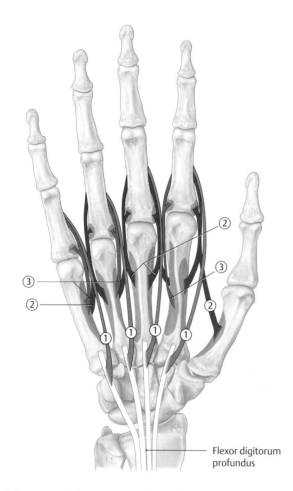

Flexor digitorum profundus

A Schematic of the metacarpal muscles

① **First through fourth lumbrical muscles**

Origin: Radial sides of the tendons of flexor digitorum profundus (variable)

Insertion:
- First lumbrical: dorsal digital expansion of the second digit (index finger)
- Second lumbrical: dorsal digital expansion of the third digit (middle finger)
- Third lumbrical: dorsal digital expansion of the fourth digit (ring finger)
- Fourth lumbrical: dorsal digital expansion of the fifth digit (little finger)

Actions:
- Metacarpophalangeal joints of the second through fifth digits: flexion
- Proximal and distal interphalangeal joints of the second through fifth digits: extension

Innervation:
- Median nerve, C 8, T 1 (first and second lumbricals)
- Ulnar nerve, C 8, T 1 (third and fourth lumbricals)

② **First through fourth dorsal interossei**

Origin: By two heads from adjacent sides of the first through fifth metacarpals

Insertion:
- Dorsal digital expansion of the second through fourth digits, base of the proximal phalanx
- First interosseus: radial side of the second proximal phalanx (index finger)
- Second interosseus: radial side of the third proximal phalanx (middle finger)
- Third interosseus: ulnar side of the third proximal phalanx (middle finger)
- Fourth interosseus: ulnar side of the fourth proximal phalanx (ring finger)

Actions:
- Metacarpophalangeal joints of the second through fourth digits: flexion
- Proximal and distal interphalangeal joints of the second through fourth digits: extension and abduction of the fingers (abduction of the index and ring fingers from the middle finger)

Innervation: Ulnar nerve (C 8, T 1)

③ **First through third palmar interossei**

Origin:
- First interosseus: ulnar side of the second metacarpal (index finger)
- Second interosseus: radial side of the fourth metacarpal (ring finger)
- Third interosseus: radial side of the fifth metacarpal (little finger)

Insertion: Dorsal digital expansion and base of the proximal phalanx of the associated finger

Actions:
- Metacarpophalangeal joints of the second, fourth, and fifth digits: flexion
- Proximal and distal interphalangeal joints of the second, fourth, and fifth digits: extension and adduction of the fingers (adduction of the second, fourth, and fifth digits toward the middle finger)

Innervation: Ulnar nerve (C 8, T 1)

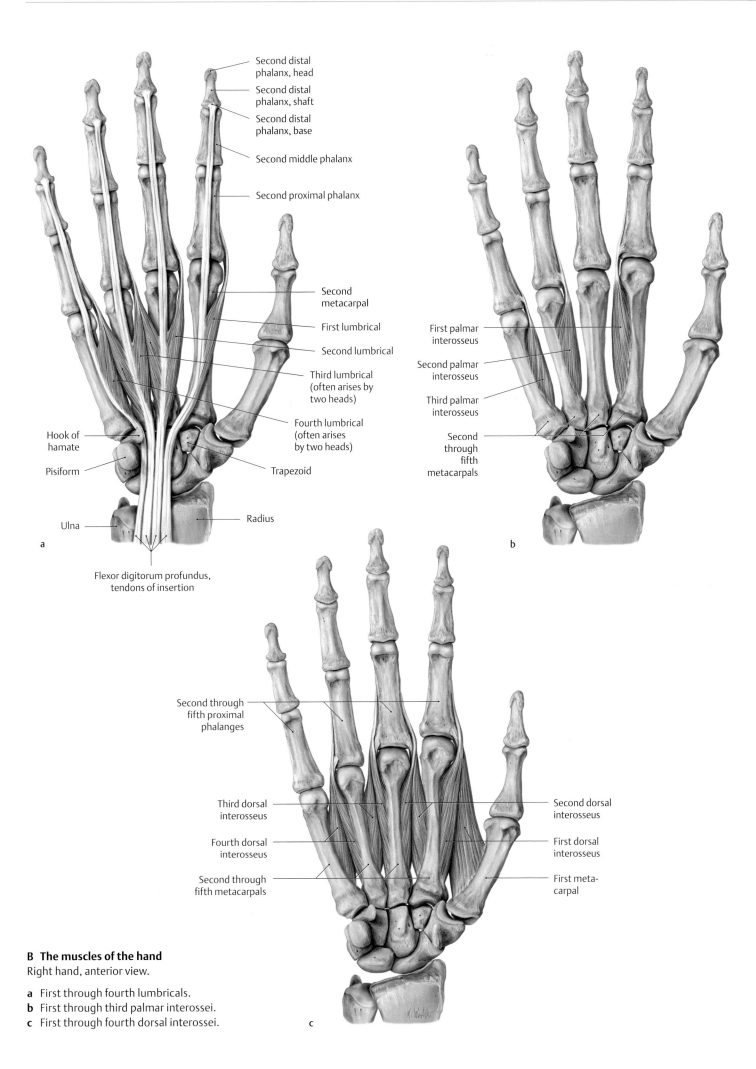

Second distal phalanx, head

Second distal phalanx, shaft

Second distal phalanx, base

Second middle phalanx

Second proximal phalanx

Second metacarpal

First lumbrical

Second lumbrical

Third lumbrical (often arises by two heads)

Fourth lumbrical (often arises by two heads)

Trapezoid

Radius

Hook of hamate

Pisiform

Ulna

a

Flexor digitorum profundus, tendons of insertion

First palmar interosseus

Second palmar interosseus

Third palmar interosseus

Second through fifth metacarpals

b

Second through fifth proximal phalanges

Third dorsal interosseus

Fourth dorsal interosseus

Second through fifth metacarpals

Second dorsal interosseus

First dorsal interosseus

First meta-carpal

c

B The muscles of the hand

Right hand, anterior view.

a First through fourth lumbricals.
b First through third palmar interossei.
c First through fourth dorsal interossei.

283

3.1 The Posterior Muscles of the Shoulder Girdle and Shoulder Joint

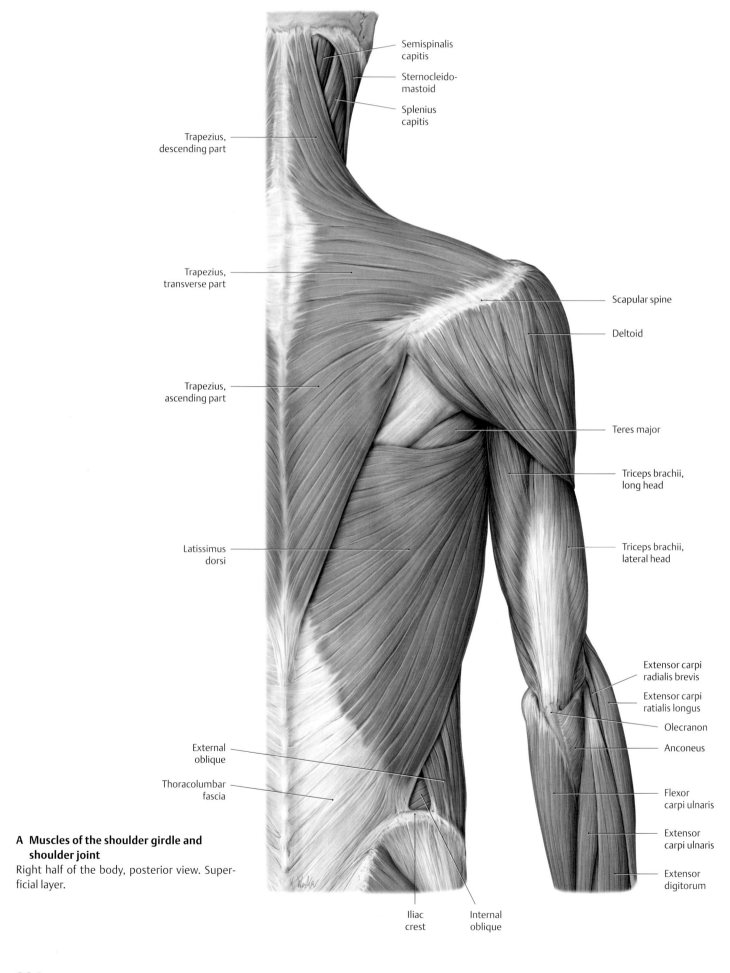

Semispinalis
capitis

Sternocleido-
mastoid

Splenius
capitis

Trapezius,
descending part

Trapezius,
transverse part

Scapular spine

Deltoid

Trapezius,
ascending part

Teres major

Triceps brachii,
long head

Triceps brachii,
lateral head

Latissimus
dorsi

Extensor carpi
radialis brevis

Extensor carpi
ratialis longus

Olecranon

Anconeus

External
oblique

Thoracolumbar
fascia

Flexor
carpi ulnaris

Extensor
carpi ulnaris

Extensor
digitorum

**A Muscles of the shoulder girdle and
shoulder joint**
Right half of the body, posterior view. Superficial layer.

Iliac
crest

Internal
oblique

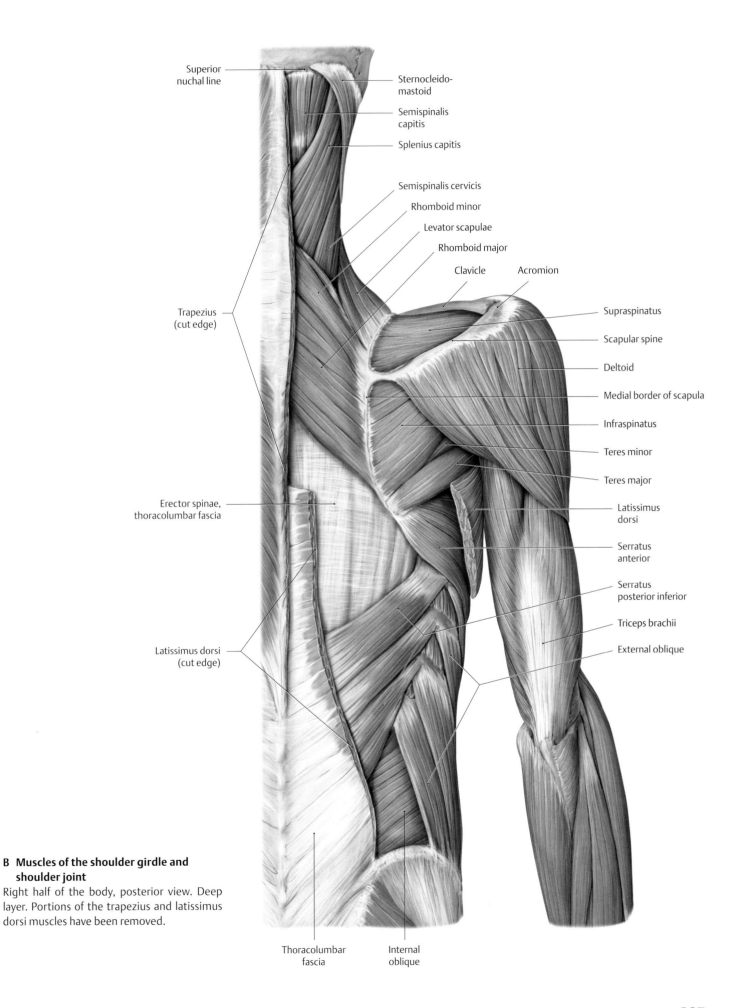

Superior
nuchal line

Sternocleido-
mastoid

Semispinalis
capitis

Splenius capitis

Semispinalis cervicis

Rhomboid minor

Levator scapulae

Rhomboid major

Clavicle   Acromion

Trapezius
(cut edge)

Supraspinatus

Scapular spine

Deltoid

Medial border of scapula

Infraspinatus

Teres minor

Teres major

Erector spinae,
thoracolumbar fascia

Latissimus
dorsi

Serratus
anterior

Serratus
posterior inferior

Triceps brachii

Latissimus dorsi
(cut edge)

External oblique

Thoracolumbar
fascia

Internal
oblique

**B Muscles of the shoulder girdle and
shoulder joint**
Right half of the body, posterior view. Deep
layer. Portions of the trapezius and latissimus
dorsi muscles have been removed.

285

3.2   The Posterior Muscles of the Shoulder Joint and Arm

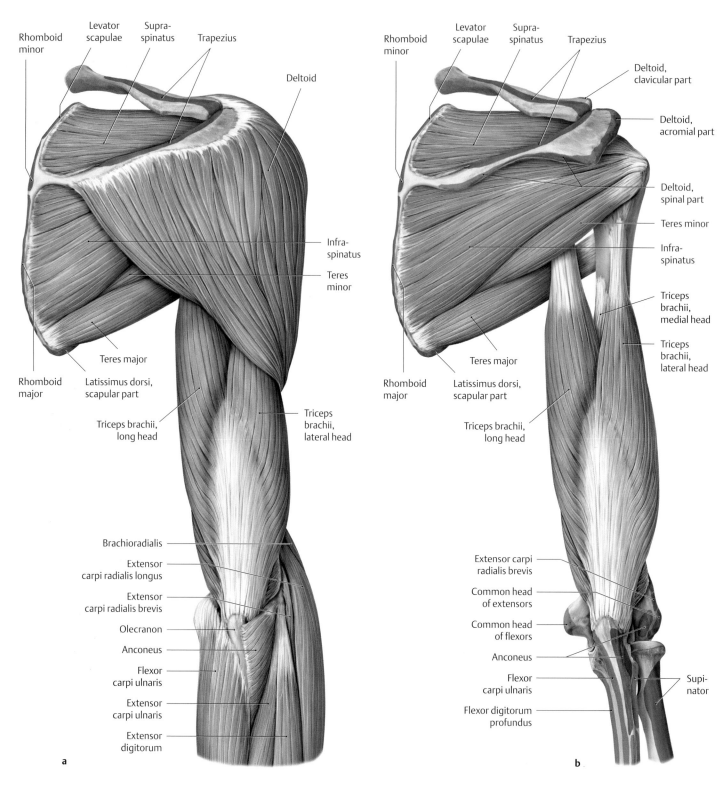

A Muscles of the right shoulder and right arm from the posterior view

The origins and insertions of the muscles are indicated by color shading (red = origin, blue = insertion).

a After removal of the trapezius.
b After removal of the deltoid and forearm muscles.

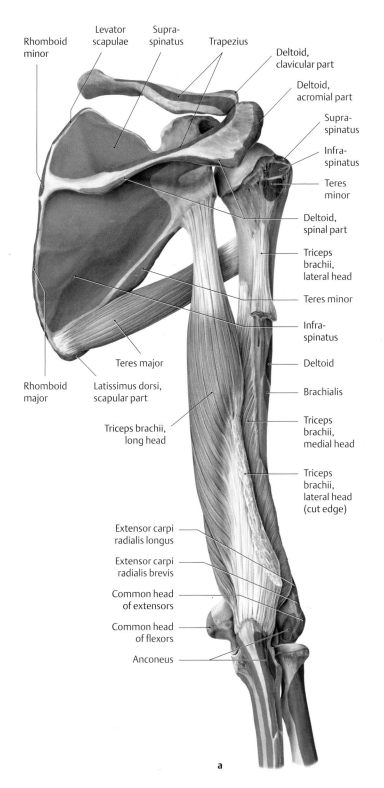

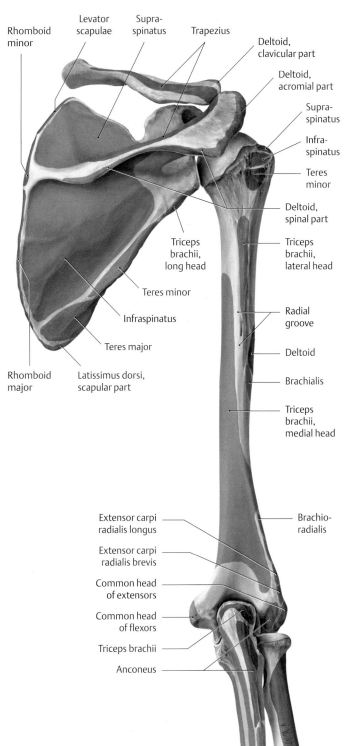

Rhomboid minor

Levator scapulae

Supra-spinatus

Trapezius

Deltoid, clavicular part

Deltoid, acromial part

Supra-spinatus

Infra-spinatus

Teres minor

Deltoid, spinal part

Triceps brachii, lateral head

Teres minor

Infra-spinatus

Deltoid

Brachialis

Triceps brachii, medial head

Triceps brachii, lateral head (cut edge)

Extensor carpi radialis longus

Extensor carpi radialis brevis

Common head of extensors

Common head of flexors

Anconeus

Rhomboid major

Latissimus dorsi, scapular part

Teres major

Triceps brachii, long head

a

Rhomboid minor

Levator scapulae

Supra-spinatus

Trapezius

Deltoid, clavicular part

Deltoid, acromial part

Supra-spinatus

Infra-spinatus

Teres minor

Deltoid, spinal part

Triceps brachii, lateral head

Radial groove

Deltoid

Brachialis

Triceps brachii, medial head

Brachio-radialis

Triceps brachii, long head

Teres minor

Infraspinatus

Teres major

Rhomboid major

Latissimus dorsi, scapular part

Extensor carpi radialis longus

Extensor carpi radialis brevis

Common head of extensors

Common head of flexors

Triceps brachii

Anconeus

b

B Muscles of the right shoulder and right arm from the posterior view

The origins and insertions of the muscles are indicated by color shading (red = origin, blue = insertion).

a The supraspinatus, infraspinatus, and teres minor have been removed. The lateral head of triceps brachii has been partially removed.

b All the muscles have been removed.

287

3.3 The Anterior Muscles of the Shoulder Girdle and Shoulder Joint

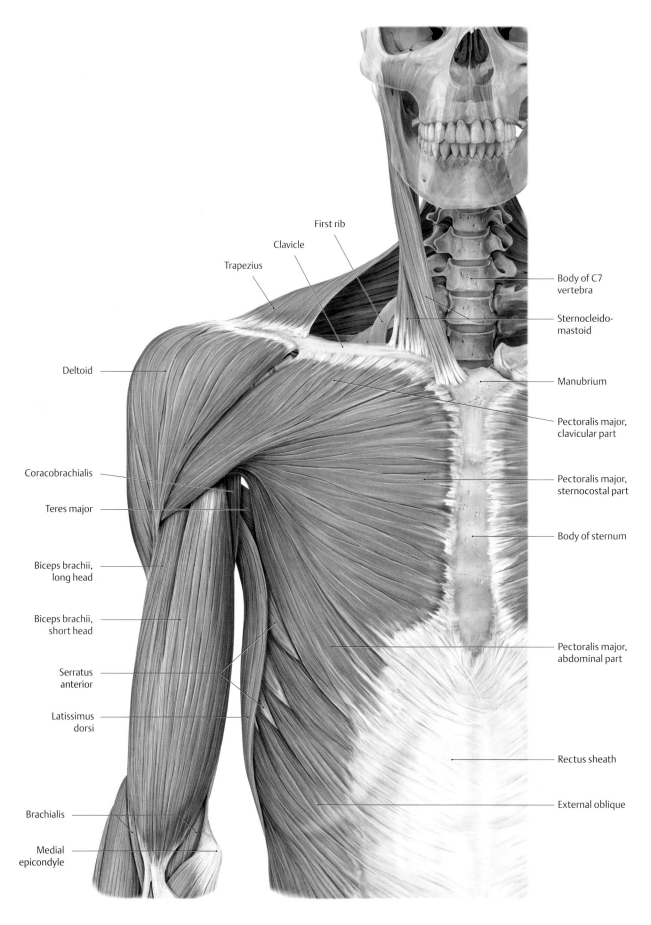

First rib

Clavicle

Trapezius

Body of C7
vertebra

Sternocleido-
mastoid

Deltoid

Manubrium

Pectoralis major,
clavicular part

Coracobrachialis

Pectoralis major,
sternocostal part

Teres major

Body of sternum

Biceps brachii,
long head

Biceps brachii,
short head

Serratus
anterior

Pectoralis major,
abdominal part

Latissimus
dorsi

Rectus sheath

External oblique

Brachialis

Medial
epicondyle

**A Muscles of the right shoulder and right arm from the anterior
view**

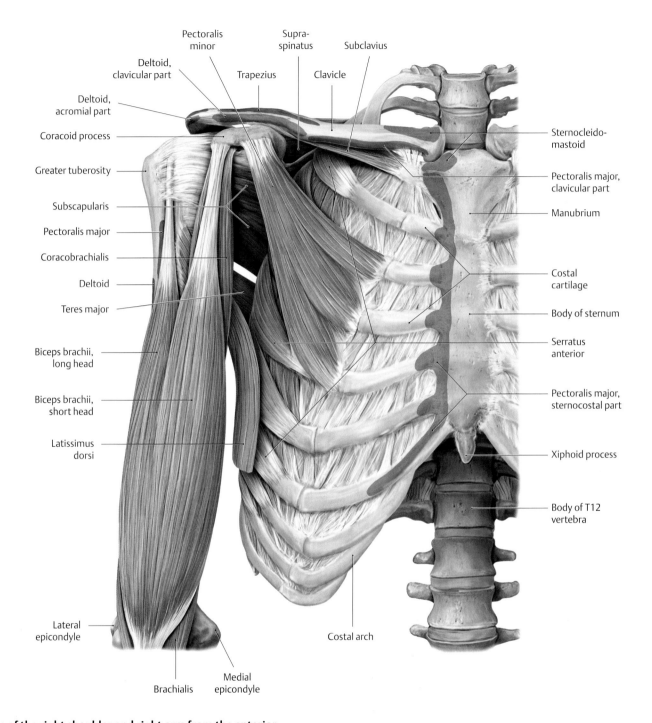

Pectoralis minor

Supra-spinatus

Subclavius

Deltoid, clavicular part

Trapezius

Clavicle

Deltoid, acromial part

Coracoid process

Sternocleido-mastoid

Greater tuberosity

Pectoralis major, clavicular part

Subscapularis

Manubrium

Pectoralis major

Coracobrachialis

Costal cartilage

Deltoid

Body of sternum

Teres major

Biceps brachii, long head

Serratus anterior

Biceps brachii, short head

Pectoralis major, sternocostal part

Latissimus dorsi

Xiphoid process

Body of T12 vertebra

Lateral epicondyle

Costal arch

Medial epicondyle

Brachialis

B Muscles of the right shoulder and right arm from the anterior view

The origins and insertions of the muscles are indicated by color shading (red = origin, blue = insertion). The sternocleidomastoid, trapezius, pectoralis major, deltoid, and external oblique muscles have been completely removed. The latissimus dorsi has been partially removed.

289

3.4 The Anterior Muscles of the Shoulder Joint and Arm

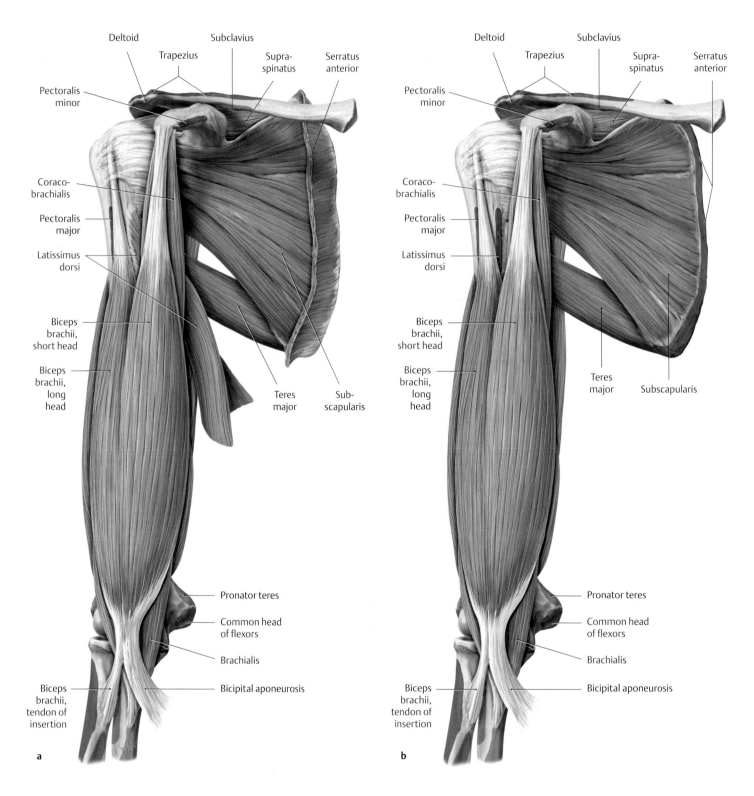

A Muscles of the right shoulder and right arm from the anterior view

The origins and insertions of the muscles are indicated by color shading (red = origin, blue = insertion).

a After removal of the thoracic skeleton. Latissimus dorsi and serratus anterior have been removed to their insertions.

b Latissimus dorsi and serratus anterior have been completely removed.

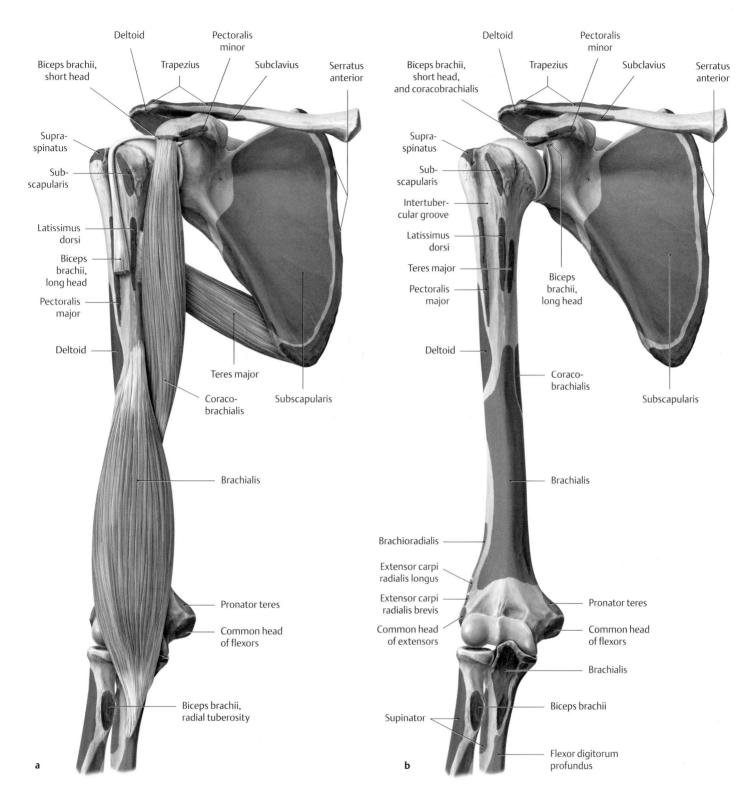

B Muscles of the right shoulder and right arm from the anterior view

The origins and insertions of the muscles are indicated by color shading (red = origin, blue = insertion).

a After removal of the thoracic skeleton and the subscapularis and supraspinatus muscles. The biceps brachii has been removed to the tendon of origin of its long head (note its course through the intertubercular groove).

b All the muscles have been removed.

3.5 The Anterior Muscles of the Forearm

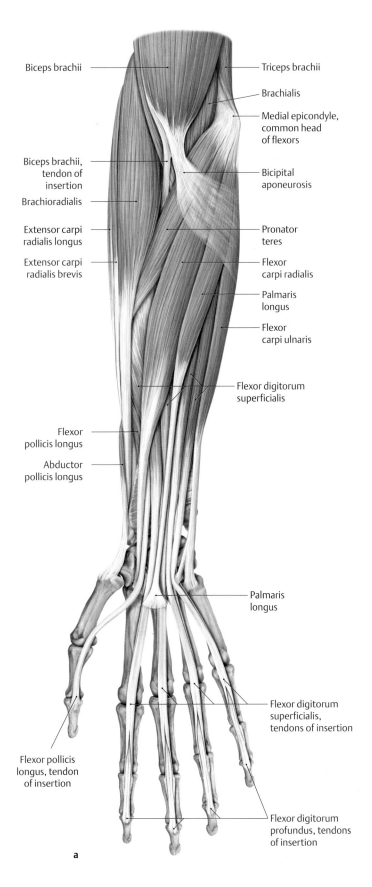

Biceps brachii

Triceps brachii

Brachialis

Medial epicondyle, common head of flexors

Biceps brachii, tendon of insertion

Bicipital aponeurosis

Brachioradialis

Extensor carpi radialis longus

Pronator teres

Extensor carpi radialis brevis

Flexor carpi radialis

Palmaris longus

Flexor carpi ulnaris

Flexor digitorum superficialis

Flexor pollicis longus

Abductor pollicis longus

Palmaris longus

Flexor digitorum superficialis, tendons of insertion

Flexor pollicis longus, tendon of insertion

Flexor digitorum profundus, tendons of insertion

a

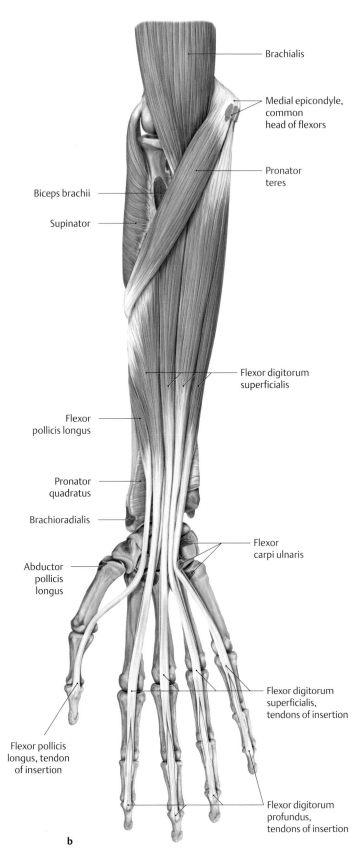

Brachialis

Medial epicondyle, common head of flexors

Biceps brachii

Pronator teres

Supinator

Flexor digitorum superficialis

Flexor pollicis longus

Pronator quadratus

Brachioradialis

Flexor carpi ulnaris

Abductor pollicis longus

Flexor digitorum superficialis, tendons of insertion

Flexor pollicis longus, tendon of insertion

Flexor digitorum profundus, tendons of insertion

b

A Muscles of the right forearm from the anterior (ventral) view
The origins and insertions of the muscles are indicated by color shading (red = origin, blue = insertion).

a The superficial flexors and the radialis group are shown.
b The radialis group (brachioradialis, extensor carpi radialis longus, extensor carpi radialis brevis) has been completely removed along with flexor carpi radialis, flexor carpi ulnaris, abductor pollicis longus, palmaris longus, and biceps brachii.

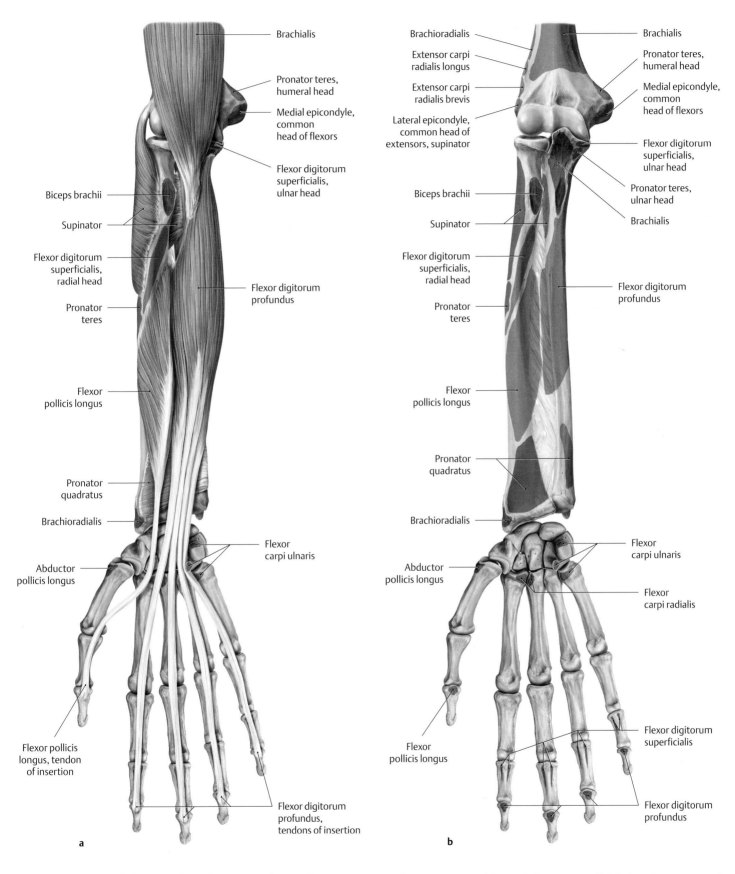

Brachialis

Pronator teres,
humeral head

Medial epicondyle,
common
head of flexors

Flexor digitorum
superficialis,
ulnar head

Biceps brachii

Supinator

Flexor digitorum
superficialis,
radial head

Pronator
teres

Flexor digitorum
profundus

Flexor
pollicis longus

Pronator
quadratus

Brachioradialis

Abductor
pollicis longus

Flexor
carpi ulnaris

Flexor pollicis
longus, tendon
of insertion

Flexor digitorum
profundus,
tendons of insertion

a

Brachioradialis

Extensor carpi
radialis longus

Extensor carpi
radialis brevis

Lateral epicondyle,
common head of
extensors, supinator

Biceps brachii

Supinator

Flexor digitorum
superficialis,
radial head

Pronator
teres

Flexor
pollicis longus

Pronator
quadratus

Brachioradialis

Abductor
pollicis longus

Flexor
pollicis longus

Brachialis

Pronator teres,
humeral head

Medial epicondyle,
common
head of flexors

Flexor digitorum
superficialis,
ulnar head

Pronator teres,
ulnar head

Brachialis

Flexor digitorum
profundus

Flexor
carpi ulnaris

Flexor
carpi radialis

Flexor digitorum
superficialis

Flexor digitorum
profundus

b

B Muscles of the right forearm from the anterior (ventral) view
The origins and insertions of the muscles are indicated by color shading
(red = origin, blue = insertion).

a Pronator teres and flexor digitorum superficialis have been removed.
b All the muscles have been removed.

3.6 The Posterior Muscles of the Forearm

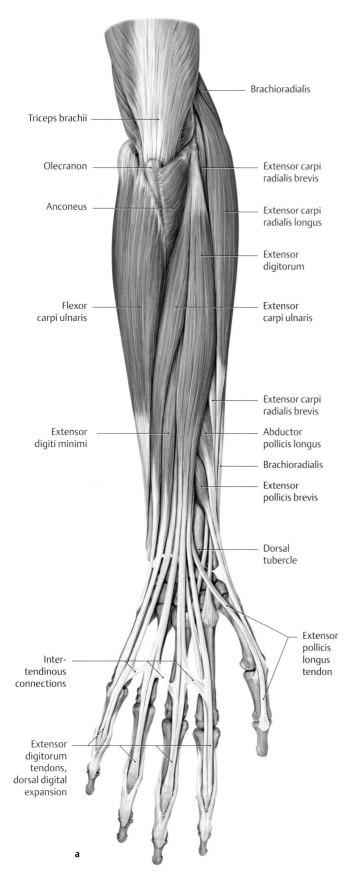

a

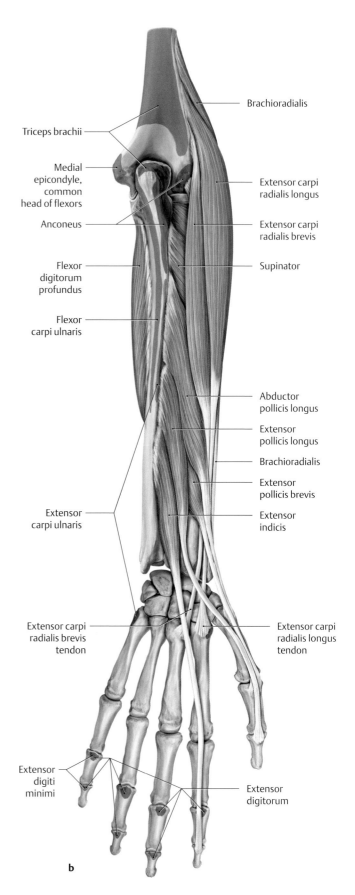

b

A Muscles of the right forearm from the posterior (dorsal) view
The origins and insertions of the muscles are indicated by color shading
(red = origin, blue = insertion).

a The superficial extensors and the radialis group are shown.
b Triceps brachii, anconeus, flexor carpi ulnaris, extensor carpi ulnaris,
and extensor digitorum have been removed.

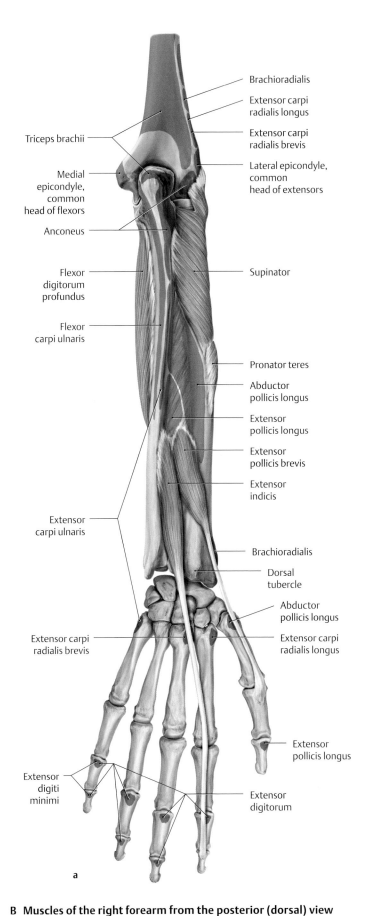

Triceps brachii

Medial epicondyle, common head of flexors

Anconeus

Flexor digitorum profundus

Flexor carpi ulnaris

Extensor carpi ulnaris

Extensor carpi radialis brevis

Extensor digiti minimi

Brachioradialis

Extensor carpi radialis longus

Extensor carpi radialis brevis

Lateral epicondyle, common head of extensors

Supinator

Pronator teres

Abductor pollicis longus

Extensor pollicis longus

Extensor pollicis brevis

Extensor indicis

Brachioradialis

Dorsal tubercle

Abductor pollicis longus

Extensor carpi radialis longus

Extensor pollicis longus

Extensor digitorum

a

Triceps brachii

Medial epicondyle, common head of flexors

Anconeus

Flexor digitorum profundus

Flexor carpi ulnaris

Extensor carpi ulnaris

Extensor carpi radialis brevis

Extensor digiti minimi

Brachioradialis

Extensor carpi radialis longus

Extensor carpi radialis brevis

Supinator, humeral head

Lateral epicondyle, common head of extensors

Supinator

Pronator teres

Abductor pollicis longus

Extensor pollicis longus

Extensor pollicis brevis

Extensor indicis

Interosseous membrane

Brachioradialis

Abductor pollicis longus

Extensor carpi radialis longus

Extensor pollicis brevis

Extensor pollicis longus

Extensor digitorum

Extensor indicis

b

B Muscles of the right forearm from the posterior (dorsal) view
The origins and insertions of the muscles are indicated by color shading (red = origin, blue = insertion).
Note the interosseous membrane, which contributes to the origin of several muscles in the forearm.

a Abductor pollicis longus, extensor pollicis longus, and the radialis group have been removed.
b All the muscles have been removed.

295

3.7 Cross Sections of the Arm and Forearm

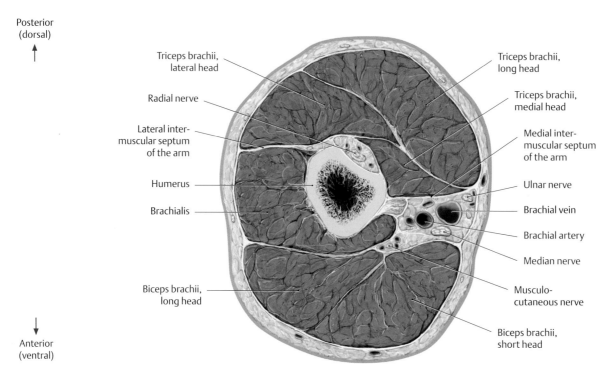

Posterior
(dorsal)

Anterior
(ventral)

Triceps brachii,
lateral head

Radial nerve

Lateral inter-
muscular septum
of the arm

Humerus

Brachialis

Biceps brachii,
long head

Triceps brachii,
long head

Triceps brachii,
medial head

Medial inter-
muscular septum
of the arm

Ulnar nerve

Brachial vein

Brachial artery

Median nerve

Musculo-
cutaneous nerve

Biceps brachii,
short head

A Cross section through the right arm
Proximal view. The location of the sectional plane is shown in **C**.

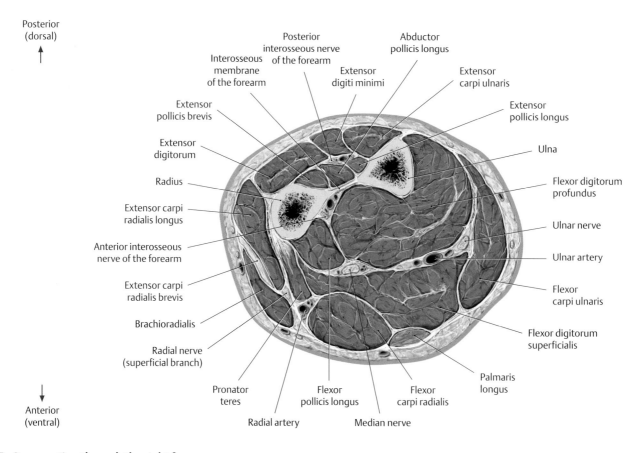

Posterior
(dorsal)

Anterior
(ventral)

Posterior
interosseous nerve
of the forearm

Interosseous
membrane
of the forearm

Extensor
pollicis brevis

Extensor
digitorum

Radius

Extensor carpi
radialis longus

Anterior interosseous
nerve of the forearm

Extensor carpi
radialis brevis

Brachioradialis

Radial nerve
(superficial branch)

Pronator
teres

Radial artery

Extensor
digiti minimi

Abductor
pollicis longus

Extensor
carpi ulnaris

Extensor
pollicis longus

Ulna

Flexor digitorum
profundus

Ulnar nerve

Ulnar artery

Flexor
carpi ulnaris

Flexor digitorum
superficialis

Palmaris
longus

Flexor
pollicis longus

Flexor
carpi radialis

Median nerve

B Cross section through the right forearm
Proximal view. The location of the plane of section is shown in **D**.

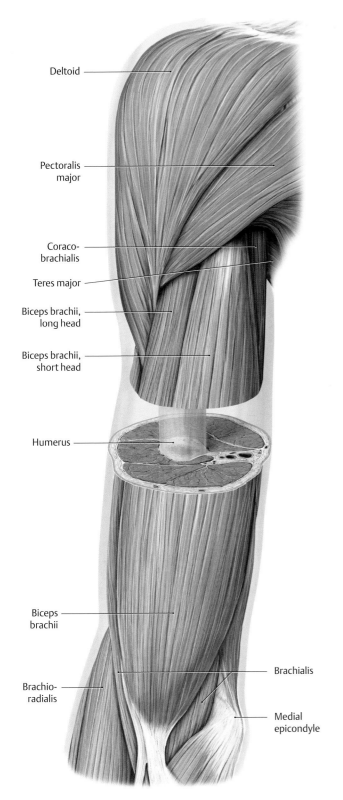

Deltoid

Pectoralis major

Coraco-brachialis

Teres major

Biceps brachii, long head

Biceps brachii, short head

Humerus

Biceps brachii

Brachio-radialis

Brachialis

Medial epicondyle

C "Windowed" dissection of the right arm
Anterior (ventral) view.

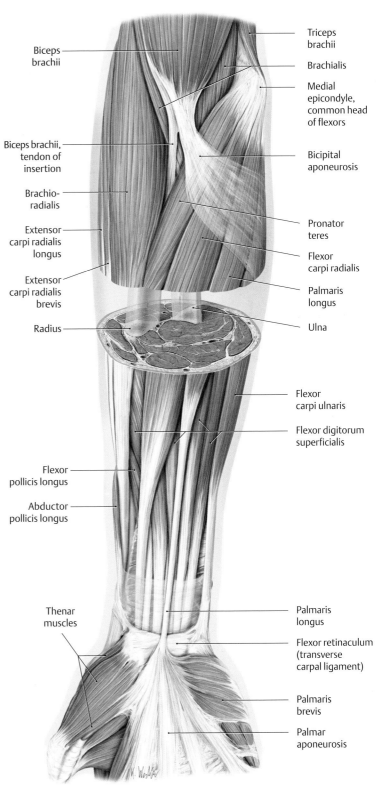

Biceps brachii

Biceps brachii, tendon of insertion

Brachio-radialis

Extensor carpi radialis longus

Extensor carpi radialis brevis

Radius

Flexor pollicis longus

Abductor pollicis longus

Thenar muscles

Triceps brachii

Brachialis

Medial epicondyle, common head of flexors

Bicipital aponeurosis

Pronator teres

Flexor carpi radialis

Palmaris longus

Ulna

Flexor carpi ulnaris

Flexor digitorum superficialis

Palmaris longus

Flexor retinaculum (transverse carpal ligament)

Palmaris brevis

Palmar aponeurosis

D "Windowed" dissection of the right forearm
Anterior (ventral) view.

297

3.8   The Tendon Sheaths of the Hand

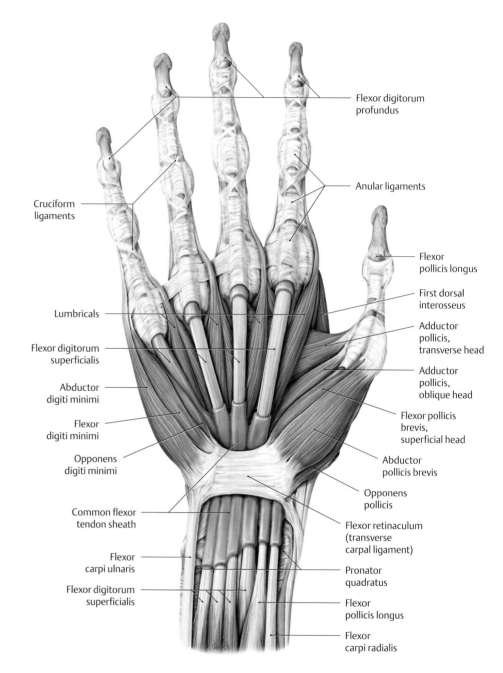

A Carpal and digital tendon sheaths on the palmar surface of the right hand

The palmar aponeurosis (see p. 302) has been removed. The tendons of flexor pollicis longus, flexor carpi radialis, and flexor digitorum superficialis and profundus run from the distal forearm through a fibro-osseous canal (carpal tunnel) to the palm, accompanied by the median nerve and protected by the palmar carpal tendon sheaths (see also p. 248 and p. 354). The carpal tendon sheath of flexor pollicis longus is consistently continuous with the digital tendon sheath of the thumb, while the digital tendon sheaths of the remaining fingers show variable communication with the carpal tendon sheaths (see **B**).

Labels (clockwise from top right):
- Flexor digitorum profundus
- Anular ligaments
- Flexor pollicis longus
- First dorsal interosseus
- Adductor pollicis, transverse head
- Adductor pollicis, oblique head
- Flexor pollicis brevis, superficial head
- Abductor pollicis brevis
- Opponens pollicis
- Flexor retinaculum (transverse carpal ligament)
- Pronator quadratus
- Flexor pollicis longus
- Flexor carpi radialis
- Flexor digitorum superficialis
- Flexor carpi ulnaris
- Common flexor tendon sheath
- Opponens digiti minimi
- Flexor digiti minimi
- Abductor digiti minimi
- Flexor digitorum superficialis
- Lumbricals
- Cruciform ligaments

B Communication between the digital and carpal tendon sheaths

Right hand, anterior view (after Schmidt and Lanz).

a In 71.4% of cases (Scheldrup 1951) the digital tendon sheath of the little finger communicates directly with the carpal tendon sheath, while the other tendon sheaths of the second through fourth digits extend only from the metacarpophalangeal joint to the distal interphalangeal joint.

b In 17.4% of cases the carpal tendon sheath does not communicate with the digital tendon sheath of the little finger.

c Besides the tendon sheath of the little finger, the carpal tendon sheath may occasionally be continuous with the digital tendon sheath of the index finger (3.5%) or of the ring finger (3%).

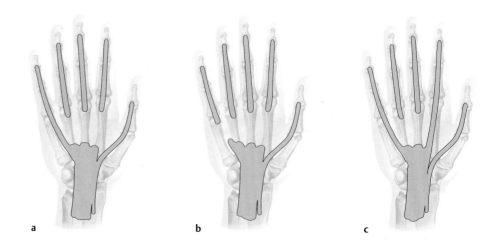

a   b   c

C Dorsal tendon compartments for the extensor tendons

First tendon compartment:	Abductor pollicis longus Extensor pollicis brevis
Second tendon compartment:	Extensor carpi radialis longus and brevis
Third tendon compartment:	Extensor pollicis longus
Fourth tendon compartment:	Extensor digitorum Extensor indicis
Fifth tendon compartment:	Extensor digiti minimi
Sixth tendon compartment:	Extensor carpi ulnaris

The location of the tendon compartments is shown in **D**.

D Extensor retinaculum and dorsal carpal tendon sheaths of the right hand

The extensor retinaculum is part of the antebrachial (forearm) fascia. Its transverse fibers strengthen the fibrous layer of the tendon sheaths and fix it to the dorsum of the hand. Deep to the extensor retinaculum are *tendon sheath compartments* which transmit the long extensor tendons singly or in groups. There are a total of six of these compartments, numbered 1–6 from the radial side to the ulnar side of the wrist (their contents are shown in **C**).

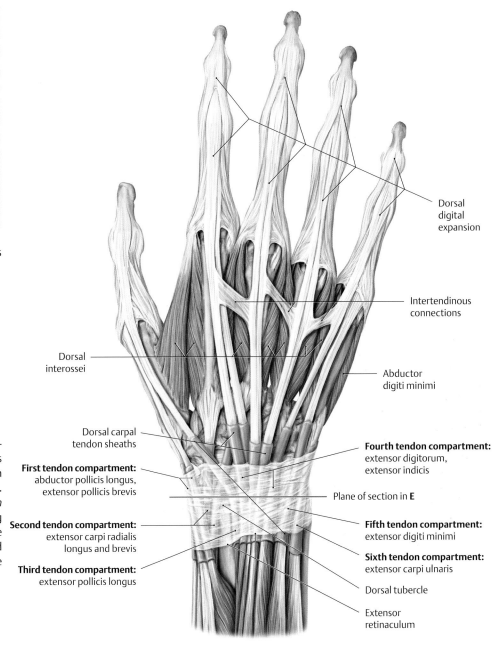

Dorsal digital expansion

Intertendinous connections

Dorsal interossei

Abductor digiti minimi

Dorsal carpal tendon sheaths

Fourth tendon compartment: extensor digitorum, extensor indicis

First tendon compartment: abductor pollicis longus, extensor pollicis brevis

Plane of section in **E**

Second tendon compartment: extensor carpi radialis longus and brevis

Fifth tendon compartment: extensor digiti minimi

Third tendon compartment: extensor pollicis longus

Sixth tendon compartment: extensor carpi ulnaris

Dorsal tubercle

Extensor retinaculum

E Schematic cross section through the forearm at the level of the distal radioulnar joint, viewed from the proximal view

(Location of the sectional plane is shown in **D**.) Vertical connective tissue septa extend anteriorly from the deep surface of the extensor retinaculum to the bone or joint capsule and form six fibro-osseous canals, the tendon sheath compartments of the extensor tendons (extensor tendon compartments). *Note* also the dorsal tubercle, which redirects the tendon of insertion of extensor pollicis longus to the thumb (see also **D**).

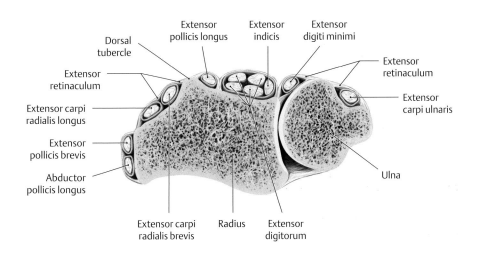

Dorsal tubercle

Extensor pollicis longus

Extensor indicis

Extensor digiti minimi

Extensor retinaculum

Extensor retinaculum

Extensor carpi radialis longus

Extensor pollicis brevis

Abductor pollicis longus

Extensor carpi ulnaris

Ulna

Extensor carpi radialis brevis

Radius

Extensor digitorum

299

3.9 The Dorsal Digital Expansion

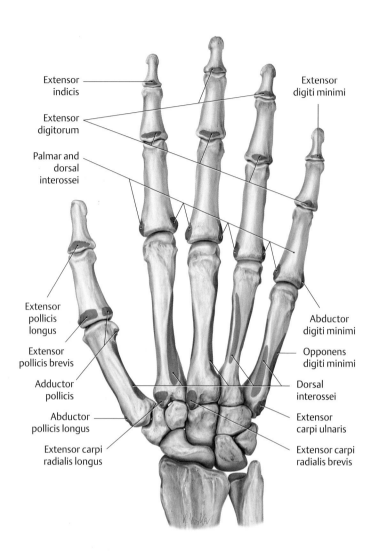

A Origins and insertions of the dorsal muscles of the right hand
The origins and insertions of the muscles are indicated by color shading (red = origin, blue = insertion).

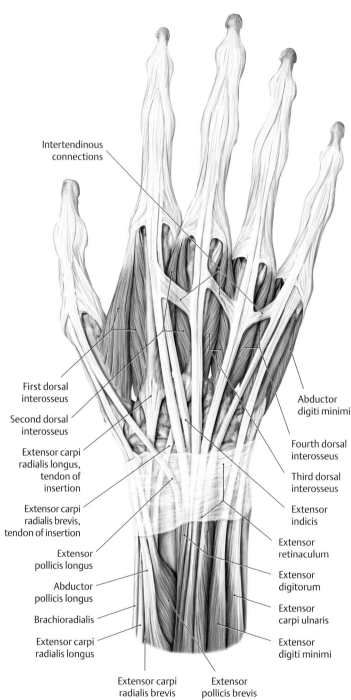

B Extensor tendons and intertendinous connections on the dorsum of the right hand
The tendons of insertion of extensor digitorum are interlinked by variable oblique bands called *intertendinous connections*. The most proximal of the intertendinous connections are those extending between the index and middle fingers. No such connection is present on the tendon of extensor indicis. The extensor digitorum inserts by a variable number of tendons. Generally, all of the fingers have at least two extensor tendon elements. In addition, the *index finger* and *little finger* have their own extensor muscles (extensor indicis and extensor digiti minimi) whose tendons always run on the ulnar side of the tendons of the common extensor digitorum. Because the index finger and little finger have their own extensors, they can more easily be moved independently of the other fingers.

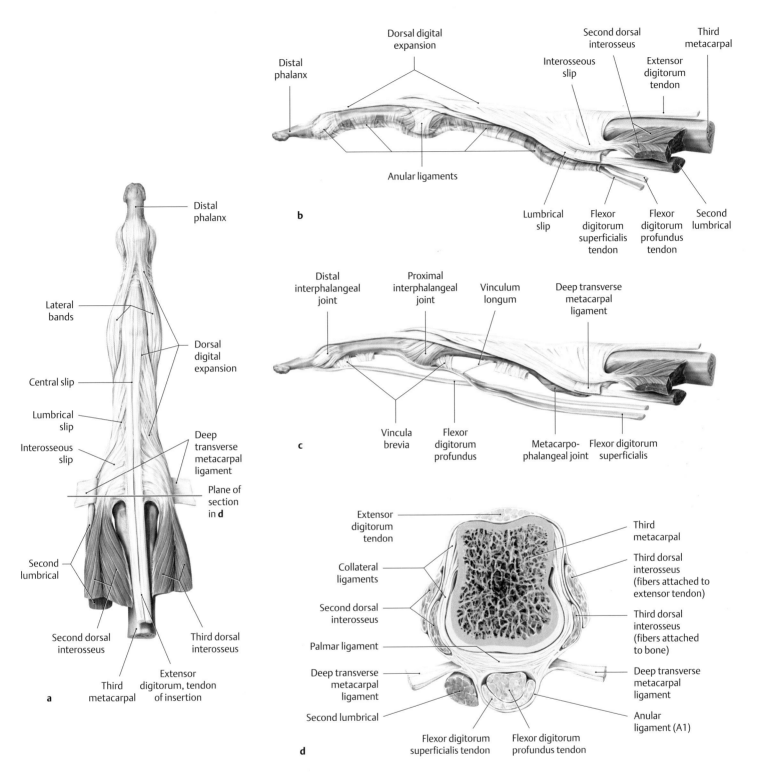

C Dorsal digital expansion

Dorsal digital expansion of the middle finger of the right hand (after Schmidt and Lanz).

a Posterior view.
b Radial view.
c After opening the common tendon sheath of the flexor digitorum superficialis and profundus muscles.
d Cross section at the level of the metacarpal head.

The dorsal digital expansion is more than an aponeurosis that incorporates slips from the extensor digitorum, lumbrical, and interosseous tendons. It is a complex system of interwoven fiber bands, joined by loose connective tissue to the periosteum of the phalanges. The dorsal digital expansion consists of a *central slip* and *lateral bands*, each of which has a *lateral part* and a *medial part*. The lateral part of the expansion receives slips from the tendons of the lumbrical 1ond interosseous muscles (see **a**). This complex arrangement makes it possible for the long digital flexors and the short hand muscles to act on all three of the finger joints.

3.10 The Intrinsic Muscles of the Hand: Superficial Layer

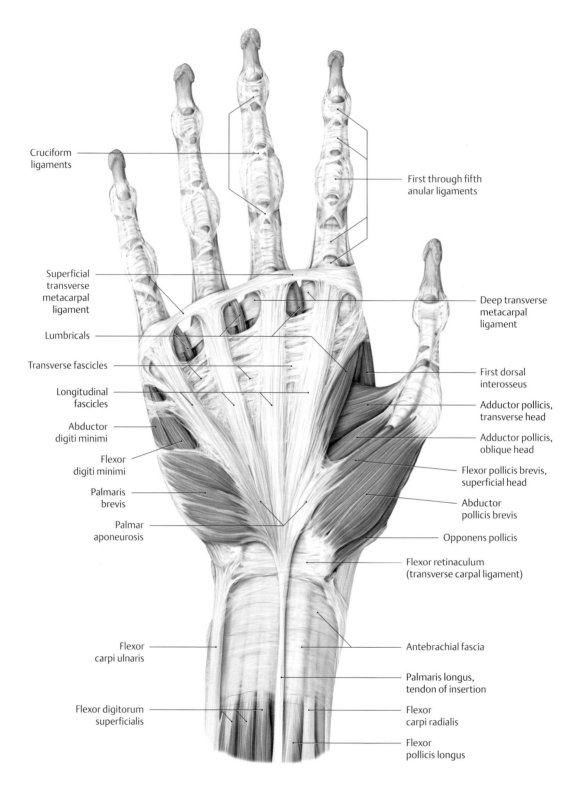

Cruciform ligaments

First through fifth anular ligaments

Superficial transverse metacarpal ligament

Lumbricals

Transverse fascicles

Longitudinal fascicles

Abductor digiti minimi

Flexor digiti minimi

Palmaris brevis

Palmar aponeurosis

Deep transverse metacarpal ligament

First dorsal interosseus

Adductor pollicis, transverse head

Adductor pollicis, oblique head

Flexor pollicis brevis, superficial head

Abductor pollicis brevis

Opponens pollicis

Flexor retinaculum (transverse carpal ligament)

Flexor carpi ulnaris

Antebrachial fascia

Palmaris longus, tendon of insertion

Flexor digitorum superficialis

Flexor carpi radialis

Flexor pollicis longus

A The palmar aponeurosis and Dupuytren's contracture
Right hand, anterior view. The muscular fascia of the palm is thickened by firm connective tissue to form the *palmar aponeurosis*, which separates the palm from the subcutaneous fat to protect the soft tissues. It is composed mainly of longitudinal fiber bundles (*longitudinal fascicles*), which give it a fan-shaped arrangement. The longitudinal fascicles are held together by transverse fiber bundles (*transverse fascicles*) at the level of the metacarpal bones and by the superficial transverse metacarpal ligament at the level of the metacarpophalangeal joints. Two muscles, the palmaris brevis and palmaris longus, keep the palmar aponeurosis tense and prevent it from contracting, especially when the hand is clenched into a fist. Gradual atrophy or contracture of the palmar

aponeurosis leads to progressive shortening of the palmar fascia that chiefly affects the little finger and ring finger (*Dupuytren's contracture*). Over a period of years, the contracture may become so severe that the fingers assume a fixed flexed position with the fingertips touching the palm; this seriously compromises the grasping ability of the hand. The causes of Dupuytren's contracture are poorly understood, but it is a relatively common condition that is most prevalent in men over 40 years of age and is associated with chronic liver disease (e.g., cirrhosis). Treatment generally consists of complete surgical removal of the palmar aponeurosis.

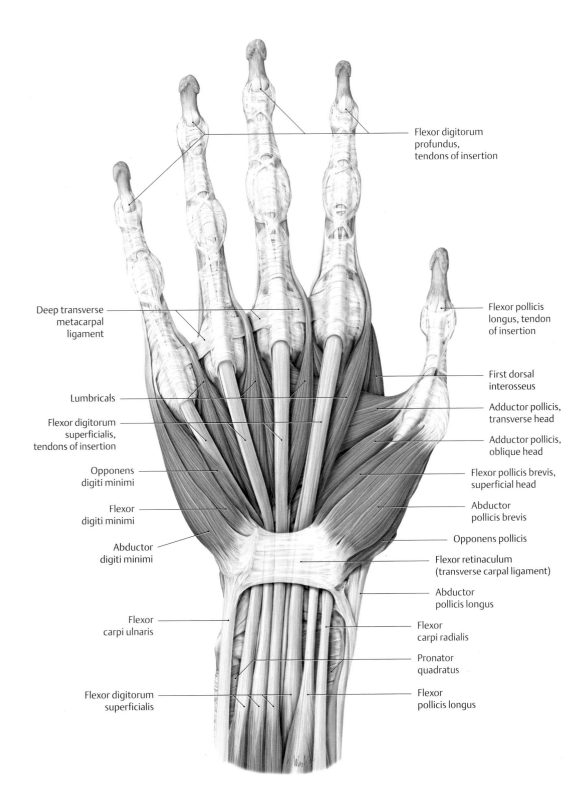

Flexor digitorum profundus, tendons of insertion

Deep transverse metacarpal ligament

Lumbricals

Flexor digitorum superficialis, tendons of insertion

Opponens digiti minimi

Flexor digiti minimi

Abductor digiti minimi

Flexor carpi ulnaris

Flexor digitorum superficialis

Flexor pollicis longus, tendon of insertion

First dorsal interosseus

Adductor pollicis, transverse head

Adductor pollicis, oblique head

Flexor pollicis brevis, superficial head

Abductor pollicis brevis

Opponens pollicis

Flexor retinaculum (transverse carpal ligament)

Abductor pollicis longus

Flexor carpi radialis

Pronator quadratus

Flexor pollicis longus

B Superficial muscles of the right hand after removal of the palmar aponeurosis

Anterior view. The palmar aponeurosis, antebrachial (forearm) fascia, and palmaris brevis and longus muscles have been removed along with the palmar and carpal tendon sheaths.

3.11 The Intrinsic Muscles of the Hand: Middle Layer

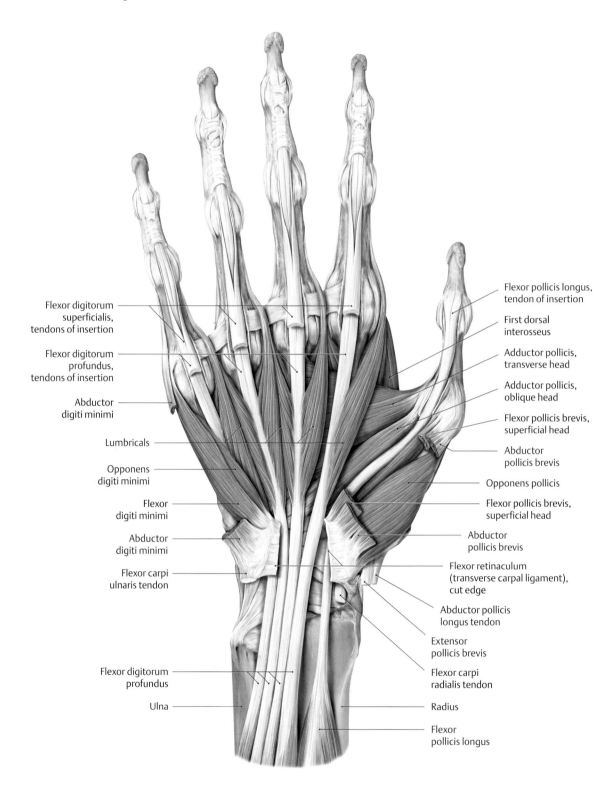

Flexor digitorum superficialis, tendons of insertion

Flexor digitorum profundus, tendons of insertion

Abductor digiti minimi

Lumbricals

Opponens digiti minimi

Flexor digiti minimi

Abductor digiti minimi

Flexor carpi ulnaris tendon

Flexor digitorum profundus

Ulna

Flexor pollicis longus, tendon of insertion

First dorsal interosseus

Adductor pollicis, transverse head

Adductor pollicis, oblique head

Flexor pollicis brevis, superficial head

Abductor pollicis brevis

Opponens pollicis

Flexor pollicis brevis, superficial head

Abductor pollicis brevis

Flexor retinaculum (transverse carpal ligament), cut edge

Abductor pollicis longus tendon

Extensor pollicis brevis

Flexor carpi radialis tendon

Radius

Flexor pollicis longus

A Muscles of the right hand

Anterior view. The flexor digitorum superficialis muscle has been removed, and its four tendons of insertion have been divided at the level of the metacarpophalangeal joints. The first through third anular ligaments have been cut open to reveal the flexor tendons on the fingers.

The flexor retinaculum (transverse carpal ligament) has been partially removed to open the carpal tunnel. Of the thenar muscles, portions of abductor pollicis brevis and flexor pollicis brevis (superficial head) have been removed. Part of the abductor digiti minimi has been resected on the hypothenar side.

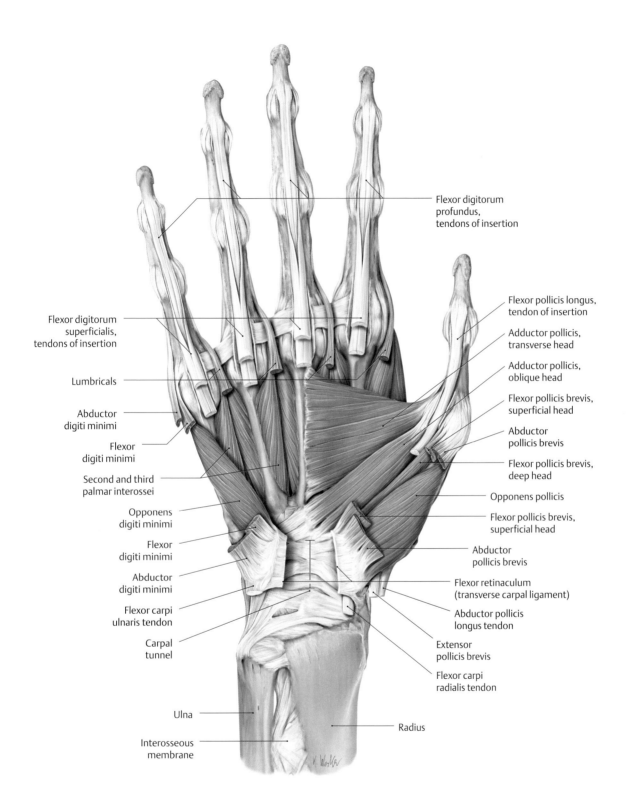

Flexor digitorum profundus, tendons of insertion

Flexor digitorum superficialis, tendons of insertion

Lumbricals

Abductor digiti minimi

Flexor digiti minimi

Second and third palmar interossei

Opponens digiti minimi

Flexor digiti minimi

Abductor digiti minimi

Flexor carpi ulnaris tendon

Carpal tunnel

Ulna

Interosseous membrane

Flexor pollicis longus, tendon of insertion

Adductor pollicis, transverse head

Adductor pollicis, oblique head

Flexor pollicis brevis, superficial head

Abductor pollicis brevis

Flexor pollicis brevis, deep head

Opponens pollicis

Flexor pollicis brevis, superficial head

Abductor pollicis brevis

Flexor retinaculum (transverse carpal ligament)

Abductor pollicis longus tendon

Extensor pollicis brevis

Flexor carpi radialis tendon

Radius

B Muscles of the right hand

Anterior view. The flexor digitorum profundus muscle has been removed, and its four tendons of insertion and the lumbricals arising from them have been divided. The flexor pollicis longus and flexor digiti minimi muscles have also been removed.

3.12 The Intrinsic Muscles of the Hand: Deep Layer

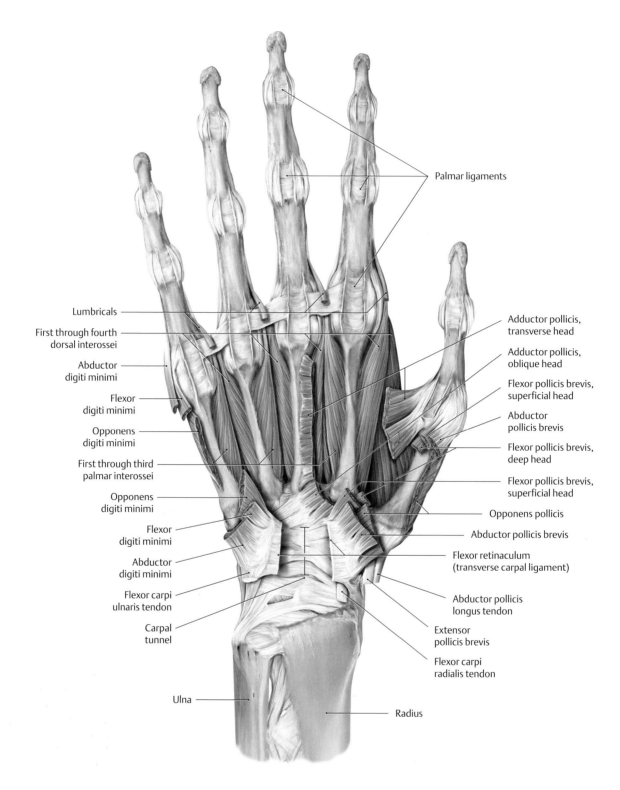

Palmar ligaments

Lumbricals

First through fourth dorsal interossei

Abductor digiti minimi

Flexor digiti minimi

Opponens digiti minimi

First through third palmar interossei

Opponens digiti minimi

Flexor digiti minimi

Abductor digiti minimi

Flexor carpi ulnaris tendon

Carpal tunnel

Ulna

Adductor pollicis, transverse head

Adductor pollicis, oblique head

Flexor pollicis brevis, superficial head

Abductor pollicis brevis

Flexor pollicis brevis, deep head

Flexor pollicis brevis, superficial head

Opponens pollicis

Abductor pollicis brevis

Flexor retinaculum (transverse carpal ligament)

Abductor pollicis longus tendon

Extensor pollicis brevis

Flexor carpi radialis tendon

Radius

A Muscles of the right hand
Anterior view. The tendons of insertion, tendon sheaths, and anular ligaments of the long digital flexors have been completely removed.
Note the exposed palmar ligaments, which combine with the tendon sheaths to form a kind of trough that directs the long flexor tendons (see p. 251).

The first dorsal interosseus and first palmar interosseus muscles have been almost completely exposed by removal of the adductor pollicis. Both the opponens pollicis and the opponens digiti minimi have been partially removed.

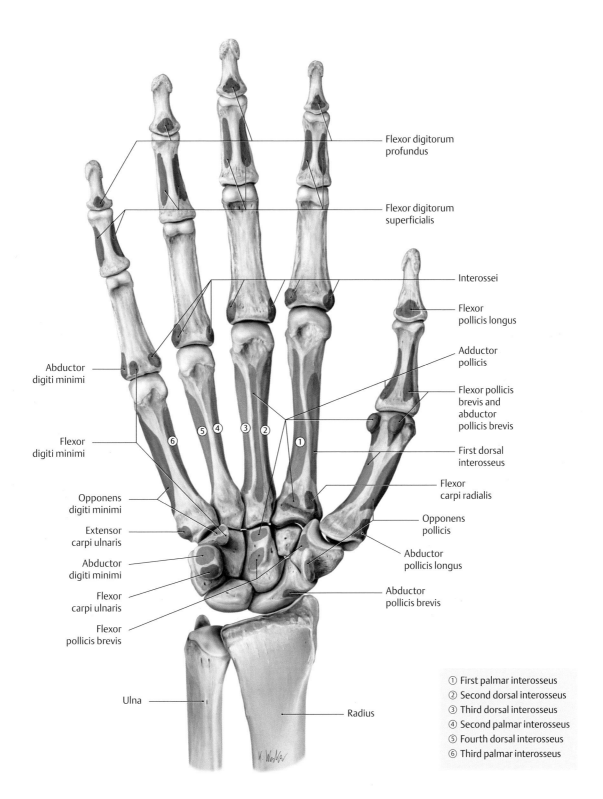

Flexor digitorum profundus

Flexor digitorum superficialis

Interossei

Flexor pollicis longus

Adductor pollicis

Flexor pollicis brevis and abductor pollicis brevis

First dorsal interosseus

Flexor carpi radialis

Opponens pollicis

Abductor pollicis longus

Abductor pollicis brevis

Abductor digiti minimi

Flexor digiti minimi

Opponens digiti minimi

Extensor carpi ulnaris

Abductor digiti minimi

Flexor carpi ulnaris

Flexor pollicis brevis

Ulna

Radius

① First palmar interosseus
② Second dorsal interosseus
③ Third dorsal interosseus
④ Second palmar interosseus
⑤ Fourth dorsal interosseus
⑥ Third palmar interosseus

B Origins and insertions of the palmar muscles of the right hand
The origins and insertions of the muscles are indicated by color shading
(red = origin, blue = insertion).

4.1   The Arteries

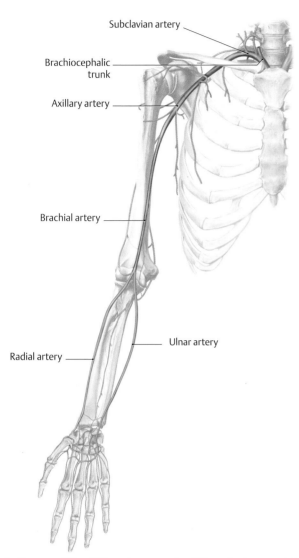

Subclavian artery

Brachiocephalic trunk

Axillary artery

Brachial artery

Radial artery

Ulnar artery

A Course of the different segments of the arteries supplying the shoulder and arm

Subclavian artery: The right subclavian artery arises from the brachiocephalic trunk (as shown here), and the left arises directly from the aortic arch. The vessel runs over the first rib between the scalenus anterior and scalenus medius (interscalene space, scalene interval) and continues as the axillary artery (see below) on reaching the lateral border of the rib. Unlike the other arteries pictured here, the subclavian artery supplies blood not only to the upper limb (i.e., the shoulder girdle and arm) but also to:

- a portion of the neck,
- the cerebral circulation, and
- the anterior chest wall.

Axillary artery: The continuation of the subclavian, the axillary artery runs from the lateral border of the first rib to the inferior border of the teres major muscle.

Brachial artery: The brachial artery is the continuation of the axillary artery. It ends at the elbow joint by dividing into the radial and ulnar arteries.

Radial artery: The radial artery runs distally on the radial side of the forearm from the division of the brachial artery, passing between the brachioradialis and flexor carpi radialis muscles on its way to the wrist. It terminates in the deep palmar arch.

Ulnar artery: This second division of the brachial artery runs below pronator teres on the ulnar side of the forearm, under cover of flexor carpi ulnaris, to the superficial palmar arch.

B Overview of the arteries of the shoulder and arm

The arteries of the shoulder and arm vary considerably in their origins and branching patterns (the principal variants are reviewed in Chapter 5, Neurovascular Systems: Topographical Anatomy). The branches are listed below in the order in which they arise from the parent vessels.

Branches of the subclavian artery
- Vertebral artery
- Internal thoracic artery (internal mammary artery)
- Thyrocervical trunk
    - Inferior thyroid artery
    - Suprascapular artery
    - Transverse cervical artery
- Costocervical trunk
    - Deep cervical artery
    - Supreme intercostal artery

Branches of the axillary artery
- Superior thoracic artery
- Thoracoacromial artery
    - Acromial branch
    - Clavicular branch
    - Deltoid branch
    - Pectoral branch
- Lateral thoracic artery
- Subscapular artery
    - Thoracodorsal artery
    - Circumflex scapular artery
- Anterior circumflex humeral artery
- Posterior circumflex humeral artery

Branches of the brachial artery
- Profunda brachii (deep brachial artery)
    - Medial collateral artery
    - Radial collateral artery
- Superior ulnar collateral artery (arterial network of the elbow)
- Inferior ulnar collateral artery (arterial network of the elbow)

Branches of the radial artery
- Radial recurrent artery (arterial network of the elbow)
- Palmar carpal branch (palmar carpal network)
- Superficial palmar branch (superficial palmar arch)
- Dorsal carpal branch (dorsal carpal network)
    - Dorsal metacarpal arteries
    - Dorsal digital arteries
- Princeps pollicis artery
- Radialis indicis artery
- Deep palmar arch
    - Palmar metacarpal arteries
    - Perforating branches

Branches of the ulnar artery
- Ulnar recurrent artery (arterial network of the elbow)
- Common interosseous artery
    - Posterior interosseous artery
    - Recurrent interosseous artery
    - Anterior interosseous artery
- Palmar carpal branch (palmar carpal network)
- Dorsal carpal branch (dorsal carpal network)
- Deep palmar branch (deep palmar arch)
- Superficial palmar arch
    - Common palmar digital arteries
    - Proper palmar digital arteries

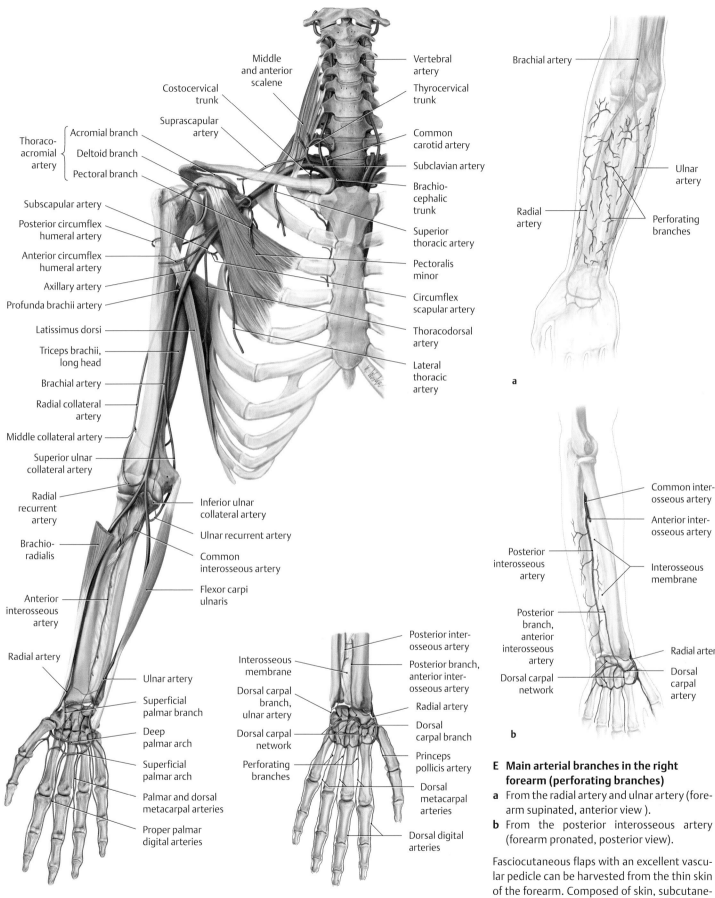

Middle and anterior scalene
Costocervical trunk
Suprascapular artery
Thoraco-acromial artery { **Acromial branch** — **Deltoid branch** — **Pectoral branch** }
Subscapular artery
Posterior circumflex humeral artery
Anterior circumflex humeral artery
Axillary artery
Profunda brachii artery
Latissimus dorsi
Triceps brachii, long head
Brachial artery
Radial collateral artery
Middle collateral artery
Superior ulnar collateral artery
Radial recurrent artery
Brachio-radialis
Anterior interosseous artery
Radial artery

Vertebral artery
Thyrocervical trunk
Common carotid artery
Subclavian artery
Brachio-cephalic trunk
Superior thoracic artery
Pectoralis minor
Circumflex scapular artery
Thoracodorsal artery
Lateral thoracic artery

Inferior ulnar collateral artery
Ulnar recurrent artery
Common interosseous artery
Flexor carpi ulnaris

Ulnar artery
Superficial palmar branch
Deep palmar arch
Superficial palmar arch
Palmar and dorsal metacarpal arteries
Proper palmar digital arteries

Brachial artery
Radial artery
Ulnar artery
Perforating branches

a

Common inter-osseous artery
Anterior inter-osseous artery
Interosseous membrane
Posterior interosseous artery
Posterior branch, anterior interosseous artery
Dorsal carpal network
Radial artery
Dorsal carpal artery

b

Posterior inter-osseous artery
Interosseous membrane
Dorsal carpal branch, ulnar artery
Dorsal carpal network
Perforating branches
Posterior branch, anterior inter-osseous artery
Radial artery
Dorsal carpal branch
Princeps pollicis artery
Dorsal metacarpal arteries
Dorsal digital arteries

C Arteries of the right upper limb
Anterior view with the forearm supinated. For clarity, some of the arteries listed in **B** are not illustrated.

D Arteries of the right hand
Posterior view.

E Main arterial branches in the right forearm (perforating branches)
a From the radial artery and ulnar artery (forearm supinated, anterior view).
b From the posterior interosseous artery (forearm pronated, posterior view).

Fasciocutaneous flaps with an excellent vascular pedicle can be harvested from the thin skin of the forearm. Composed of skin, subcutaneous tissue and fascia, these flaps are supplied by branches of major arteries and their accompanying veins. The skin flaps carry this vascular supply with them when they are transferred to the recipient site.

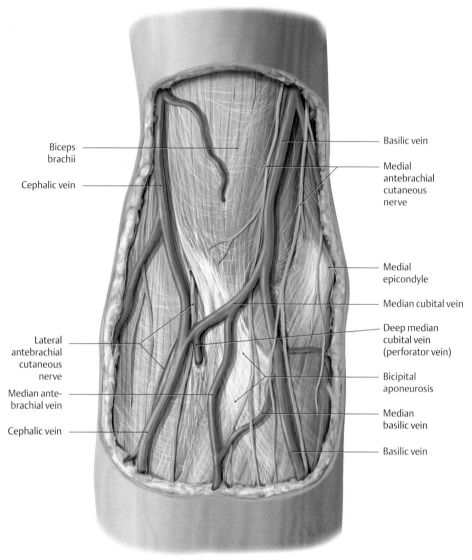

Biceps brachii

Cephalic vein

Lateral antebrachial cutaneous nerve

Median antebrachial vein

Cephalic vein

Basilic vein

Medial antebrachial cutaneous nerve

Medial epicondyle

Median cubital vein

Deep median cubital vein (perforator vein)

Bicipital aponeurosis

Median basilic vein

Basilic vein

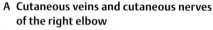

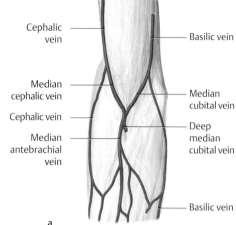

Cephalic vein

Median cephalic vein

Cephalic vein

Median antebrachial vein

Basilic vein

Median cubital vein

Deep median cubital vein

Basilic vein

a

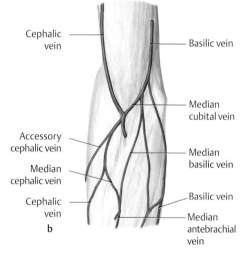

Cephalic vein

Accessory cephalic vein

Median cephalic vein

Cephalic vein

Basilic vein

Median cubital vein

Median basilic vein

Basilic vein

Median antebrachial vein

b

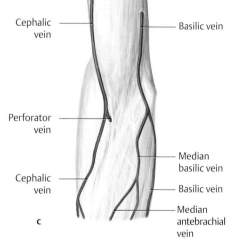

Cephalic vein

Perforator vein

Cephalic vein

Basilic vein

Median basilic vein

Basilic vein

Median antebrachial vein

c

A Cutaneous veins and cutaneous nerves of the right elbow

Anterior view. The subcutaneous veins of the elbow are excellent sites for administering intravenous injections and drawing blood owing to their size and accessibility and the relatively thin skin in that region. But given their close relationship to the cutaneous nerves, as illustrated by the proximity of the basilic vein to the medial antebrachial cutaneous nerve, injections into these veins may cause severe transient pain, as in cases where an accidental "paravascular" injection irritates the surrounding connective tissue. "Rolling veins" refers to a condition in which the subcutaneous veins are exceptionally mobile within the subcutaneous fat. In approximately 3% of cases the ulnar artery may pass over the surface of the flexor muscles (superficial ulnar artery, see also p. 347). An unintended intra-*arterial* injection can have devastating consequences with certain medications. This complication can be avoided by palpating the vessel and confirming arterial-type pulsations before giving the injection and always drawing a small amount of blood back into the syringe (dark red = venous blood, bright red = arterial blood) before depressing the plunger.

B Cubital fossa of the right arm: variable course of the subcutaneous veins

a M-shaped venous pattern above the median antebrachial vein.

b Presence of an accessory cephalic vein from the venous plexuses on the extensor side of the forearm.

c Absence of the median cubital vein.

All of the illustrated variants are common.

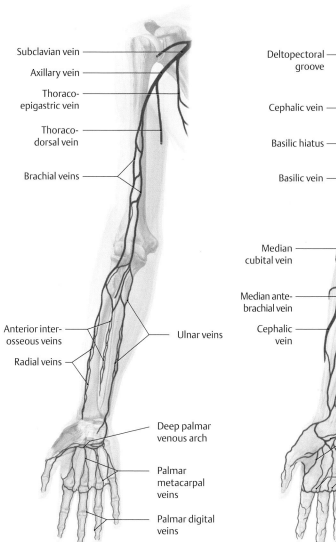

C Deep veins of the right upper limb
Anterior view.

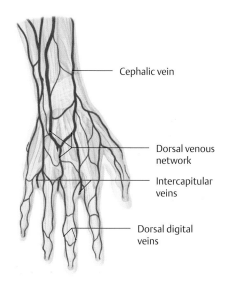

E Superficial veins of the dorsum of the right hand

D Superficial veins of the right upper limb
Anterior view. The main longitudinal trunks of the subcutaneous venous network of the arm are the median antebrachial vein, the basilic vein, and the cephalic vein.

Median antebrachial vein: This vein, unlike the cephalic and basilic, receives blood mainly from the cutaneous veins on the dorsum of the hand, draining the *flexor side of the forearm*. The *variable* median antebrachial vein opens into the corresponding longitudinal veins at the elbow, usually by way of the median cephalic vein and median basilic vein (see p. 333).

Basilic vein: This vein begins at the *elbow*, first ascending in the *epifascial* plane in the medial bicipital groove to the basilic hiatus, where it pierces the fascia in the middle of the arm. It terminates in a *subfascial* plane at the ulnar brachial vein.

Cephalic vein: In the *arm* the cephalic vein first ascends on the lateral side of the biceps brachii, then enters a groove between the deltoid and pectoralis major muscles (the deltopectoral groove). It finally opens into the axillary vein in the clavipectoral triangle (see p. 334).

F Overview of the main superficial and deep veins of the upper limb
Numerous connections exist between the deep and superficial veins of the arm—the perforator veins. Valves are incorporated into the veins at regular intervals, increasing the efficiency of venous return (see p. 47).

Deep veins of the upper limb
- Subclavian vein
- Axillary vein
- Brachial veins
- Ulnar veins
- Radial veins
- Anterior interosseous veins
- Posterior interosseous veins
- Deep palmar venous arch
- Palmar metacarpal veins

Superficial veins of the upper limb
- Cephalic vein
- Accessory cephalic vein
- Basilic vein
- Median cubital vein
- Median antebrachial vein
- Median cephalic vein
- Median basilic vein
- Dorsal venous network of the hand
- Superficial palmar venous arch

311

4.3   The Lymphatic Vessels and Lymph Nodes

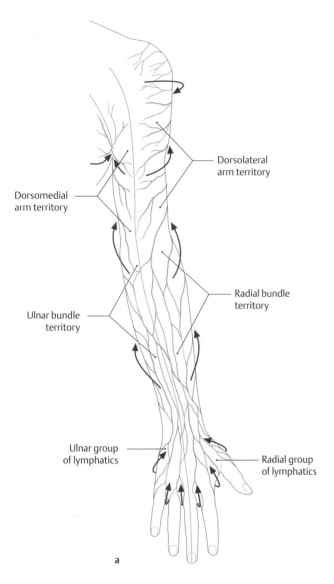

Dorsolateral arm territory

Dorsomedial arm territory

Radial bundle territory

Ulnar bundle territory

Ulnar group of lymphatics

Radial group of lymphatics

a

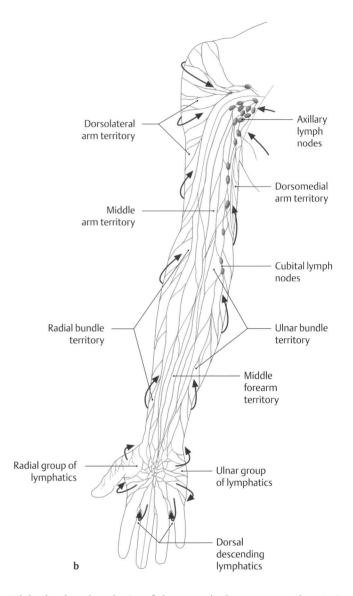

Dorsolateral arm territory

Axillary lymph nodes

Dorsomedial arm territory

Middle arm territory

Cubital lymph nodes

Radial bundle territory

Ulnar bundle territory

Middle forearm territory

Radial group of lymphatics

Ulnar group of lymphatics

Dorsal descending lymphatics

b

A Lymph vessels of the upper limb (after Schmidt and Lanz)
a Posterior view, **b** anterior view. The lymph vessels (lymphatics) in the upper limb are of two types:

- Superficial (epifascial) lymphatics
- Deep lymphatics

While the deep lymphatics of the upper limb accompany the arteries and deep veins, the superficial lymphatics lie in the subcutaneous tissue. In the forearm, they are most closely related to the cephalic and basilic veins. Numerous anastomoses exist between the deep and superficial systems. The arrows in the diagrams indicate the main directions of lymphatic drainage. Inflammations and infections of the hand generally incite a painful swelling of the axillary lymph nodes. When the lymph vessels are also involved, they are visible as red streaks beneath the skin (lymphangitis).

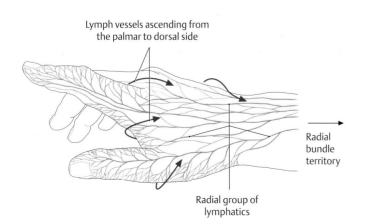

Lymph vessels ascending from the palmar to dorsal side

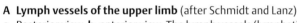
Radial bundle territory

Radial group of lymphatics

B Lymphatic drainage of the thumb, index finger, and dorsum of the hand (after Schmidt and Lanz)
The thumb, index finger, and part of the middle finger are drained by a radial group of lymph vessels that pass directly to the axillary lymph nodes. The other fingers are drained by an ulnar group of lymphatics (not shown here) that end at the cubital lymph nodes.

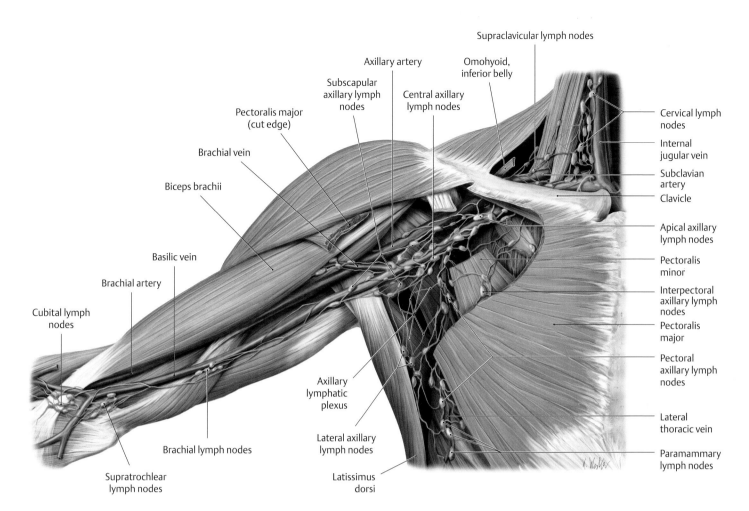

C Regional lymph nodes of the right upper limb
Anterior view. The lymph nodes of the axilla (*axillary lymph nodes*) are important collecting stations for the arm, shoulder girdle, and anterior chest wall. The 30 to 60 lymph nodes of the axilla are divided into several groups or levels, numbered I–III (see **E**), which are interconnected by lymph vessels. Taken together, the lymphatics in this region form an *axillary lymphatic plexus* lying within the fatty tissue. Lymphatic drainage from the axilla is collected in the subclavian trunk (not shown here). On the right side, the lymph is conveyed by the right jugular trunk and right bronchomediastinal trunk to the right lymphatic duct, which opens into the junction of the right subclavian and internal jugular veins (see p. 166).

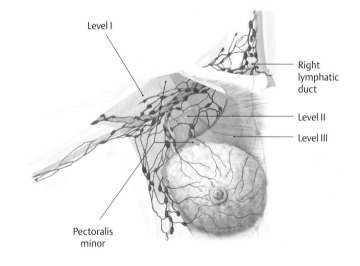

D The axillary lymph nodes, grouped by levels
(after Henne-Bruns, Dürig, and Kremer)

Level I: lower axillary group
(lateral to pectoralis minor)
- Pectoral axillary lymph nodes
- Subscapular axillary lymph nodes
- Lateral axillary lymph nodes
- Paramammary lymph nodes

Level II: middle axillary group
(at the level of pectoralis minor)
- Interpectoral axillary lymph nodes
- Central axillary lymph nodes

Level III: upper, infraclavicular group
(medial to pectoralis minor)
- Apical axillary lymph nodes

E Classification of axillary lymph nodes by level
The axillary lymph nodes have major clinical importance in breast cancer. A malignant breast tumor will metastasize (seed tumor cells) to the axillary nodes as it grows. As a guide for surgical removal, the axillary lymph nodes can be segregated into groups arranged in three levels, based on their relationship to the pectoralis minor muscle.

- Level I: all the lymph nodes lateral to pectoralis minor.
- Level II: all the lymph nodes at the level of pectoralis minor.
- Level III: all the lymph nodes medial to pectoralis minor (see p. 260).

313

4.4 The Brachial Plexus: Structure

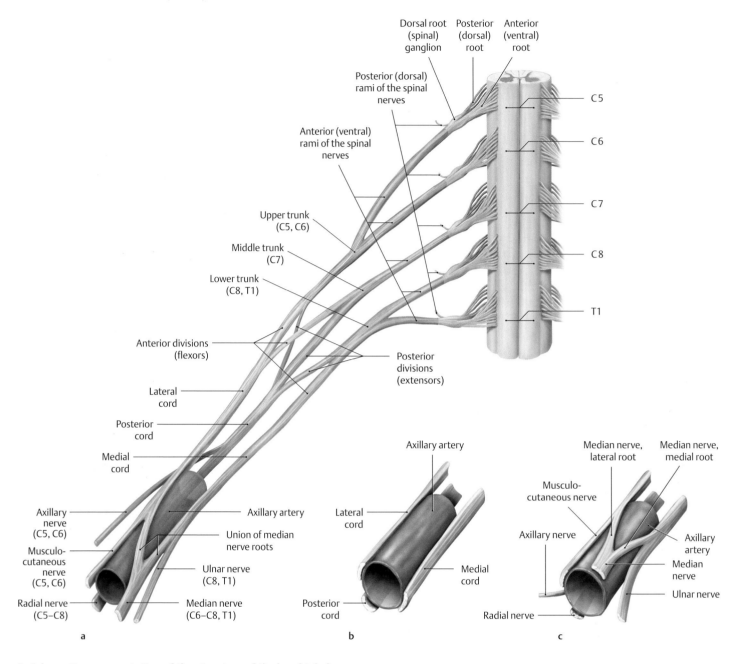

Dorsal root (spinal) ganglion — Posterior (dorsal) root — Anterior (ventral) root

Posterior (dorsal) rami of the spinal nerves

Anterior (ventral) rami of the spinal nerves

C5
C6
C7
C8
T1

Upper trunk (C5, C6)

Middle trunk (C7)

Lower trunk (C8, T1)

Anterior divisions (flexors)

Posterior divisions (extensors)

Lateral cord

Posterior cord

Medial cord

Axillary nerve (C5, C6)

Axillary artery

Union of median nerve roots

Musculo-cutaneous nerve (C5, C6)

Ulnar nerve (C8, T1)

Radial nerve (C5–C8)

Median nerve (C6–C8, T1)

a

Axillary artery

Lateral cord

Medial cord

Posterior cord

b

Median nerve, lateral root — Median nerve, medial root

Musculo-cutaneous nerve

Axillary nerve

Axillary artery

Median nerve

Ulnar nerve

Radial nerve

c

A Schematic representation of the structure of the brachial plexus
a Names and sequence of the various elements of the brachial plexus.
b Relationship of the lateral, medial, and posterior cords of the brachial plexus to the axillary artery.
c Subdivision of the brachial plexus cords into their main branches.

B Number and location of the main components of the brachial plexus

Components	Number	Location
1. Plexus roots (anterior rami of the spinal nerves from cord segments C5–T1)	5	Between scalenus anterior and scalenus medius (interscalene space)
2. The primary trunks: upper, middle, and lower	3	Lateral to the interscalene space and above the clavicle
3. The three anterior and three posterior divisions	6	Posterior to the clavicle
4. The lateral, medial, and posterior cords	3	In the axilla, posterior to pectoralis minor

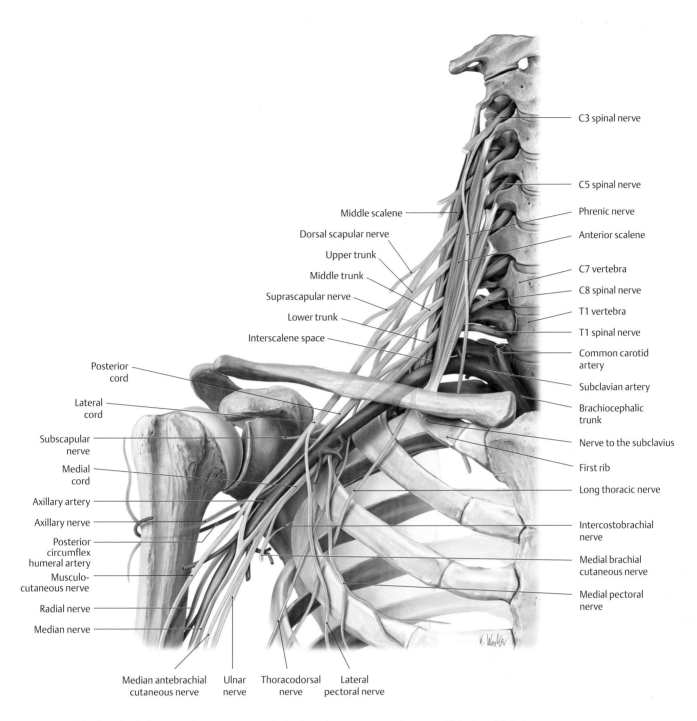

C3 spinal nerve
C5 spinal nerve
Phrenic nerve
Anterior scalene
C7 vertebra
C8 spinal nerve
T1 vertebra
T1 spinal nerve
Common carotid artery
Subclavian artery
Brachiocephalic trunk
Nerve to the subclavius
First rib
Long thoracic nerve
Intercostobrachial nerve
Medial brachial cutaneous nerve
Medial pectoral nerve

Middle scalene
Dorsal scapular nerve
Upper trunk
Middle trunk
Suprascapular nerve
Lower trunk
Interscalene space

Posterior cord
Lateral cord
Subscapular nerve
Medial cord
Axillary artery
Axillary nerve
Posterior circumflex humeral artery
Musculo-cutaneous nerve
Radial nerve
Median nerve

Median antebrachial cutaneous nerve
Ulnar nerve
Thoracodorsal nerve
Lateral pectoral nerve

C Course of the brachial plexus and its relation to the thorax after passing through the interscalene space
Right side, anterior view.

D Spinal cord segments and nerves of the brachial plexus

Brachial plexus trunks and associated spinal cord segments
- Upper trunk C5 + C6
- Middle trunk C7
- Lower trunk C8 + T1

Brachial plexus cords and associated spinal cord segments
- Lateral cord C5–C7
- Medial cord C8 + T1
- Posterior cord C5–T1

Nerves of the supraclavicular part of the brachial plexus (direct branches from the anterior rami or plexus trunks)
- Dorsal scapular nerve
- Long thoracic nerve
- Suprascapular nerve
- Nerve to the subclavius

Nerves of the infraclavicular part of the brachial plexus (short and long branches from the plexus cords)
- Lateral cord
  – Musculocutaneous nerve
  – Lateral pectoral nerve
  – Median nerve (lateral root)
- Medial cord
  – Median nerve (medial root)
  – Ulnar nerve
  – Medial pectoral nerve
  – Medial brachial cutaneous nerve
  – Median antebrachial cutaneous nerve
- Posterior cord
  – Radial nerve
  – Axillary nerve
  – Subscapular nerve
  – Thoracodorsal nerve

4.5 The Brachial Plexus: Supraclavicular Part

A Supraclavicular part of the brachial plexus

The supraclavicular part of the brachial plexus includes all nerves that arise directly from the plexus roots (anterior rami of the spinal nerves) or from the plexus trunks in the lateral cervical triangle between the scalenus anterior and scalenus medius muscles. The different nerves of the supraclavicular plexus are predisposed to paralysis and/or compression in varying degrees based on their location and course (see **B–D**).

Nerve	Segment	Innervated muscle
Dorsal scapular nerve	C3–5	• Levator scapulae • Rhomboid major • Rhomboid minor
Suprascapular nerve	C4–6	• Supraspinatus • Infraspinatus
Long thoracic nerve	C5–7	• Serratus anterior
Nerve to the subclavius	C5, 6	• Subclavius

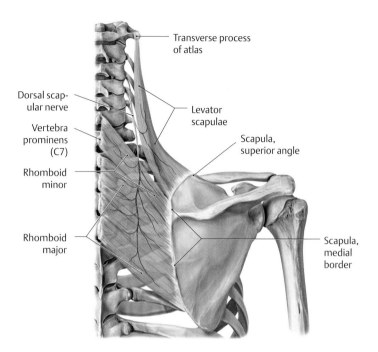

B The dorsal scapular nerve

Isolated paralysis of the dorsal scapular nerve is extremely rare owing to the protected location of the nerve between the deep nuchal muscles, the levator scapulae, and the rhomboids.

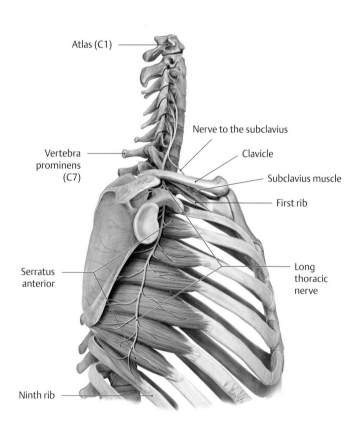

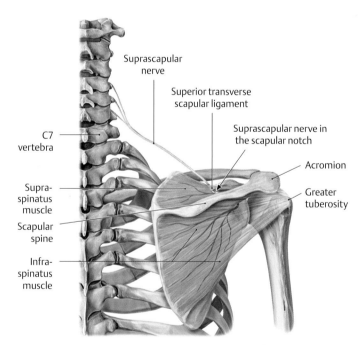

C The long thoracic nerve and nerve to the subclavius

Its long, superficial course on the serratus anterior along the lateral chest wall makes the long thoracic nerve susceptible to mechanical injury. The prolonged wearing of a heavy backpack is a common mechanism for this type of lesion. In iatrogenic cases, the nerve may be damaged by an axillary lymphadenectomy performed for a metastatic breast tumor. Clinically, loss of the serratus anterior muscle causes the medial scapular border to become elevated from the chest wall. This "winging" of the scapula is most conspicuous when the arm is raised forward, and generally the arm cannot be elevated past 90°.

D The suprascapular nerve

Injuries and chronic compression of the suprascapular nerve are uncommon conditions that lead to atrophy of the supraspinatus and infraspinatus muscles with weakness of arm abduction (especially during the initial phase owing to the "starter" function of the supraspinatus) and external rotation of the arm. Besides an isolated injury, the nerve may become compressed in the fibro-osseous canal between the scapular notch and the superior transverse scapular ligament (which is occasionally ossified to form a bony canal). The resulting symptoms are known collectively as "scapular notch syndrome" (see p. 213).

E Brachial plexus compression syndrome based on narrow anatomical passages in the shoulder region

In its course from the intervertebral foramina to the nerves of the upper limb, the brachial plexus must negotiate several narrow passages in which it may become compressed by surrounding structures. There are also extrinsic factors, such as carrying heavy loads, that may exert direct pressure on the brachial plexus. Several types of compression syndrome are distinguished:

1. Scalene syndrome or cervical rib syndrome:
   neurovascular compression in the interscalene space caused by a cervical rib or ligamentous structure (see **F**)

2. Costoclavicular syndrome:
   narrowing of the space between the first rib and clavicle (see **G**)

3. Hyperabduction syndrome:
   compression of the brachial plexus by the pectoralis minor muscle and coracoid process when the upper arm is raised above the head (see **H**)

4. Chronic heavy load on the shoulder girdle (e.g., "backpack paralysis")

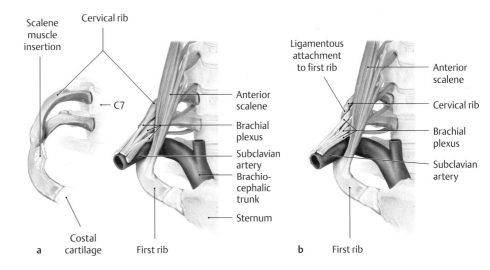

F Scalene syndrome due to narrowing of the interscalene space by a cervical rib

In approximately 1% of the population, cervical ribs may narrow the interscalene space bounded by the anterior and middle scalene muscles and the first rib. In this condition the trunks of the brachial plexus that pass through the interscalene space along with the subclavian artery are compressed from behind and below, placing varying degrees of tension on the neurovascular bundle. If there is no bony contact between a short cervical rib and the first rib (**b**), that site is often occupied by a ligamentous structure which can also cause neurovascular compression. The main clinical manifestations are pain radiating down the arm, chiefly to the ulnar side of the hand, and circulatory impairment caused by mechanical irritation of the periarterial sympathetic plexus of the subclavian artery.

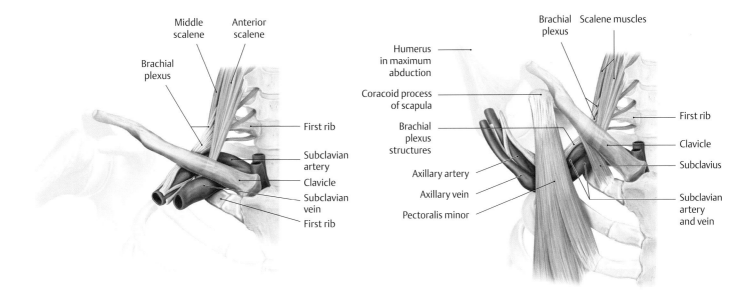

G Costoclavicular syndrome due to compression of the neurovascular bundle between the first rib and clavicle

Narrowing of the costoclavicular space is a rare condition that is most common in persons with drooping shoulders, a flat back, retracted shoulders (from carrying heavy loads), a deformed first rib, or a previous clavicular fracture. Any narrowing of the costoclavicular space can be aggravated by lowering and retracting the shoulder girdle. The complaints are similar to those in scalene syndrome and may be accompanied by signs of venous stasis caused by impaired return through the subclavian vein.

H Hyperabduction syndrome due to compression of the neurovascular bundle below the pectoralis minor and coracoid process

This rare syndrome is caused by neurovascular compression beneath the tendon of the pectoralis minor under the coracoid process. It is precipitated by maximum abduction or elevation of the arm on the affected side. A simple clinical test consists of pulling the arm upward and backward and holding it there. In normal cases, a definite radial artery pulse should still be palpable after 1–2 minutes, and the patient should not complain of radiating pain.

317

4.6 Infraclavicular Part of the Brachial Plexus: Overview and Short Branches

A Infraclavicular part of the brachial plexus
The infraclavicular part of the brachial plexus includes all the nerves that leave the plexus at the level of the plexus cords—the *short branches*— and those that continue down the arm as terminal branches of the individual plexus cords—the *long branches*. These nerves are reviewed below, beginning with the short branches.

Nerve	Segment	Innervated muscle	Cutaneous branches
Part I: Short branches			
• Subscapular nerve	C5, C6	• Subscapularis • Teres major	–
• Thoracodorsal nerve	C6–C8	• Latissimus dorsi	–
• Medial and lateral pectoral nerves	C5–T1	• Pectoralis major • Pectoralis minor	–
• Medial brachial cutaneous nerve	T1	–	• Medial brachial cutaneous nerve
• Medial antebrachial cutaneous nerve	C8, T1	–	• Medial antebrachial cutaneous nerve
• Intercostobrachial nerves*	T1, T2	–	• Lateral cutaneous branches
Part II: Long branches			
• Musculocutaneous nerve (see p. 320)	C5–C7	• Coracobrachialis • Biceps brachii • Brachialis	• Lateral antebrachial cutaneous nerve
• Axillary nerve (see p. 320)	C5, C6	• Deltoid • Teres minor	• Superior lateral brachial cutaneous nerve
• Radial nerve (see p. 322)	C5–T1	• Brachialis (contribution) • Triceps brachii • Anconeus • Supinator • Brachioradialis • Extensor carpi radialis longus • Extensor carpi radialis brevis • Extensor digitorum • Extensor digiti minimi • Extensor carpi ulnaris • Extensor pollicis longus • Extensor pollicis brevis • Extensor indicis • Abductor pollicis longus	• Inferior lateral brachial cutaneous nerve • Posterior brachial cutaneous nerve • Posterior antebrachial cutaneous nerve • Superficial branch of radial nerve
• Median nerve (see p. 326)	C6–T1	• Pronator teres • Pronator quadratus • Palmaris longus • Flexor carpi radialis • Flexor pollicis longus • Flexor digitorum profundus (½) • Flexor digitorum superficialis • Abductor pollicis brevis • Opponens pollicis • Flexor pollicis brevis (superficial head) • First and second lumbricals	• Palmar branch of median nerve • Common and proper palmar digital nerves
• Ulnar nerve (see p. 324)	C8, T1	• Flexor carpi ulnaris • Flexor digitorum profundus (½) • Palmaris brevis • Flexor digiti minimi • Abductor digiti minimi • Opponens digiti minimi • Adductor pollicis • Flexor pollicis brevis (deep head) • Palmar and dorsal interosseous muscles • Third and fourth lumbricals	• Palmar branch of ulnar nerve • Dorsal branch of ulnar nerve • Dorsal digital nerves • Common and proper palmar digital nerves

* These are the cutaneous branches of the intercostal nerves 2 and 3, which accompany the medial brachial cutaneous nerve.

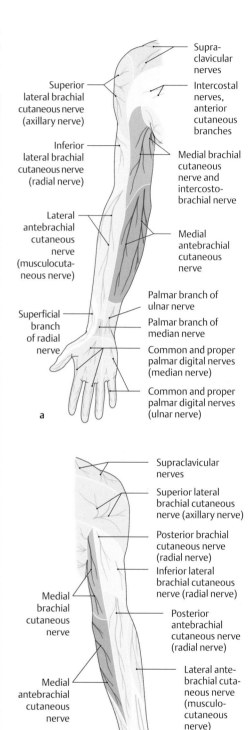

B Sensory distribution of the medial brachial cutaneous nerve and medial antebrachial cutaneous nerve of the right arm
a Anterior view, **b** posterior view.

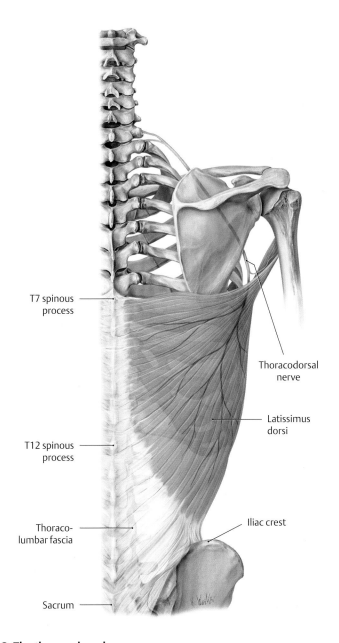

C **The thoracodorsal nerve**
Right side, posterior view.

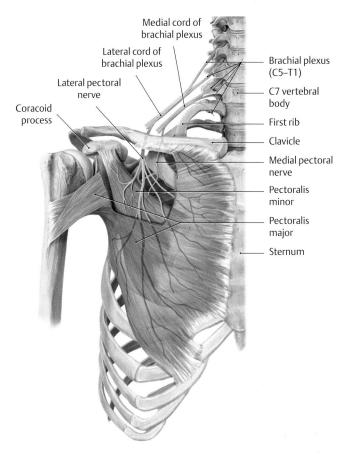

D **The medial and lateral pectoral nerves**
Right side, anterior view.

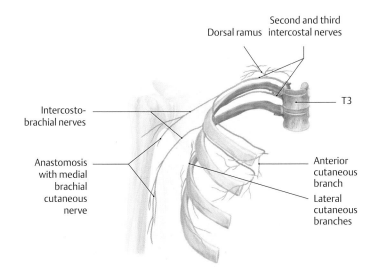

E **Origin and cutaneous distribution of the intercostobrachial
nerves of the right arm**
Anterior view.

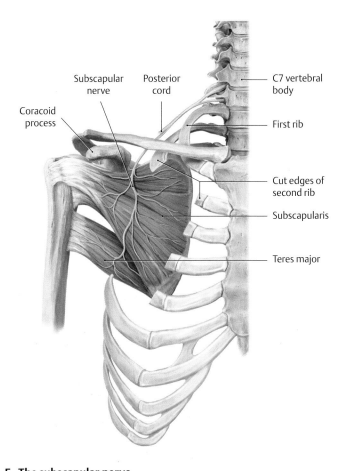

F **The subscapular nerve**
Right side, anterior view. The ribs have been partially removed.

4.7 Infraclavicular Part of the Brachial Plexus: The Musculocutaneous Nerve and Axillary Nerve

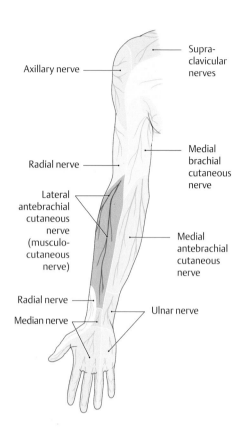

A Sensory distribution of the lateral antebrachial cutaneous nerve
Anterior view.

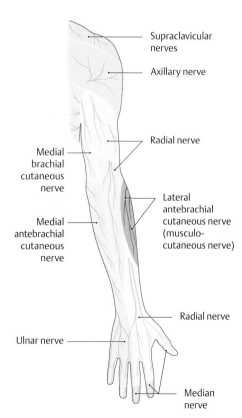

B Sensory distribution of the lateral antebrachial cutaneous nerve
Posterior view.

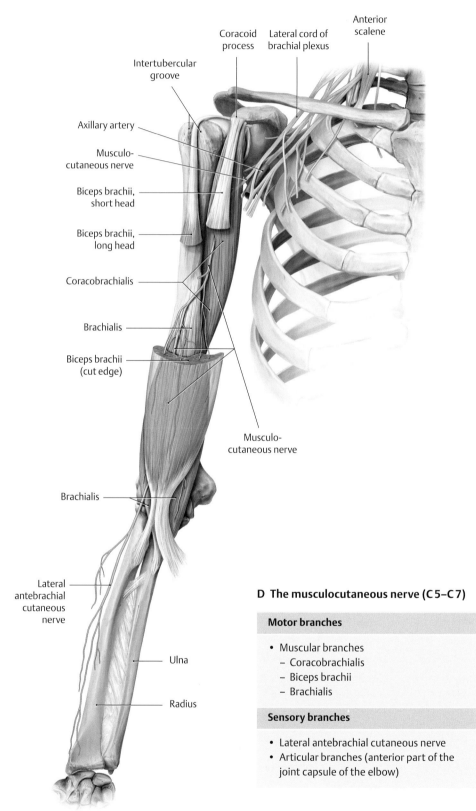

C Course of the musculocutaneous nerve after leaving the lateral cord of the brachial plexus
Right upper limb, anterior view. The musculocutaneous nerve leaves the lateral cord of the brachial plexus as a mixed nerve (one with motor and sensory branches) at the level of the lateral border of the pectoralis minor (not shown here) and runs a short course before piercing the coracobrachialis. It then runs between the biceps brachii and brachialis muscles to the elbow, where its terminal sensory branch supplies the skin on the radial side of the forearm.

D The musculocutaneous nerve (C 5–C 7)

Motor branches
• Muscular branches – Coracobrachialis – Biceps brachii – Brachialis

Sensory branches
• Lateral antebrachial cutaneous nerve • Articular branches (anterior part of the joint capsule of the elbow)

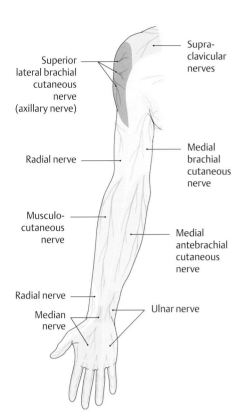

E Sensory distribution of the superior lateral brachial cutaneous nerve
Anterior view.

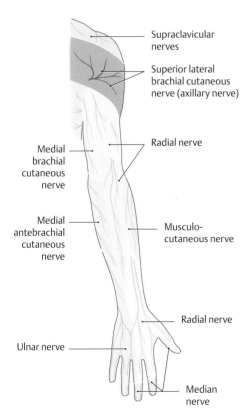

F Sensory distribution of the superior lateral brachial cutaneous nerve
Posterior view.

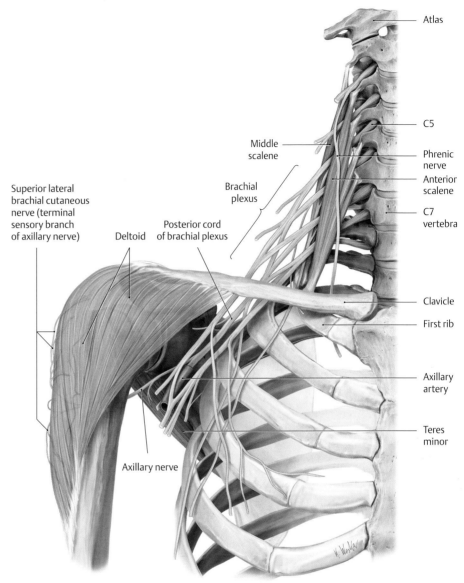

G Course of the axillary nerve after leaving the posterior cord of the brachial plexus
Right upper limb, anterior view. The axillary nerve leaves the posterior cord of the brachial plexus as a mixed nerve and runs backward through the deep part of the axilla, passing directly below the shoulder joint. It courses through the quadrangular space of the axilla (with the posterior circumflex humeral artery) and along the surgical neck to the posterior side of the proximal humerus. Its terminal sensory branch supplies the skin over the deltoid muscle. Isolated *axillary nerve palsy* may occur following an anteroinferior shoulder dislocation (or a traumatic reduction attempt), a humeral fracture at the level of the surgical neck, or prolonged pressure from an improperly adjusted crutch in the axilla.

H The axillary nerve (C 5 and C 6)

Motor branches

• Muscular branches
  – Deltoid
  – Teres minor

Sensory branch
• Superior lateral brachial cutaneous nerve

4.8 Infraclavicular Part of the Brachial Plexus: The Radial Nerve

A The radial nerve (C 5–T 1)

Motor branches

- Muscular branches (from the radial nerve)
  - Brachialis (contribution)
  - Triceps brachii
  - Anconeus
  - Brachioradialis
  - Extensor carpi radialis longus
  - Extensor carpi radialis brevis
- Deep branch (terminal branch: posterior interosseous nerve)
  - Supinator
  - Extensor digitorum
  - Extensor digiti minimi
  - Extensor carpi ulnaris
  - Extensor pollicis longus
  - Extensor pollicis brevis
  - Extensor indicis
  - Abductor pollicis longus

Sensory branches

- Articular branches (from the radial nerve)
  - Capsule of the shoulder joint
- Articular branches (from the posterior interosseous nerve)
  - Joint capsule of the wrist and the four radial metacarpophalangeal joints
- Posterior brachial cutaneous nerve
- Inferior lateral brachial cutaneous nerve
- Posterior antebrachial cutaneous nerve
- Superficial branches
  - Dorsal digital nerves
  - Ulnar communicating branch

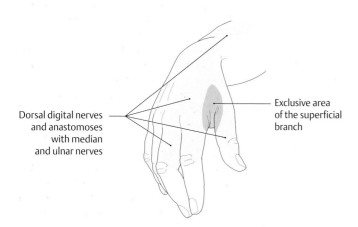

Dorsal digital nerves and anastomoses with median and ulnar nerves

Exclusive area of the superficial branch

C Wrist drop due to proximal and midlevel radial nerve lesions

When the radial nerve is damaged, the patient can no longer actively extend the hand at the wrist, and *wrist drop* (drop hand) is said to be present. Besides the dropped position of the wrist, clinical examination reveals areas of sensory loss on the radial surface of the dorsum and on the extensor surface of the thumb, index finger, and the radial half of the middle finger extending to the proximal interphalangeal joint. The sensory deficits are often confined to the area of the hand that receives sensory innervation exclusively from the radial nerve (the interosseous space between the thumb and index finger).

B Traumatic lesions and compression syndromes involving the radial nerve

The radial nerve may be damaged anywhere in its course as a result of injury or chronic compression. The clinical features depend critically on the *site of the lesion*. As a general rule, the more proximal the site of the lesion, the greater the number of extensor muscles that are affected. The characteristic feature of a proximal ("high") radial nerve lesion is *wrist drop* (see **C**), in which the patient in unable to extend the wrist or the metacarpophalangeal joints. Lesions at some sites may additionally cause sensory disturbances (pain, paresthesia, numbness), particularly in the exclusive sensory territory of the superficial branch on the radial side of the dorsum (first interosseous space between the thumb and index finger).

Proximal radial nerve lesion

- Chronic pressure in the axilla (e.g., due to prolonged crutch use). **Clinical features:** typical dropped wrist with loss of the triceps brachii (and sensory disturbances).
- Traumatic lesion due to a humeral shaft fracture at the level of the radial groove (spiral canal). **Clinical features:** usually a typical dropped wrist *without involvement of the triceps brachii,* since the muscular branches that supply the triceps brachii leave the radial nerve just before it enters the radial groove (sensory disturbances are present, however).
- Chronic compression of the radial nerve against the bony floor of the radial groove (e.g., during sleep or due to improper positioning of the patient during general anesthesia, exuberant callus formation after a fracture, or a tendon expansion from the lateral head of triceps brachii). "Park bench palsy" is a common form caused by draping the arm over the back of a park bench. **Clinical features:** dropped wrist *without involvement of the triceps brachii.* Sensory disturbances are present. The prognosis is usually favorable, and the palsy should resolve in a few days.

Midlevel radial nerve lesion

- Chronic compression of the radial nerve in its passage through the lateral intermuscular septum and in the radial tunnel (e.g., by bridging vessels and connective-tissue septa). **Clinical features:** dropped wrist with sensory disturbances.

Distal radial nerve lesion

- Compression of the deep branch of the radial nerve at its entry into the supinator canal by a sharp-edged tendon of the superficial part of the supinator muscle: supinator syndrome or distal radial nerve compression syndrome. **Clinical features:** no typical wrist drop and no sensory disturbances involving the hand (before entering the supinator canal, the deep branch gives off the purely sensory superficial branch and muscular branches for the supinator, brachioradialis, and extensor carpi radialis longus and brevis). There are palsies involving the extensor pollicis brevis and longus, abductor pollicis longus, extensor digitorum, extensor indicis, and extensor carpi ulnaris.
- Trauma to the deep radial nerve branch caused by a fracture or dislocation of the radius. **Clinical features:** no wrist drop and no sensory disturbances.

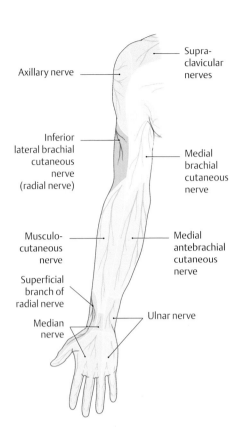

D Sensory distribution of the radial nerve
Anterior view.

Axillary nerve

Supra-clavicular nerves

Inferior lateral brachial cutaneous nerve (radial nerve)

Medial brachial cutaneous nerve

Musculo-cutaneous nerve

Medial antebrachial cutaneous nerve

Superficial branch of radial nerve

Median nerve

Ulnar nerve

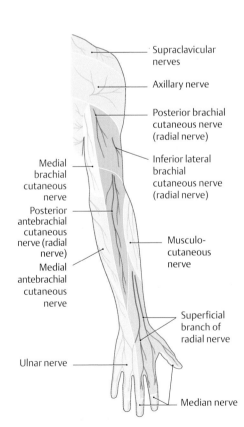

E Sensory distribution of the radial nerve
Posterior view.

Supraclavicular nerves

Axillary nerve

Posterior brachial cutaneous nerve (radial nerve)

Inferior lateral brachial cutaneous nerve (radial nerve)

Medial brachial cutaneous nerve

Posterior antebrachial cutaneous nerve (radial nerve)

Medial antebrachial cutaneous nerve

Musculo-cutaneous nerve

Superficial branch of radial nerve

Ulnar nerve

Median nerve

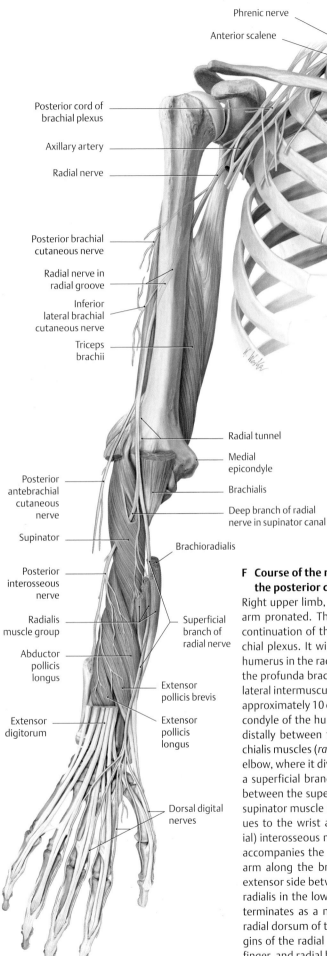

Phrenic nerve

Anterior scalene

Posterior cord of brachial plexus

Axillary artery

Radial nerve

Posterior brachial cutaneous nerve

Radial nerve in radial groove

Inferior lateral brachial cutaneous nerve

Triceps brachii

Radial tunnel

Medial epicondyle

Brachialis

Deep branch of radial nerve in supinator canal

Posterior antebrachial cutaneous nerve

Supinator

Brachioradialis

Posterior interosseous nerve

Radialis muscle group

Abductor pollicis longus

Superficial branch of radial nerve

Extensor pollicis brevis

Extensor digitorum

Extensor pollicis longus

Dorsal digital nerves

F Course of the radial nerve after leaving the posterior cord of the brachial plexus

Right upper limb, anterior view with the forearm pronated. The radial nerve is the direct continuation of the posterior cord of the brachial plexus. It winds around the back of the humerus in the radial groove, accompanied by the profunda brachii artery. After piercing the lateral intermuscular septum (not shown here) approximately 10 cm proximal to the radial epicondyle of the humerus, the radial nerve runs distally between the brachioradialis and brachialis muscles (*radial tunnel*, see p. 344) to the elbow, where it divides into a deep branch and a superficial branch. The deep branch passes between the superficial and deep parts of the supinator muscle (*supinator canal*) and continues to the wrist as the posterior (antebrachial) interosseous nerve. The superficial branch accompanies the radial artery down the forearm along the brachioradialis, passes to the extensor side between the radius and brachioradialis in the lower third of the forearm, and terminates as a main sensory branch on the radial dorsum of the hand and the dorsal margins of the radial 2½ digits (the thumb, index finger, and radial half of the middle finger).

4.9 Infraclavicular Part of the Brachial Plexus: The Ulnar Nerve

A The ulnar nerve (C 8 + T 1)

Motor branches

- Muscular branches (directly from the ulnar ½)
  - Flexor carpi ulnaris
  - Flexor digitorum profundus (ulnar ½)
- Muscular branch (from the superficial ulnar nerve branch)
  - Palmaris brevis
- Muscular branches (from the deep ulnar nerve branch)
  - Abductor digiti minimi
  - Flexor digiti minimi
  - Opponens digiti minimi
  - Third and fourth lumbricals
  - Palmar and dorsal interosseous muscles
  - Adductor pollicis
  - Flexor pollicis brevis (deep head)

Sensory branches

- Articular branches
  - Capsule of the elbow joint and of the carpal and metacarpophalangeal joints
- Dorsal branch of the ulnar nerve (terminal branches: dorsal digital nerves)
- Palmar branch of the ulnar nerve
- Proper palmar digital nerve (from the superficial branch)
- Common palmar digital nerve (from the superficial branch; terminal branches: proper palmar digital nerves)

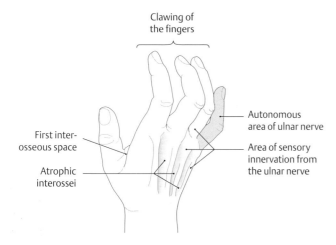

Clawing of the fingers

First interosseous space

Atrophic interossei

Autonomous area of ulnar nerve

Area of sensory innervation from the ulnar nerve

C Claw hand due to an ulnar nerve lesion

Besides the typical clawlike appearance of the hand, atrophy of the interossei leads to hollowing of the interosseous spaces in the metacarpus. Sensory abnormalities are frequently confined to the little finger (exclusive sensory territory of the ulnar nerve).

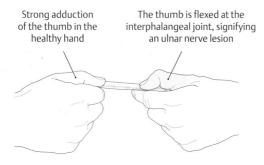

Strong adduction of the thumb in the healthy hand

The thumb is flexed at the interphalangeal joint, signifying an ulnar nerve lesion

B Traumatic lesions and compression syndromes involving the ulnar nerve

Ulnar nerve palsy is the *most common peripheral nerve paralysis*. The characteristic feature of an ulnar nerve lesion is a "*claw hand*" deformity (see **C**), in which *loss of the interosseous muscles* causes the fingers to be hyperextended at the metacarpophalangeal joints and slightly flexed at the proximal and distal interphalangeal joints. The deformity is least pronounced in the index and middle fingers because the first and second lumbrical muscles, which are innervated by the median nerve, can partially compensate for the clawing of those fingers. The thumb is markedly hyperextended due to the loss of adductor pollicis and the dominance of extensor pollicis longus and abductor pollicis. The interossei muscles become atrophic in 2–3 months; this is most conspicuous in the first interosseous space and is accompanied by hypothenar atrophy. Sensory disturbances affect the ulnar portion of the hand, the ulnar half of the ring finger, and the entire little finger.

Proximal ulnar nerve lesion

- Traumatic lesions, usually occurring at the elbow joint due to the exposed position of the nerve in the ulnar groove (e.g., pressure from resting on the arm), displacement of the nerve from its groove, or articular injuries due to fractures.
- Chronic pressure on the nerve in the ulnar groove due to degenerative or inflammatory changes in the elbow joint, or chronic traction on the nerve caused by repetitive flexion and extension at the elbow joint (sulcus ulnaris syndrome).
- Possible compression between the tendons of origin of flexor carpi ulnaris (cubital tunnel syndrome).
  Clinical features: claw hand and sensory disturbances.

Midlevel ulnar nerve lesion

- Traumatic lesions at the wrist (e.g., lacerations).
- Chronic compression of the nerve in the ulnar tunnel, a fibro-osseous canal between the palmar carpal ligament, pisiform bone, and flexor retinaculum (ulnar tunnel syndrome, see p. 357).
  Clinical features: claw hand and sensory disturbances that spare the hypothenar region (palmar branch is intact).

Distal ulnar nerve lesion

- Compression of the deep branch of the ulnar nerve in the palm due to chronic pressure (e.g., from an air hammer or other tools).
  Clinical features: claw hand with no sensory disturbances (superficial branch is intact).

D Positive "Froment sign" in the left hand

A positive Froment sign indicates palsy of the adductor pollicis muscle. When the patient is told to hold a piece of paper firmly between the thumb and index finger, he or she must use the flexor pollicis longus, which is innervated by the *median nerve*, rather than the paralyzed adductor pollicis, which is innervated by the *ulnar nerve*. Flexing the thumb at the interphalangeal joint signifies a positive test.

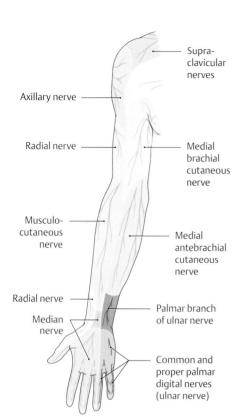

Supra-
clavicular
nerves

Axillary nerve

Radial nerve

Medial
brachial
cutaneous
nerve

Musculo-
cutaneous
nerve

Medial
antebrachial
cutaneous
nerve

Radial nerve

Palmar branch
of ulnar nerve

Median
nerve

Common and
proper palmar
digital nerves
(ulnar nerve)

E Sensory distribution of the ulnar nerve
Anterior view.

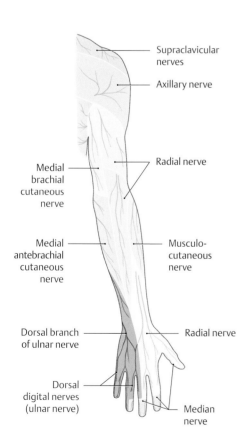

Supraclavicular
nerves

Axillary nerve

Medial
brachial
cutaneous
nerve

Radial nerve

Medial
antebrachial
cutaneous
nerve

Musculo-
cutaneous
nerve

Dorsal branch
of ulnar nerve

Radial nerve

Dorsal
digital nerves
(ulnar nerve)

Median
nerve

F Sensory distribution of the ulnar nerve
Posterior view.

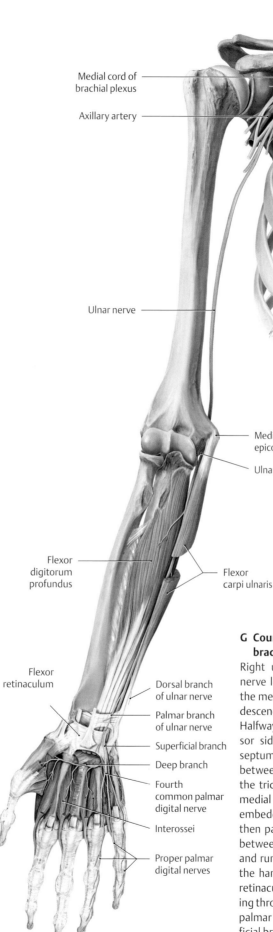

Medial cord of
brachial plexus

Axillary artery

Ulnar nerve

Medial
epicondyle

Ulnar groove

Flexor
digitorum
profundus

Flexor
carpi ulnaris

Flexor
retinaculum

Dorsal branch
of ulnar nerve

Palmar branch
of ulnar nerve

Superficial branch

Deep branch

Fourth
common palmar
digital nerve

Interossei

Proper palmar
digital nerves

**G Course of the ulnar nerve from the
brachial plexus**

Right upper limb, anterior view. The ulnar
nerve leaves the axilla as the continuation of
the medial cord of the brachial plexus, initially
descending in the medial bicipital groove.
Halfway down the arm it crosses to the extensor side, piercing the medial intermuscular
septum (see p. 338). It reaches the elbow joint
between the septum and the medial head of
the triceps and crosses over the joint on the
medial side below the medial epicondyle,
embedded in the bony ulnar groove. The nerve
then passes to the flexor side of the forearm
between the two heads of flexor carpi ulnaris
and runs beneath that muscle to the wrist. In
the hand, the ulnar nerve runs on the flexor
retinaculum radial to the pisiform bone, passing through the ulnar tunnel (see p. 357) to the
palmar surface, where it divides into a superficial branch and a deep motor branch.

325

4.10 Infraclavicular Part of the Brachial Plexus: The Median Nerve

A The median nerve (C 6–T 1)

Motor branches

- Muscular branches (directly from the median nerve)
  - Pronator teres
  - Flexor carpi radialis
  - Palmaris longus
  - Flexor digitorum superficialis
- Muscular branches (from the anterior antebrachial interosseous nerve)
  - Pronator quadratus
  - Flexor pollicis longus
  - Flexor digitorum profundus (radial ½)
- Thenar muscular branch ("thenar branch")
  - Abductor pollicis brevis
  - Flexor pollicis brevis (superficial head)
  - Opponens pollicis
- Muscular branches (from the common palmar digital nerves)
  - First and second lumbricals

Sensory branches

- Articular branches
  - Capsules of the elbow joint and wrist joints
- Palmar branch of median nerve (thenar eminence)
- Communicating branch to ulnar nerve
- Common palmar digital nerves
- Proper palmar digital nerves (fingers)

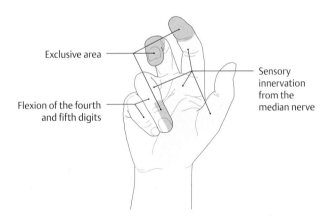

Exclusive area

Flexion of the fourth and fifth digits

Sensory innervation from the median nerve

C "Hand of benediction" following a proximal median nerve lesion

When patients try to make a fist, they can flex only the ulnar fingers. This is the "hand of benediction" deformity. There may be associated sensory disturbances, particularly in the autonomous area of the nerve (tips of the radial 3½ digits).

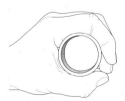

In a healthy hand, the thumb can be abducted to fully grasp a cylindrical object

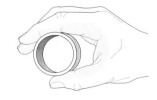

With a proximal median nerve lesion, the thumb cannot be fully abducted

B Traumatic lesions and compression syndromes involving the median nerve

Median nerve lesions in the arm caused by an acute injury or chronic pressure are among the most common peripheral nerve lesions. The clinical manifestations depend on the *site of the lesion*. The two main categories are proximal and distal nerve lesions, as illustrated by the *pronator teres syndrome* and the *carpal tunnel syndrome*. The hallmark of a proximal median nerve lesion is the "*hand of benediction*," which occurs when the patient tries to clench the hand into a fist (loss of the long digital flexors except for the part of flexor digitorum profundus supplied by the ulnar nerve). This contrasts with distal median nerve lesions, which present selectively with thenar atrophy and sensory disturbances, as in carpal tunnel syndrome.

Proximal median nerve lesion

- Traumatic injury caused by a fracture or dislocation of the elbow joint.
- Chronic pressure injury from an anomalous supracondylar process connected to the medial epicondyle by a ligament ("Struther's ligament," see p. 345), pressure from a tight bicipital aponeurosis, or a *pronator teres syndrome* in which the nerve is squeezed between the two heads of pronator teres.
  Clinical features: Typical "hand of benediction" when fist closure is attempted, with incomplete pronation, loss of thumb opposition, impaired grasping ability, atrophy of the thenar muscles, and sensory disturbances affecting the radial part of the palm and radial 3½ digits (also autonomic trophic disturbances such as decreased sweat secretion and increased cutaneous blood flow). The patient also has a positive "*bottle sign*" in which the fingers and thumb cannot fully close around a cylindrical object due to weakness of the abductor pollicis brevis.

Distal median nerve lesion

- The superficial location of the nerve in the distal forearm makes it vulnerable to cuts and lacerations (e.g., in attempted suicide).
- Chronic compression of the median nerve in the carpal tunnel (most common compression syndrome affecting the median nerve: carpal tunnel syndrome). Compression or entrapment of the nerve within the carpal tunnel can have various causes such as fractures and dislocations of the carpal bones, inflammatory changes in the tendon sheaths, muscle variants (e.g., lumbricals passing through the carpal tunnel), and connective tissue proliferation due to endocrine hormonal changes (diabetes mellitus, pregnancy, menopause).
  Clinical features: Oath hand is not present. Initial signs consist of sensory disturbances (paresthesias and dysasthesias), chiefly affecting the tips of the index and middle fingers and thumb due to increased carpal tunnel pressure resulting from prolonged flexion or extension of the wrist during sleep ("brachialgia paraesthetica nocturna"). Chronic or severe damage leads to motor deficits involving the thenar muscles (thenar atrophy) with preservation of thenar sensation (intact palmar branch of the median nerve) and a positive bottle sign (see **D**).

D Positive "bottle sign" in the right hand

When proximal and distal median nerve lesions are present, the thumb and fingers cannot completely encircle a cylindrical vessel with the affected hand due to weakness or loss of the abductor pollicis brevis.

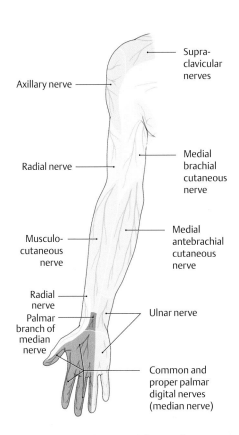

E Sensory distribution of the median nerve.
Anterior view.

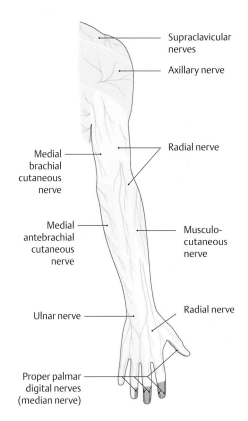

F Sensory distribution of the median nerve
Posterior view.

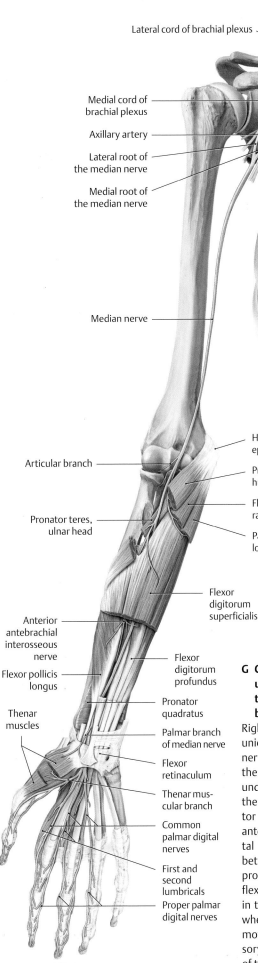

G Course of the median nerve after the union of its medial and lateral roots from the medial and lateral cords of the brachial plexus

Right upper limb, anterior view. Distal to the union of its brachial plexus roots, the median nerve runs in the medial bicipital groove above the brachial artery to the elbow and passes under the bicipital aponeurosis and between the two heads (humeral and ulnar) of pronator teres to the forearm. After giving off the anterior antebrachial interosseous nerve distal to pronator teres, the median nerve runs between the flexor digitorum superficialis and profundus to the wrist and passes beneath the flexor retinaculum (transverse carpal ligament) in the carpal tunnel to the palm of the hand, where it divides into its terminal branches (a motor branch for the thenar muscles and sensory branches for the skin on the palmar side of the radial 3½ digits).

327

5.1 Surface Anatomy and Superficial Nerves and Vessels: Anterior View

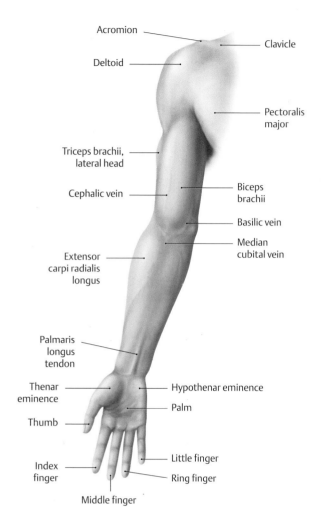

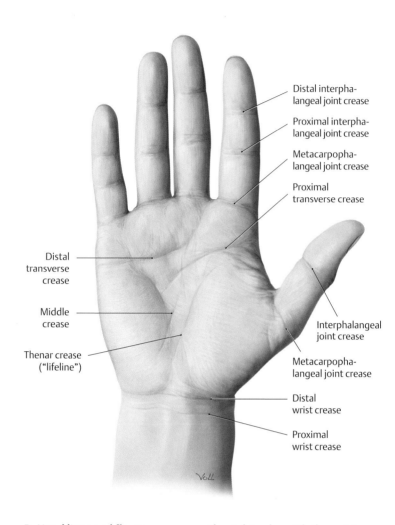

A Surface anatomy of the right upper limb
Anterior view. The palpable bony landmarks of the upper limb are reviewed on p. 209.

B Hand lines and flexion creases on the right palm with the wrist in slight flexion (after Schmidt and Lanz)
The *proximal wrist crease*, located approximately one fingerwidth from the palm, coincides with the distal epiphyseal lines of the radius and ulna. The *distal wrist crease* usually overlies the midcarpal joint.

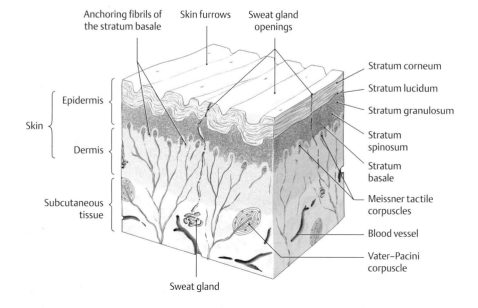

C Schematic structure of the ridged skin on the palm of the hand
The smooth, thin skin of the forearm gives way to the thicker, ridged skin on the palm of the hand. The papillary ridges are particularly high on the palmar skin of the fingers and, at 0.1–0.4 mm, are distinctly visible. The ridge pattern (dermatoglyphs) found on the bulbs of the fingers is unique for each individual. The tactile sensitivity of the fingertips is closely linked to the spatial distribution of tactile corpuscles and free nerve endings (e.g., 75–80 Vater–Pacini corpuscles per finger and approximately 100 free nerve endings per square millimeter).

328

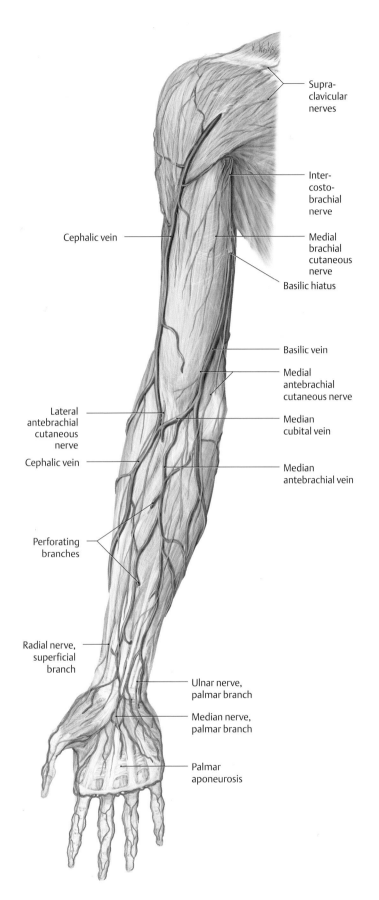

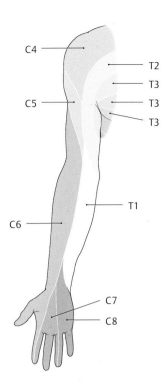

E Segmental, radicular cutaneous innervation pattern (dermatomes) in the right upper limb

Anterior view. With the outgrowth of the upper limb during development, the sensory cutaneous segments become elongated in varying degrees to form narrow bands. In the process, segments C 5–C 7 become separated from the body wall.

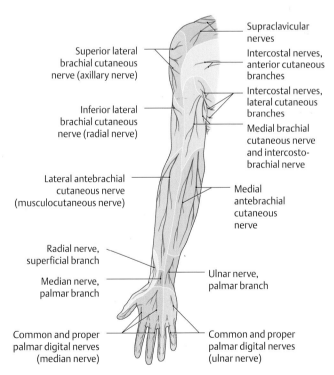

D Superficial cutaneous veins (subcutaneous veins) and cutaneous nerves of the right upper limb

Anterior view. The arrangement of cutaneous veins about the elbow can vary considerably (see p. 310). This dissection does not show the cutaneous arteries that perforate the antebrachial fascia (particularly those arising from the radial artery, see also p. 309).

F Pattern of peripheral sensory cutaneous innervation in the right upper limb

Anterior view. The territories supplied by the peripheral cutaneous nerves (cutaneous branches) correspond to the areas of cutaneous nerve branching in the subcutaneous connective tissue that are demonstrable by dissection. The area served exclusively by a single nerve and thus rendered completely anesthetic by a lesion is much smaller, because the individual sensory territories overlap extensively. *Note:* The sensory loss following damage to a *peripheral nerve* shows a completely different pattern to that of a damaged *nerve root*.

5.2 Surface Anatomy and Superficial Nerves and Vessels: Posterior View

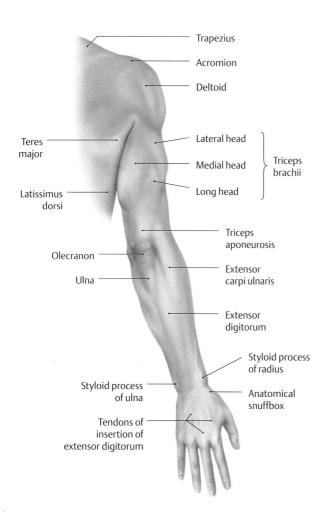

Trapezius

Acromion

Deltoid

Teres major

Lateral head

Medial head — Triceps brachii

Long head

Latissimus dorsi

Triceps aponeurosis

Olecranon

Extensor carpi ulnaris

Ulna

Extensor digitorum

Styloid process of radius

Styloid process of ulna

Anatomical snuffbox

Tendons of insertion of extensor digitorum

Extensor pollicis longus

Anatomical snuffbox

Distal extension crease

Proximal extension crease

Extensor digitorum, tendons of insertion

Styloid process of ulna

Extensor retinaculum

A Surface anatomy of the right upper limb
Posterior view. The palpable bony landmarks of the upper limb are reviewed on p. 209.

B Extension creases on the dorsum of the right hand (after Schmidt and Lanz)
In contrast to the palm, the dorsal surfaces of the hand and fingers bear indistinct extension creases that deepen with maximum dorsiflexion of the hand. The most proximal crease overlies the styloid process of the ulna, while the most distal crease approximately overlies the distal margin of the extensor retinaculum. Unlike the hairless ridged skin of the palm, the dorsum of the hand is covered by smooth, thin, hair-bearing skin.

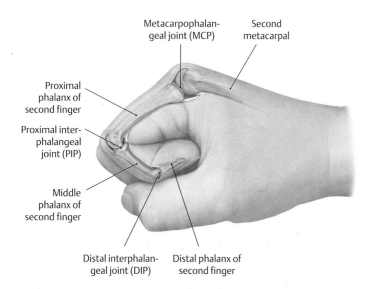

Metacarpophalangeal joint (MCP)

Second metacarpal

Proximal phalanx of second finger

Proximal interphalangeal joint (PIP)

Middle phalanx of second finger

Distal interphalangeal joint (DIP)

Distal phalanx of second finger

C Location of the MCP, PIP, and DIP joint spaces
Right hand closed into a fist, radial view.

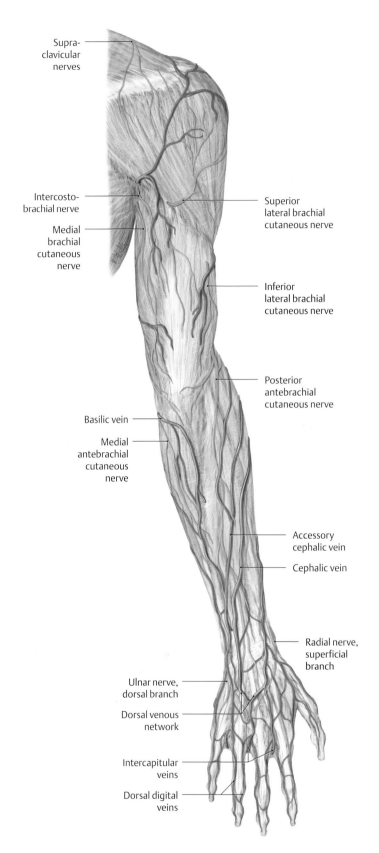

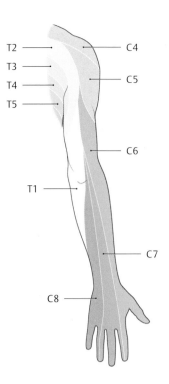

E Segmental, radicular cutaneous innervation pattern (dermatomes) in the right upper limb

Posterior view. With the outgrowth of the limb during development, the sensory cutaneous segments become elongated in varying degrees to form narrow bands. As this occurs, segments C 5–C 7 become separated from the body wall.

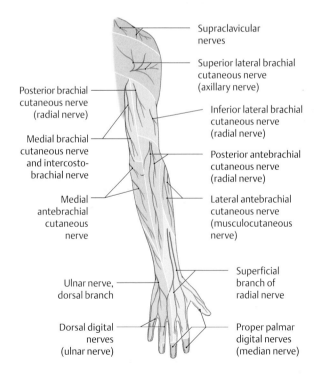

D Superficial cutaneous veins (subcutaneous veins) and cutaneous nerves of the right upper limb

Posterior view. The epifascial veins of the dorsum of the hand (dorsal venous network) display a highly variable branching pattern. Generally the epifascial veins are clearly visible beneath the skin, receiving tributaries that include perforating veins from the palmar side of the hand. The cephalic vein on the radial side of the hand provides for most of the dorsal venous drainage, while the basilic vein provides for a lesser degree on the ulnar side. This dissection does not show the main branches of the posterior interosseous artery that perforate the antebrachial fascia on the back of the forearm (see also p. 309).

F Peripheral sensory cutaneous innervation topography pattern in the right upper limb

Posterior view. The color-coded areas that are supplied by the peripheral cutaneous nerves (cutaneous branches) correspond to the areas of cutaneous nerve branching in the subcutaneous connective tissue that are demonstrable by dissection. The areas of exclusive non-overlapping innervation of a specific nerve is much smaller.

Note that the sensory loss following damage to a *peripheral nerve* shows a completely different pattern from that caused by damage to a *nerve root* (see **E**).

5.3 The Shoulder Region: Anterior View

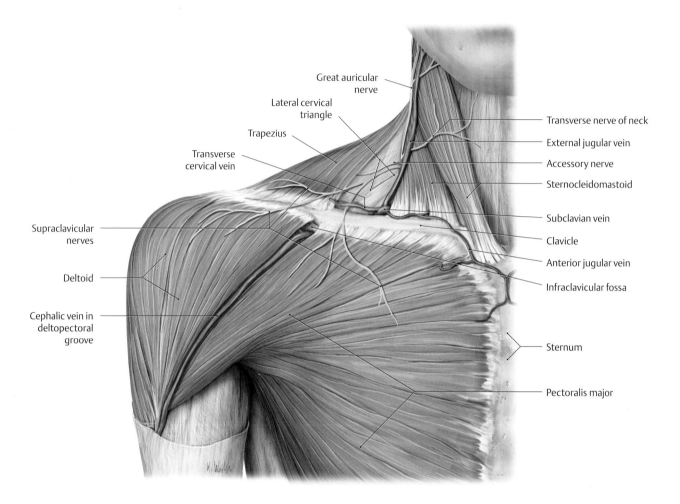

A Superficial veins and nerves of the right shoulder and neck region

Anterior view. The skin, platysma, muscle fasciae, and superficial layer of the cervical fascia have been removed in this dissection to demonstrate the branches of the cervical plexus (e.g., the great auricular nerve) and the superficial veins of the lateral and anterior neck. The *external jugular vein* and *anterior jugular vein* are visible through the skin when the patient is lying supine and the veins are well filled. When *right-sided heart failure* is present, these veins may be engorged due to the damming back of venous blood and may be visible even when the patient is sitting upright. The *cephalic vein* crosses the shoulder in the groove between the pectoralis major and deltoid muscles (*deltopectoral groove*) and empties into the subclavian vein. This site of entry into the subclavian vein, and thus into the deep veins, is visible and palpable on the skin as the infraclavicular fossa.

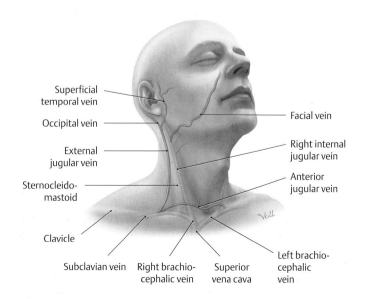

B Relationship of major superficial and deep veins in the neck to the sternocleidomastoid muscle

Anterior view. The internal jugular vein runs almost straight downward from the jugular foramen and unites with the subclavian vein just lateral to the sternoclavicular joint to form the brachiocephalic vein. When its course is projected onto the side of the neck, it follows a line drawn from the earlobe to the medial end of the clavicle. The *internal* jugular vein is crossed obliquely in its lower third by the sternocleidomastoid muscle, while the *external* jugular vein runs obliquely downward on the muscle and opens into the subclavian vein.

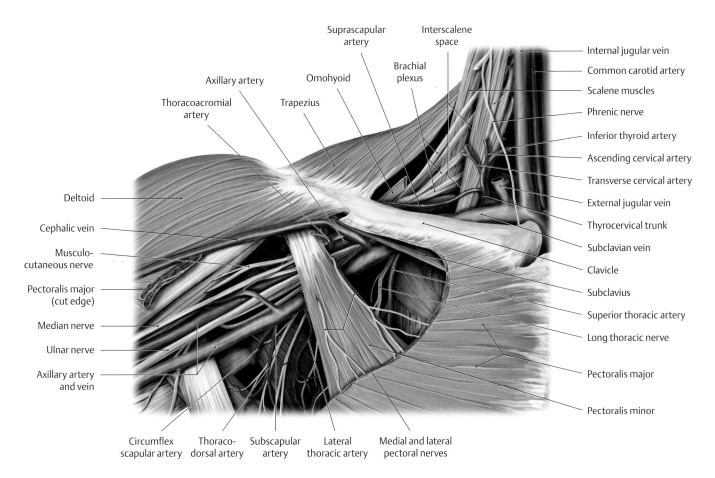

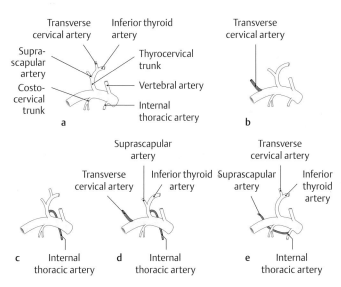

C Course of the right subclavian artery in the lateral neck region

Anterior view. The sternocleidomastoid and omohyoid muscles and all layers of the cervical fasciae have been removed to demonstrate the deep lateral cervical triangle and the passage of the subclavian artery and brachial plexus through the interval between the anterior and middle scalene muscles (interscalene space). At the level of the first rib the subclavian artery becomes the axillary artery, which enters the axilla below the tendon of insertion of pectoralis minor.

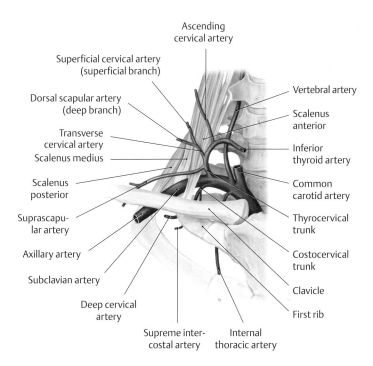

D Origin and branches of the right subclavian artery

Anterior view.

E Branches of the subclavian artery: normal anatomy and variants
(after Lippert and Pabst)

a Normally (30%) the subclavian artery gives off the following branches:
- Thyrocervical trunk with the inferior thyroid artery, suprascapular artery, and transverse cervical artery
- Vertebral artery
- Internal thoracic artery
- Costocervical trunk

b–e Variants:

b The transverse cervical artery arises separately from the subclavian artery (30%).

c The internal thoracic artery arises from the thyrocervical trunk (10%).

d The thyrocervical trunk is made up of the inferior thyroid artery, suprascapular artery, and internal thoracic artery (8%).

e The subclavian artery gives off two main branches:
1. One with the inferior thyroid and transverse cervical arteries.
2. One with the internal thoracic and suprascapular artieries (4%).

333

5.4 The Axilla: Anterior Wall

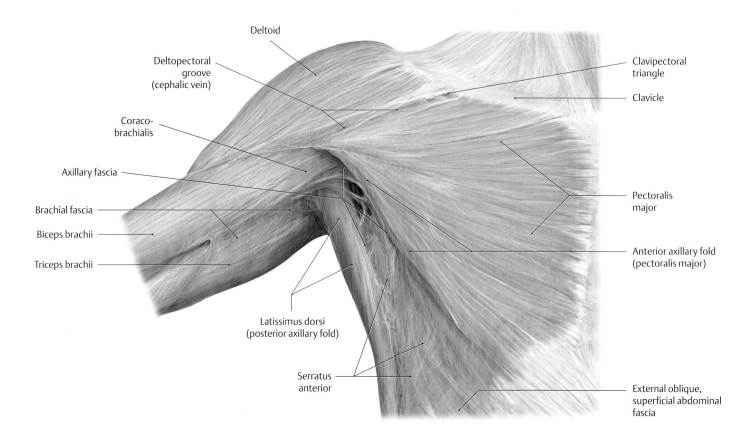

A The walls and fasciae of the right axilla

Anterior view. With the arm abducted, the axilla (axillary fossa) resembles a four-sided pyramid whose apex is approximately at the center of the clavicle and whose base is represented by the axillary *fascia*. The walls of the axilla are formed by various muscles and their fasciae:

Anterior wall: The anterior wall of the axilla consists of the pectoralis major and minor and the clavipectoral fascia (the pectoralis minor is not shown here; see **C** and **D**).

Posterior wall: This consists of the subscapularis, teres major (not shown here, see p. 266), and latissimus dorsi.

Lateral wall: This is narrow and formed by the intertubercular groove of the humerus.

Medial wall: This is formed by the lateral thoracic wall (ribs 1–4 and associated intercostal muscles) and the serratus anterior.

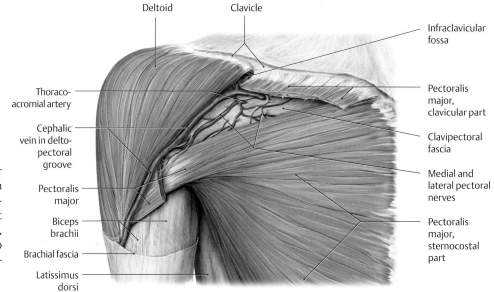

B The clavipectoral triangle and clavipectoral fascia

Right shoulder, anterior view. The clavicular part of pectoralis major has been removed. In the clavipectoral triangle bounded by the deltoid, pectoralis major, and clavicle, the cephalic vein runs upward in the deltopectoral groove, pierces the clavipectoral fascia, and drains into the subclavian vein at the level of the infraclavicular fossa.

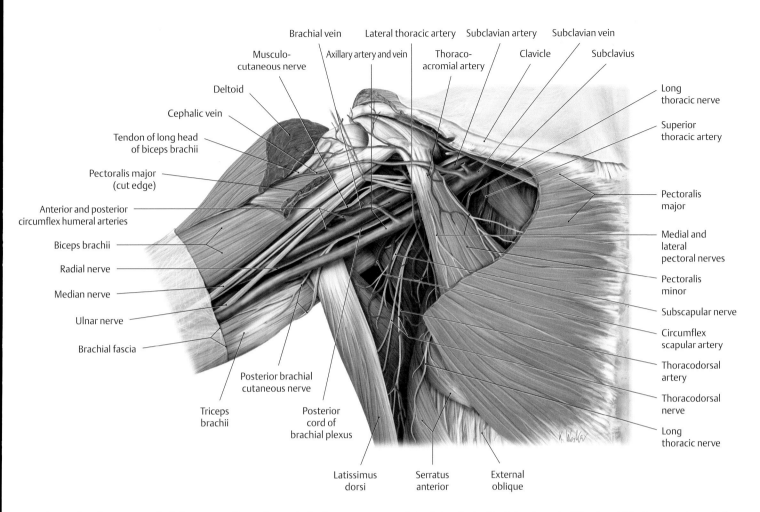

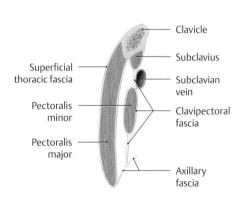

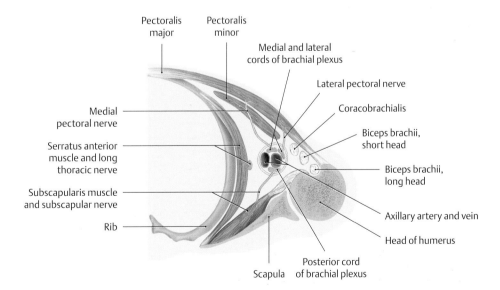

C The axilla after removal of the pectoralis major and clavipectoral fascia

Right shoulder, anterior view. The axillary artery runs approximately 2 cm below the coracoid process and behind the pectoralis minor. It relates laterally to the lateral cord of the brachial plexus and medially to the medial cord (both are retracted slightly upward in the drawing). The posterior cord of the brachial plexus, which runs behind the axillary artery, is just visible.

D Location of the superficial and deep thoracic fasciae

Sagittal section through the anterior wall of the right axilla. The clavipectoral fascia, known also as the "deep" thoracic fascia, encloses the pectoralis minor and subclavius muscles and covers the subclavian vein while being fused to its wall. The fascia is made tense by the pectoralis minor. The clavipectoral fascia exerts traction on the vein wall that can keep its lumen patent, thus facilitating venous return to the superior vena cava.

E Schematic transverse section through the right axilla

Superior view. The three muscular walls and the bony lateral wall of the axilla are clearly delineated in this view. Neurovascular structures (axillary artery and vein plus the medial, lateral, and posterior cords of the brachial plexus) traverse the axilla, invested by a fibrous sheath and embedded in the axillary fat.

5.5 The Axilla: Posterior Wall

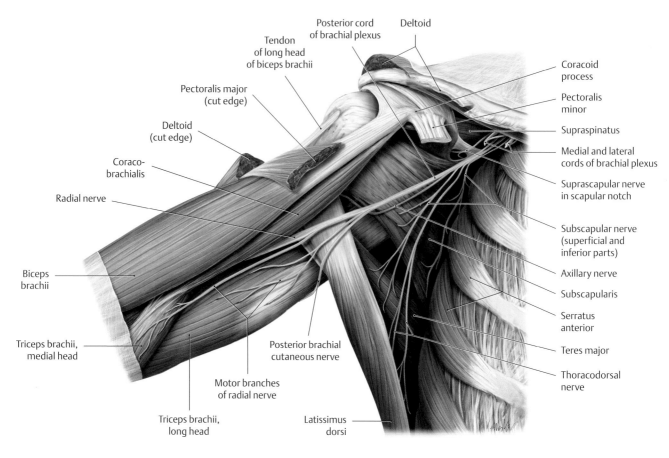

A Posterior wall of the axilla with the posterior cord and its branches

Right shoulder, anterior view. The medial and lateral cords of the brachial plexus and the axillary vessels have been removed to demonstrate the course of the *posterior* cord and its branches in the posterior axilla.

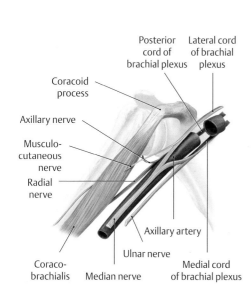

B Relationship of the medial, lateral, and posterior cords of the brachial plexus to the axillary artery

Note that the musculocutaneous nerve passes through the coracobrachialis, which aids in locating the nerve. Very rarely, this nerve may be compressed as it pierces the muscle.

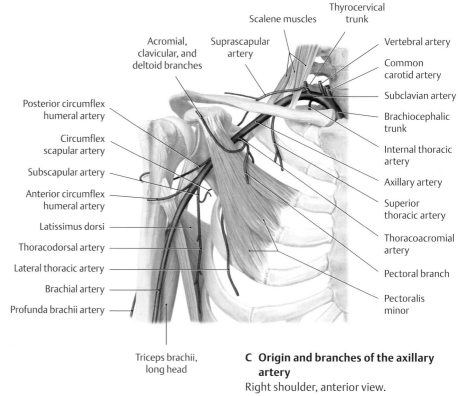

C Origin and branches of the axillary artery

Right shoulder, anterior view.

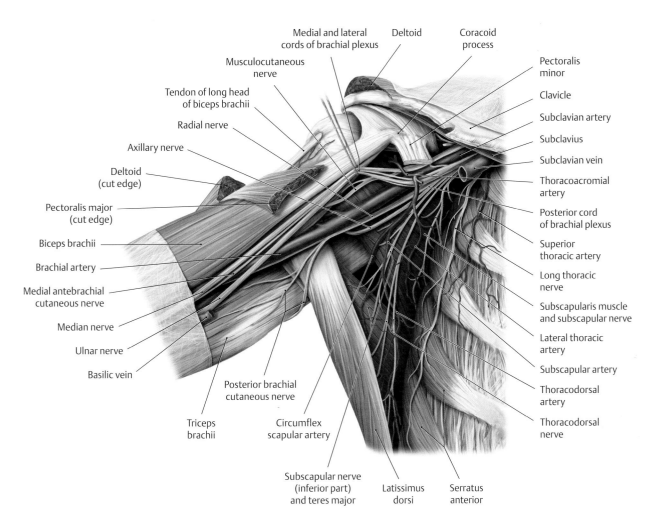

D Axilla with the entire anterior wall removed
Right shoulder, anterior view. The axillary vein has been removed and the medial and lateral cords of the brachial plexus have been retracted upward to show more clearly the location and course of the posterior cord and its terminal branches, the radial nerve and axillary nerve.

Note the superficial course of the long thoracic nerve on the serratus anterior.

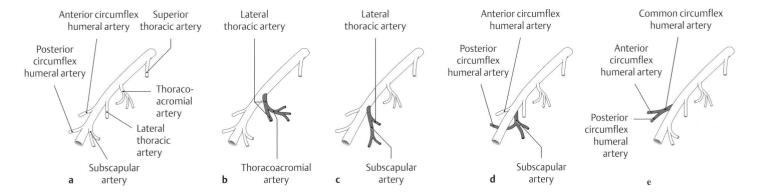

E Branches of the axillary artery: normal anatomy and variants
(after Lippert and Pabst)

a Normally (40 % of cases) the subclavian artery gives off the following branches:
Superior thoracic artery, thoracoacromial artery, lateral thoracic artery, subscapular artery, anterior circumflex humeral artery, and posterior circumflex humeral artery.

b–e Variants:
b The thoracoacromial artery arises from the lateral thoracic artery (10 % of cases).

c Common origin of the lateral thoracic artery and suprascapular artery (10 % of cases).

d The posterior circumflex humeral artery arises from the subscapular artery (20 % of cases).

e Common origin of the anterior and posterior circumflex humeral arteries (20 % of cases). The common segment formed by both arteries is termed the common circumflex humeral artery.

5.6 The Anterior Brachial Region

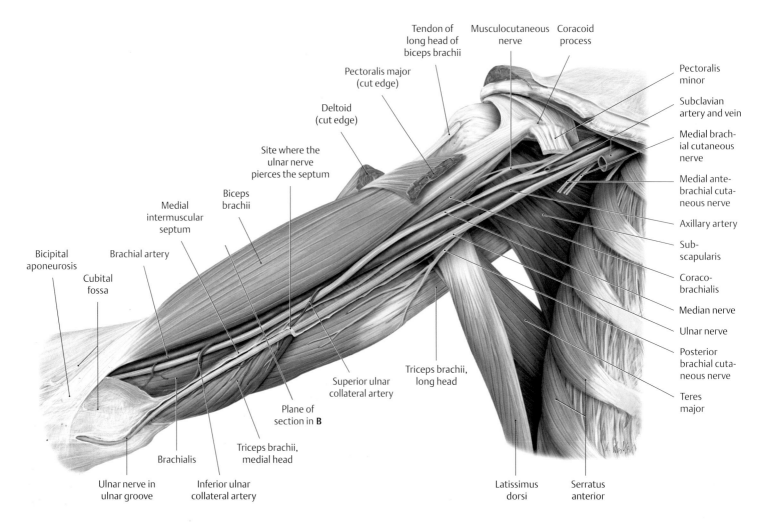

Tendon of long head of biceps brachii

Musculocutaneous nerve

Coracoid process

Pectoralis major (cut edge)

Pectoralis minor

Deltoid (cut edge)

Subclavian artery and vein

Site where the ulnar nerve pierces the septum

Medial brachial cutaneous nerve

Biceps brachii

Medial antebrachial cutaneous nerve

Medial intermuscular septum

Axillary artery

Brachial artery

Subscapularis

Bicipital aponeurosis

Cubital fossa

Coracobrachialis

Median nerve

Ulnar nerve

Posterior brachial cutaneous nerve

Triceps brachii, long head

Teres major

Superior ulnar collateral artery

Plane of section in **B**

Brachialis

Triceps brachii, medial head

Ulnar nerve in ulnar groove

Inferior ulnar collateral artery

Latissimus dorsi

Serratus anterior

A Main neurovascular tract of the arm: the medial bicipital groove
The right arm has been abducted and slightly rotated externally and is viewed from the anterior view. The deltoid, pectoralis major, and pectoralis minor muscles have been removed. The medial bicipital groove is a subcutaneous longitudinal groove on the medial side of the arm that is bounded deeply by the biceps brachii and brachialis muscles and the medial intermuscular septum of the arm. It marks the location of the main neurovascular tract of the arm extending from the axilla to the cubital fossa. The *most superficial* structure of the tract is the *medial antebrachial cutaneous nerve*, which leaves the medial bicipital groove at the basilic hiatus in company with the basilic vein (see p. 329). The *most medial* structure is the *ulnar nerve*, which initially courses on the medial intermuscular septum. In the lower third of the arm, the ulnar nerve pierces the intermuscular septum and passes to the back of the septum, entering the ulnar groove on the medial epicondyle of the humerus. The *deep part of the medial bicipital groove* transmits the principal artery of the arm, the *brachial artery*, which extends from the axilla to the elbow accompanied by the *median nerve*.

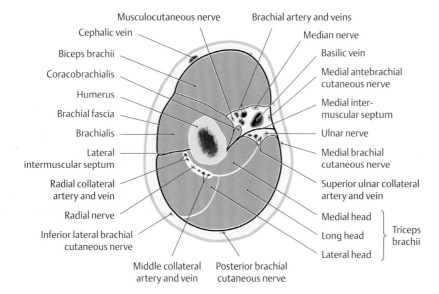

Musculocutaneous nerve

Brachial artery and veins

Cephalic vein

Median nerve

Biceps brachii

Basilic vein

Coracobrachialis

Medial antebrachial cutaneous nerve

Humerus

Medial intermuscular septum

Brachial fascia

Brachialis

Ulnar nerve

Lateral intermuscular septum

Medial brachial cutaneous nerve

Radial collateral artery and vein

Superior ulnar collateral artery and vein

Radial nerve

Medial head

Inferior lateral brachial cutaneous nerve

Long head

Triceps brachii

Lateral head

Middle collateral artery and vein

Posterior brachial cutaneous nerve

B Cross section through the middle third of the right arm
Note for orientation that the basilic hiatus (where the basilic vein perforates the deep fascia medial to the biceps) is distal to (below) the level of this section. Thus the basilic vein and medial antebrachial cutaneous nerve are subfascial. The ulnar nerve and ulnar collateral artery have left the medial bicipital groove and have pierced the medial intermuscular septum, and thus lie posterior to it, in this section. Proximal to (above) this level, the profunda brachii artery has split into its two terminal branches, the radial collateral and middle collateral arteries, which are seen here posterior to the humerus.

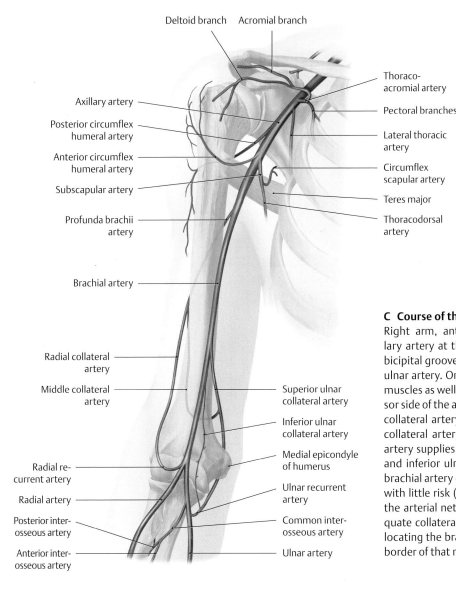

Deltoid branch   Acromial branch

Axillary artery

Posterior circumflex humeral artery

Anterior circumflex humeral artery

Subscapular artery

Profunda brachii artery

Brachial artery

Radial collateral artery

Middle collateral artery

Radial recurrent artery

Radial artery

Posterior interosseous artery

Anterior interosseous artery

Thoraco-acromial artery

Pectoral branches

Lateral thoracic artery

Circumflex scapular artery

Teres major

Thoracodorsal artery

Superior ulnar collateral artery

Inferior ulnar collateral artery

Medial epicondyle of humerus

Ulnar recurrent artery

Common interosseous artery

Ulnar artery

C Course of the brachial artery in the arm

Right arm, anterior view. The brachial artery arises from the axillary artery at the level of the teres major and descends in the medial bicipital groove to the elbow. There it divides into the radial artery and ulnar artery. On its way down the arm, it gives off branches to the arm muscles as well as the profunda brachii artery, which runs on the extensor side of the arm and divides distal to the radial groove into the middle collateral artery (to the medial head of triceps brachii) and the radial collateral artery (to the arterial network of the elbow). The brachial artery supplies the arterial network of the elbow through the superior and inferior ulnar collateral arteries. It is significant clinically that the brachial artery can be ligated distal to the origin of the profunda brachii with little risk (e.g., to control heavy posttraumatic bleeding) because the arterial network of the elbow (see **C**, p. 345) can establish an adequate collateral circulation. The biceps brachii is a useful landmark for locating the brachial artery, whose pulse is palpable all along the ulnar border of that muscle.

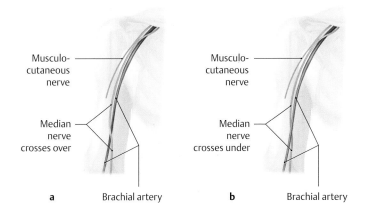

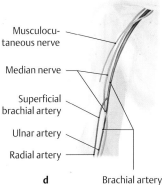

Musculocutaneous nerve

Median nerve crosses over

a   Brachial artery

Musculocutaneous nerve

Median nerve crosses under

b   Brachial artery

High division of the vessel

Musculocutaneous nerve

Superficial brachial artery

Median nerve

Ulnar artery

Radial artery

c   Brachial artery

Musculocutaneous nerve

Median nerve

Superficial brachial artery

Ulnar artery

Radial artery

d   Brachial artery

D Course of the brachial artery in the arm:
normal anatomy and variants (after von Lanz and Wachsmuth)
Right shoulder, anterior view.

a   Usually (74% of cases) the median nerve *crosses over* the brachial artery in the lower third of the arm.

b–d   Variants:

b   The median nerve *crosses under* the brachial artery (very rare, 1% of cases).

c, d   The brachial artery divides into a *superficial* brachial artery and a brachial artery while still in the arm ("high division" pattern, 25% of cases). Both of these arteries may be well developed and may flank the union of the median nerve roots and the median nerve itself. In this case the radial artery arises from the superficial brachial artery ("high origin of the radial artery") while the ulnar artery is the continuation of the brachial artery (see p. 347).

5.7 The Shoulder Region: Posterior and Superior Views

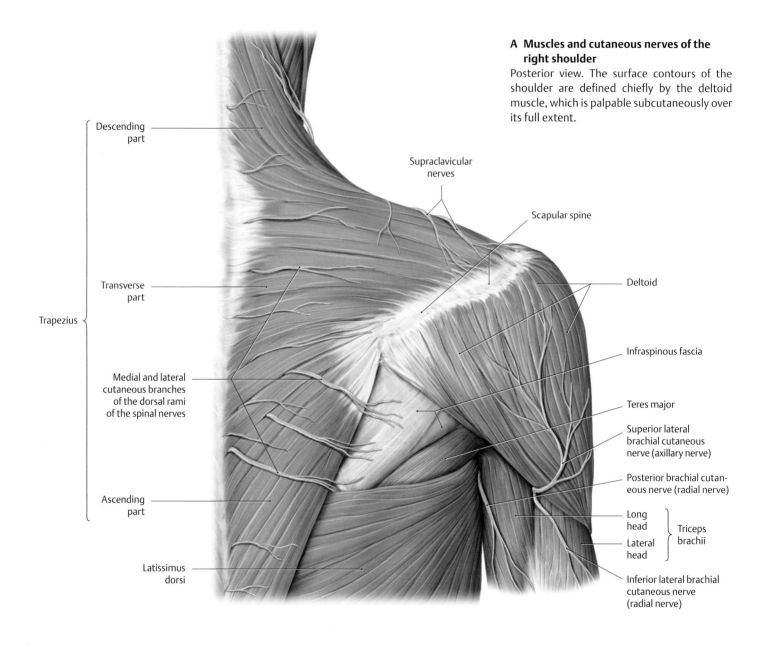

A Muscles and cutaneous nerves of the right shoulder

Posterior view. The surface contours of the shoulder are defined chiefly by the deltoid muscle, which is palpable subcutaneously over its full extent.

Labels (clockwise):
- Descending part
- Transverse part
- Trapezius
- Medial and lateral cutaneous branches of the dorsal rami of the spinal nerves
- Ascending part
- Latissimus dorsi
- Supraclavicular nerves
- Scapular spine
- Deltoid
- Infraspinous fascia
- Teres major
- Superior lateral brachial cutaneous nerve (axillary nerve)
- Posterior brachial cutaneous nerve (radial nerve)
- Long head / Lateral head } Triceps brachii
- Inferior lateral brachial cutaneous nerve (radial nerve)

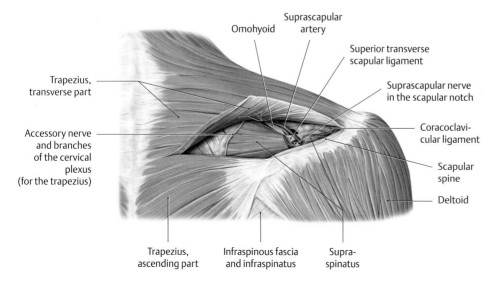

Labels:
- Trapezius, transverse part
- Accessory nerve and branches of the cervical plexus (for the trapezius)
- Omohyoid
- Suprascapular artery
- Superior transverse scapular ligament
- Suprascapular nerve in the scapular notch
- Coracoclavicular ligament
- Scapular spine
- Deltoid
- Trapezius, ascending part
- Infraspinous fascia and infraspinatus
- Supraspinatus

B Suprascapular region of the right shoulder from the posterior view

A flap from the transverse part of the trapezius muscle has been raised to demonstrate the suprascapular region, the central portion of the supraspinatus has been removed.

Note the course of the suprascapular nerve in its fibro-osseous canal *below* the superior transverse scapular ligament in the scapular notch. Compression of this nerve in its canal, especially on extreme external rotation of the shoulder, can lead to paralysis of the supra- and infraspinatus muscles (*scapular notch syndrome*). Ossification of the superior transverse scapular ligament creates a scapular foramen that can also cause suprascapular nerve compression (see p. 213).

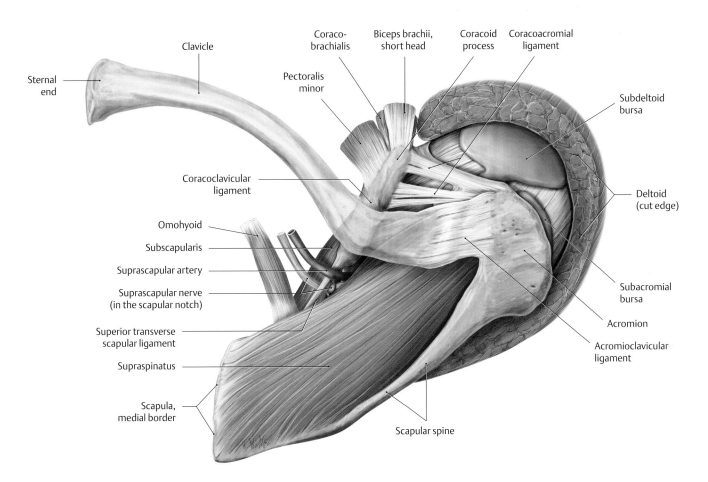

Sternal end

Clavicle

Coraco-brachialis

Biceps brachii, short head

Coracoid process

Coracoacromial ligament

Pectoralis minor

Subdeltoid bursa

Coracoclavicular ligament

Deltoid (cut edge)

Omohyoid

Subscapularis

Suprascapular artery

Suprascapular nerve (in the scapular notch)

Superior transverse scapular ligament

Supraspinatus

Subacromial bursa

Acromion

Acromioclavicular ligament

Scapula, medial border

Scapular spine

C Suprascapular region of the right shoulder, viewed from above
The trapezius and deltoid muscles have been removed to demonstrate the *supraspinatus*, which originates in the supraspinous fossa and passes laterally beneath the humeral fornix to its insertion on the greater tuber-osity. The suprascapular artery and nerve run along the anterior border of the supraspinatus at the level of the superior transverse scapular ligament, just lateral to the omohyoid insertion—the artery above the ligament and the nerve below it (see **B** and **D**).

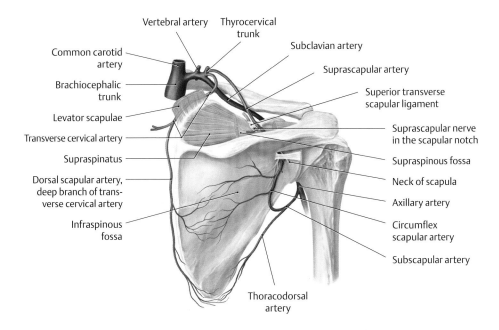

Vertebral artery

Thyrocervical trunk

Common carotid artery

Brachiocephalic trunk

Levator scapulae

Transverse cervical artery

Supraspinatus

Dorsal scapular artery, deep branch of trans-verse cervical artery

Infraspinous fossa

Subclavian artery

Suprascapular artery

Superior transverse scapular ligament

Suprascapular nerve in the scapular notch

Supraspinous fossa

Neck of scapula

Axillary artery

Circumflex scapular artery

Subscapular artery

Thoracodorsal artery

D Scapular arcade
Right scapula, posterior view. The suprascapular artery arises from the thyrocervical trunk and passes *over* the *superior* transverse scapular ligament to enter the supraspinous fossa. From there it runs past the neck of the scapula, passing *under* the *inferior* transverse scapular ligament (often absent), and enters the infraspinous fossa where it communicates with the circumflex scapular artery (from the subscapular artery) and the deep branch (dorsal scapular artery) of the transverse cervical artery.
Note the anastomosis between the suprascapular artery and the circumflex scapular artery (*scapular arcade*). It is important clinically because it can provide a collateral circulation in response to ligation or occlusion of the axillary artery (see also p. 342).

341

5.8   The Posterior Brachial Region

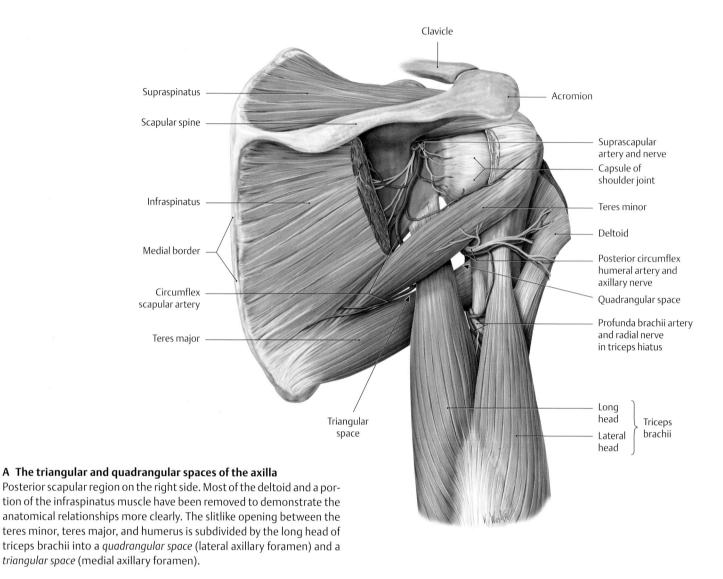

A The triangular and quadrangular spaces of the axilla

Posterior scapular region on the right side. Most of the deltoid and a portion of the infraspinatus muscle have been removed to demonstrate the anatomical relationships more clearly. The slitlike opening between the teres minor, teres major, and humerus is subdivided by the long head of triceps brachii into a *quadrangular space* (lateral axillary foramen) and a *triangular space* (medial axillary foramen).

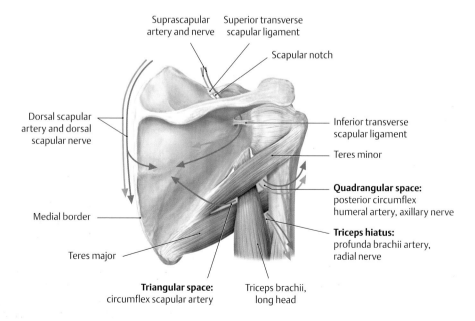

B Neurovascular tracts associated with the scapula

The triangular and quadrangular spaces of the axilla and the triceps hiatus provide important passageways that transmit neurovascular structures from the anterior to the posterior scapular region.

Passageways	Structures transmitted
• Triangular space	Circumflex scapular artery
• Quadrangular space	Posterior circumflex humeral artery and axillary nerve
• Triceps hiatus	Profunda brachii artery and radial nerve

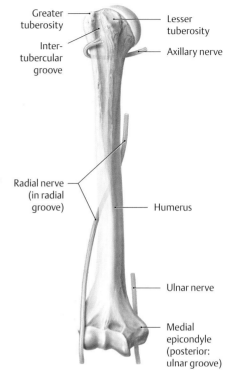

E Nerves that are closely related to the humerus
Right humerus, anterior view.

C Course of the radial nerve in the radial groove

Right shoulder and upper arm, posterior view. The lateral head of triceps brachii has been divided to show how the radial nerve spirals around the humerus. The dissection shows the bony radial groove between the origins of the medial and lateral heads of triceps brachii. At the distal end of the groove, the radial nerve passes through the lateral intermuscular septum to the front of the humerus and contin-

ues in the radial tunnel to the cubital fossa (not shown here; see also p. 344).

Note that the radial nerve branches for the triceps brachii arise proximal to the radial groove. Thus the triceps brachii may still be functional after a humeral shaft fracture at the level of the radial groove, even though the radial nerve has been damaged, because the muscular branches to the triceps arise proximal to the site of the lesion.

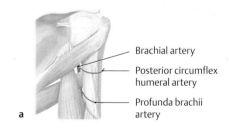

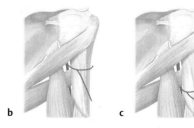

F Branches of the brachial artery: normal anatomy and variants (after von Lanz and Wachsmuth)

a Typically (77% of cases) the profunda brachii artery and posterior circumflex humeral artery arise from the brachial artery.

b, c Variants:

b The profunda brachii artery arises from the posterior circumflex humeral artery (7%).

c As in **b**, but the posterior circumflex humeral artery runs through the triceps hiatus rather than the quadrangular space (16%).

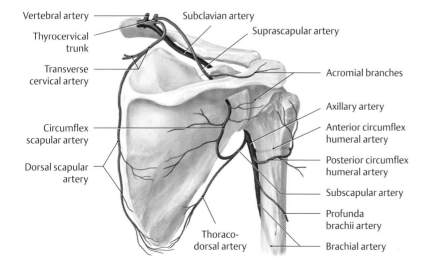

D Arterial supply to the scapular region
Right shoulder, posterior view.

343

5.9 The Elbow (Cubital Region)

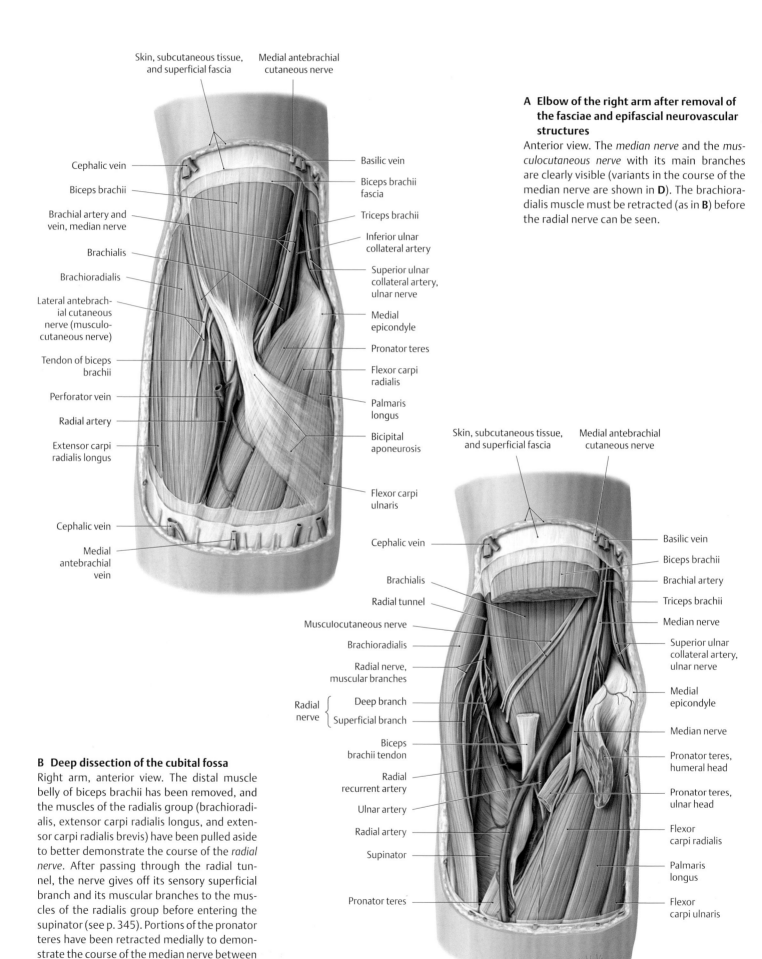

Skin, subcutaneous tissue, and superficial fascia

Medial antebrachial cutaneous nerve

Cephalic vein

Biceps brachii

Brachial artery and vein, median nerve

Brachialis

Brachioradialis

Lateral antebrachial cutaneous nerve (musculocutaneous nerve)

Tendon of biceps brachii

Perforator vein

Radial artery

Extensor carpi radialis longus

Cephalic vein

Medial antebrachial vein

Basilic vein

Biceps brachii fascia

Triceps brachii

Inferior ulnar collateral artery

Superior ulnar collateral artery, ulnar nerve

Medial epicondyle

Pronator teres

Flexor carpi radialis

Palmaris longus

Bicipital aponeurosis

Flexor carpi ulnaris

A Elbow of the right arm after removal of the fasciae and epifascial neurovascular structures

Anterior view. The *median nerve* and the *musculocutaneous nerve* with its main branches are clearly visible (variants in the course of the median nerve are shown in **D**). The brachioradialis muscle must be retracted (as in **B**) before the radial nerve can be seen.

Skin, subcutaneous tissue, and superficial fascia

Medial antebrachial cutaneous nerve

Cephalic vein

Brachialis

Radial tunnel

Musculocutaneous nerve

Brachioradialis

Radial nerve, muscular branches

Radial nerve { Deep branch / Superficial branch

Biceps brachii tendon

Radial recurrent artery

Ulnar artery

Radial artery

Supinator

Pronator teres

Basilic vein

Biceps brachii

Brachial artery

Triceps brachii

Median nerve

Superior ulnar collateral artery, ulnar nerve

Medial epicondyle

Median nerve

Pronator teres, humeral head

Pronator teres, ulnar head

Flexor carpi radialis

Palmaris longus

Flexor carpi ulnaris

B Deep dissection of the cubital fossa

Right arm, anterior view. The distal muscle belly of biceps brachii has been removed, and the muscles of the radialis group (brachioradialis, extensor carpi radialis longus, and extensor carpi radialis brevis) have been pulled aside to better demonstrate the course of the *radial nerve*. After passing through the radial tunnel, the nerve gives off its sensory superficial branch and its muscular branches to the muscles of the radialis group before entering the supinator (see p. 345). Portions of the pronator teres have been retracted medially to demonstrate the course of the median nerve between the two heads of that muscle.

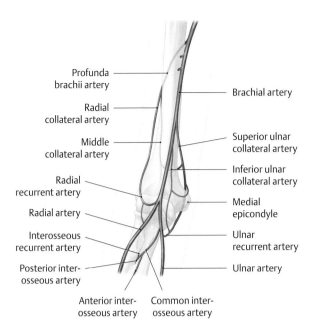

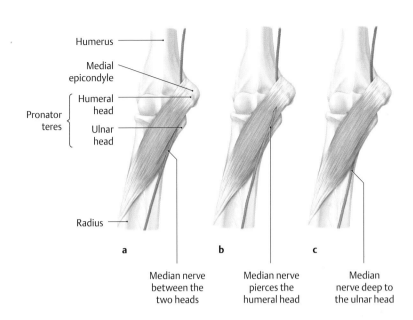

a Median nerve between the two heads

b Median nerve pierces the humeral head

c Median nerve deep to the ulnar head

C Arterial anastomoses about the elbow joint: the arterial network of the elbow

Right arm, anterior view. The arterial anastomoses in the elbow region form a vascular network that is fed by several arteries:

- The middle collateral artery and radial collateral artery from the profunda brachii artery (communicate with the radial artery via the radial recurrent artery and interosseous recurrent artery)
- The superior ulnar collateral artery and inferior ulnar collateral artery from the brachial artery (communicate with the ulnar artery via the ulnar recurrent artery)

Because of this arterial network, the brachial artery can be ligated distal to the origin of the profunda brachii without compromising the blood supply to the elbow region.

D Relationship of the median nerve to pronator teres: normal anatomy and variants (after von Lanz and Wachsmuth)

Right arm, anterior view.

a In the great majority of cases (95 %) the median nerve runs between the two heads of pronator teres.

b, c Variants:

b The median nerve pierces the humeral head of pronator teres (2 % of cases).

c The median nerve runs on the bone beneath the ulnar head (3 % of cases).

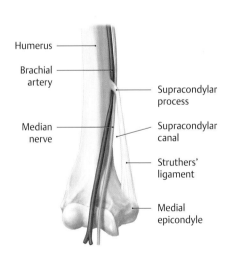

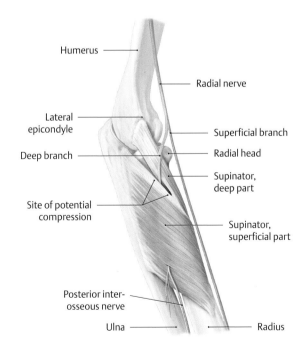

E Supracondylar process of the humerus

Distal humerus, right arm, anterior view. The *supracondylar process* is an unusual anomaly (0.7 % of the population), a bony outgrowth above the medial epicondyle (see p. 214). When present, it can serve as an attachment for a connective tissue band referred to as Struthers' ligament, which ends on the medial epicondyle. The resulting fibro-osseous *supracondylar canal* can entrap and compress the brachial artery and median nerve.

F Relationship of the radial nerve to the supinator

Right elbow region, radial view. Just proximal to the supinator muscle, the radial nerve divides into its deep motor branch and superficial sensory branch. This arrangement can lead to entrapment and compression of the deep motor branch, with resulting selective palsy of the extensor muscles (and abductor pollicis longus) served by this nerve.

345

5.10 The Anterior Forearm Region

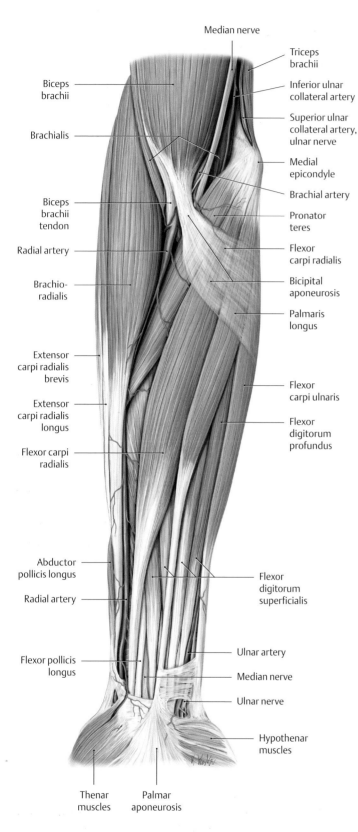

A Right forearm, anterior view, superficial layer
The fasciae and superficial neurovascular structures have been removed. Most of the forearm's neurovascular structures are obscured in this view. (The superficial veins are shown in **D**, p. 329.)

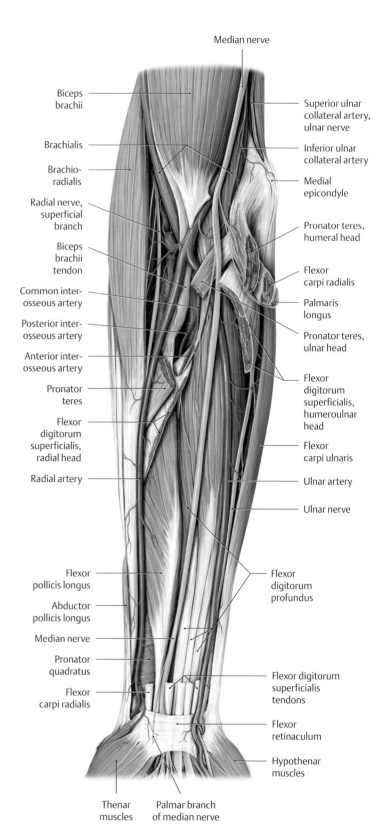

B Right forearm, anterior view, deep layer
The pronator teres, flexor digitorum superficialis, palmaris longus, and flexor carpi radialis have been partially removed to demonstrate the median nerve, the superficial branch of the radial nerve, and the radial and ulnar arteries (variants in the course of the arteries are shown in **D**).

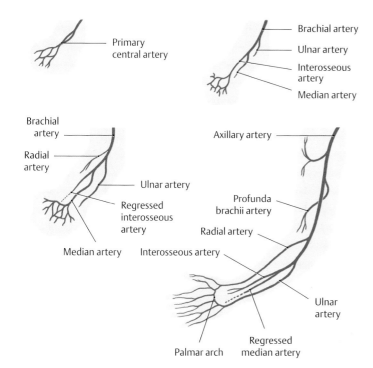

C Development of the arteries of the upper limb (after Stark)

The vascular system in the embryonic arm does not develop directly into the mature anatomy but undergoes several basic changes. The early limb bud is supplied by a central vascular trunk that develops distally into the *common interosseous artery*. As development proceeds, a second longitudinal trunk, called the *median artery*, is formed parallel to the median nerve. That vessel provides most of the blood supply to the forearm and hand, while the interosseous artery regresses. Finally the initially small muscular branches enlarge on the ulnar and radial sides to form the *ulnar artery* and the *radial artery*, which replace the median artery in primates and assume its functions. The interosseous artery remains the principal vessel of the arm in nonmammals, while the median artery is the dominant vessel in lower mammals. The interosseous and median arteries may persist in humans as well-developed atavistic anomalies (see **D**), providing most of the blood supply to the palm of the hand.

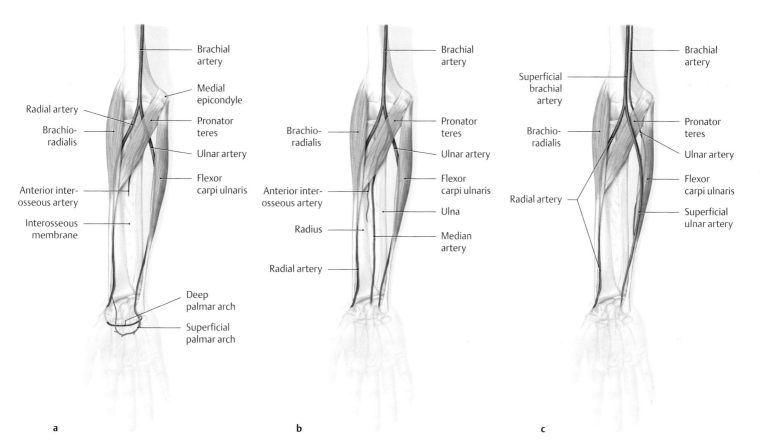

D Arteries of the forearm: normal anatomy and variants
(after Lippert and Pabst)
Right forearm, anterior view.

a Typical arterial anatomy in the forearm (84% of cases).

b, c Variants:

b A persistent median artery is present, often arising from the ulnar artery distal to the origin of the common interosseous artery (8% of cases).

c Accessory superficial arteries are present in the forearm (superficial antebrachial arteries, 8% of cases), such as a superficial ulnar artery arising from a superficial brachial artery, which runs over the surface of the flexor muscles and may unite distally with the ulnar artery. The presence of this vessel is a potential hazard during intravenous injections in the cubital area (see p. 310). Accessory superficial arteries most commonly develop in cases where the brachial artery divides in the arm into a superficial brachial artery (which becomes the radial artery in the forearm) and a brachial artery (which becomes the ulnar artery in the forearm; see "high division" pattern, p. 339).

5.11 The Posterior Forearm Region and the Dorsum of the Hand

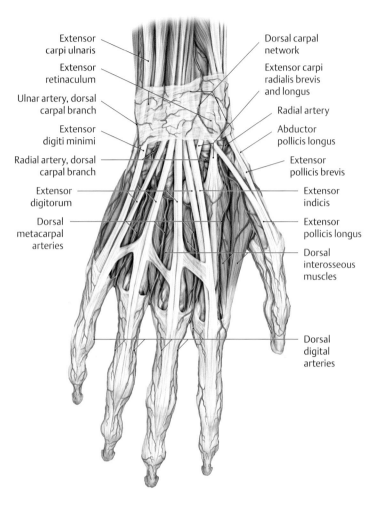

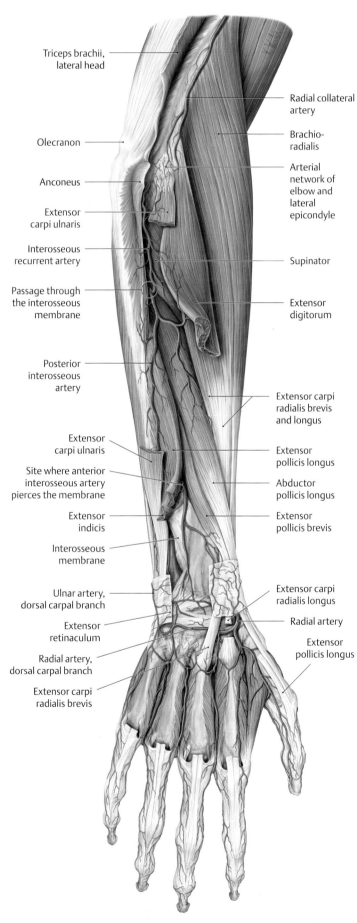

A Arteries of the dorsum of the hand and the extensor sides of the fingers in the right hand

The skin, subcutaneous tissue, and dorsal fascia of the hand have been removed to demonstrate the dorsal arteries (for clarity, the veins and nerves have also been removed). The dorsum of the hand receives most of its blood supply from the radial artery, while the ulnar artery contributes only one small vessel (the dorsal carpal branch). The perforating branches, however, create numerous connections between the palmar and dorsal arteries of the hand. In the fingers, these connections are provided by lateral anastomoses between the dorsal digital arteries and the proper palmar digital arteries (not seen here).

B Deep dissection of the arteries on the extensor side of the forearm and the dorsum of the hand in the right arm

In the elbow region the anconeus muscle has been released from its origin and reflected to the side. The triceps brachii has also been released from its origin at a more proximal level. On the extensor side of the forearm, the extensor carpi ulnaris and extensor digitorum have been partially resected.

Note how the posterior interosseous artery pierces the interosseous membrane just below the lower border of the supinator and enters the extensor compartment of the forearm. In the distal forearm, parts of the extensor pollicis longus and extensor indicis have been removed to demonstrate the site where the anterior interosseous artery pierces the interosseous membrane to reach the back of the forearm. Both arteries are important sources of blood to the extensor compartment.

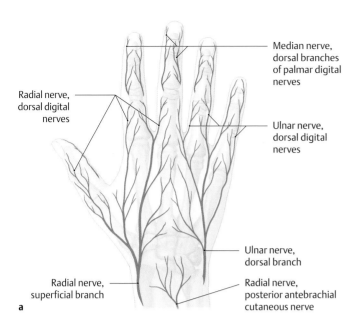

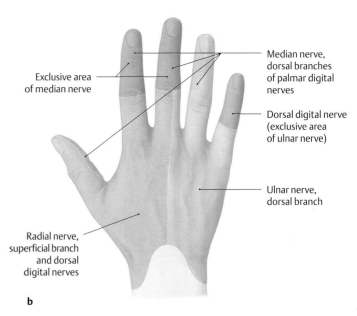

C Nerve supply to the dorsum of the hand
Right hand, posterior view.

a The cutaneous nerves on the dorsum of the hand. *Note* that the index and middle fingers and the radial part of the ring finger are supplied by different nerves in their proximal and distal portions.

- *Distal:* by the dorsal branches of the palmar digital nerves from the *median nerve*.
- *Proximal:* by the dorsal digital nerves from the *radial nerve* (to about the proximal interphalangeal joints of the index and middle fingers) and from the *ulnar nerve* (also to the level of the proximal interphalangeal joints of the middle and ring fingers).

b Exclusive and overlapping areas of sensory innervation on the dorsum of the hand, for ulnar, median, and radial nerves. In lighter shading, areas are indicated that receive sensory innervation mostly from the corresponding nerve. Because the sensory distribution of each nerve in actuality overlaps extensively with the adjacent sensory territories of the other nerves, an isolated nerve lesion does not render its entire territory anesthetic. Instead, extensive or complete loss of sensation is restricted to areas where there is little or no overlap, depicted in heavier shading.

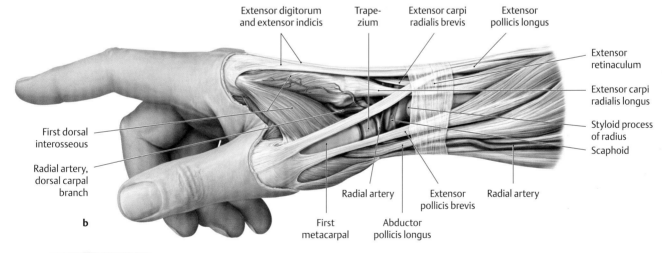

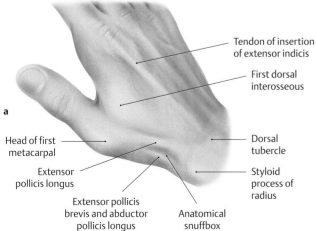

D Boundaries of the anatomical snuffbox
a Surface anatomy of the dorsum of the right hand, posteriolateral view.
b Muscles and tendons of the dorsum of the right hand, radial view. The three-sided "anatomical snuffbox" is bounded on the palmar side by the tendons of insertion of abductor pollicis longus and extensor pollicis brevis and dorsally by the tendon of insertion of extensor pollicis longus. The floor is formed mostly by the scaphoid and trapezium carpal bones. Fractures of the scaphoid bone are thus often associated with deep tenderness in the snuffbox. The snuffbox is bounded proximally by the extensor retinaculum.

Note that the radial artery runs deep in the snuffbox between the trapezium and scaphoid, providing a landmark for dissection.

349

5.12 The Palm of the Hand: Epifascial Nerves and Vessels

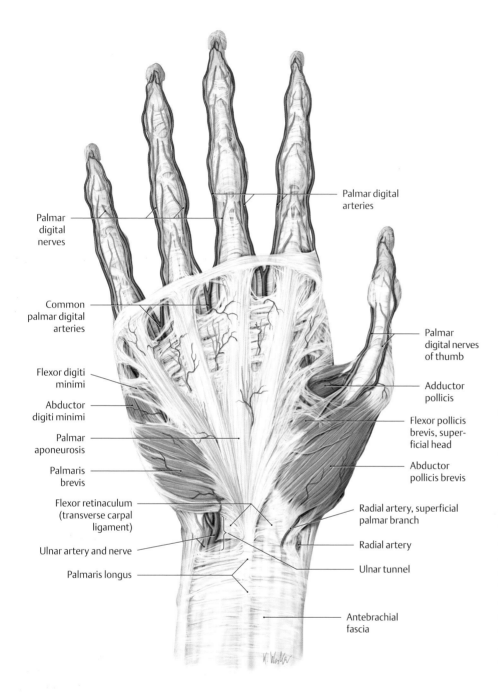

Palmar digital nerves

Common palmar digital arteries

Flexor digiti minimi

Abductor digiti minimi

Palmar aponeurosis

Palmaris brevis

Flexor retinaculum (transverse carpal ligament)

Ulnar artery and nerve

Palmaris longus

Palmar digital arteries

Palmar digital nerves of thumb

Adductor pollicis

Flexor pollicis brevis, superficial head

Abductor pollicis brevis

Radial artery, superficial palmar branch

Radial artery

Ulnar tunnel

Antebrachial fascia

A Superficial arteries and nerves of the palm

Right hand, anterior view. All of the fasciae except the palmar aponeurosis have been removed to demonstrate the superficial neurovascular structures of the palm. The palmar carpal ligament has also been removed to demonstrate the neurovascular structures that pass through the ulnar tunnel (the ulnar artery and nerve; see p. 357).

Note the superficial palmar branch of the radial artery, which is highly variable in its course. In the case shown, it runs between the origins of abductor and flexor pollicis brevis to the palm of the hand. In approximately 30% of cases it combines with the ulnar artery to form the superficial palmar arch (not shown here; see also p. 352).

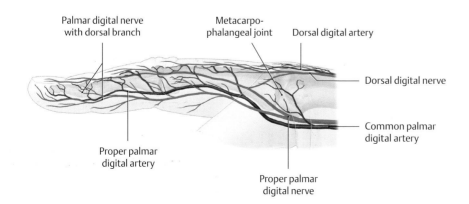

Palmar digital nerve with dorsal branch

Metacarpo-phalangeal joint

Dorsal digital artery

Dorsal digital nerve

Common palmar digital artery

Proper palmar digital artery

Proper palmar digital nerve

B Nerves and vessels of the right middle finger

Lateral view. The arteries of the palm are anterior to the nerves, but they are dorsal to the nerves in the fingers (generally crossing at the level of the metacarpophalangeal joint). The lateral and distal dorsal surfaces of the fingers are supplied by branches of the proper palmar digital nerves (from the median nerve).

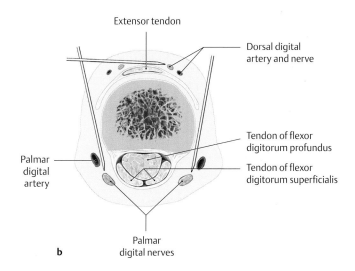

C Nerve supply to the palm of the hand
Right hand, anterior view.

a–c Innervation patterns in the palm of the hand (after Schmidt and Lanz). The sensory innervation pattern is marked by the presence of connecting branches between the median nerve and ulnar nerve. The following innervation patterns are most frequently encountered:

a Most commonly (46 % of cases) the median nerve and ulnar nerve are interconnected by an ulnar communicating branch.

b Variant 1 (20 % of cases): The median nerve and ulnar nerve are cross-connected by an ulnar communicating branch and a median communicating branch.

c Variant 2 (20 % of cases): There are no communicating branches between the median and ulnar nerves.

d **Exclusive and overlapping areas of sensory innervation of the hand, palmar view.** Non-overlapping areas of exclusive innervation are indicated by darker shading. Compare with the dorsal aspect (**C**, p. 349). .

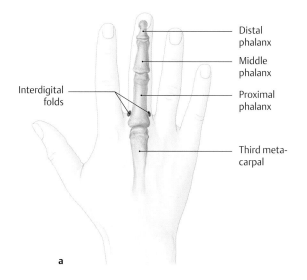

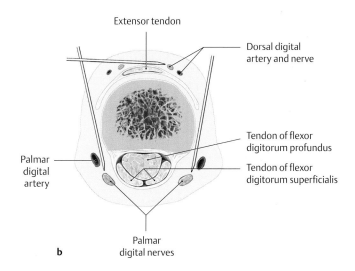

D The Oberst nerve block
Right hand, posterior view. This type of local anesthesia is clinically useful for injuries of the fingers, specifically for wounds that require suturing.

a The injection sites are located in the interdigital folds.

b After the dorsal nerve branches have been numbed, the needle is advanced on both the radial and ulnar sides toward the palmar nerves, and a subcutaneous bolus of 1–2 mL of local anesthetic is injected at each site.

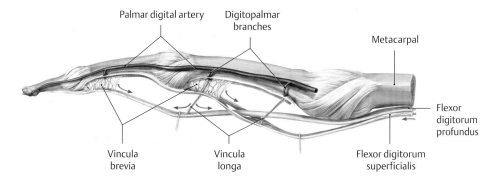

E Blood supply to the flexor tendons of the finger within the tendon sheath
(after Lundborg)

Right middle finger, lateral view. The flexor tendons are supplied within their sheath by branches of the palmar digital arteries that are transmitted to the tendons through the mesotendineum (vinculum longum and vinculum breve).

5.13 The Palm of the Hand: Vascular Supply

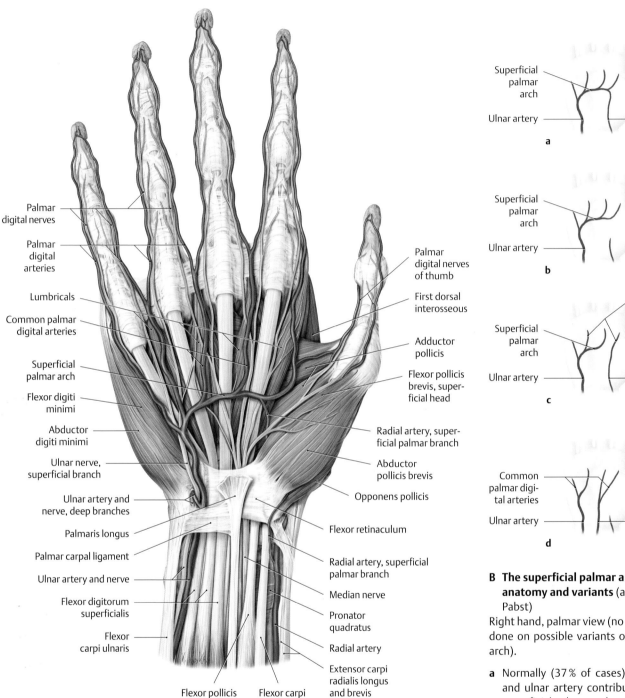

A The superficial palmar arch and its branches

Right hand, anterior view. The palmar aponeurosis and other fasciae have been removed to demonstrate the *superficial palmar arch* (variants are shown in **B**).

B The superficial palmar arch: normal anatomy and variants (after Lippert and Pabst)

Right hand, palmar view (no studies have been done on possible variants of the *deep* palmar arch).

a Normally (37% of cases) the radial artery and ulnar artery contribute equally to the superficial palmar arch.

b–d Variants:

b The palmar arch arises entirely from the ulnar artery (37% of cases).

c All of the common palmar digital arteries arise from the ulnar artery except for the first, which arises from the radial artery (13%).

d The ulnar artery and a median artery give off the common palmar digital arteries (very rare).

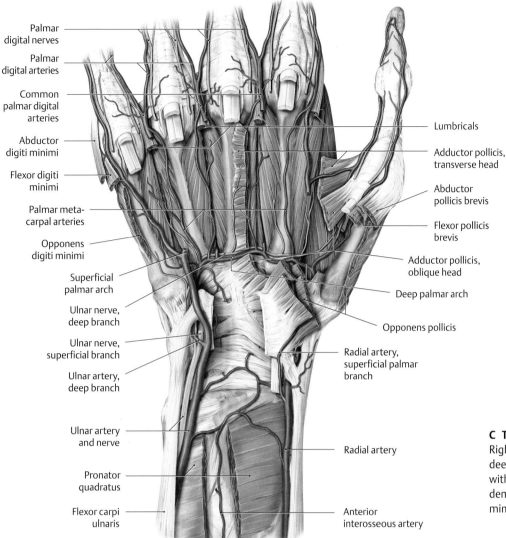

Palmar digital nerves
Palmar digital arteries
Common palmar digital arteries
Abductor digiti minimi
Flexor digiti minimi
Palmar metacarpal arteries
Opponens digiti minimi
Superficial palmar arch
Ulnar nerve, deep branch
Ulnar nerve, superficial branch
Ulnar artery, deep branch
Ulnar artery and nerve
Pronator quadratus
Flexor carpi ulnaris

Lumbricals
Adductor pollicis, transverse head
Abductor pollicis brevis
Flexor pollicis brevis
Adductor pollicis, oblique head
Deep palmar arch
Opponens pollicis
Radial artery, superficial palmar branch
Radial artery
Anterior interosseous artery

C The deep palmar arch and its branches
Right hand, anterior view. The superficial and deep flexor tendons have been removed along with the thenar and hypothenar muscles to demonstrate the *deep palmar arch* as the terminal branch of the radial artery.

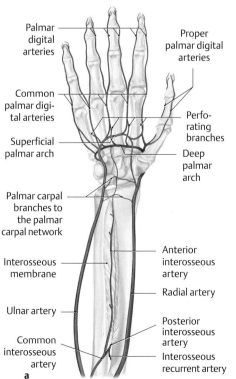

Palmar digital arteries
Common palmar digital arteries
Superficial palmar arch
Palmar carpal branches to the palmar carpal network
Interosseous membrane
Ulnar artery
Common interosseous artery
a

Proper palmar digital arteries
Perforating branches
Deep palmar arch
Anterior interosseous artery
Radial artery
Posterior interosseous artery
Interosseous recurrent artery

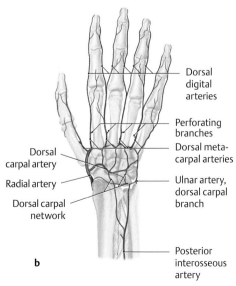

Dorsal carpal artery
Radial artery
Dorsal carpal network
b

Dorsal digital arteries
Perforating branches
Dorsal metacarpal arteries
Ulnar artery, dorsal carpal branch
Posterior interosseous artery

D Arterial anastomoses in the hand
The ulnar artery and radial artery are interconnected by the superficial and deep palmar arch, the perforating branches, and the dorsal carpal network.

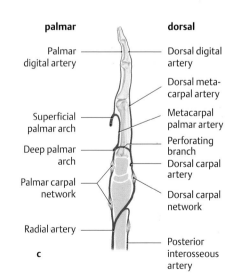

palmar   **dorsal**

Palmar digital artery
Superficial palmar arch
Deep palmar arch
Palmar carpal network
Radial artery
c

Dorsal digital artery
Dorsal metacarpal artery
Metacarpal palmar artery
Perforating branch
Dorsal carpal artery
Dorsal carpal network
Posterior interosseous artery

a Right hand, anterior view.
b Right hand, posterior view.
c Right middle finger, lateral view.

353

5.14   The Carpal Tunnel

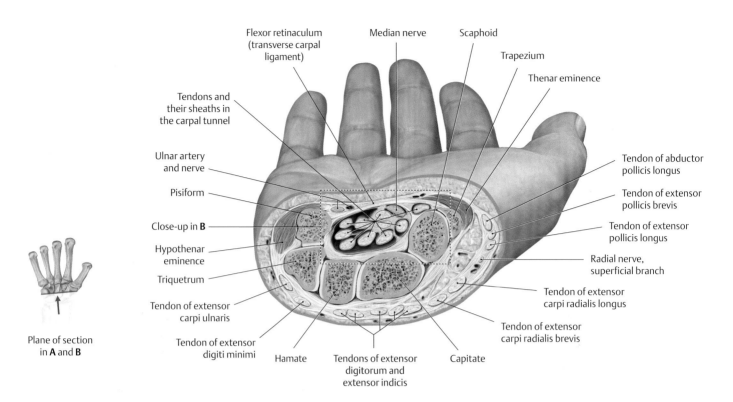

Plane of section
in **A** and **B**

A   Cross section through the right wrist (see also **B**)
Distal view. The *carpal tunnel* is a fibro-osseous canal (see p. 248) through which pass the median nerve and the tendons of insertion of flexor digitorum superficialis, flexor digitorum profundus, flexor pollicis longus, and flexor carpi radialis. Its dorsal boundary is formed by the carpal sul- cus on the front surface of the carpal bones, and its palmar boundary is the flexor retinaculum (also known clinically as the transverse carpal ligament). The ulnar artery and ulnar nerve pass through the *ulnar tunnel* on the palmar view of the retinaculum (see p. 357).

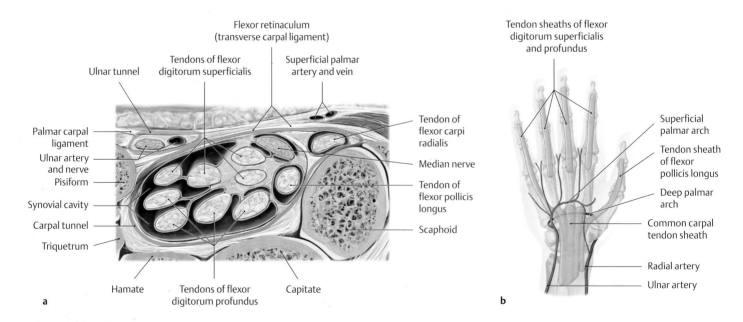

B   Relationship of the palmar arches to the carpal and digital tendon sheaths (after Schmidt and Lanz)
a   Tendon sheaths in the carpal tunnel (detail from **A**). The long flexor tendons pass through the carpal tunnel, encased in their palmar ten- don sheaths. The tendons of flexor digitorum superficialis and pro- fundus are contained in their own ulnar synovial sheath. Radial to this sheath is the tendon of flexor pollicis longus. The common mesoten- dineum of all the digital flexor tendons is attached to the radial and palmar walls of the carpal tunnel. The median nerve generally occu- pies a separate space just deep to the flexor retinaculum (the variable course of the tendon sheaths is described on p. 298).
b   Relationship of the carpal and digital tendon sheaths to the palmar arches.

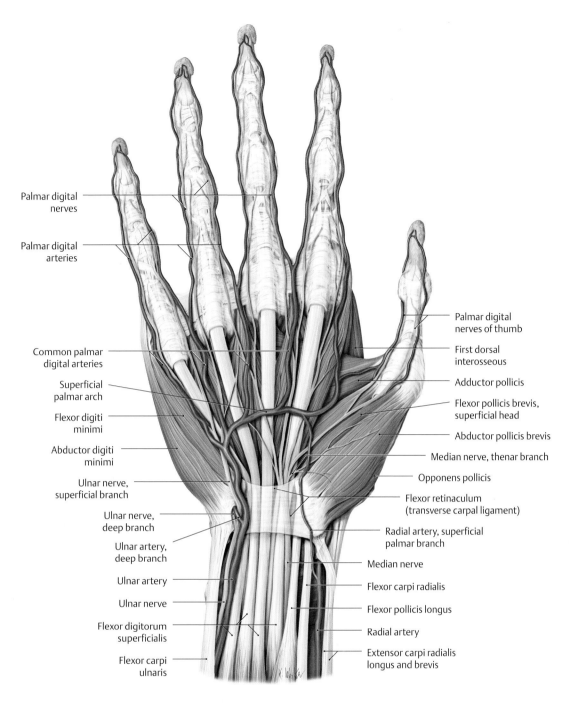

Palmar digital
nerves

Palmar digital
arteries

Common palmar
digital arteries

Superficial
palmar arch

Flexor digiti
minimi

Abductor digiti
minimi

Ulnar nerve,
superficial branch

Ulnar nerve,
deep branch

Ulnar artery,
deep branch

Ulnar artery

Ulnar nerve

Flexor digitorum
superficialis

Flexor carpi
ulnaris

Palmar digital
nerves of thumb

First dorsal
interosseous

Adductor pollicis

Flexor pollicis brevis,
superficial head

Abductor pollicis brevis

Median nerve, thenar branch

Opponens pollicis

Flexor retinaculum
(transverse carpal ligament)

Radial artery, superficial
palmar branch

Median nerve

Flexor carpi radialis

Flexor pollicis longus

Radial artery

Extensor carpi radialis
longus and brevis

C View into the carpal tunnel of the right hand
Anterior view. The transverse carpal ligament is shown in light shading.
The ulnar tunnel has been opened to display the ulnar artery and nerve.
Note the superficial course of the median nerve in the carpal tunnel
and the origin of its thenar motor branch just distal to the retinaculum
(variants are shown in **D**). During surgical division of the flexor retinacu-

lum for carpal tunnel syndrome, the hand surgeon must be aware of its
variable course to avoid cutting the thenar branch.
The superficial palmar branch of the radial artery runs on the flexor
retinaculum in the case shown here, but frequently it passes through
the thenar muscles (see p. 280).

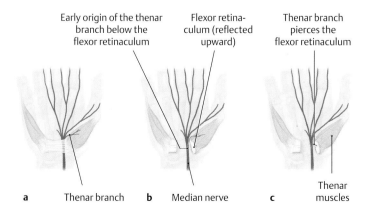

Early origin of the thenar
branch below the
flexor retinaculum

Flexor retina-
culum (reflected
upward)

Thenar branch
pierces the
flexor retinaculum

a Thenar branch **b** Median nerve **c** Thenar
muscles

**D Origin of the thenar motor branch of the median nerve: normal
anatomy and variants** (after Schmidt and Lanz)
a Normally (46 % of cases) the median nerve gives off its thenar branch
distal to the flexor retinaculum (transverse carpal ligament).

b, c Variants:
b The thenar branch has a subligamentous origin and course (31% of
cases).
c The thenar branch pierces the flexor retinaculum (transverse carpal
ligament; approximately 23 % of all cases), making it vulnerable during surgical division of the retinaculum.

5.15 The Ulnar Tunnel and Anterior Carpal Region

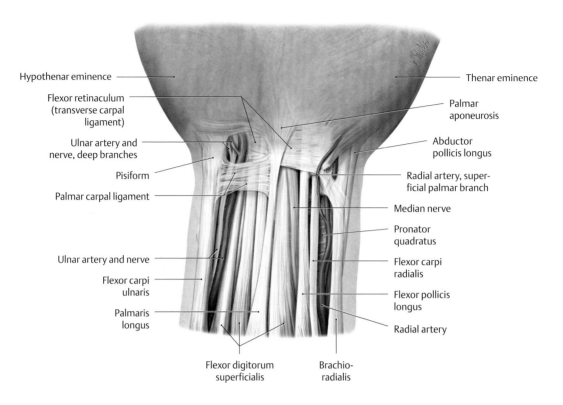

Hypothenar eminence

Flexor retinaculum
(transverse carpal
ligament)

Ulnar artery and
nerve, deep branches

Pisiform

Palmar carpal ligament

Ulnar artery and nerve

Flexor carpi
ulnaris

Palmaris
longus

Thenar eminence

Palmar
aponeurosis

Abductor
pollicis longus

Radial artery, super-
ficial palmar branch

Median nerve

Pronator
quadratus

Flexor carpi
radialis

Flexor pollicis
longus

Radial artery

Flexor digitorum
superficialis

Brachio-
radialis

A Superficial structures of the anterior carpal region
Right hand, anterior view. The skin and antebrachial fascia have been removed to demonstrate the superficial structures of the anterior carpal region, which is bounded distally by the flexor retinaculum (transverse carpal ligament). The tendons of insertion of flexor carpi ulnaris, palmaris longus, and flexor carpi radialis in particular are clearly visible and palpable beneath the skin, especially when the fist is tightly clenched

and the wrist is in slight flexion (see **B**). The tendon of flexor carpi radialis is a useful landmark for locating the *radial artery pulse*. The flexor carpi ulnaris tendon is palpable proximally over the pisiform bone.
Note: Due to their superficial course, the median and ulnar nerves and the radial and ulnar arteries are particularly susceptible to injury from lacerations of the wrist.

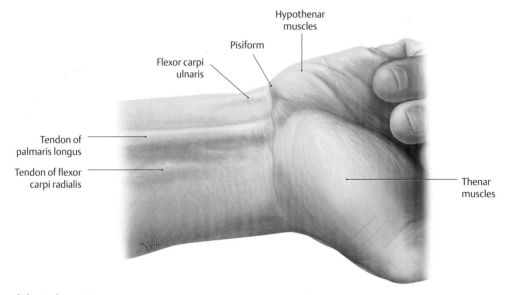

Hypothenar
muscles

Pisiform

Flexor carpi
ulnaris

Tendon of
palmaris longus

Tendon of flexor
carpi radialis

Thenar
muscles

B Surface anatomy of the right wrist
Anterior view.

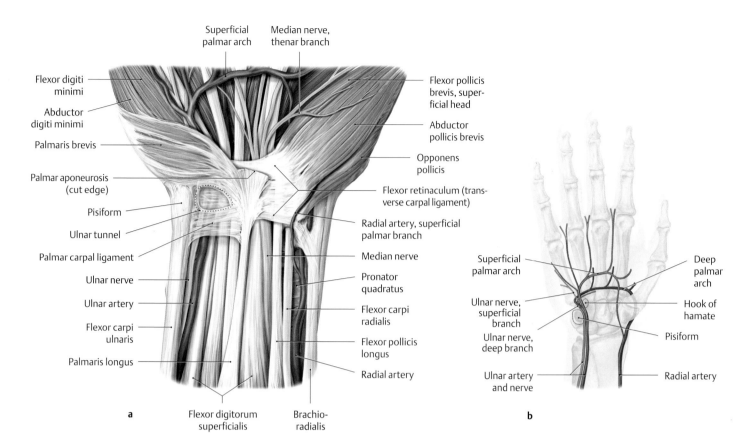

Superficial palmar arch
Median nerve, thenar branch
Flexor digiti minimi
Abductor digiti minimi
Palmaris brevis
Palmar aponeurosis (cut edge)
Pisiform
Ulnar tunnel
Palmar carpal ligament
Ulnar nerve
Ulnar artery
Flexor carpi ulnaris
Palmaris longus
Flexor pollicis brevis, superficial head
Abductor pollicis brevis
Opponens pollicis
Flexor retinaculum (transverse carpal ligament)
Radial artery, superficial palmar branch
Median nerve
Pronator quadratus
Flexor carpi radialis
Flexor pollicis longus
Radial artery
Flexor digitorum superficialis
Brachioradialis

a

Superficial palmar arch
Ulnar nerve, superficial branch
Ulnar nerve, deep branch
Ulnar artery and nerve
Deep palmar arch
Hook of hamate
Pisiform
Radial artery

b

C Course of the ulnar artery and nerve in the ulnar tunnel and deep palm
Right hand, anterior view.

a The palmar aponeurosis and antebrachial fascia have been removed to demonstrate the course of the ulnar artery and nerve through the ulnar tunnel.

b Bony landmarks within the ulnar tunnel. The pisiform bone on the ulnar side of the wrist and the hook of the hamate bone, which lies more distally and radially, provide the bony landmarks between which the ulnar artery and nerve pass through the ulnar tunnel.

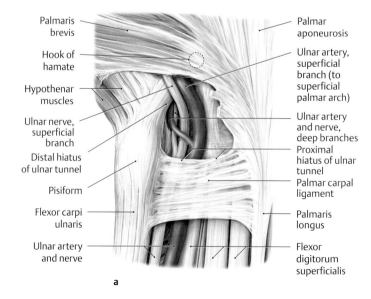

Palmaris brevis
Hook of hamate
Hypothenar muscles
Ulnar nerve, superficial branch
Distal hiatus of ulnar tunnel
Pisiform
Flexor carpi ulnaris
Ulnar artery and nerve
Palmar aponeurosis
Ulnar artery, superficial branch (to superficial palmar arch)
Ulnar artery and nerve, deep branches
Proximal hiatus of ulnar tunnel
Palmar carpal ligament
Palmaris longus
Flexor digitorum superficialis

a

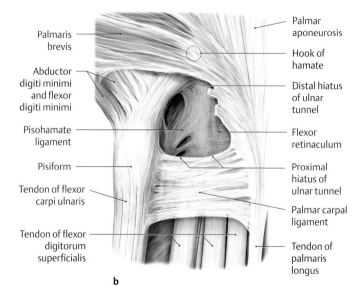

Palmaris brevis
Abductor digiti minimi and flexor digiti minimi
Pisohamate ligament
Pisiform
Tendon of flexor carpi ulnaris
Tendon of flexor digitorum superficialis
Palmar aponeurosis
Hook of hamate
Distal hiatus of ulnar tunnel
Flexor retinaculum
Proximal hiatus of ulnar tunnel
Palmar carpal ligament
Tendon of palmaris longus

b

D Apertures and walls of the ulnar tunnel with (a) and without (b) the nerves and vessels (after Schmidt and Lanz)
Anterior view. The *palmar* roof of the ulnar tunnel is formed by skin and subcutaneous fat, the palmar carpal ligament (proximal), and the palmaris brevis muscle (distal). The ulnar tunnel is bounded *dorsally* by the flexor retinaculum (transverse carpal ligament) and the pisohamate ligament. The *entrance* to the tunnel begins at the level of the pisiform bone below the palmar carpal ligament (proximal hiatus). The *outlet* is at the level of the hook of the hamate, marked by a taut, transverse, crescent-shaped tendinous arch between the pisiform and the hook of the hamate (distal hiatus), the latter giving attachment to the flexor digiti minimi. The *deep branches* of the ulnar artery and nerve reach the central compartment of the palm on the pisohamate ligament, passing deep to the tendinous arch. The *superficial branches* of the artery and nerve run distally above the tendinous arch, passing deep to the palmaris brevis.

357

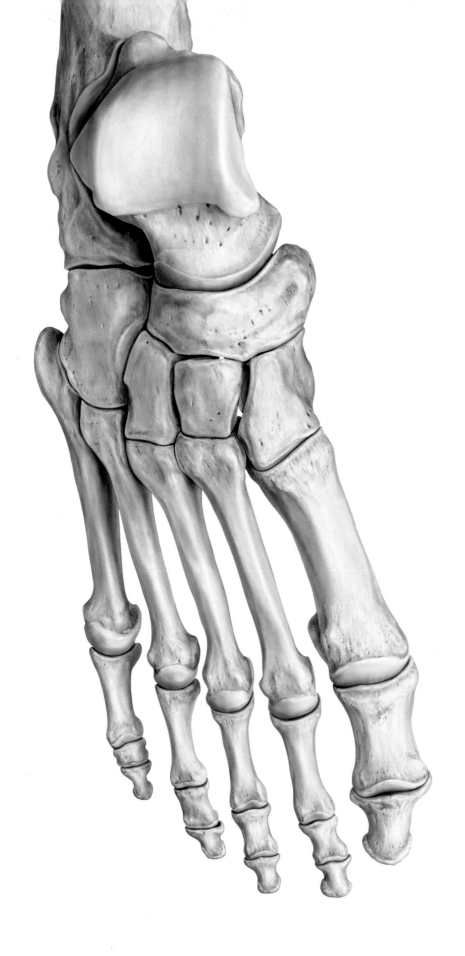

The Lower Limb

A Unique features and specialized function of the human lower limb

Coupled with the specialization of the upper limb for visually-guided manipulation, the evolution of the lower limb into a mechanism specifically adapted for bipedal locomotion has created a distinctive feature of the anatomy of the human primate. The uniquely human conformation of shapes and proportions is the end result of a process that rearranged the primate center of gravity and the positions of internal organs, dramatically altering the form and biomechanics of the trunk to produce a progressively more efficient bipedal gait. Other primates have the capacity to assume an erect body posture and to walk upright, but only for short periods and at a much greater relative expenditure of energy. The habitual upright gait of humans has been achieved through a series of anatomical adaptations of the musculoskeletal system. The most critical of these adaptations occurred in the vertebral column and pelvis. The design of the human vertebral column differs markedly from that of other primates – the simple "arch and chord" construction of the chimpanzee spine has been abandoned in favor of the human double-S-shaped curve, which allows the human axial skeleton to act as a shock-absorbing spring (see p. 77), while shifting the entire weight of the trunk over the load-bearing surface of the feet. This shift to an upright posture has imposed the full weight of the abdominal viscera upon the pelvis. Concomitantly, the iliac wings of the pelvis have spread farther apart and the sacrum has broadened, to generate a structure in humans that is now specialized for bearing the load of the viscera. The efficiency of upright gait has been improved further by stabilization of the pelvis and secure anchoring to the spine via the sacrum. The unique proportions of the human lower limb provide a dramatic demonstration of the extent of this specialization. Because their function is more exclusively directed toward support and locomotion, the legs are exceptionally long and powerful in humans. While the leg length is 111 % of trunk length in orangutans and 128 % in chimpanzees, it measures 171 % of trunk length in humans. The specialization of the human lower limb for bipedal gait is also reflected in the substantial changes in function of certain muscles, particularly the gluteal muscles, the knee-joint extensors, and the muscles of the calf.

B Overview of the skeleton of the lower limb

a Right lower limb, anterior view.
b Right lower limb, posterior view (the foot is in maximum plantar flexion in both views).

As in the upper limb, the skeleton of the lower limb consists of a limb girdle and the attached free limb.

- The pelvic girdle in adults is formed by the paired hip bones (ossa coxae, innominate bones). They differ from the shoulder girdle in that they are firmly integrated into the axial skeleton through the sacroiliac joints (see p. 116). The two hip bones combine with the sacrum and pubic symphysis to form the *pelvic ring* (see p. 365).
- The free limb consists of the thigh (femur), the leg (tibia and fibula), and the foot. It is connected to the pelvic girdle by the hip joint.

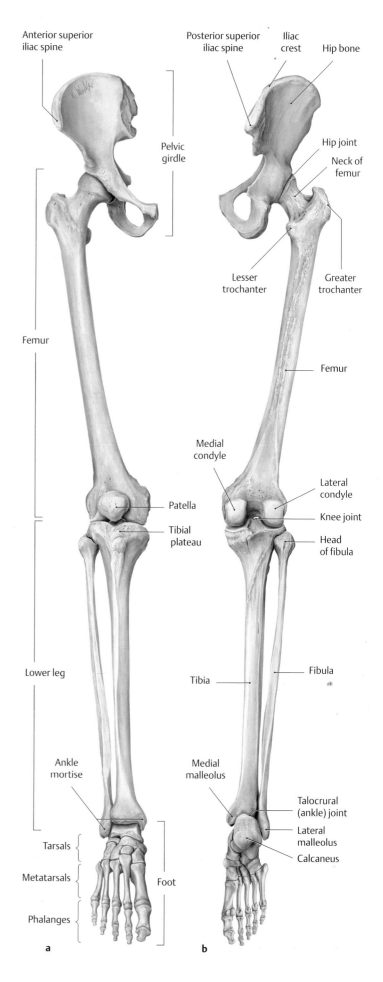

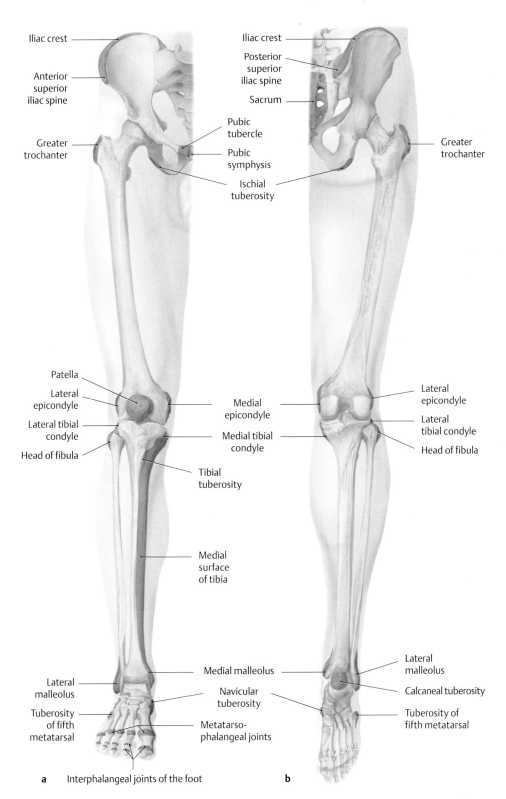

Iliac crest

Anterior superior iliac spine

Greater trochanter

Iliac crest

Posterior superior iliac spine

Sacrum

Pubic tubercle

Pubic symphysis

Ischial tuberosity

Greater trochanter

Patella

Lateral epicondyle

Lateral tibial condyle

Head of fibula

Medial epicondyle

Medial tibial condyle

Tibial tuberosity

Lateral epicondyle

Lateral tibial condyle

Head of fibula

Medial surface of tibia

Lateral malleolus

Tuberosity of fifth metatarsal

Medial malleolus

Navicular tuberosity

Metatarso-phalangeal joints

Lateral malleolus

Calcaneal tuberosity

Tuberosity of fifth metatarsal

a Interphalangeal joints of the foot

b

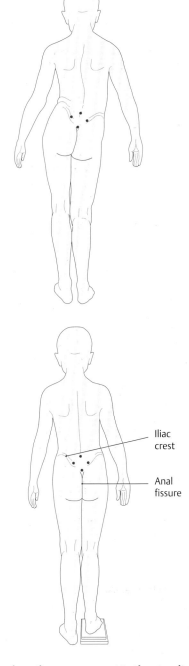

Iliac crest

Anal fissure

D Leg length measurement in the standing position

Leg length discrepancy can be measured with reasonable accuracy in the standing patient by placing wooden blocks of known thickness (0.5 cm, 1 cm, 2 cm) beneath the foot of the shorter leg until the pelvis is horizontal. Horizontal position is confirmed when noting that both iliac crests are at the same level when palpated from behind and the anal fissure is vertical. If the pelvis cannot be leveled by placing blocks under the apparently shorter limb, then a "functional" leg length discrepancy is present rather than a "true" discrepancy. Most cases of this kind are caused by a fixed pelvic tilt secondary to a hip joint contracture or scoliosis. The measured leg lengths in these cases may actually be equal, and the pelvic tilt only mimics a length discrepancy.

C Palpable bony prominences of the right lower limb

a Anterior view, **b** posterior view.

Almost all the skeletal elements of the lower limb have bony prominences, margins, or surfaces (e.g., the medial tibial surface) that can be palpated through the skin and soft tissues. The only exceptions are structures that are largely covered by muscle, such as the hip joint, the neck and shaft of the femur, and large portions of the fibular shaft. Several standard anatomical landmarks have been defined in the lower limb for use in measuring the length of

the leg and certain skeletal elements. They are the anterior superior iliac spine, the greater trochanter of the femur, the medial joint space of the knee (superior margin of the medial tibial condyle), and the medial malleolus. The clinical evaluation of leg length discrepancy is important because "true" shortening of the leg (a disparity of anatomical leg lengths) as well as functional leg shortening (e.g., due to muscle contractures) can lead to *pelvic tilt* as well as scoliotic deformity of the spine (see p. 106).

361

1.2 The Anatomical and Mechanical Axes of the Lower Limb

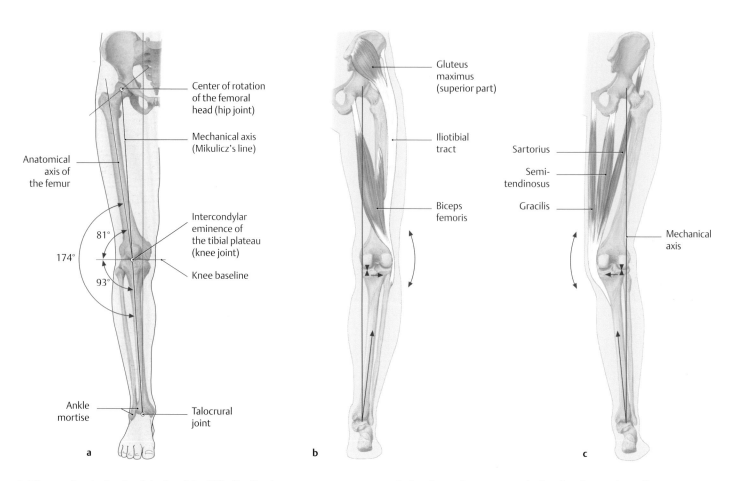

a

b

c

A The mechanical axis of the leg (the Mikulicz line)
a Normal mechanical axis, anterior view.
b Mechanical axis in genu varum, posterior view.
c Mechanical axis in genu valgum, posterior view.

In an individual with normal axial alignment, the large joints of the lower limb (the hip, knee, and ankle) lie on a straight line which represents the mechanical longitudinal axis of the leg (the *Mikulicz line*). This mechanical axis extends from the center of rotation of the femoral head through the intercondylar eminence of the tibial plateau and down through the center of the ankle *mortise* (the pocket created by the fibula and tibia for the talus in the ankle joint, from Arabic, *murtazz*, fastened). While the mechanical axis and anatomical axis coincide in the *tibial shaft*, the anatomical and mechanical axes of the *femoral shaft* diverge at a 6° angle. Thus the longitudinal anatomical axes of the femur

and tibia do not lie on a straight line but form a laterally open angle of 174° at the level of the knee joint in the coronal plane (the *femorotibial angle*). In genu varum (**b**) the center of the knee joint is lateral to the mechanical axis, and in genu valgum (**c**) it is medial to the mechanical axis. Both conditions impose abnormal, unbalanced loads on the joints (see **B**) that gradually cause degenerative changes to develop in the bone and cartilage (osteoarthritis of the knee) accompanied by stretching of the associated joint capsule, ligaments, and muscles. In genu varum (**b**), for example, the medial joint complex of the knee is subjected to abnormal pressure while the lateral joint structures (e.g., the lateral collateral ligament), iliotibial tract, and biceps femoris muscle are subjected to abnormal tension. Genu varum also places greater stress on the lateral border of the foot, resulting in a fallen pedal arch.

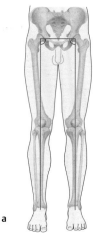

a

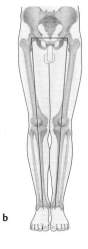

b

B Position of the mechanical axes with the feet slightly apart and together
Anterior view.

a In upright stance with the feet placed slightly apart, the mechanical axis runs almost vertically through the center of the three large joints.
b The legs are generally considered "straight" if, when the feet are together, the opposing medial malleoli and knees are touching. Accordingly, the intercondylar distance and the intermalleolar distance between the legs provide an index for the measurement of genu varum and genu valgum. When this stance is attempted, an intercondylar distance greater than 3 cm or an intermalleolar distance greater than 5 cm is considered abnormal (see **C**).

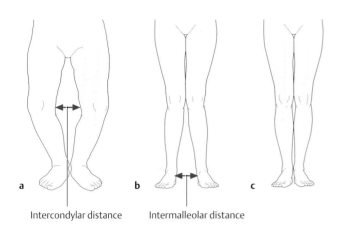

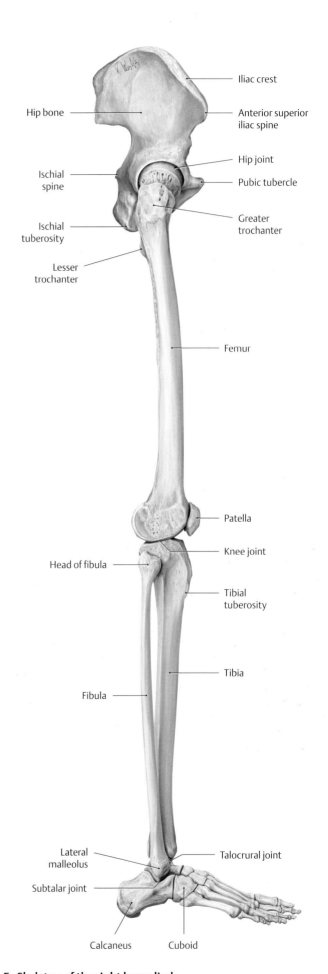

C The normal leg axes at different ages

a Infant, **b** small child, **c** school-age child.

Up to about 20° of genu varum is considered normal during the first year of life. Up to about 10° of genu valgum is also considered normal through 2 years of age. By the time the child enters school, the legs are essentially straight as a result of musculoskeletal growth.

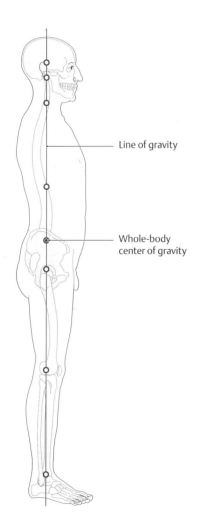

D Normal anatomical position in relation to the line of gravity

Right lateral view. The *line of gravity* runs vertically from the whole-body center of gravity to the ground. In normal upright humans, it intersects the external auditory canal, the dens of the axis (dental process C 2), the inflection points between the normal curves in the vertebral column (between the cervical and thoracic curves, and thoracic and lumbar curves), the whole-body center of gravity, and the hip, knee, and ankle joints. Chronic deviation of any reference point from this line imposes abnormal stresses on different clusters of musculoskeletal elements.

E Skeleton of the right lower limb

Right lateral view.

363

1.3 The Bones of the Pelvic Girdle

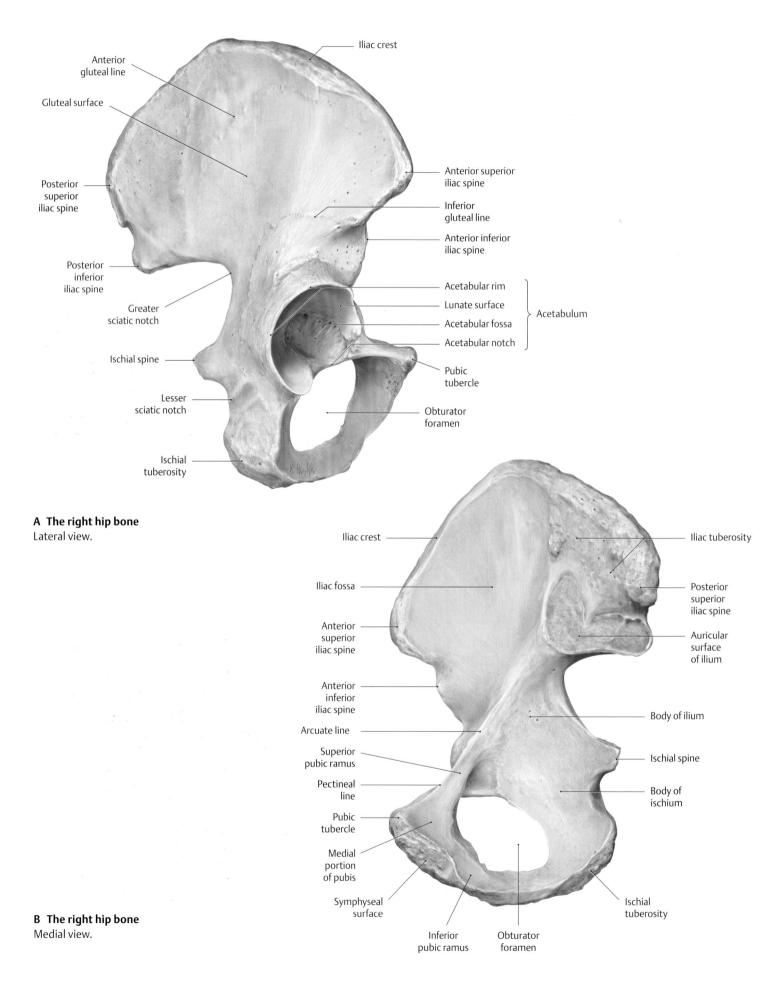

Iliac crest

Anterior gluteal line

Gluteal surface

Posterior superior iliac spine

Posterior inferior iliac spine

Greater sciatic notch

Ischial spine

Lesser sciatic notch

Ischial tuberosity

Anterior superior iliac spine

Inferior gluteal line

Anterior inferior iliac spine

Acetabular rim

Lunate surface

Acetabular fossa

Acetabular notch

Acetabulum

Pubic tubercle

Obturator foramen

A The right hip bone
Lateral view.

Iliac crest

Iliac fossa

Anterior superior iliac spine

Anterior inferior iliac spine

Arcuate line

Superior pubic ramus

Pectineal line

Pubic tubercle

Medial portion of pubis

Symphyseal surface

Inferior pubic ramus

Obturator foramen

Iliac tuberosity

Posterior superior iliac spine

Auricular surface of ilium

Body of ilium

Ischial spine

Body of ischium

Ischial tuberosity

B The right hip bone
Medial view.

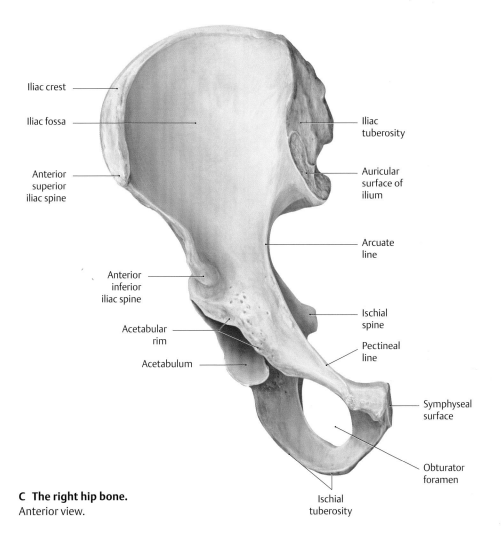

Iliac crest

Iliac fossa

Anterior superior iliac spine

Anterior inferior iliac spine

Acetabular rim

Acetabulum

Iliac tuberosity

Auricular surface of ilium

Arcuate line

Ischial spine

Pectineal line

Symphyseal surface

Obturator foramen

Ischial tuberosity

C The right hip bone.
Anterior view.

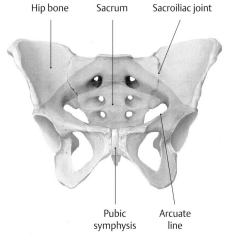

Hip bone   Sacrum   Sacroiliac joint

Pubic symphysis   Arcuate line

D The pelvic girdle and pelvic ring
Anterior view. The paired hip bones that make up the pelvic girdle are connected to each other at the cartilaginous pubic symphysis and to the sacrum at the sacroiliac joints (see p. 116). This creates a stable ring, the bony pelvic ring (shaded in red), that permits very little motion. This stability throughout the pelvic ring is an important prerequisite for the transfer of trunk loads to the lower limb necessary for normal gait.

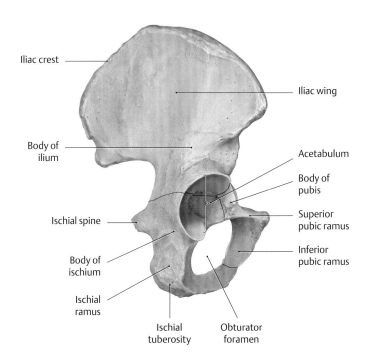

Iliac crest

Body of ilium

Ischial spine

Body of ischium

Ischial ramus

Ischial tuberosity

Obturator foramen

Iliac wing

Acetabulum

Body of pubis

Superior pubic ramus

Inferior pubic ramus

E The triradiate cartilage of a right hip bone: the junction of the ilium, ischium, and pubis.
Lateral view.

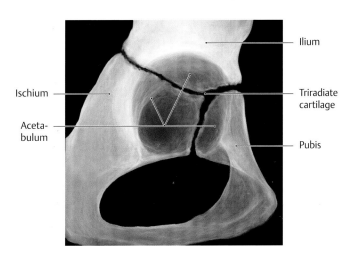

Ischium

Aceta- bulum

Ilium

Triradiate cartilage

Pubis

F Schematic radiograph of the right acetabulum of a child
Lateral view (lateral projection). The bony elements of the hip bone come together in the acetabulum, with the ilium and ischium each comprising two-fifths of the acetabulum and the pubis one-fifth. Definitive fusion of the Y-shaped growth plate (triradiate cartilage) occurs between the 14th and 16th years of life.

1.4 The Femur: Importance of the Femoral Neck Angle

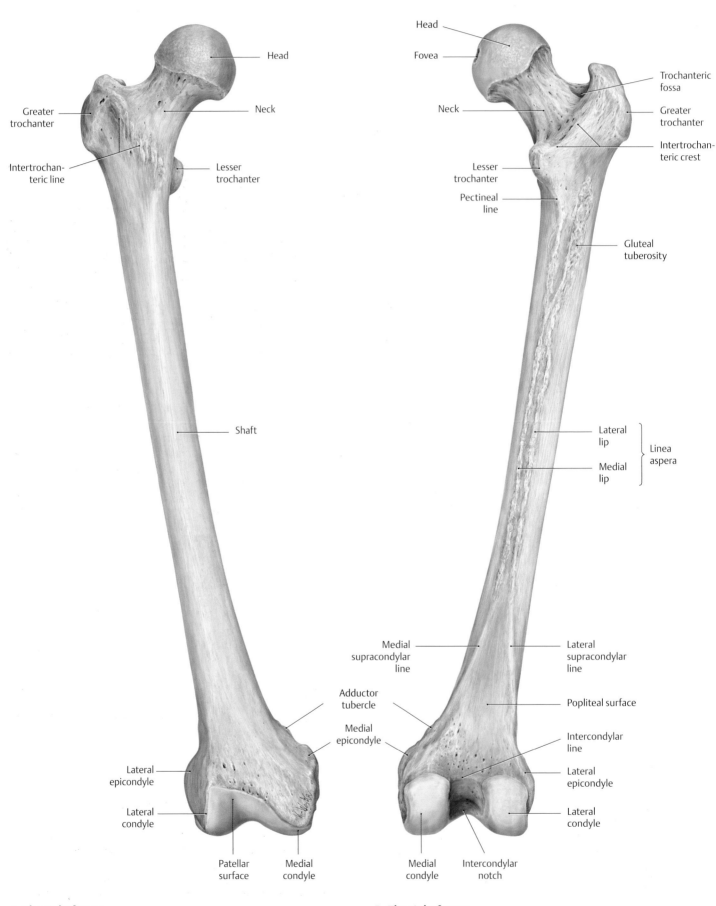

A The right femur
Anterior view.

B The right femur
Posterior view.

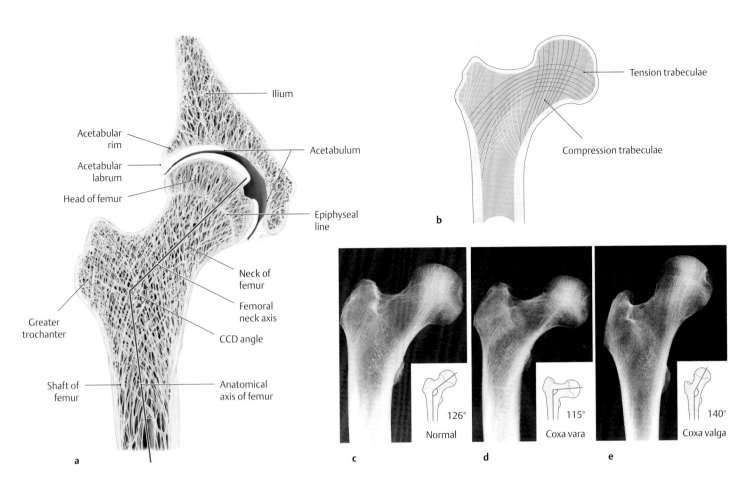

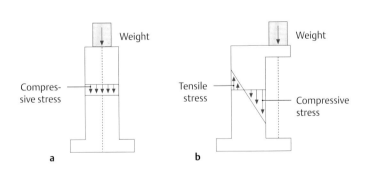

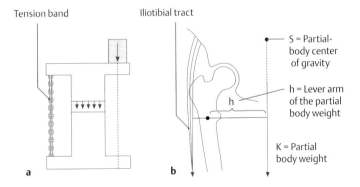

C The arrangement and prominence of tension trabeculae and compression trabeculae as a function of the femoral neck angle
Right femur, anterior view.

a Coronal section through the right hip joint at the level of the fovea on the femoral head. The angle between the longitudinal axis of the femoral neck and the axis of the femoral shaft is called the femoral neck angle or CCD angle (caput-collum-diaphyseal angle). This angle normally measures approximately 126° in adults and 150° in newborns. It decreases continually during growth due to the constant bone remodeling that occurs in response to the changing stress patterns across the hip.

b The trabecular pattern associated with a normal femoral neck angle.
c–e Radiographs in the sagittal projection.
c Normal femoral neck angle with a normal bending load.
d A *decreased* femoral neck angle (coxa vara) leads to a greater bending load with higher tensile stresses, thereby stimulating the formation of more tension trabeculae.
e An *increased* femoral neck angle (coxa valga) leads to a greater pressure load with higher compressive stresses, stimulating the formation of more compression trabeculae.

D Compressive and tensile stresses in a bone model
a An *axial* (centered) weight placed atop a Plexiglas model of a pillar creates a uniform pressure load that is evenly distributed over the cross section of the pillar and whose sum is equal to the applied weight.
b A *nonaxial* (eccentric) weight placed on an overhang creates a bending load that generates both tensile and compressive stresses in the pillar.

E The principle of the tension band (after Pauwels)
a The bending load acting on an I-beam model can be reduced by placing a high-tensile-strength member (chain) on the side opposite the bending force. This added member transforms the bending load into a pure compressive load.
b In the leg, the fascia lata on the lateral side of the thigh is thickened to form the iliotibial tract (see p. 425). By functioning as a tension band, the iliotibial tract reduces the bending loads on the proximal femur.

367

1.5 The Femoral Head and Deformities of the Femoral Neck

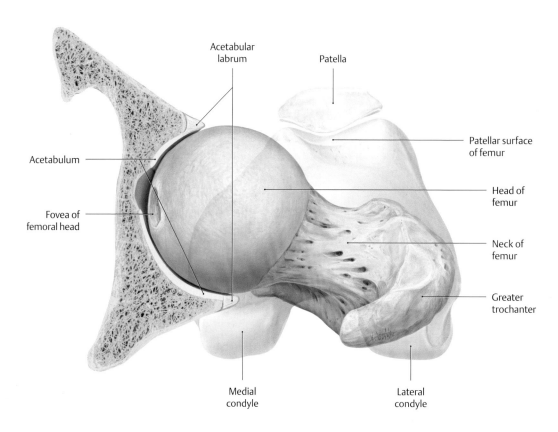

Acetabular labrum

Patella

Patellar surface of femur

Head of femur

Neck of femur

Greater trochanter

Acetabulum

Fovea of femoral head

Medial condyle

Lateral condyle

A The right femur
Proximal view. For clarity, the acetabulum has been sectioned in the horizontal plane. The distal end of the femur (with patella) has been added in light shading.
Note the orientation of the acetabulum, which is angled forward by approximately 17°. This anterior angle affects the stability and "seat-

ing" of the femoral head in the hip joint (see p. 378). When the femoral head is centered in the acetabulum and there is normal anteversion of the femoral neck, the patella is directed forward.

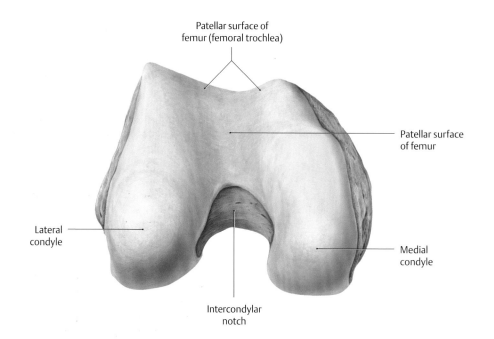

Patellar surface of femur (femoral trochlea)

Patellar surface of femur

Lateral condyle

Medial condyle

Intercondylar notch

B The right femur
Distal view.
Note the reversal of perspective from **A**.

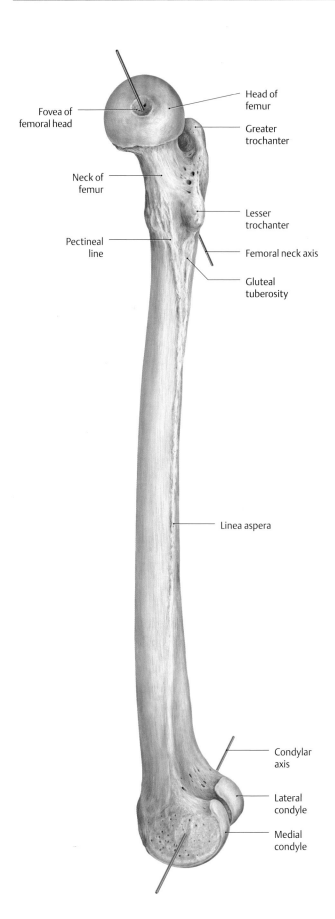

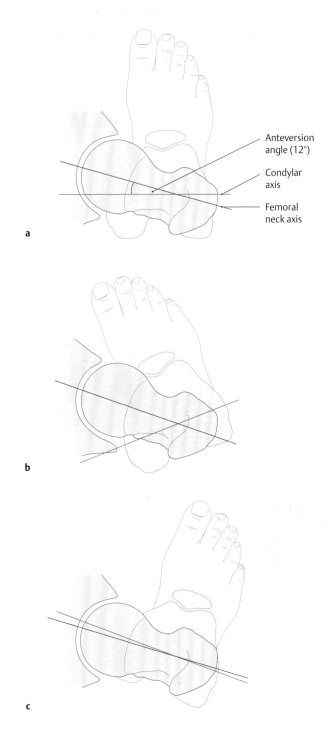

C The right femur.
Medial view.

Note the transverse condylar axis and the femoral neck axis. When the axes are superimposed, the two lines intersect each other at a 12° angle in adults (anteversion angle, see also **D** and **A**). This angle is considerably larger at birth, measuring 30–40°, but decreases to the normal adult value by the end of the second decade.

D Rotational deformities of the femoral neck
Right hip joint, superior view. Increased or decreased torsion of the femoral shaft results in torsion angles of varying size. When the hip is centered, this leads to increased internal or external rotation of the leg with a corresponding change in gait (a "toeing-in" or "toeing-out" gait). When the condylar axis is taken as the reference point, femoral torsion may be described as normal (**a**), increased (**b**), or decreased (**c**).

a A normal anteversion angle of approximately 12° with the foot directed forward.

b An increased anteversion angle (*coxa anteverta*) typically leads to a toeing-in gait accompanied by a pronounced limitation of external rotation.

c The femoral neck is retroverted (points backward in relation to the condylar axis). The result is *coxa retroverta* with a toeing-out gait.

1.6 The Patella

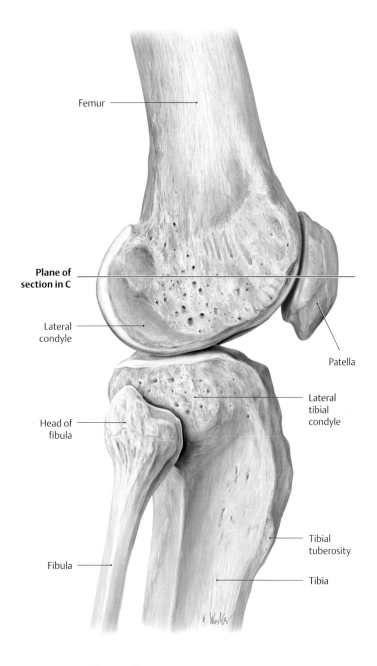

A Location of the patella
Right knee joint, lateral view. The red line indicates the plane of section in **C**.

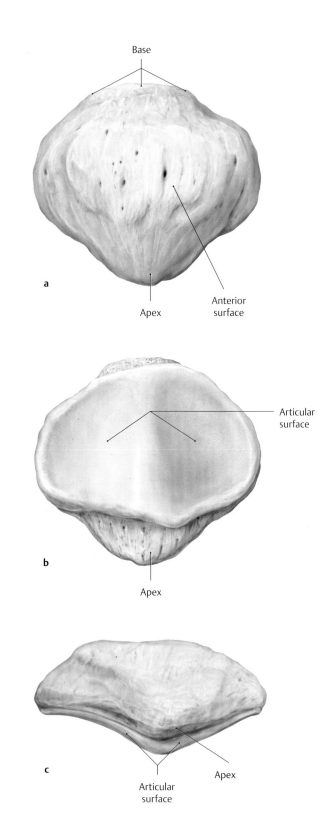

B Right patella
a Anterior view, **b** posterior view, **c** distal view.
Note that the *apex* of the patella points downward.

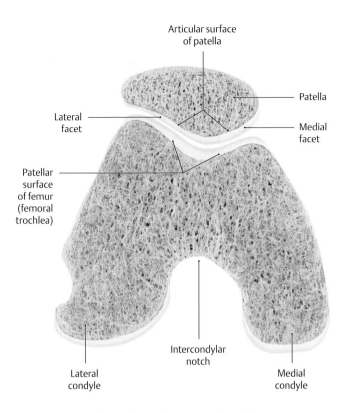

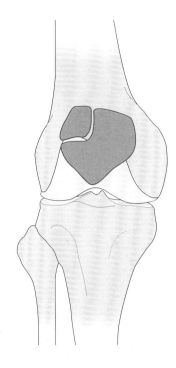

C Cross section through the femoropatellar joint

Right knee, distal view. The level of the cross section is shown in **A**. The femoropatellar joint is the site where the patellar surface of the femur, often called the femoral trochlea (by analogy with the distal humerus), articulates with the posterior articular surface of the patella. The patella is a sesamoid bone (the largest sesamoid), embedded in the quadriceps tendon. The patella is well centered when the ridge on the undersurface of the patella is seated within the groove of the femoral trochlea. The main functional role of the patella is to lengthen the effective lever arm of the quadriceps femoris muscle (the only extensor muscle of the knee), thereby reducing the force required to extend the knee joint (see also p. 428).

D Bipartite patella

Because the patella develops from multiple ossification centers, the failure of an ossification center to fuse results in a two-part (bipartite) patella. The upper lateral quadrant of the patella is most commonly affected. A fracture should always be considered in the radiographic differential diagnosis of a bipartite patella.

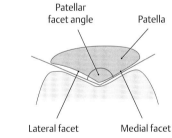 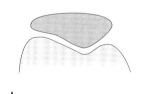 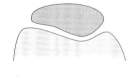 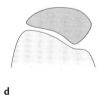

E The evaluation of patellar shape

Diagrams of tangential radiographs of the patella ("sunrise" view: supine position, knee flexed 60°, caudocranial beam directed parallel to the posterior patellar surface). Each diagram shows the relation of the patella to the femoral trochlea in a horizontal plane through the right knee joint. The posterior articular surface of the patella bears a vertical ridge dividing it into a lateral facet and a medial facet. Generally the lateral facet is slightly concave while the medial facet is slightly convex. The angle between the lateral and medial facets, called the patellar facet angle, is normally 130° ± 10°. Wiberg, Baumgart, and Ficat devised the following scheme for the classification of patellar shape based on the facet angle:

a Patella with medial and lateral facets of approximately equal size and a facet angle within the normal range.
b Most common patellar shape with a slightly smaller medial facet.
c A distinctly smaller medial facet ("medial hypoplasia").
d Patellar dysplasia with a very steep medial facet ("hunter's hat" configuration).

Besides the various patellar shapes, the patellar surface of the femur (the femoral trochlea) also has a variable morphology (described in the Hepp classification system). Developmental dysplasias of the patella and femoral trochlea lead to patellar instability marked by recurrent lateral or medial subluxation or dislocation of the patella.

371

1.7 The Tibia and Fibula

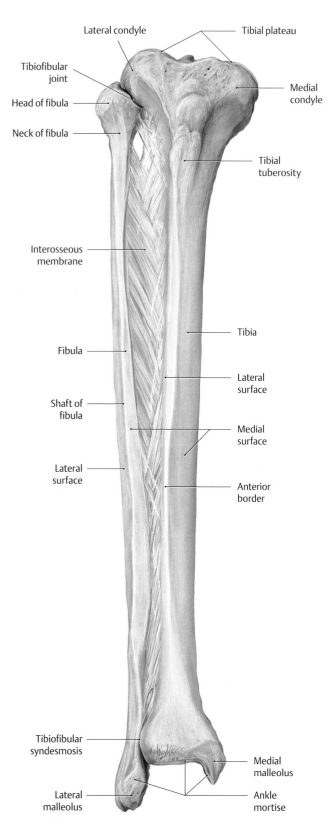

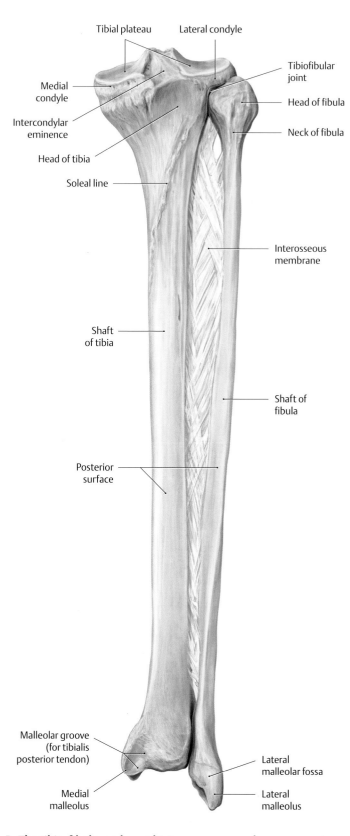

A The tibia, fibula, and crural interosseous membrane
Right leg, anterior view. The tibia and fibula articulate at two joints that allow only very limited motion (rotation). Proximally, near the knee, is the synovial tibiofibular joint; distally, at the ankle, is the tibiofibular *syndesmosis* (fibrous joint with bony elements united by ligaments). The crural interosseous membrane (see also **F**) is a sheet of tough connective tissue that serves as an origin for several muscles in the leg. Additionally, it acts with the tibiofibular syndesmosis to stabilize the ankle mortise.

B The tibia, fibula, and crural interosseous membrane
Right leg, posterior view.

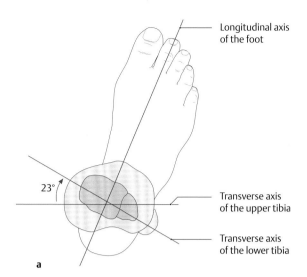

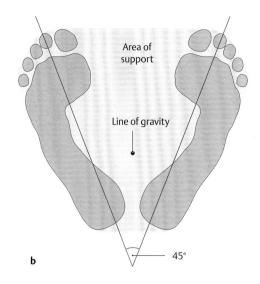

C Normal orientation of the tibia and its role in stability

When the transverse axes of the upper tibia (tibial plateau) and lower tibia (ankle mortise) are superimposed, they form an angle of approximately 23°, i. e., the transverse axis of the ankle joint is rotated 23° laterally relative to the transverse axis of the tibial plateau (*normal tibial*

orientation, **a**). As a result of this, the longitudinal anatomical axis of the foot does not lie in the sagittal plane, and the toes point outward when the upper tibia is directed forward (**b**). This significantly improves the stability of bipedal stance by placing the line of gravity close to the center of the area of support (see p. 363).

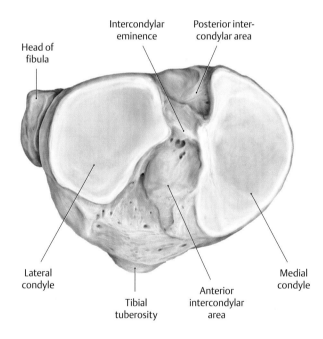

D The right tibial plateau
Proximal view.

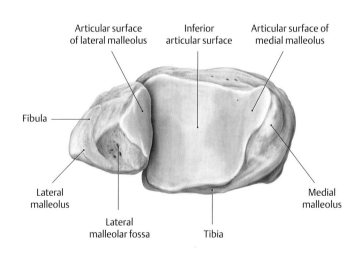

E The right ankle mortise
Distal view.

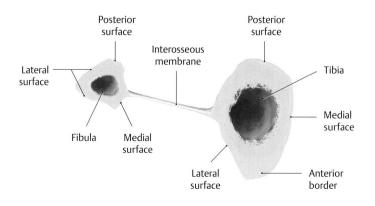

F Cross section through the middle third of the right leg
Proximal view.

1.8 The Bones of the Foot from the Dorsal and Plantar Views

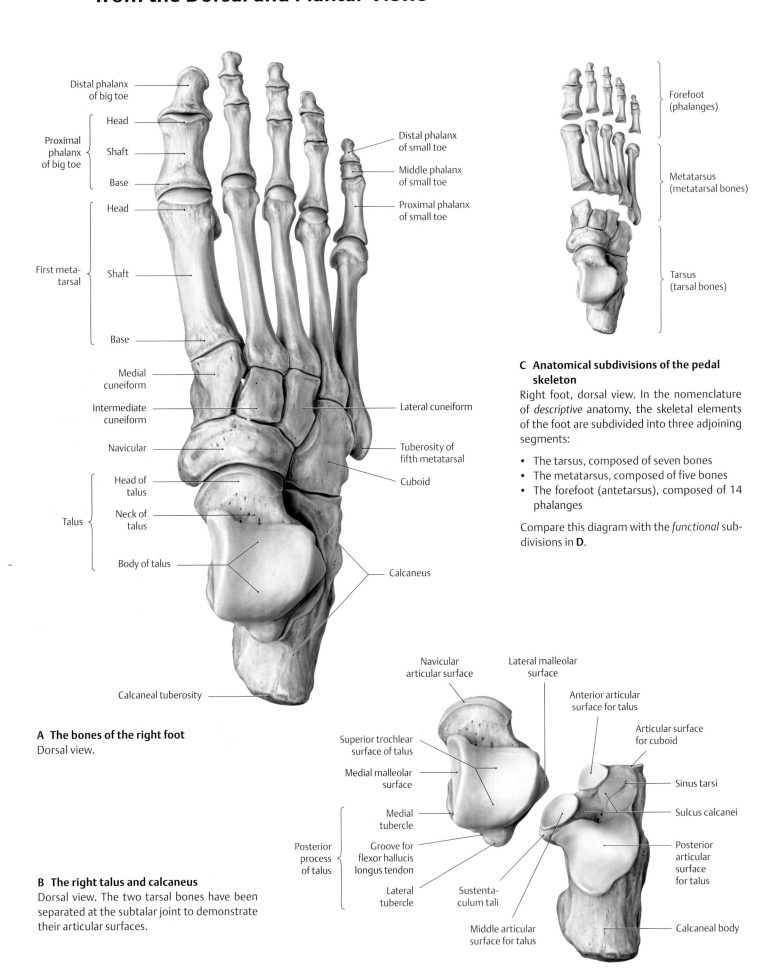

Distal phalanx of big toe

Proximal phalanx of big toe { Head / Shaft / Base

First meta-tarsal { Head / Shaft / Base

Medial cuneiform

Intermediate cuneiform

Navicular

Talus { Head of talus / Neck of talus / Body of talus

Calcaneal tuberosity

Distal phalanx of small toe

Middle phalanx of small toe

Proximal phalanx of small toe

Lateral cuneiform

Tuberosity of fifth metatarsal

Cuboid

Calcaneus

A The bones of the right foot
Dorsal view.

B The right talus and calcaneus
Dorsal view. The two tarsal bones have been separated at the subtalar joint to demonstrate their articular surfaces.

Forefoot (phalanges)

Metatarsus (metatarsal bones)

Tarsus (tarsal bones)

C Anatomical subdivisions of the pedal skeleton

Right foot, dorsal view. In the nomenclature of *descriptive* anatomy, the skeletal elements of the foot are subdivided into three adjoining segments:

- The tarsus, composed of seven bones
- The metatarsus, composed of five bones
- The forefoot (antetarsus), composed of 14 phalanges

Compare this diagram with the *functional* subdivisions in **D**.

Navicular articular surface

Lateral malleolar surface

Superior trochlear surface of talus

Medial malleolar surface

Posterior process of talus { Medial tubercle / Groove for flexor hallucis longus tendon / Lateral tubercle

Anterior articular surface for talus

Articular surface for cuboid

Sinus tarsi

Sulcus calcanei

Posterior articular surface for talus

Sustenta-culum tali

Middle articular surface for talus

Calcaneal body

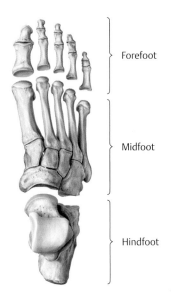

Forefoot

Midfoot

Hindfoot

D Functional subdivisions of the pedal skeleton

Right foot, dorsal view. The skeleton of the foot is often subdivided as follows based on functional and clinical criteria:

- The hindfoot (calcaneus and talus)
- The midfoot (cuboid, navicular, cuneiforms, and metatarsals)
- The forefoot (the proximal, middle and distal phalanges)

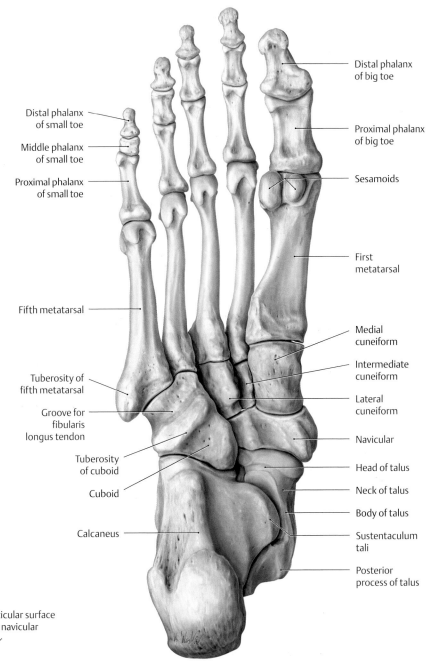

Distal phalanx of small toe

Middle phalanx of small toe

Proximal phalanx of small toe

Distal phalanx of big toe

Proximal phalanx of big toe

Sesamoids

First metatarsal

Fifth metatarsal

Tuberosity of fifth metatarsal

Groove for fibularis longus tendon

Tuberosity of cuboid

Cuboid

Calcaneus

Medial cuneiform

Intermediate cuneiform

Lateral cuneiform

Navicular

Head of talus

Neck of talus

Body of talus

Sustentaculum tali

Posterior process of talus

E The bones of the right foot
Plantar view.

Anterior articular surface for calcaneus

Articular surface for navicular

Sinus tarsi

Articular surface for cuboid

Groove for flexor hallucis longus tendon

Medial process of calcaneal tuberosity

Lateral process of calcaneal tuberosity

Calcaneal tuberosity

Middle articular surface for calcaneus

Sulcus tali

Posterior articular surface for calcaneus

Medial tubercle

Groove for flexor hallucis longus tendon

Lateral tubercle

F The right talus and calcaneus
Plantar view. The two tarsal bones have been separated at the subtalar joint to demonstrate their articular surfaces.

375

1.9 The Bones of the Foot from the Lateral and Medial Views; Accessory Tarsal Bones

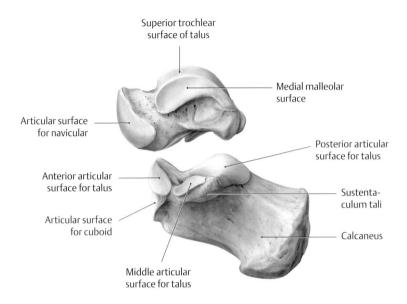

Superior trochlear
surface of talus

Medial malleolar
surface

Articular surface
for navicular

Posterior articular
surface for talus

Anterior articular
surface for talus

Sustenta-
culum tali

Articular surface
for cuboid

Calcaneus

Middle articular
surface for talus

A The right talus and calcaneus
Medial view. The two tarsal bones have been separated at the subtalar
joint to demonstrate their articular surfaces.

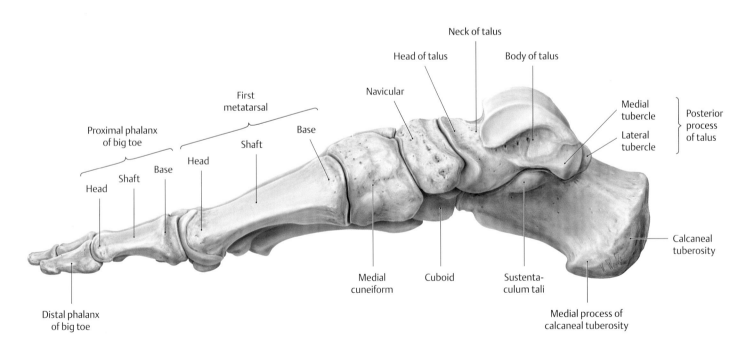

Neck of talus

Head of talus

Body of talus

First
metatarsal

Navicular

Medial
tubercle

Posterior
process
of talus

Proximal phalanx
of big toe

Base

Lateral
tubercle

Head

Shaft

Base

Head

Shaft

Base

Head

Shaft

Head

Calcaneal
tuberosity

Medial
cuneiform

Cuboid

Sustenta-
culum tali

Distal phalanx
of big toe

Medial process of
calcaneal tuberosity

B The bones of the right foot
Medial view.

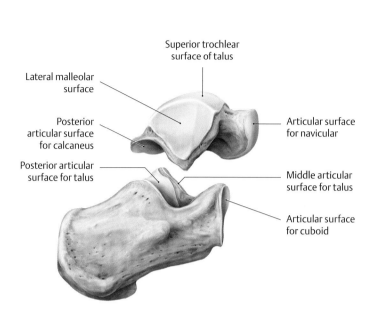

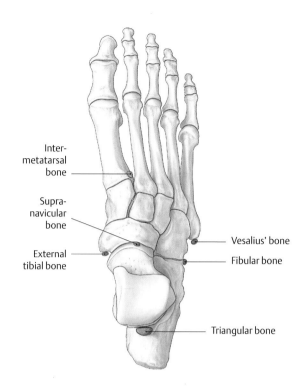

C The right talus and calcaneus
Lateral view. The two tarsal bones have been separated at the subtalar joint to demonstrate their articular surfaces.

E Accessory tarsal bones
Right foot, dorsal view. A number of accessory (inconstant) ossicles are sometimes found in the foot. While they rarely cause complaints, they do require differentiation from fractures. A clinically important accessory bone is the external tibial bone, which can be a source of discomfort when tight shoes are worn.

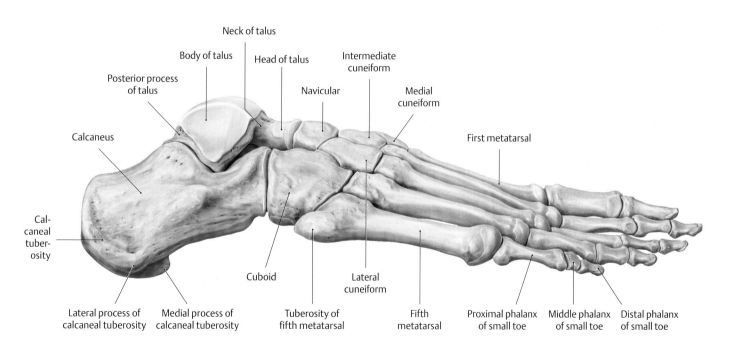

D The bones of the right foot
Lateral view.

1.10 The Hip Joint: Articulating Bones

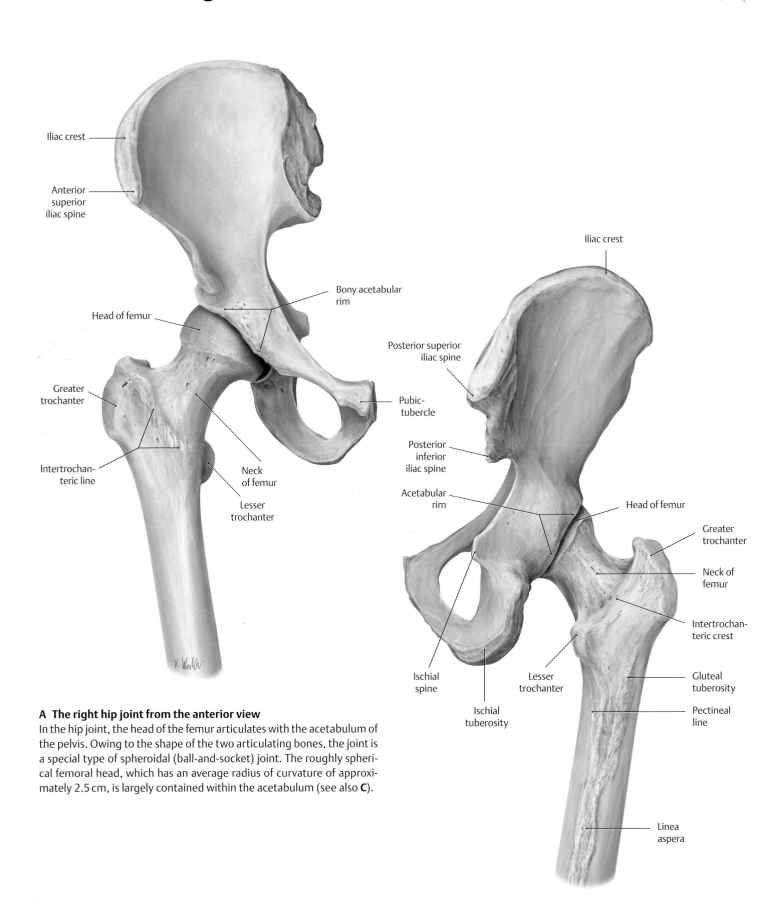

Iliac crest

Anterior superior iliac spine

Head of femur

Greater trochanter

Intertrochanteric line

Lesser trochanter

Neck of femur

Bony acetabular rim

Iliac crest

Posterior superior iliac spine

Pubic-tubercle

Posterior inferior iliac spine

Acetabular rim

Head of femur

Greater trochanter

Neck of femur

Intertrochanteric crest

Gluteal tuberosity

Pectineal line

Ischial spine

Ischial tuberosity

Lesser trochanter

Linea aspera

A The right hip joint from the anterior view
In the hip joint, the head of the femur articulates with the acetabulum of the pelvis. Owing to the shape of the two articulating bones, the joint is a special type of spheroidal (ball-and-socket) joint. The roughly spherical femoral head, which has an average radius of curvature of approximately 2.5 cm, is largely contained within the acetabulum (see also **C**).

B The right hip joint from the posterior view

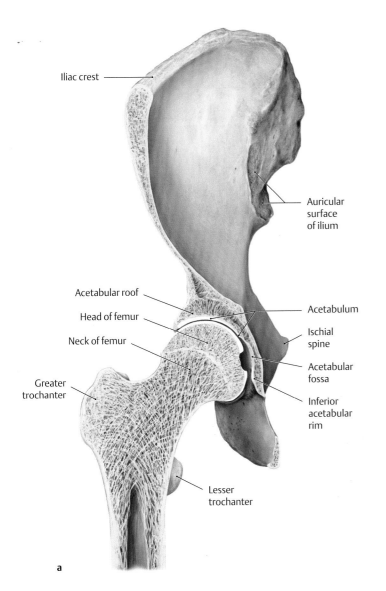

Iliac crest

Auricular
surface
of ilium

Acetabular roof

Head of femur

Neck of femur

Greater
trochanter

Acetabulum

Ischial
spine

Acetabular
fossa

Inferior
acetabular
rim

Lesser
trochanter

a

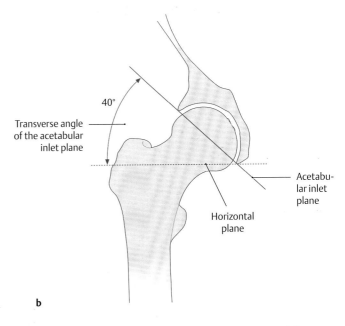

40°

Transverse angle
of the acetabular
inlet plane

Acetabu-
lar inlet
plane

Horizontal
plane

b

C Transverse angle of the acetabular inlet plane in the adult

Right hip joint, anterior view. Coronal section at the level of the acetabular fossa. The acetabular inlet plane, or bony acetabular rim, faces inferolaterally (*transverse angle*) and also anteroinferiorly (*sagittal angle*; see **D**). The inferolateral tilt of the acetabulum can be determined by drawing a line from the superior acetabular rim to the inferior acetabular rim (lowest point of the acetabular notch) and measuring the angle between that line and the true horizontal. This transverse angle normally measures approximately 51° at birth, 45° at 10 years of age, and 40° in adults (after Ullmann and Sharp). The value of the transverse angle affects several parameters, including the degree of lateral coverage of the femoral head by the acetabulum (the *center-edge angle* of Wiberg, see p. 389).

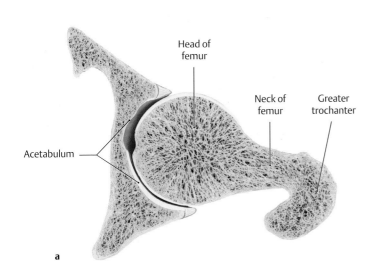

Head of
femur

Neck of
femur

Greater
trochanter

Acetabulum

a

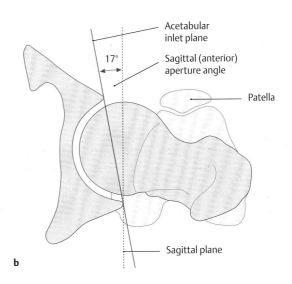

Acetabular
inlet plane

17°

Sagittal (anterior)
aperture angle

Patella

Sagittal plane

b

D Sagittal angle of the acetabular inlet plane in the adult

Right hip joint, superior view. Horizontal section through the center of the femoral head.

The bony acetabular rim is angled anteroinferiorly relative to the sagittal plane (compare this with the horizontal plane in **C**). This aperture angle measures approximately 7° at birth and increases to 17° by adulthood (after Chassard and Lapine).

1.11 The Ligaments of the Hip Joint: Stabilization of the Femoral Head

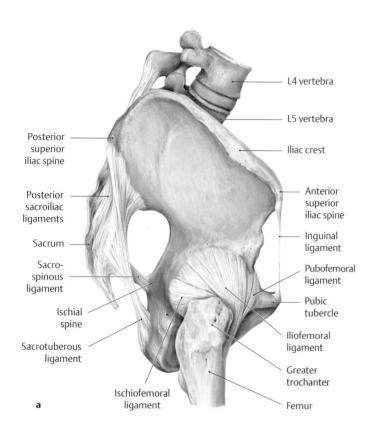

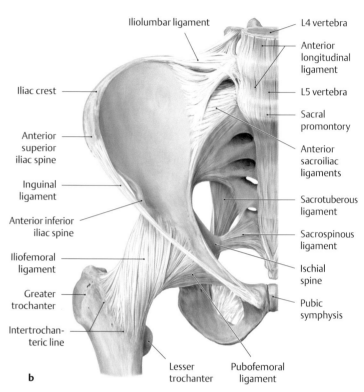

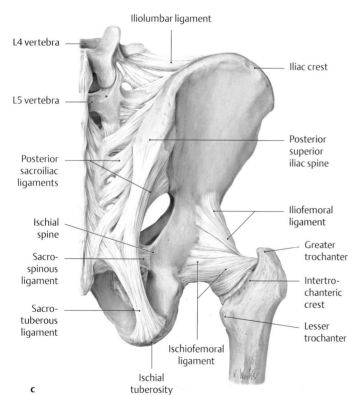

A The ligaments of the right hip joint

a Lateral view, **b** anterior view, **c** posterior view.

The strongest of the three ligaments, the iliofemoral ligament, arises from the anterior inferior iliac spine and fans out at the front of the hip, attaching along the intertrochanteric line (see **b**). With a tensile strength greater than 350 N, it is the most powerful ligament in the human body and provides an important constraint for the hip joint: It keeps the pelvis from tilting posteriorly in upright stance, without the need for muscular effort. It also limits adduction of the extended limb (particularly the lateral elements of the ligament) and it stabilizes the pelvis on the stance side during gait, i.e., it acts with the small gluteal muscles to keep the pelvis from tilting toward the swing side.

B The ligaments of the hip joint

- Iliofemoral ligament
- Pubofemoral ligament
- Ischiofemoral ligament
- Zona orbicularis (anular ligament)*
- Ligamentum teres (of the femoral head)**

* Not visible externally, it encircles the femoral neck like a button-hole.

** Has no mechanical function, but transmits vessels that supply the femoral head (see also p. 383).

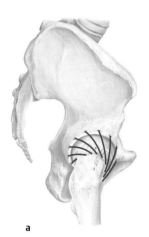
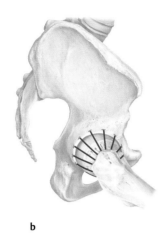
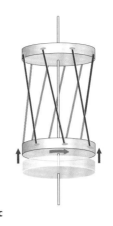
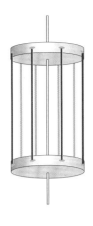

a   **b**   **c**   **d**

C Actions of the ligaments as a function of joint position
a Right hip joint in extension, lateral view. The capsular ligaments of the hip joint (see facing page) form a ringlike collar that encircles the femoral neck. When the hip is extended, these ligaments become twisted upon themselves (as shown here), pushing the femoral head more firmly into the acetabulum (joint-stabilizing function of the ligaments).
b Right hip joint in flexion, lateral view. During flexion (anteversion), the ligament fibers are lax and press the femoral head less firmly into the acetabulum, allowing a greater degree of femoral mobility.

c, d The twisting mechanism of the capsular ligaments can be represented by a model consisting of two disks interconnected by parallel bands. The situation in **c** represents the position of the ligaments when the hip joint is extended. When one of the two disks rotates (blue arrow), the bands become twisted and draw the two disks closer together (red arrows). Panel **d** models the situation in the flexed hip. The ligaments are no longer twisted, and so the distance between the two disks is increased (after Kapandji).

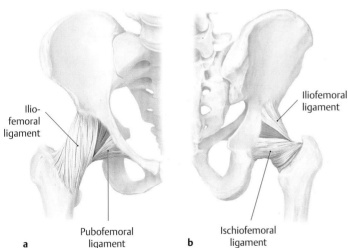

Ilio-femoral ligament — Iliofemoral ligament — Pubofemoral ligament — Ischiofemoral ligament

a   **b**

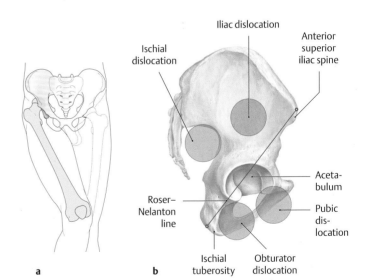

Iliac dislocation — Ischial dislocation — Anterior superior iliac spine — Roser–Nelanton line — Aceta-bulum — Pubic dis-location — Ischial tuberosity — Obturator dislocation

a   **b**

D Weak spots in the capsule of the right hip joint
a Anterior view, **b** posterior view.
There are weak spots in the joint capsule (color-shaded areas) located between the ligaments that strengthen the fibrous membrane (see **A**). External trauma may cause the femoral head to dislocate from the acetabulum at these sites (see **E**).
The combination of great ligament strength and the close congruity of the femoral head in the acetabulum make the hip joint very stable, and dislocations relatively rare. The situation is different, however, following a hip replacement arthroplasty. The hip joint ligaments must be at least partially divided to implant the prosthesis, and the risk of dislocation is markedly increased.

E Traumatic dislocation of the hip
a It is most common for the femoral head to dislocate upward and backward from the acetabulum (iliac dislocation) between the iliofemoral ligament and ischiofemoral ligament. Typically this is caused by a fall from a great height, a motor vehicle accident (front-end collision), etc. In this type of dislocation the leg assumes a position of adduction and slight internal rotation.
b Lateral view. Position of the femoral head in various types of dislocation. The greater trochanter may be above or below the Roser–Nélanton line.

381

1.12 The Ligaments of the Hip Joint: Nutrition of the Femoral Head

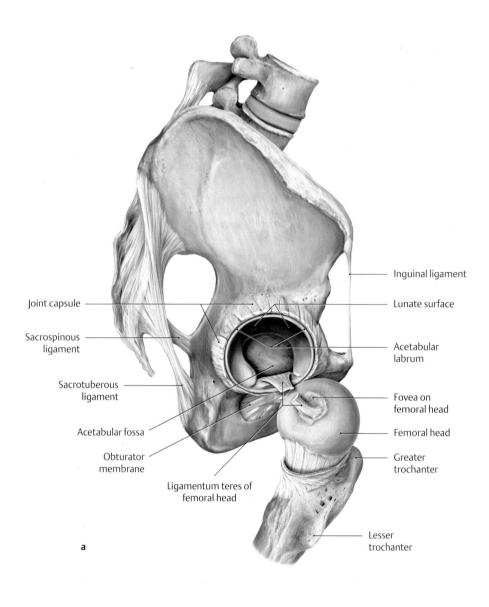

a

A The ligaments of the right hip joint

a Lateral view. The joint capsule has been divided at the level of the acetabular labrum and the femoral head has been dislocated to expose the divided *ligamentum teres* of the femoral head. This ligament transmits important nutrient blood vessels for the femoral head.

b Anterior view. The fibrous membrane of the joint capsule has been removed at the level of the femoral neck to show the conformation of the synovial membrane. This membrane extends laterally from the acetabular rim and, about 1 cm proximal to the attachment of the fibrous membrane, it is reflected onto the femoral neck within the joint cavity. It continues up the femoral neck to the chondro-osseous junction of the femoral head (see also the coronal section in **C**).

c Posterior view.

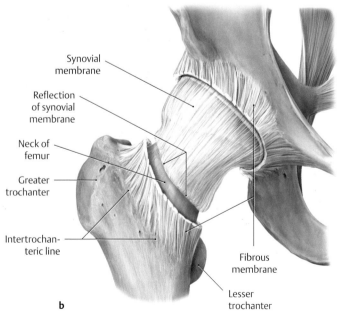

b

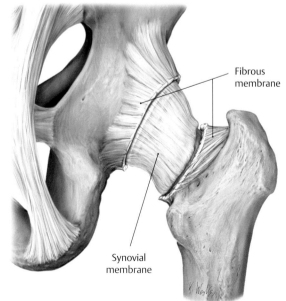

c

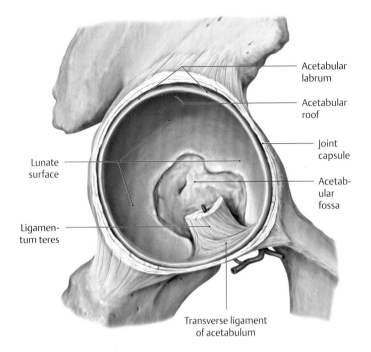

B The acetabulum of the right hip joint with the femoral head removed

Lateral view. The cartilage-covered articular surface of the acetabulum is crescent-shaped (lunate surface) and is broadest and thickest over the acetabular roof. The lunate surface is bounded externally by the slightly protruding bony rim of the acetabulum, which is extended by a lip (the acetabular labrum) composed of tough connective tissue and fibrocartilage. The cartilaginous articular surface lines much of the acetabular fossa, which is occupied by loose, fibrofatty tissue and is bounded inferiorly by the transverse acetabular ligament in the area of the acetabular notch (not visible here). The ligamentum teres, which has been sectioned in the drawing, transmits blood vessels that nourish the femoral head (see **C**).

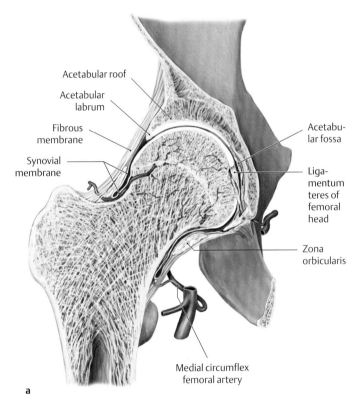

a

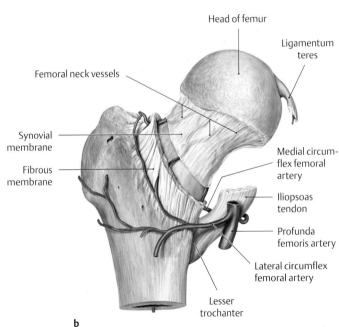

b

C The blood supply to the femoral head

a Coronal section through the right hip joint, anterior view.
b Course of the femoral neck vessels in relation to the joint capsule (right femur, anterior view).

The femoral head derives its blood supply from the lateral and medial circumflex femoral arteries and the artery of the ligamentum teres,

which branches from the obturator artery (see p. 490). If the anastomoses between the vessels of the ligamentum teres and the femoral neck vessels are absent or deficient due to the avulsion of blood vessels caused by a dislocation or femoral neck fracture, the bony tissue in the head of the femur may become necrotic (avascular necrosis of the femoral head).

383

1.13 Cross-Sectional Anatomy of the Hip Joint

A knowledge of cross-sectional anatomy is important for the interpretation of MR images of the hip joint. Because the bones of the hip joint are not accessible to direct examination by palpation, the examiner must be familiar with the relationships of the muscles to the hip joint.

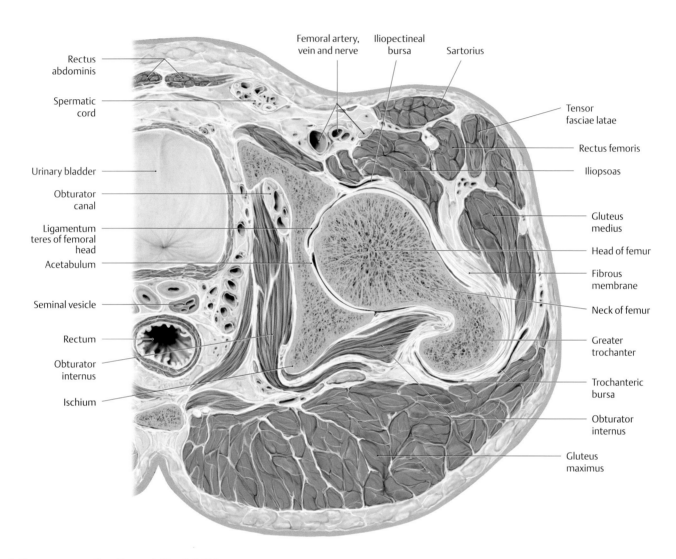

A Transverse section through the right hip joint
Superior view (drawing based on a specimen from the Anatomical Collection of Kiel University).

B MRI of the hip region: axial (transverse) T1-weighted SE image at the level of the femoral neck (from Vahlensieck and Reiser: MRT des Bewegungsapparates, 2nd ed. Thieme, Stuttgart 2001).
Note: The bursae illustrated in **A** are not seen here because bursae always have low signal intensity on T1-weighted MR images, making them very difficult to distinguish from the musculature, which has similar signal intensity.

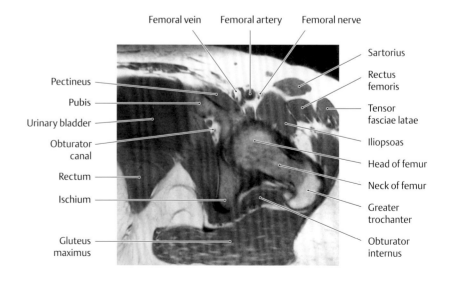

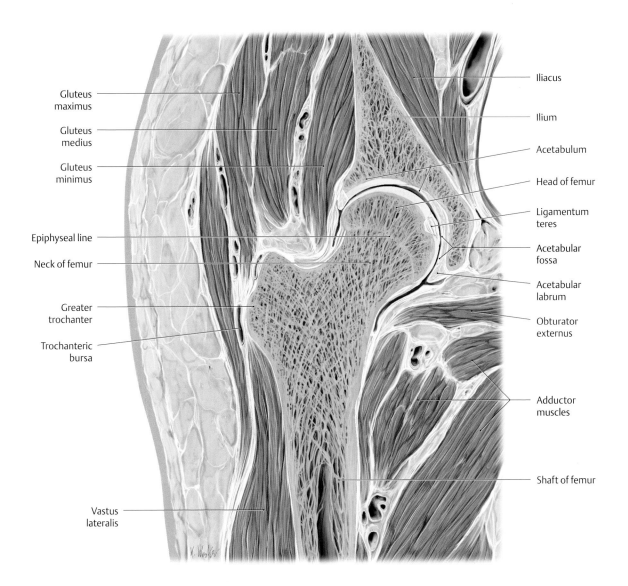

Gluteus maximus

Gluteus medius

Gluteus minimus

Epiphyseal line

Neck of femur

Greater trochanter

Trochanteric bursa

Vastus lateralis

Iliacus

Ilium

Acetabulum

Head of femur

Ligamentum teres

Acetabular fossa

Acetabular labrum

Obturator externus

Adductor muscles

Shaft of femur

C Coronal section through the right hip joint
Anterior view (drawing based on a specimen from the Anatomical Collection of Kiel University).

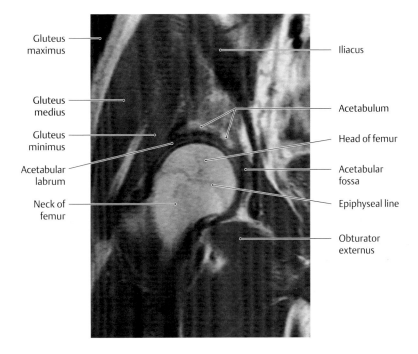

Gluteus maximus

Gluteus medius

Gluteus minimus

Acetabular labrum

Neck of femur

Iliacus

Acetabulum

Head of femur

Acetabular fossa

Epiphyseal line

Obturator externus

D MRI of the hip region: coronal T1-weighted SE image at the level of the acetabular fossa (from Vahlensieck and Reiser: MRT des Bewegungsapparates, 2nd ed. Thieme, Stuttgart 2001).

385

1.14 The Movements and Biomechanics of the Hip Joint

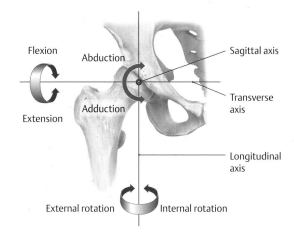

Flexion, Abduction, Sagittal axis, Transverse axis, Extension, Adduction, Longitudinal axis, External rotation, Internal rotation

A The axes of motion in the hip joint
Right hip joint, anterior view. As a spheroidal joint, the hip has three principal axes of motion, all of which pass through the center of the femoral head (the rotational center of the hip) and are mutually perpendicular. Accordingly, the joint has three degrees of freedom allowing movement in six principal directions:

1. Transverse axis: flexion (anteversion) and extension (retroversion)
2. Sagittal axis: abduction and adduction
3. Longitudinal axis: internal rotation and external rotation

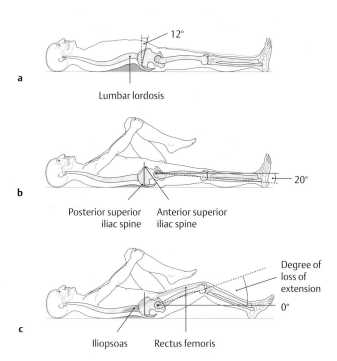

a 12° Lumbar lordosis

b 20° Posterior superior iliac spine, Anterior superior iliac spine

c Degree of loss of extension 0°, Iliopsoas, Rectus femoris

B Range of extension of the right hip joint determined with the Thomas maneuver
The Thomas maneuver is used to measure the range of hip extension while the patient lies supine on a hard surface.

a Starting position with a slight degree of anterior pelvic tilt (approximately 12°). In this position it cannot be determined whether or not there is a flexion contraction of the hip joint. This is because the patient can compensate for any limitation of extension by increasing lumbar lordosis (arching the lower back to hyperlordosis) and increasing the degree of anterior pelvic tilt.

b Pelvic tilt can be temporarily eliminated by drawing the opposite hip joint (in this case the left hip) into a position of maximum flexion. If the right thigh remains flat on the table, the right hip joint will be in approximately 20° of extension (*normal extension*).

c If hip extension is limited (e.g., due to a shortened rectus femoris or iliopsoas muscle) and the opposite (left) hip is placed in maximum flexion, the femur of the affected leg will be raised from the table by an amount equal to the loss of extension. Increased lumbar lordosis is generally present when hip extension is limited and is easily detected clinically by palpating the lower back.

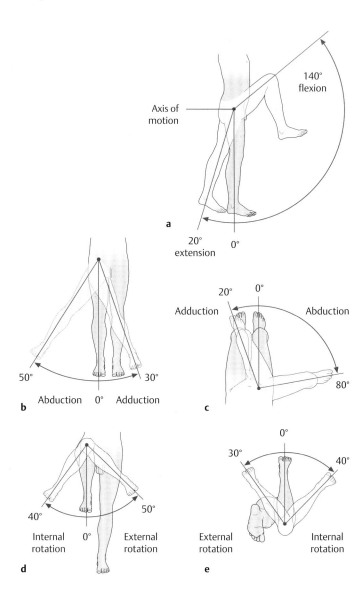

a 140° flexion, Axis of motion, 20° extension, 0°

b Abduction 50°, Adduction 30°, Abduction 0° Adduction

c Adduction 20°, Abduction 0°, 80°

d Internal rotation 40°, External rotation 50°, 0°

e External rotation 30°, Internal rotation 40°, 0°

C Range of motion of the hip joint from the neutral (zero-degree) position (0°) (after Debrunner)
The range of motion of the hip joint is measured using the neutral-zero method (see p. 39).

a Range of flexion/extension.
b Range of abduction/adduction with the hip extended.
c Range of abduction/adduction with the hip flexed 90°.
d Range of internal rotation/external rotation with the hip flexed 90°.
e Range of internal rotation/external rotation in the prone position with the hip extended (when measuring rotation, the examiner uses the leg, flexed 90°, as a pointer to determine the range of motion).

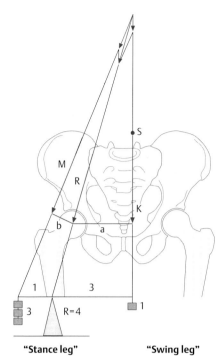

"Stance leg"   "Swing leg"

D Loads on the right hip joint during the stance phase of gait
Anterior view. In one-legged stance or during the stance phase of gait, the partial-body center of gravity (S) is shifted toward the opposite swing side so that the partial body weight (K) acts along a line that runs medial to the hip joint. This eccentric load produces a rotational moment, or *torque*, which tends to tilt the part of the body above the joint toward the side of the swing leg. To maintain stable balance, a counterforce must be applied (e.g., by muscles and ligaments) that is sufficient to counteract the torque. In the hip joint, this force is supplied mainly by the muscular force (M) of the hip abductors (gluteus medius and minimus). This force, however, acts upon the hip joint with a lever arm that is only about one-third the lever arm of the partial body weight, i.e., the ratio of the lever arm of the muscular force (b) to that of the partial body weight (a) is approximately 1:3. Consequently, the *muscular force* needed to stabilize the hip *in one-legged stance* is equal to about three times the body weight. This means that the *compressive force* that the hip joint must be able to withstand (e.g., *during walking*) is approximately four times greater than the partial body weight K (according to Pauwels). As a result, the hip is constantly subjected to extreme loads which predispose the joint to osteoarthritic changes.

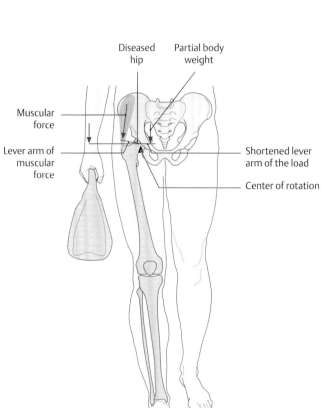

Diseased hip
Partial body weight
Muscular force
Lever arm of muscular force
Shortened lever arm of the load
Center of rotation

a

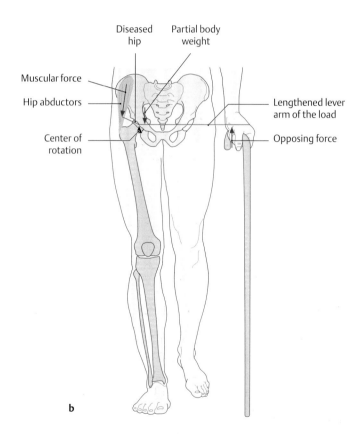

Diseased hip
Partial body weight
Muscular force
Hip abductors
Lengthened lever arm of the load
Center of rotation
Opposing force

b

E Reducing the stresses on an osteoarthritic right hip
Anterior view. In patients with advanced osteoarthritis of the hip, various measures can be taken to alleviate the stresses, and thus the pain, on the affected side.

a Shift the partial-body center of gravity (see above) toward the affected side. One way to do this is by carrying a shopping bag *on the affected right side*, as shown here. This moves the partial-body center of gravity closer to the center of the femoral head, thereby *shortening* the lever arm of the load (in this case the partial body weight)

and also reducing the torque generated by the partial body weight. The same effect is produced by adopting a *Duchenne limp*—an unconscious response in which the patient leans over the affected side with the upper body during the stance phase of gait (see also p. 476).

b Use a cane *on the unaffected (left) side*. While this *lengthens* the lever arm of the load (the partial body weight), it also provides a force (the cane) which counteracts the body load at the end of that lever arm. This reduces the torque generated by the load (as in **a**).

1.15 The Development of the Hip Joint

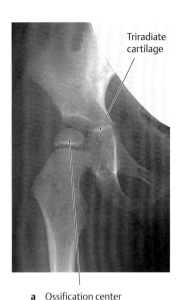
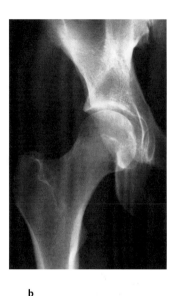

a Ossification center   **b**

A Radiographic appearance of the right hip joint
Anteroposterior projection.

a Boy, 2 years of age (original film from the Department of Diagnostic Radiology, Schleswig-Holstein University Hospital, Kiel Campus, Prof. S. Müller-Hülsbeck, M.D.).
Note: The ossification center for the femoral head is already visible.
b Man 25 years of age (from Möller and Reif: *Pocket Atlas of Radiographic Anatomy*, 2nd ed. Thieme, Stuttgart 2000).

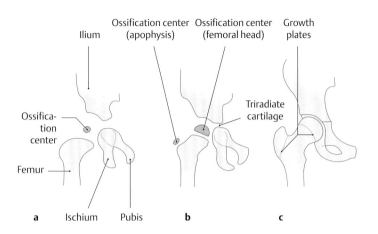

a Ischium   Pubis   **b**   **c**

B Stages in the radiographic development of the hip joint
Schematic representations of AP radiographs taken at various stages in the development of the right hip joint. The ossification centers are indicated by dark shading.

a The ossification center for the femoral head can be identified at 6 months of age.
b Ossification centers for the femoral head and greater trochanter are visible at 4 years of age.
c At 15 years of age, the growth plates have not yet fused.

The anatomical differentiation of all structures that comprise the hip joint is largely complete by the 12th week of development (crown–rump length 80 mm). Whereas ossification of the acetabulum begins between the third and sixth months of fetal development, the ossification center for the capital femoral epiphysis (femoral head) does not appear until about 5–6 months after birth. The ossification center for the apophysis of the greater trochanter appears during the fourth year of life. Fusion of the growth plates takes place between 16 and 18 years of age in the proximal femur and at about 15 years of age in the triradiate cartilage.

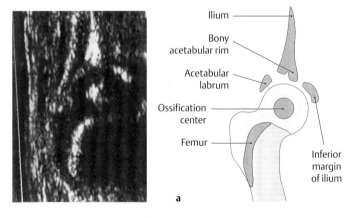
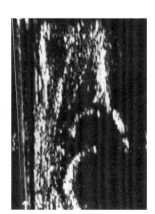
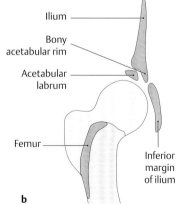

a   **b**

C Ultrasound evaluation of the infant hip (from Niethard and Pfeil: *Orthopädie*. 4th ed. Thieme, Stuttgart 2003).
a Normal hip joint in a 5-month-old child.
b Hip dislocation (type IV) in a 3-month-old child.

Ultrasonography is the most important imaging method for screening the infant hip, demonstrating potential morphological changes during the first year of life without exposure to ionizing radiation. The child is examined in the lateral decubitus position (on his or her side, other hip on the examination table) with the ultrasound transducer placed

longitudinally over the hip joint and perpendicular to the skin. The key landmark is the superior acetabular rim, i.e., the bony and cartilaginous roof of the acetabulum (see **D**). Infant hips are classified into four types based on their sonographic features:

- Type I   Normal hip
- Type II   Physiologically immature hip
- Type III   Subluxated hip
- Type IV   Dislocated hip

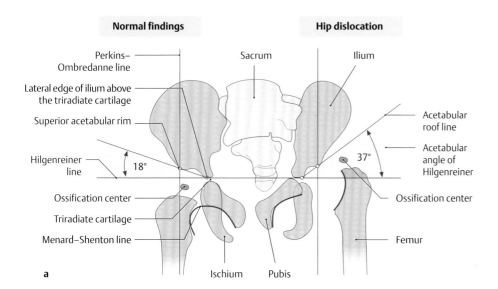

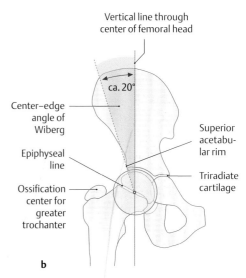

D Radiographic evaluation of the pediatric hip

Schematic representations of AP pelvic radiographs. Radiographic evaluation of the infant hip is feasible after three months of age, by which time there has been sufficient ossification of the joint. Both hips should always be imaged on the same radiograph.

a Normal findings (left half of figure) contrasted with findings in congenital hip dislocation (right half of figure) in a two-year-old child. The following standard reference lines are used in the radiographic analysis of the infant hip:

- *Hilgenreiner line:* connects the inferolateral edge of the ilium above the triradiate cartilage on both sides.
- *Perkins–Ombredanne line:* drawn from the most lateral edge of the acetabular roof, perpendicular to the Hilgenreiner line.
- *Menard–Shenton line:* curved line drawn from the superior border of the obturator foramen along the medial border of the femoral neck.
- *Acetabular angle of Hilgenreiner (AC angle):* angle formed by the intersection of the Hilgenreiner line and a line connecting the

superior acetabular rim with the lowest part of the ilium at the triradiate cartilage (see p. 365). This angle measures approximately 35° at birth, approximately 25° at 1 year of age, and should be less than 10° by 15 years of age.

Typically the acetabular angle of Hilgenreiner is increased on the affected (left) side while the center-edge angle of Wiberg (see below) is decreased. Additionally, there is a discontinuity in the Menard–Shenton line and the Perkins–Ombredanne line runs medial to the femoral shaft.

b Evaluation of lateral femoral head coverage based on the center-edge angle of Wiberg (drawing of a radiograph of the right hip in a 5-year-old child). The angle is formed by a vertical line through the center of the femoral head (within the future epiphyseal line) and a line drawn from the center of the femoral head to the superior acetabular rim. The center–edge angle should not be less than 10° between 1 and 4 years of age, and it should be in the range of 15–20° at 5 years of age.

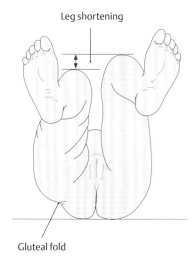

E Clinical examination of congenital dysplasia and dislocation of the hip

Hip dysplasia is characterized by an abnormal development of the acetabulum (acetabular dysplasia) in which the steep, flattened acetabular roof provides insufficient coverage for the femoral head (see also **D**). The principal complication is dislocation of the hip, since the femoral head is poorly contained in the dysplastic acetabulum and may be displaced upward and backward as a result of muscular traction or external loads. The *etiology* of hip dysplasia and dislocation is related to endogenous factors (familial disposition, maternal hormone status) as well as exogenous factors. The overall *incidence* of acetabular dysplasia in Germany is 2–4 %, while the incidence of hip

dislocation is 0.2 % (with a 7 : 1 ratio of girls to boys). The following *clinical signs* may direct attention to a dysplastic or dislocated hip:

- Instability of the hip joint: paucity of kicking activity or a positive Ortolani click caused by subluxation of the femoral head. The Ortolani test requires a very experienced examiner. While still considered part of the clinical examination, it is performed less often today owing to the availability of ultrasound.
- Leg shortening with asymmetry of the posterior leg folds and gluteal folds.
- Limitation of abduction due to increased reflex tension from the hip adductors.

389

1.16 The Knee Joint: Articulating Bones

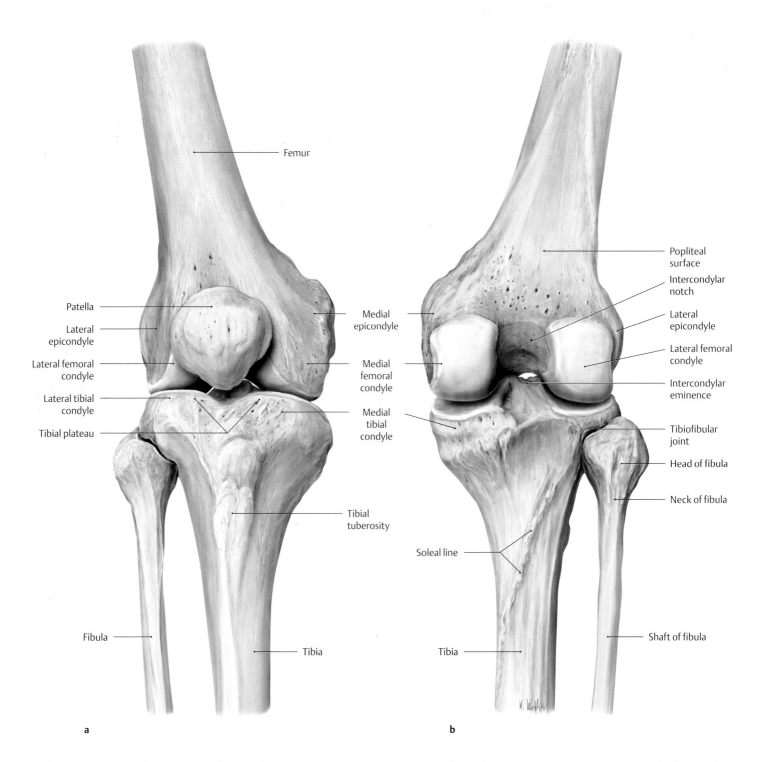

a

b

A The right knee joint from the anterior view (a) and posterior view (b)

Three bones articulate at the knee joint: the femur, tibia, and patella. The femur and tibia form the *femorotibial joint*, while the femur and patella form the *femoropatellar joint*. Both joints are contained within a com-

mon capsule and have communicating articular cavities (see p. 400). Contrasting with the elbow joint, where the forearm bones articulate with the humerus, the fibula is *not* included in the knee joint. It forms a separate, rigid articulation with the tibia called the *tibiofibular joint*.

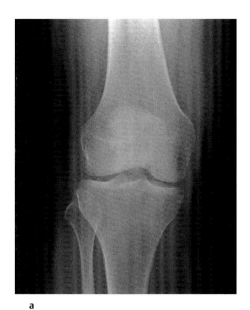

a

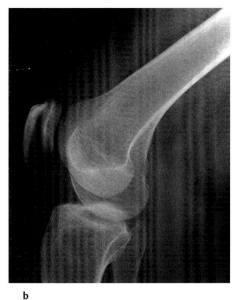

b

B The knee joint

Right knee joint: **a** anteroposterior projection, **b** lateral projection (original films from the Department of Diagnostic Radiology, Schleswig-Holstein University Hospital, Kiel Campus, Prof. S. Müller-Hülsbeck, M.D.).

There are three standard radiographic views of the knee that demonstrate the joint in three planes: anteroposterior, lateral, and tangential. The *anteroposterior view* is particularly useful for evaluating the width of the joint space and the contours of the tibial plateau. *Lateral views* are good for evaluating the shape of the femoral condyles and the height of the patella. The *tangential (sunrise) view* is used mainly for examining the femoropatellar joint and evaluating the position of the patella in the femoral trochlea (see **C**).

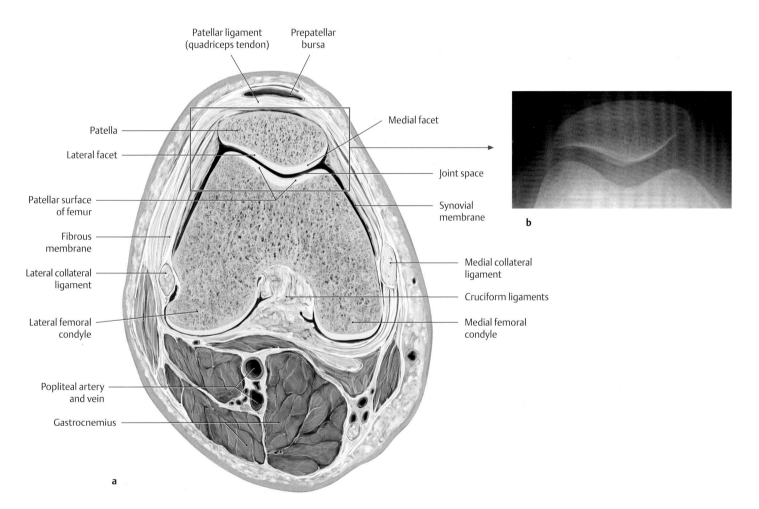

Patellar ligament (quadriceps tendon)
Prepatellar bursa
Patella
Lateral facet
Patellar surface of femur
Fibrous membrane
Lateral collateral ligament
Lateral femoral condyle
Popliteal artery and vein
Gastrocnemius
Medial facet
Joint space
Synovial membrane
Medial collateral ligament
Cruciform ligaments
Medial femoral condyle

a

b

C The femoropatellar joint

a Transverse section at the level of the femoropatellar joint. Right knee joint in slight flexion, distal view (drawn from a specimen in the Anatomical Collection of Kiel University).

b Tangential radiographic view of the patella and femoral trochlea ("sunrise" view of the right knee joint in 60° flexion with the beam parallel to the posterior patellar surface). This view is excel-

lent for evaluating the articular surface of the patella and the femoral trochlea. The radiographic "joint space" appears particularly wide owing to the relatively thick articular cartilage in this region (articular cartilage is not visible on radiographs). (Original film from the Department of Diagnostic Radiology, Schleswig-Holstein University Hospital, Kiel Campus, Prof. S. Müller-Hülsbeck, M.D.)

391

1.17 The Ligaments of the Knee Joint: An Overview

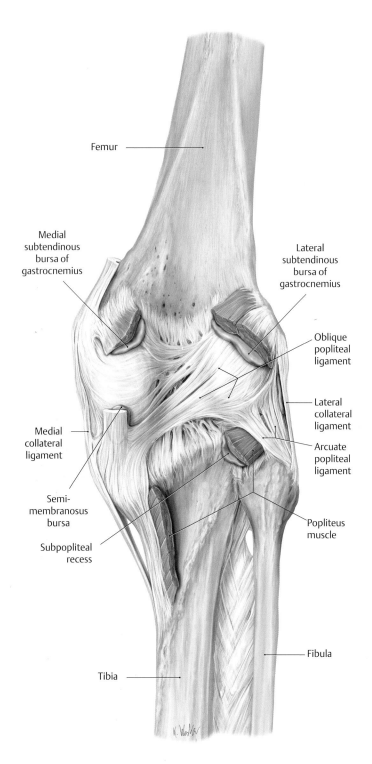

Femur

Medial subtendinous bursa of gastrocnemius

Lateral subtendinous bursa of gastrocnemius

Oblique popliteal ligament

Medial collateral ligament

Lateral collateral ligament

Arcuate popliteal ligament

Semi-membranosus bursa

Subpopliteal recess

Popliteus muscle

Fibula

Tibia

A The capsule, ligaments, and periarticular bursae of the popliteal fossa

Right knee, posterior view. Besides the ligaments that reinforce the joint capsule (the oblique popliteal ligament and arcuate popliteal ligament), the capsule is also strengthened posteriorly by the tendinous attachments of the muscles in the popliteal region. There are several sites where the joint cavity communicates with periarticular bursae—these include the subpopliteal recess, the semimembranosus bursa, and the medial subtendinous bursa of the gastrocnemius.

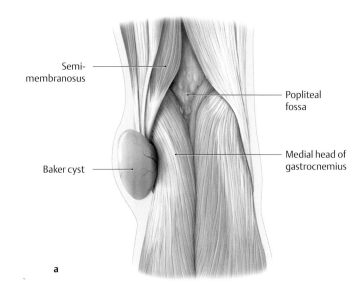

Semi-membranosus

Popliteal fossa

Medial head of gastrocnemius

Baker cyst

a

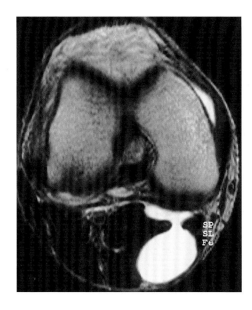

b

B Gastrocnemio-semimembranosus bursa ("Baker cyst") in the popliteal region

a Depiction of a Baker cyst in the right popliteal fossa. A painful swelling behind the knee may be caused by a cystic outpouching of the joint capsule ("synovial popliteal cyst"). This frequently results from a joint effusion (e.g., in rheumatoid arthritis) causing a rise of intra-articular pressure. A common *Baker cyst* is a cystic protrusion occurring in the medial part of the popliteal fossa between the semimembranosus tendon and the medial head of gastrocnemius at the level of the posteromedial femoral condyle (gastrocnemio-semimembranosus bursa = communication between the semimembranosus bursa and the medial subtendinous bursa of the gastrocnemius).

b Axial MR image of a knee with a Baker cyst. The cystic mass in the popliteal fossa and its communication with the joint cavity appear as conspicuous areas of high signal intensity in the T2-weighted image (from Vahlensieck and Reiser: MRT des Bewegungsapparates, 2nd ed. Thieme, Stuttgart 2001).

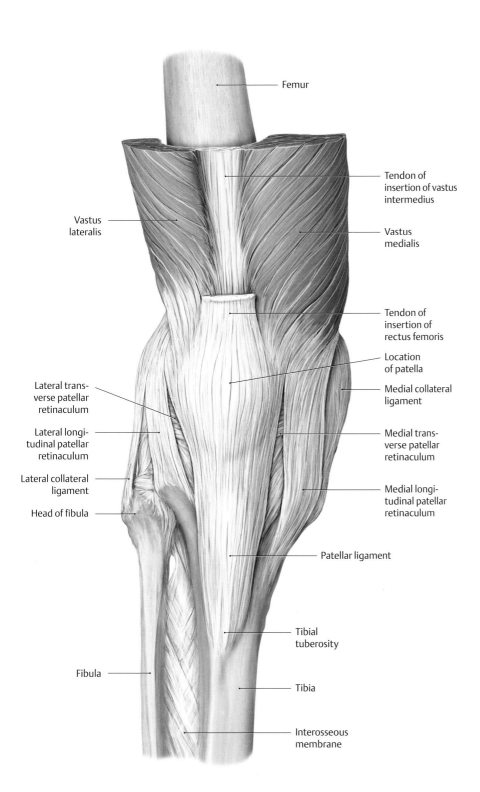

Femur

Tendon of insertion of vastus intermedius

Vastus lateralis

Vastus medialis

Tendon of insertion of rectus femoris

Location of patella

Lateral transverse patellar retinaculum

Medial collateral ligament

Lateral longitudinal patellar retinaculum

Medial transverse patellar retinaculum

Lateral collateral ligament

Medial longitudinal patellar retinaculum

Head of fibula

Patellar ligament

Tibial tuberosity

Fibula

Tibia

Interosseous membrane

C The anterior and lateral capsule and ligaments of the right knee joint

Anterior view. The capsule and ligaments at the front of the knee serve mainly to stabilize the patella. The key stabilizers for this purpose are the tendons of insertion of rectus femoris and of vastus medialis and lateralis, the longitudinal and transverse patellar retinacula, and, at a deeper level, the meniscopatellar ligaments.

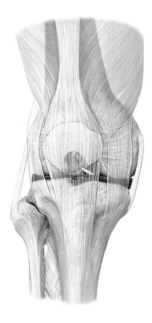

D Location of the cruciform ligaments and menisci in the knee joint

Anterior view of the right knee, in which the capsule and patella are shown in light shading. The cruciform ligaments are colored dark blue, the menisci red.

E Overview of the ligaments of the knee joint

Because its articulating bony surfaces are not closely apposed over a large area, the knee must rely upon a group of strong and extensive ligaments for stability. These ligaments of the knee joint can be segregated into two groups, extrinsic and intrinsic.

Extrinsic ligaments
• Anterior side – Patellar ligament – Medial longitudinal patellar retinaculum – Lateral longitudinal patellar retinaculum – Medial transverse patellar retinaculum – Lateral transverse patellar retinaculum • Medial and lateral sides – Medial collateral ligament (tibial collateral ligament) – Lateral collateral ligament (fibular collateral ligament) • Posterior side – Oblique popliteal ligament – Arcuate popliteal ligament

Intrinsic ligaments
– Anterior cruciform ligament – Posterior cruciform ligament – Transverse ligament of the knee – Posterior meniscofemoral ligament

393

1.18 The Knee Joint: The Cruciform and Collateral Ligaments

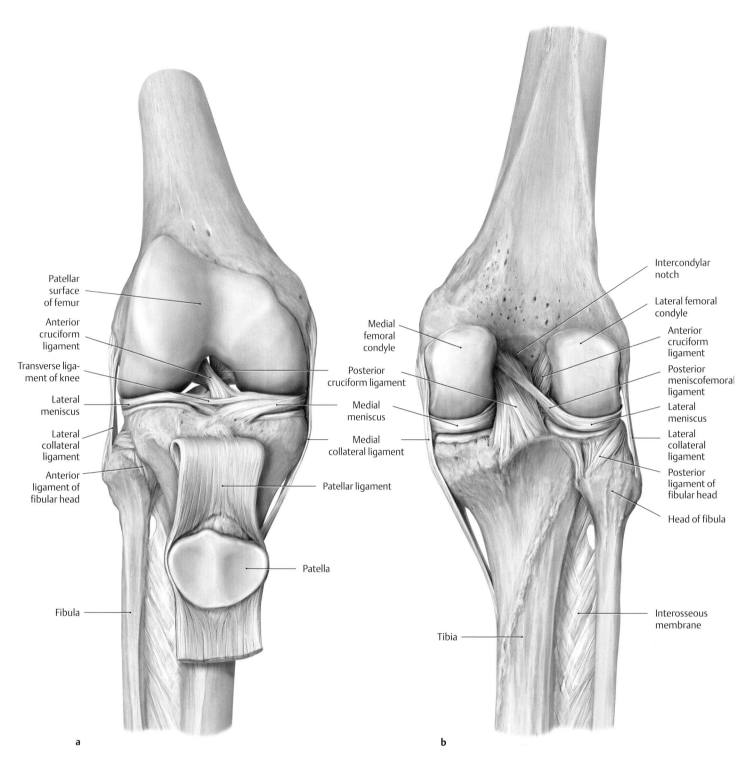

Patellar surface of femur

Anterior cruciform ligament

Transverse ligament of knee

Lateral meniscus

Lateral collateral ligament

Anterior ligament of fibular head

Fibula

Medial femoral condyle

Posterior cruciform ligament

Medial meniscus

Medial collateral ligament

Patellar ligament

Patella

Intercondylar notch

Lateral femoral condyle

Anterior cruciform ligament

Posterior meniscofemoral ligament

Lateral meniscus

Lateral collateral ligament

Posterior ligament of fibular head

Head of fibula

Interosseous membrane

Tibia

a

b

A The cruciform ligaments of the right knee joint

a Anterior view. The patellar ligament has been reflected downward with the attached patella.

b Posterior view.

The cruciform ligaments of the knee stretch between the anterior and posterior intercondylar areas of the tibia (not visible here; see p. 396) and the intercondylar notch of the femur.

- The anterior cruciform ligament runs from the anterior intercondylar area of the tibia to the medial surface of the lateral femoral condyle.

- The posterior cruciform ligament is thicker than the anterior ligament and runs approximately at right angles to it, passing from the posterior intercondylar area to the lateral surface of the medial femoral condyle.

The cruciform ligaments keep the articular surfaces of the femur and tibia in contact while stabilizing the knee joint primarily in the sagittal plane. Some portions of the cruciform ligaments are taut in every position of the joint (see p. 398).

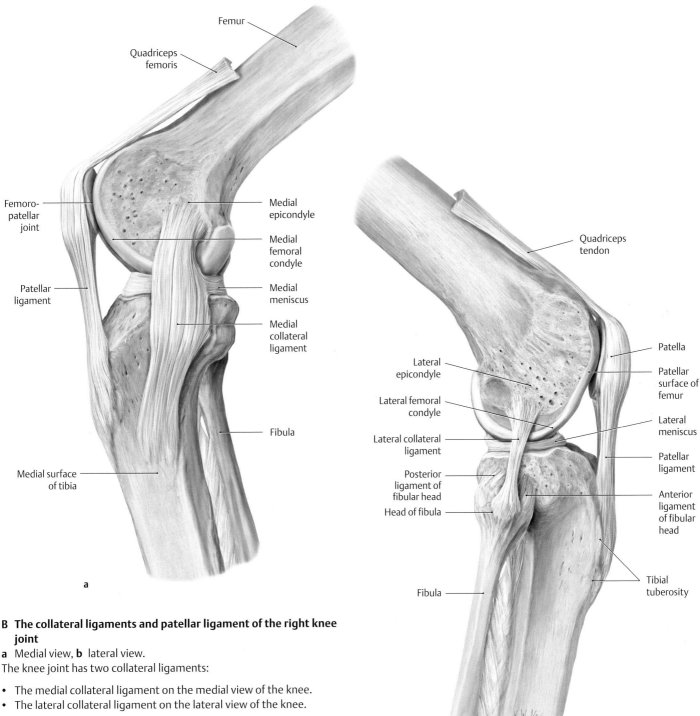

a

b

B The collateral ligaments and patellar ligament of the right knee joint

a Medial view, **b** lateral view.

The knee joint has two collateral ligaments:

- The medial collateral ligament on the medial view of the knee.
- The lateral collateral ligament on the lateral view of the knee.

The *medial collateral ligament* (tibial collateral ligament) is the broader of the two ligaments. It runs obliquely downward and forward from the medial epicondyle of the femur to the medial surface of the upper tibia approximately 7–8 cm below the tibial plateau. The *lateral collateral ligament* (fibular collateral ligament) is a round cord that runs obliquely downward and backward from the lateral epicondyle of the femur to the head of the fibula. Both of the collateral ligaments are taut when the knee is in *extension* (see **A**). When the knee is in *flexion*, the radius of curvature is decreased and the origins and insertions of the collateral ligaments move closer together, causing the ligaments to become lax. Both collateral ligaments stabilize the knee joint in the coronal plane. Thus, damage or rupture of these ligaments can be diagnosed by examining the mediolateral stability of the knee and the extent of medial and lateral opening of the joint space with manipulation.

Note the different relationship of each collateral ligament to the joint capsule and associated meniscus: The *medial* collateral ligament is firmly attached both to the capsule and the medial meniscus, whereas the *lateral* collateral ligament has no direct contact with the capsule or the lateral meniscus. As a result, the medial meniscus is less mobile than the lateral meniscus and is thus far more susceptible to injury (see also p. 397).

1.19 The Knee Joint: The Menisci

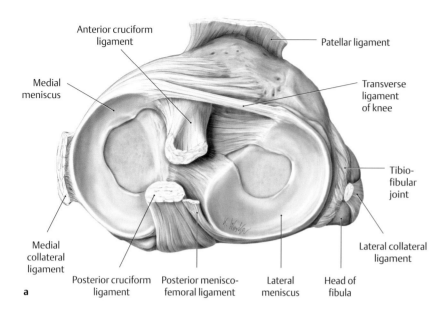

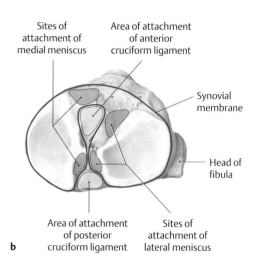

a — Anterior cruciform ligament · Patellar ligament · Medial meniscus · Transverse ligament of knee · Medial collateral ligament · Tibio-fibular joint · Lateral collateral ligament · Posterior cruciform ligament · Posterior menisco-femoral ligament · Lateral meniscus · Head of fibula

b — Sites of attachment of medial meniscus · Area of attachment of anterior cruciform ligament · Synovial membrane · Head of fibula · Area of attachment of posterior cruciform ligament · Sites of attachment of lateral meniscus

A The tibial plateau with the medial and lateral menisci and the sites of attachment of the menisci and cruciform ligaments

Right tibial plateau, proximal view with the cruciform and collateral ligaments divided and the femur removed.

a Shape and attachments of the menisci: The medial and lateral menisci are both crescent-shaped when viewed from above (L. *meniscus* = crescent). Their ends (the anterior and posterior horns) are attached by short ligaments to the bone of the anterior and posterior intercondylar areas of the tibia. The *lateral meniscus* forms almost a complete ring, while the *medial meniscus* has a more semicircular shape. On the whole, the medial meniscus is less mobile than the lateral meniscus because its points of attachment to the bone are spaced farther

apart (see **b**) and it is also firmly attached peripherally to the medial collateral ligament. The lateral meniscus, by contrast, has no attachment to the lateral collateral ligament (see **E**).

b Sites of attachment of the medial and lateral menisci and the cruciform ligaments: The red line indicates the tibial attachment of the synovial membrane, which covers the cruciform ligaments anteriorly and at the sides. The cruciform ligaments lie in the subsynovial connective tissue of the joint capsule and are covered posteriorly by the heavy fibrous membrane. Because the cruciform ligaments migrate forward into the knee joint during development, they are extracapsular but intra-articular in their location, and they derive their blood supply from the popliteal fossa (middle genicular artery, see p. 501).

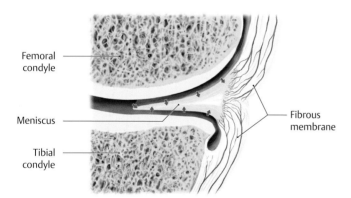

Femoral condyle · Meniscus · Tibial condyle · Fibrous membrane

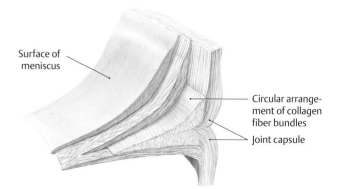

Surface of meniscus · Circular arrangement of collagen fiber bundles · Joint capsule

B Blood supply to the menisci

Schematic coronal section through the femorotibial joint. The fibrous portions of the menisci located adjacent to the capsule have a rich blood supply (the medial and lateral inferior articular arteries from the popliteal artery, see p. 501). But the more central portions of the menisci, composed of fibrocartilage, are avascular and are nourished entirely by the synovial fluid (arrows).

C Structure of the meniscus

The meniscus has a wedge-shaped cross section, the base of the wedge being directed toward the periphery and attached to the joint capsule. The surface facing the tibial plateau is flat, while the upper surface facing the femoral condyles is concave. The central, inner two thirds of the menisci are composed of fibrocartilage and the outer third of tough connective tissue. The bundles of collagen fibers in both the fibrocartilage and the connective tissue have a predominantly circular arrangement reflecting the high tensile stresses that develop in the menisci. The ability of the meniscal tissue to move outward in response to loading is similar to that found in intervertebral disks (converting pressure to tensile forces) (after Petersen and Tillmann).

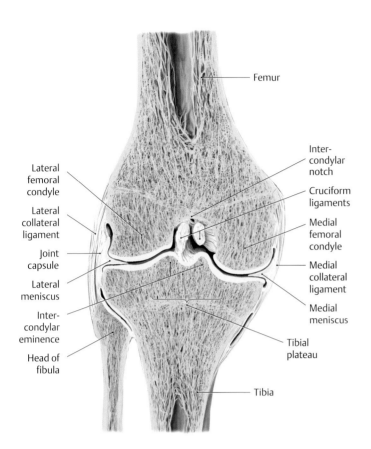

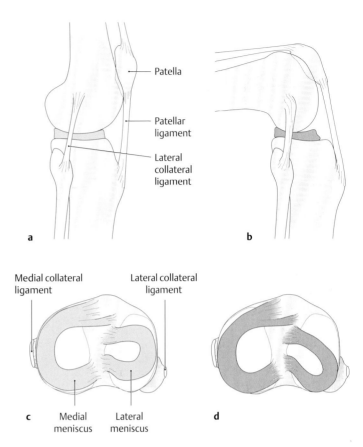

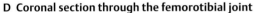

D Coronal section through the femorotibial joint

Right knee, anterior view. An essential task of the menisci is to increase the surface area available for load transfer across the knee joint. With their different curvatures, the menisci compensate for the mismatch in the articulating surfaces of the femur and tibia. They absorb approximately one-third of the loads imposed on the knee, and they help to distribute the pressures more evenly within the femorotibial joint.

E Movements of the menisci during flexion of the knee

The drawings show a right knee joint from the lateral view in extension (**a**) and flexion (**b**) and the associated tibial plateau viewed from above in extension (**c**) and flexion (**d**).

Note that the medial meniscus, which is anchored more securely than the lateral meniscus, undergoes considerably less displacement during knee flexion.

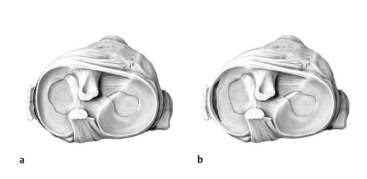

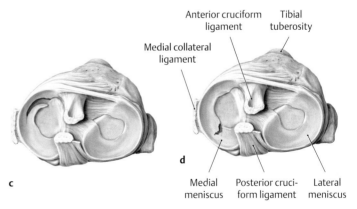

F Different patterns of meniscal tears

Right tibial plateau, proximal view.

a Peripheral tear.
b Bucket-handle tear.
c Longitudinal or flap tear of the anterior horn.
d Radial tear of the posterior horn.

The medial meniscus, being less mobile, is injured far more often than the lateral meniscus. Meniscal injuries most commonly result from sudden extension or rotational movements of the flexed knee (external and internal rotation) while the leg is fixed, as may occur while skiing or playing soccer. The resultant shearing forces can tear the substance of the meniscus or avulse it from its peripheral attachment. The cardinal feature of a fresh meniscal injury is a painful limitation of active and passive knee extension immediately after the trauma, while the patient favors the knee by keeping it slightly flexed. Degenerative changes in the menisci occur with aging and are exacerbated by excessive loads and angular deformities of the knee (genu varum or valgum, see p. 362).

1.20 The Movements of the Knee Joint

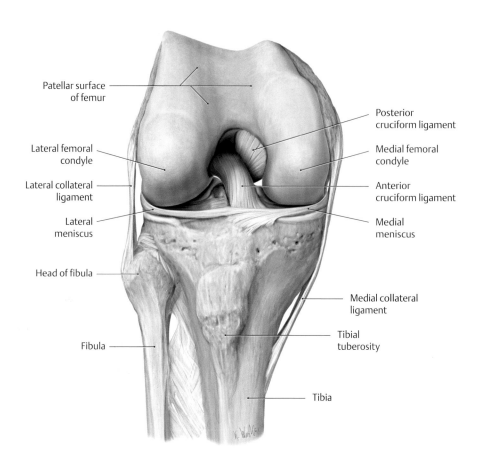

Patellar surface of femur

Lateral femoral condyle

Lateral collateral ligament

Lateral meniscus

Head of fibula

Fibula

Posterior cruciform ligament

Medial femoral condyle

Anterior cruciform ligament

Medial meniscus

Medial collateral ligament

Tibial tuberosity

Tibia

A The right knee joint in flexion
Anterior view with the joint capsule and patella removed.

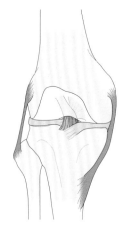

a

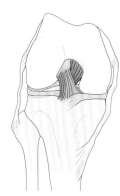

b

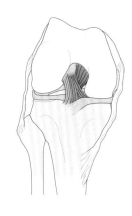

c

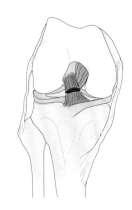

a

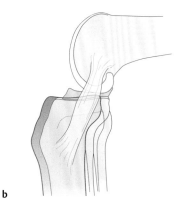

b

B Condition after rupture of the anterior cruciform ligament
a Right knee joint in flexion, anterior view.
b Right knee joint in flexion, medial view.

The instability that results from a cruciform ligament rupture allows the tibia to be moved forward or backward like a drawer relative to the femur, depending on whether the anterior or posterior cruciform ligament has been torn ("anterior or posterior drawer sign," elic-

ited with the Lachman test. A rupture of the anterior cruciform ligament, as shown in the diagram, is approximately ten times more common than a rupture of the posterior ligament. The most common mechanism of injury is an internal rotation trauma with the leg fixed (see **D**). A lateral blow to the fully extended knee, with foot planted, tends to cause concomitant rupture of the anterior cruciform ligament and the medial collateral ligament, and tearing of the attached medial meniscus, referred to colloquially as the "unhappy triad."

C Behavior of the cruciform and collateral ligaments in flexion and extension
Right knee, anterior view. Ligament fibers that are taut are colored red.

a Extension.
b Flexion.
c Flexion and internal rotation.

While the collateral knee ligaments are taut *only in extension* (a), the cruciform ligaments, or at least portions of them, are taut *in every joint position*: the medial portions of both cruciform ligaments in extension (a), the lateral part of the anterior cruciform ligament and the entire posterior cruciform ligament in flexion (b), the medial part of the anterior ligament and the entire posterior ligament in flexion and internal rotation (c). The cruciform ligaments thus help stabilize the knee in any joint position.

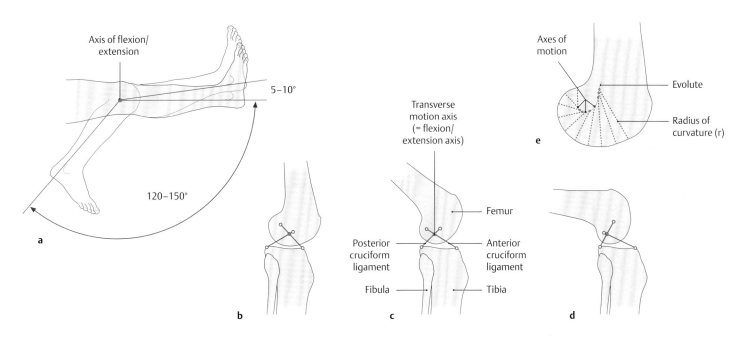

D Flexion and extension of the knee joint

Right knee joint, lateral view.

Flexion and extension of the knee joint take place about a transverse axis (**a**) that passes through the dynamic center of rotation in any joint position. That center is located at the point where both the collateral ligaments and the cruciform ligaments intersect (**b**). With increasing flex-ion of the knee (**c, d**), the dynamic flexion axis moves upward and back-ward along a curved line (the evolute, **e**). The momentary distance from that curve to the articular surface of the femur is equal to the chang-ing radius of curvature (r) of the femoral condyle. The total range of motion, especially in flexion, depends on various parameters (soft-tis-sue restraints, active insufficiency or hamstring tightness, see p. 431).

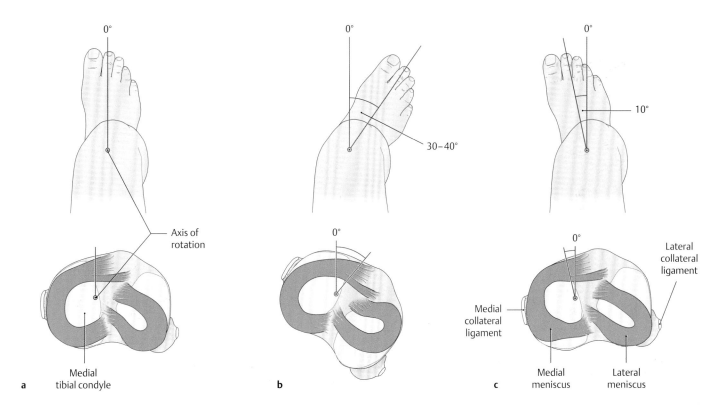

E Rotational movements of the tibia relative to the femur with the knee flexed 90°

Right knee joint, proximal view of the flexed knee and corresponding tibial plateau.

a Neutral (zero-degree) position.
b External rotation.
c Internal rotation.

The axis of tibial rotation runs vertically through the medial part of the medial tibial condyle. Because the cruciform ligaments (not shown here) twist around each other during internal rotation, the range of internal rotation in the knee (approximately 10°) is considerably smaller than the range of external rotation (30–40°). As a result, the majority of cruciform ligament tears occur during internal rotation and involve the anterior cruciform ligament.

Note the different degrees of displacement of the lateral and medial menisci.

399

1.21 The Knee Joint: Capsule and Joint Cavity

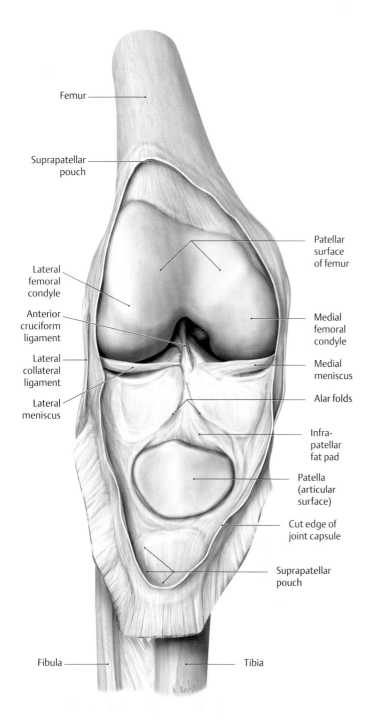

Femur

Suprapatellar pouch

Lateral femoral condyle

Anterior cruciform ligament

Lateral collateral ligament

Lateral meniscus

Patellar surface of femur

Medial femoral condyle

Medial meniscus

Alar folds

Infra-patellar fat pad

Patella (articular surface)

Cut edge of joint capsule

Suprapatellar pouch

Fibula

Tibia

A The right knee with the joint capsule opened
The patella has been reflected downward. In the anterior meniscofemoral portion of the joint capsule, variable folds of the capsule project into the joint cavity (alar folds on both sides of the infrapatellar fat pad), increasing its capacity.

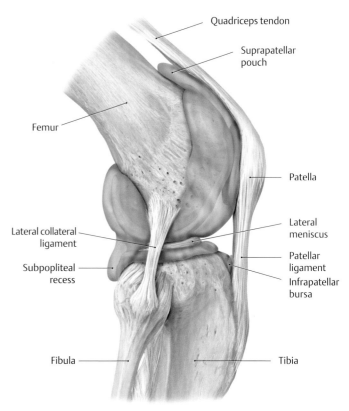

Quadriceps tendon

Suprapatellar pouch

Femur

Patella

Lateral collateral ligament

Subpopliteal recess

Lateral meniscus

Patellar ligament

Infrapatellar bursa

Fibula

Tibia

B Extent of the joint cavity
Right knee joint, lateral view. The joint cavity was demonstrated by injecting a liquid plastic into the knee joint and later removing the capsule after the plastic had cured.

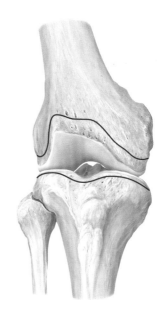

C Anterior femoral and tibial attachments of the joint capsule
Right knee joint, anterior view.

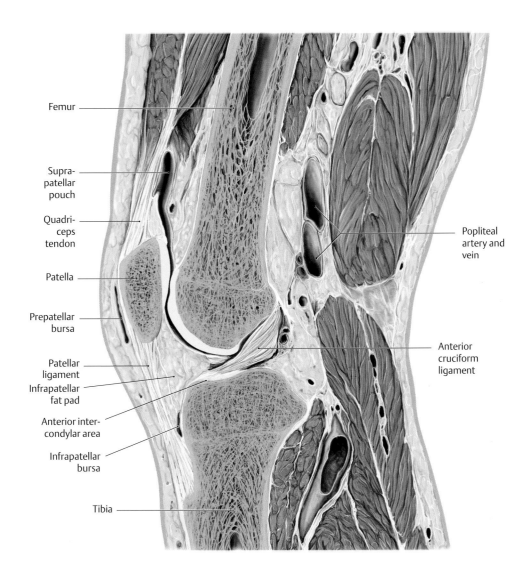

Femur

Supra-
patellar
pouch

Quadri-
ceps
tendon

Patella

Prepatellar
bursa

Patellar
ligament

Infrapatellar
fat pad

Anterior inter-
condylar area

Infrapatellar
bursa

Tibia

Popliteal
artery and
vein

Anterior
cruciform
ligament

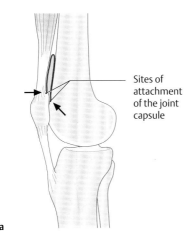

Sites of
attachment
of the joint
capsule

a

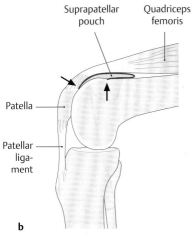

Suprapatellar
pouch

Quadriceps
femoris

Patella

Patellar
liga-
ment

b

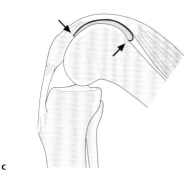

c

D Mid-sagittal section through the right knee joint

Note the extent of the suprapatellar pouch (also called the suprapatellar *bursa*) and compare it with **F**. Note also the placement of the infrapatellar fat pad between the anterior intercondylar area and the deep surface of the patellar ligament. A fall onto the knee or chronic mechanical irritation due to frequent kneeling can cause pain and inflammation of the bursae about the patella: infrapatellar bursitis ("clergyman's knee") and prepatellar bursitis (drawn from a specimen in the Anatomical Collection of Kiel University).

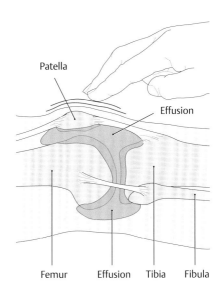

Patella

Effusion

Femur   Effusion   Tibia   Fibula

E The "ballottable patella sign" of knee effusion

When an effusion develops in the knee joint due to inflammatory changes or injury, various degrees of joint swelling may be seen. To differentiate an intra-articular effusion from swelling of the joint capsule itself, the leg is placed in a position of maximum extension. This will force the (potentially increased) intra-articular fluid out of the suprapatellar pouch and into the space between the patella and femur. The examiner then pushes the patella downward with the index finger. If there is excessive fluid in the joint, the patella will rebound when released, signifying a positive test.

F Unfolding of the suprapatellar pouch during flexion

Right knee joint, medial view.

a Neutral (zero-degree) position.
b 80° of flexion.
c 130° of flexion.

The suprapatellar pouch extends proximally from the superior pole of the patella, turns back distally, and inserts at the chondro-osseous junction on the patellar surface of the femur. This redundant fold provides a reserve capacity when the knee is flexed, opening up completely past about 130° of flexion.

401

1.22 The Joints of the Foot: Overview of the Articulating Bones and Joints

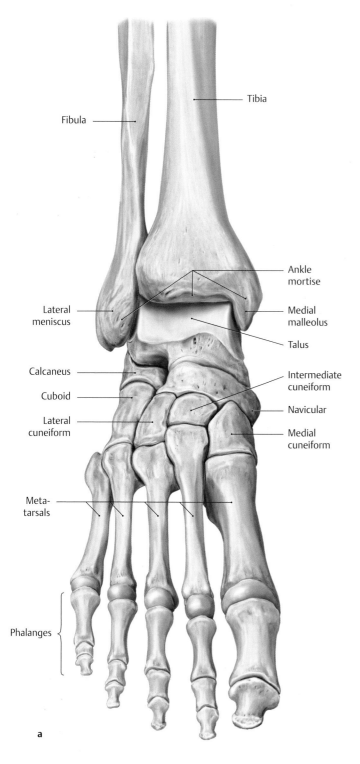

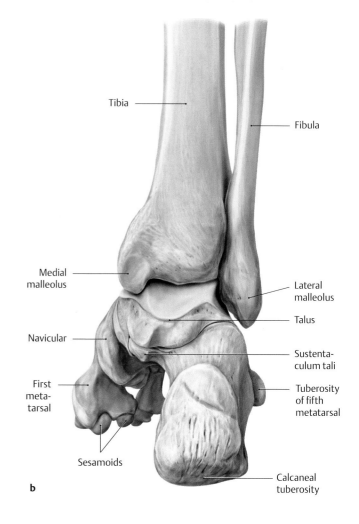

b

A The articulating bones in different joints of the right foot

a Anterior view with the talocrural joint in plantar flexion.
b Posterior view with the foot in the neutral (zero-degree) position.

B Overview of the joints in the foot

- Talocrural joint (ankle joint)
- Subtalar joint (talocalcanean joint and talocalcaneonavicular joint)*
- Calcaneocuboid joint (between the calcaneus and cuboid bone)
- Talonavicular joint (between the talus and navicular bone)
- Transverse tarsal joint**
- Cuneonavicular joint (between the cuneiform and navicular bones)
- Intercuneiform joints (between the cuneiform bones)
- Cuneocuboid joint (between the lateral cuneiform and cuboid bones)
- Tarsometatarsal joints
- Intermetatarsal joints (between the bases of the metatarsal bones)
- Metatarsophalangeal joints
- Proximal interphalangeal joints
- Distal interphalangeal joints

* In the subtalar joint the talus articulates with the calcaneus and the navicular bone to form two separate articulations: the talocalcanean joint posteriorly and the talocalcaneonavicular joint anteriorly. Both are often referred to collectively as the "subtalar joint."
** Consists of the calcaneocuboid joint and talonavicular joint.

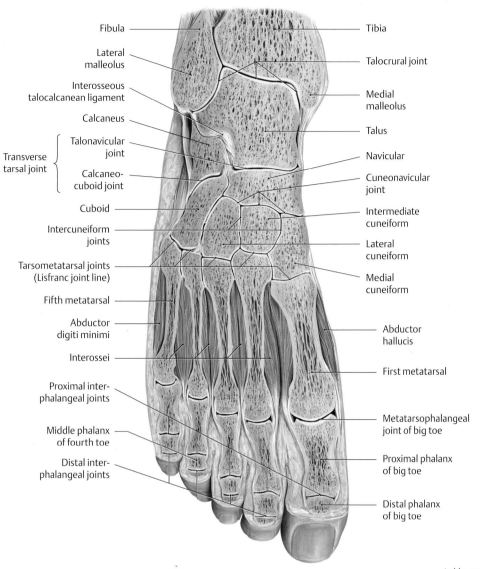

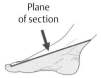

C Oblique transverse section through the foot

Right foot, superior view. The foot is plantar flexed at the talocrural (ankle) joint (drawn from a specimen in the Anatomical Collection of Kiel University).

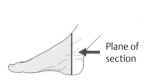

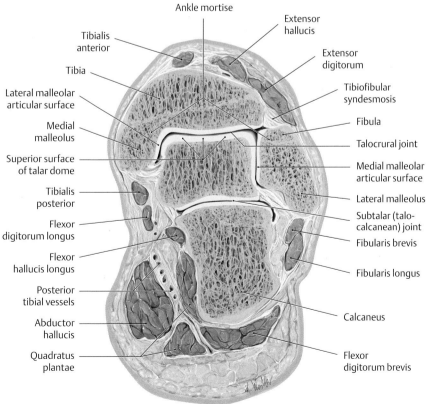

D Coronal section through the talocrural and subtalar joints

Right foot, proximal view. The talocrural joint is plantar flexed, and the subtalar joint is sectioned through its posterior compartment (drawn from a specimen in the Anatomical Collection of Kiel University).

1.23 The Joints of the Foot: Articular Surfaces

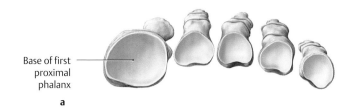

Base of first proximal phalanx

a

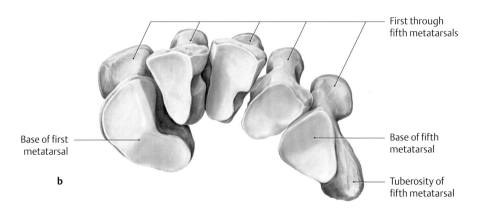

First through fifth metatarsals

Base of first metatarsal

Base of fifth metatarsal

b

Tuberosity of fifth metatarsal

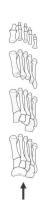

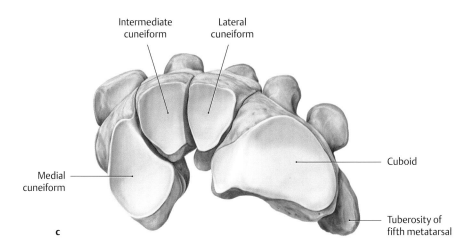

Intermediate cuneiform

Lateral cuneiform

Medial cuneiform

Cuboid

Tuberosity of fifth metatarsal

c

A Proximal articular surfaces
Right foot, proximal view.

a Metatarsophalangeal joints: bases of the first through fifth proximal phalanges.

b Tarsometatarsal joints: bases of the first through fifth metatarsals.

c Cuneonavicular joint and calcaneocuboid joint: proximal articular surfaces of the medial, intermediate, and lateral cuneiform bones and the cuboid.

d Talonavicular joint and calcaneocuboid joint: proximal articular surfaces of the navicular and cuboid bones.

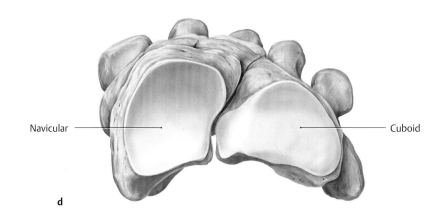

Navicular

Cuboid

d

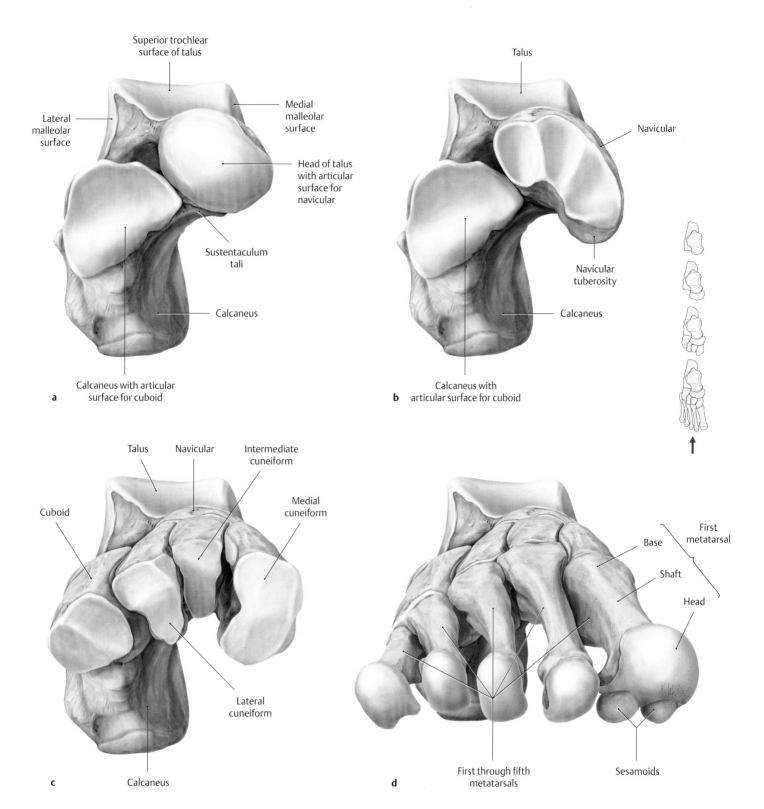

a

Superior trochlear surface of talus

Lateral malleolar surface

Medial malleolar surface

Head of talus with articular surface for navicular

Sustentaculum tali

Calcaneus

Calcaneus with articular surface for cuboid

b

Talus

Navicular

Navicular tuberosity

Calcaneus

Calcaneus with articular surface for cuboid

c

Talus   Navicular   Intermediate cuneiform

Cuboid

Medial cuneiform

Lateral cuneiform

Calcaneus

d

Base

First metatarsal

Shaft

Head

First through fifth metatarsals

Sesamoids

B Distal articular surfaces
Right foot, distal view.

a The talonavicular joint and calcaneocuboid joint: distal articular surfaces of the calcaneus and talus.

b The cuneonavicular joint and calcaneocuboid joint: distal articular surfaces of the navicular and calcaneus.

c The tarsometatarsal joints: distal articular surfaces of the medial, intermediate, and lateral cuneiform and the cuboid.

d Metatarsophalangeal joints: heads of the first through fifth metatarsals.

405

1.24 The Joints of the Foot: The Talocrural and Subtalar Joints

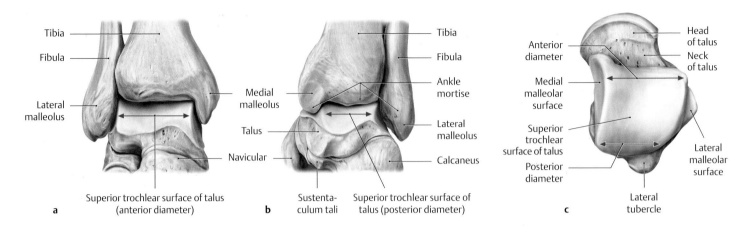

a Superior trochlear surface of talus (anterior diameter)

b Sustenta-culum tali Superior trochlear surface of talus (posterior diameter)

c

A The articulating skeletal elements of the talocrural joint
a Right foot, anterior view.
b Right foot, posterior view.
c Trochlea of the right talus, superior view.

The talocrural joint, called also the ankle joint, is formed by the distal ends of the tibia and fibula (the ankle mortise, see also **B**) articulating with the trochlea of the talus. This provides the talocrural joint with good bony and ligamentous stability and helps to stabilize the body in an erect posture. However, due to the shape of the talar trochlea (the anterior part, the superior surface, is approximately 5–6 mm broader

than the posterior part), the bony stability of the talocrural joint differs in flexion and extension. When the broader anterior part of the trochlea articulates with the ankle mortise in *dorsiflexion* (where the foot moves closer to the leg, as in squatting), the syndesmotic ligaments (see p. 409) are tightly stretched and there is excellent bony stability. But when the narrower posterior part of the trochlea comes in contact with the ankle mortise in *plantar flexion* (e.g., standing on the toes), the talus no longer provides a high degree of bony stability within the ankle mortise.

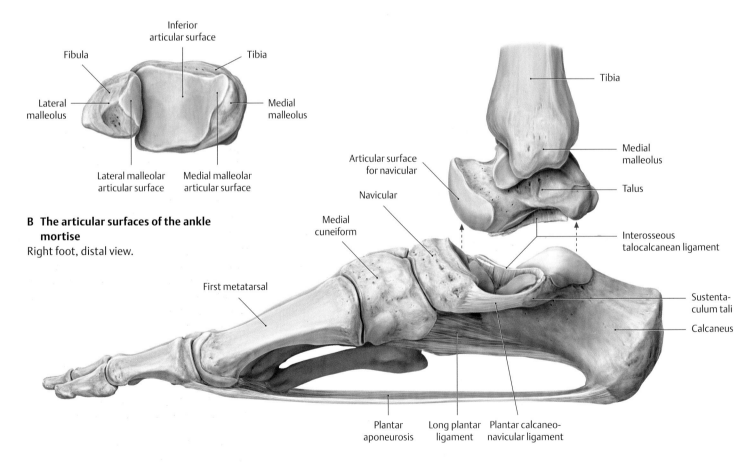

B The articular surfaces of the ankle mortise
Right foot, distal view.

C Overview of an opened subtalar joint
Right foot, medial view. The interosseous talocalcanean ligament has been divided and the talus has been displaced upward to demonstrate the articular surfaces of the subtalar joint.

Note the course of the plantar calcaneonavicular ligament, which functions with the long plantar ligament and plantar aponeurosis to support the longitudinal arch of the foot (see also **D** and p. 414).

D Course of the plantar calcaneonavicular ligament
Right foot, plantar view. The plantar calcaneonavicular (spring) ligament stretches between the sustentaculum tali and the navicular. It
completes the bony socket of the talocalcanean joint from the plantar
side.

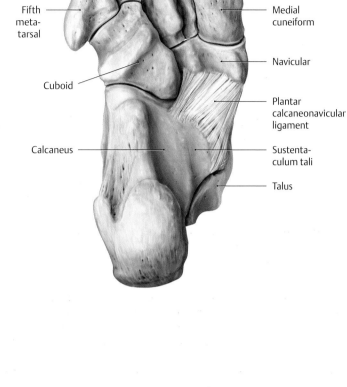

Fifth
meta-
tarsal

Cuboid

Calcaneus

Medial
cuneiform

Navicular

Plantar
calcaneonavicular
ligament

Sustenta-
culum tali

Talus

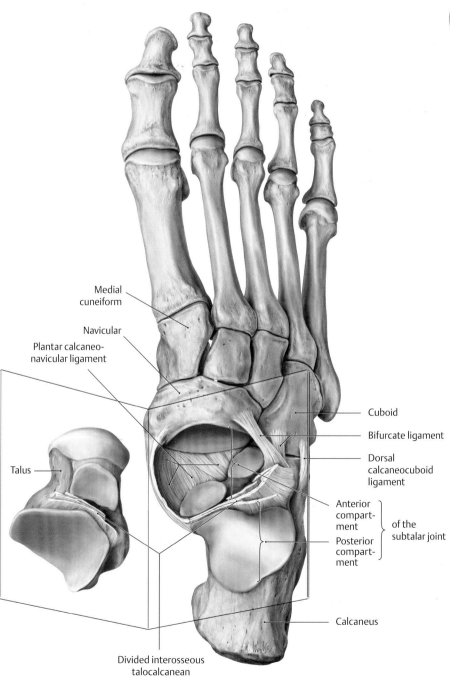

Medial
cuneiform

Navicular

Plantar calcaneo-
navicular ligament

Talus

Cuboid

Bifurcate ligament

Dorsal
calcaneocuboid
ligament

Anterior
compart-
ment
Posterior
compart-
ment
of the
subtalar joint

Calcaneus

Divided interosseous
talocalcanean
ligament

**E The articular surfaces of an opened
subtalar joint**
Right foot, dorsal view (after separation of the
talus). In the subtalar joint the talus articulates
with the calcaneus and the navicular. It consists of two completely separate articulations:

- a posterior compartment (the talocalcanean joint) and
- an anterior compartment (the talocalcaneonavicular joint).

The boundary between the two compartments is formed by the interosseous talocalcanean ligament located in the tarsal canal (bony
canal formed by the sulcus tali and sulcus calcanei; its entrance is the sinus tarsi). The plantar calcaneonavicular ligament, which has cartilage cells in its medial surface, loops like a
tendon around the plantar head of the talus,
which acts as a fulcrum. It stabilizes the position of the talus on the calcaneus and helps
to support the apex of the longitudinal pedal
arch (see p. 414). Overstretching of the plantar calcaneonavicular (spring) ligament due to
flattening of the plantar vault promotes the
development of flat foot.

407

1.25 The Ligaments of the Foot

A The ligaments of the right foot, medial view
The medial and lateral collateral ligaments, along with the syndesmotic ligaments (see **E**), are of major importance in stabilizing and guiding the subtalar joint, because portions of these ligaments are taut in every joint position and thus in every movement. The ligaments of the foot are classified by their location as belonging to the talocrural or subtalar joint, the metatarsus, the forefoot, or the sole of the foot.

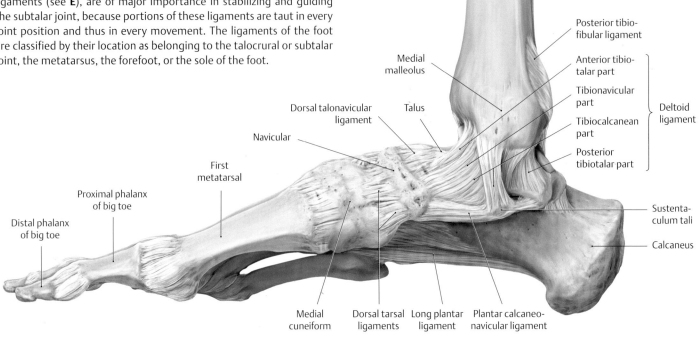

B The ligaments of the right foot, lateral view
Sprains of the ankle joint and especially of its lateral ligaments (usually supination trauma = buckling of the ankle in a supinated position) are extremely common injuries. They often occur during plantar flexion of the foot, a position that provides less bony stability to the talocrural joint (see p. 406). Most of these injuries occur during sports and other leisure activities when the ankle gives way on uneven ground. Typically the trauma will cause stretching or tearing of the anterior talofibular ligament, the calcaneofibular ligament, or both. If the leg is twisted violently while the foot is fixed, there may also be separation of the ankle mortise with disruption of the tibiofibular syndesmosis (see **D**).

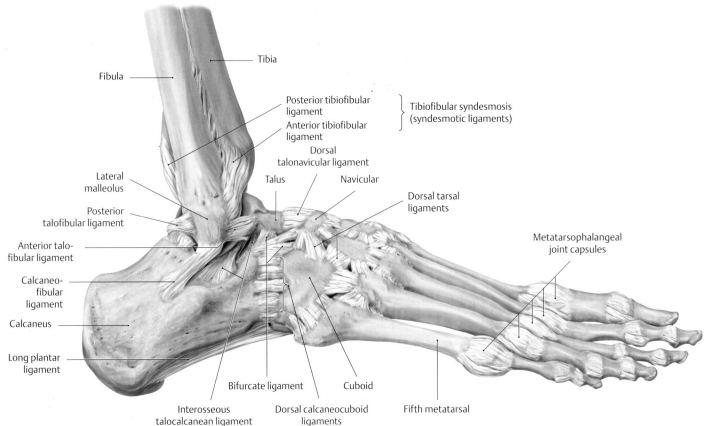

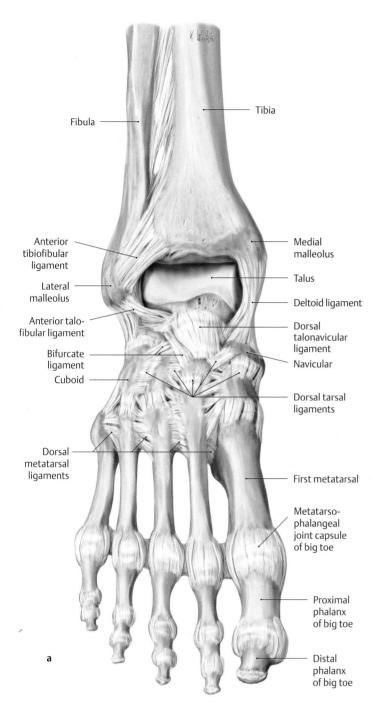

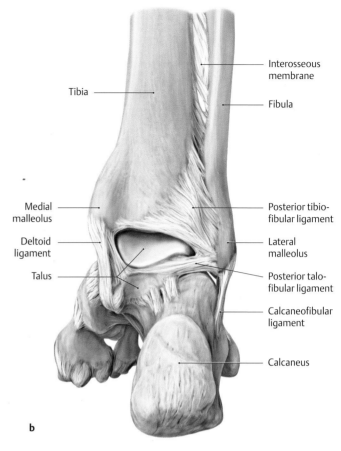

a

b

C The ligaments of the right foot

a Anterior view (talocrural joint in plantar flexion).
b Posterior view (plantigrade foot position).

The anterior and posterior portions of the talocrural joint capsule have been removed to demonstrate more clearly the placement of the ligaments.

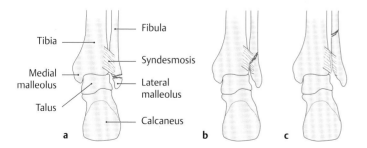

a   b   c

D Weber fractures

A Weber fracture is an avulsion fracture of the lateral malleolus from the fibula. Weber fractures are classified as type A, B, or C depending on whether the fibula is fractured below, level with, or above the syndesmosis. The syndesmosis *may* be torn in a Weber type B fracture (as shown here), but it is *always* torn in a Weber type C fracture.

E The ligaments of the talocrural joint (the ligaments of the subtalar joint are reviewed on p. 407).

Lateral ligaments*
• Anterior talofibular ligament
• Posterior talofibular ligament
• Calcaneofibular ligament

Medial ligaments*
• Deltoid ligament
  – Anterior tibiotalar part
  – Posterior tibiotalar part
  – Tibionavicular part
  – Tibiocalcanean part

Syndesmotic ligaments of the ankle mortise
• Anterior tibiofibular ligament
• Posterior tibiofibular ligament

*The medial and lateral ligaments are also termed the medial and lateral collateral ligaments.

1.26 The Movements of the Foot

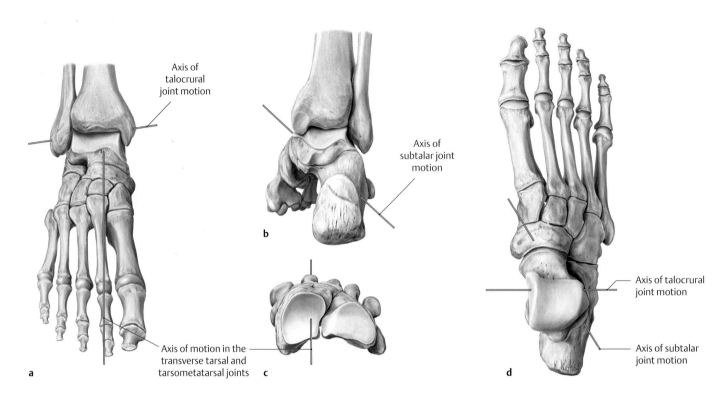

a — Axis of talocrural joint motion

b — Axis of subtalar joint motion

Axis of motion in the transverse tarsal and tarsometatarsal joints — **c**

d — Axis of talocrural joint motion / Axis of subtalar joint motion

A The principal axes of motion in the right foot
a Anterior view with the talocrural joint in plantar flexion.
b Posterior view in the functional position (see **B**).
c Isolated right forefoot, proximal view.
d Superior view.

The axes of articular motion in the foot are complex, and the descriptions of movements in the pedal joints are often inconsistent and confusing. The following axes of motion are important in clinical parlance and for the testing of joint motion (compare with the facing page):

- **Axis of talocrural joint motion (plantarflexion/dorsiflexion):** This axis runs almost transversely through the lateral and medial malleoli. It forms an approximately 82° angle with the tibial shaft axis in the

frontal plane, and it forms a 10° angle with the frontal plane on the medial side (**a, d**).
- **Axis of subtalar joint motion (inversion/eversion):** This axis runs obliquely upward through the foot in a posterolateral-to-anteromedial direction, i.e., from the lateral calcaneus through the medial portion of the tarsal canal to the center of the navicular bone. It forms an approximately 30° angle with the horizontal plane and a 20° angle with the sagittal plane (**b, d**).
- **Axis of forefoot motion in the transverse tarsal joint and tarsometatarsal joints (pronation/supination):** This axis lies approximately in the sagittal plane, running from the calcaneus through the navicular and along the second ray (**a, c**).

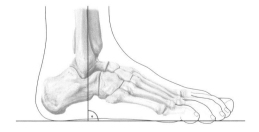

B The functional position of the foot
Right foot, lateral view. In the neutral (zero-degree) position, the skeleton of the foot is angled approximately 90° relative to the skeleton of the leg. This *plantigrade foot position* is termed the "functional position" and is an important basis for normal standing and walking.

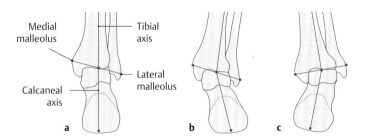

Medial malleolus — Tibial axis
Calcaneal axis — Lateral malleolus
a   **b**   **c**

C Axis of the hindfoot
Distal right leg and hindfoot, posterior view.

a With normal axial alignment in the hindfoot, the tibial axis and calcaneal axis lie on a vertical line (pes rectus). The calcaneal axis bisects a line drawn between the two malleoli.
b Pes valgus: The foot is in an everted position.
c Pes varus: The foot is in an inverted position.

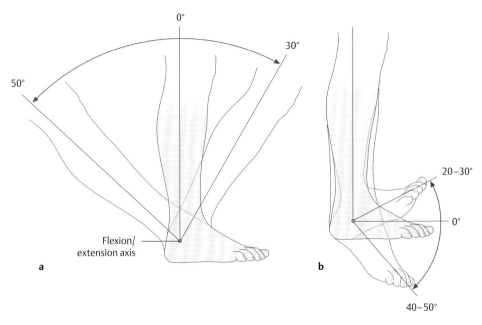
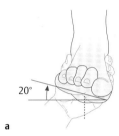
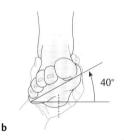

D Normal range of motion of the talocrural joint
Lateral view.

a Right foot on the ground (stance leg).
b Right foot off the ground (swing leg).

Starting from the neutral (zero-degree) (plantigrade) position, the non-weightbearing foot has an approximately 40–50° range of plantar flexion and an approximately 20–30° range of dorsiflexion (extension). When the foot is planted on the ground (in the stance phase of gait), the leg can be moved approximately 50° backward (plantar flexion) and 30° forward (dorsiflexion).

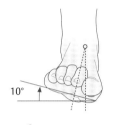
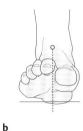
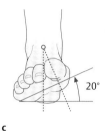

E Range of motion of the subtalar joint
Right foot, anterior view.

a Everted by 10°.
b Neutral (zero-degree) position.
c Inverted by 20°.

Rotation of the calcaneus medially (inversion) and laterally (eversion) is measured from the neutral (zero-degree) position. This is done clinically by holding the leg stationary and moving the calcaneus back and forth. Estimation of the range of inversion/eversion is based on the calcaneal axis.

F Range of pronation/supination of the transverse tarsal and tarsometatarsal joints.
Right foot, anterior view.

a Range of pronation of the forefoot: 20°.
b Range of supination of the forefoot: 40°.

Range of motion is tested with the hindfoot fixed. Pronation/supination of the forefoot is tested by rotating the forefoot outward relative to the hindfoot (raising the lateral border of the foot), or inward (raising the medial border of the foot).

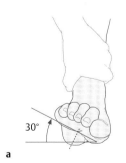
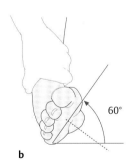
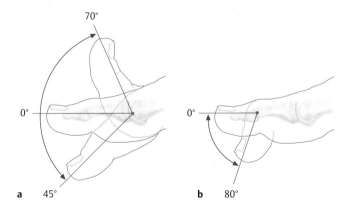

G Total range of motion of the forefoot and hindfoot
Right foot, anterior view.

a Eversion and pronation of the forefoot: 30°.
b Inversion and supination of the forefoot: 60°.

Because the movements in the joints are complex, and different joint movements are almost always mechanically coupled, the range of all joint movements can be assessed by holding the leg stationary and raising the entire foot in the medial and lateral directions.

H Range of motion of the joints of the big toe
Lateral view.

a Flexion/extension of the first metatarsophalangeal joint.
b Flexion of the first interphalangeal joint.

The toes, and especially the big toe, can be passively extended to approximately 90°. This is an important prerequisite for walking, especially during the phase between heel take-off and toe strike.

1.27 Overview of the Plantar Vault and the Transverse Arch

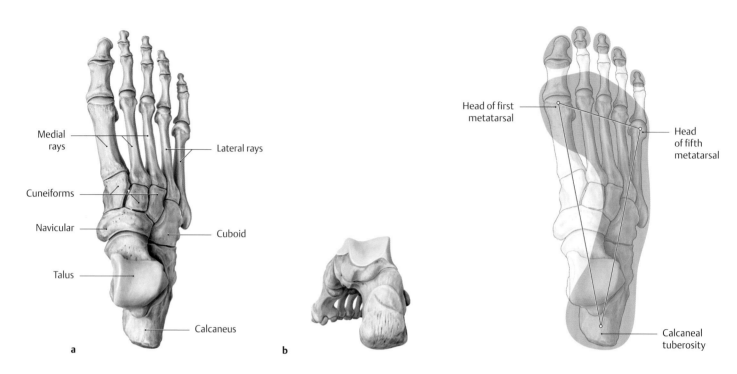

A The plantar vault

a Right foot, superior view.

b Right foot, posteromedial view.

From the perspective of structural engineering, the forces borne by the foot are distributed among two lateral (fibular) rays and three medial (tibial) rays. The lateral rays extend across the cuboid bone to the calcaneus, while the medial rays extend across the cuneiform and navicular bones to the talus. The arrangement of these rays—adjacent distally and overriding proximally—creates a lon-

gitudinal arch and a transverse arch in the sole of the foot. These plantar arches enable the foot to adapt optimally to uneven terrain, ensuring that the compressive forces can be transmitted under optimum mechanical conditions in any situation. The arches thus perform a kind of shock-absorber function, creating a springy flexibility that helps the foot absorb vertical loads. The deficient arches in a flat foot or splayfoot, for example, can lead to considerable pain during walking.

B The plantar architecture of the right foot

Superior view showing the bony points of support for the plantar vault and the associated footprint. The area that is outlined by interconnecting the bony supports (the calcaneal tuberosity and the heads of the first and fifth metatarsals) has the shape of a triangle. By contrast, the area of ground contact defined by the plantar soft tissues (the footprint or *podogram*) is considerably larger. The calluses typically found on the heel and the balls of the large and little toes confirm that these areas bear the brunt of the loads.

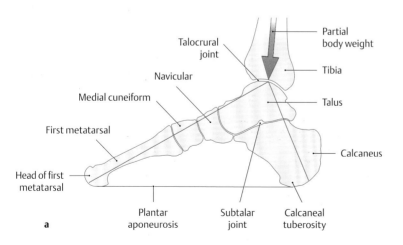

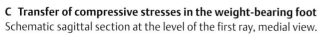

C Transfer of compressive stresses in the weight-bearing foot
Schematic sagittal section at the level of the first ray, medial view.

a During stance, the partial body weight on the talocrural joint is transferred across the talus to the forefoot and hindfoot.

b A schematic radiograph illustrates the parallel arrangement of the cancellous bony trabeculae. The pattern conforms to the compressive stresses (indicated by color shading) that result from the loads acting on the forefoot and hindfoot (**a**) (after Rauber and Kopsch).

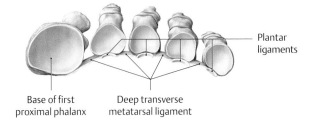

Plantar
ligaments

Base of first
proximal phalanx

Deep transverse
metatarsal ligament

a

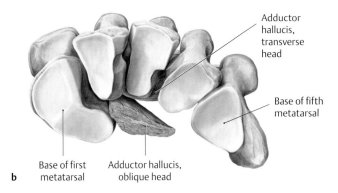

Adductor
hallucis,
transverse
head

Base of fifth
metatarsal

Base of first
metatarsal

Adductor hallucis,
oblique head

b

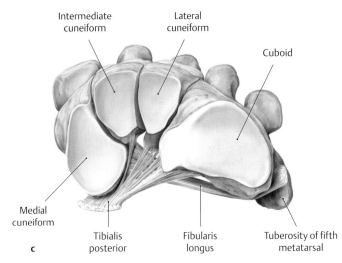

Intermediate
cuneiform

Lateral
cuneiform

Cuboid

Medial
cuneiform

Tibialis
posterior

Fibularis
longus

Tuberosity of fifth
metatarsal

c

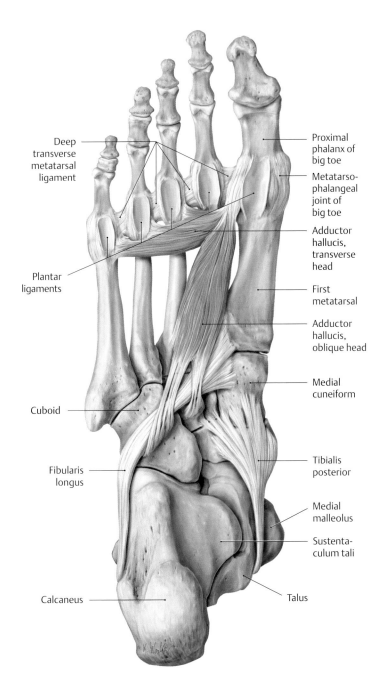

Deep transverse metatarsal ligament

Proximal phalanx of big toe

Metatarsophalangeal joint of big toe

Adductor hallucis, transverse head

First metatarsal

Adductor hallucis, oblique head

Plantar ligaments

Medial cuneiform

Cuboid

Tibialis posterior

Fibularis longus

Medial malleolus

Sustentaculum tali

Calcaneus

Talus

D Active and passive stabilizers of the transverse arch, plantar view

Right foot. Both active and passive stabilizing structures maintain the curvature of the transverse pedal arch. The passive stabilizers are ligaments, and the active stabilizers are muscles. In the foot, ligamentous structures are usually able to maintain the pedal arches without assistance from the muscles. But when the loads on the foot are increased, as during walking or running on uneven ground, active muscular forces are also recruited to give additional support.

E Active and passive stabilizers of the transverse arch, proximal view

Right foot.

a Arch stabilizers in the forefoot (anterior arch). The deep transverse metatarsal ligament stabilizes the anterior arch at the level of the metatarsal heads. The arch of the forefoot thus relies entirely on *passive* stabilizers, while the arches of the metatarsus and tarsus (**b, c**) have only *active* stabilizers.

b Stabilizers of the metatarsal arch. The transverse head of adductor hallucis is the primary muscular stabilizer of the metatarsal arch.

c The principal arch-supporting muscle in the tarsal region is the fibularis longus. After winding around the cuboid, its tendon of insertion runs from the lateral border of the foot and across the sole to the medial cuneiform bone and the base of the first metatarsal. Another active stabilizer in this region is the tibialis posterior, whose tendon of insertion gives off expansions to the cuneiform bones. Like the fibularis longus, its oblique course enables it to support the longitudinal arch in addition to its transverse component.

413

1.28 The Longitudinal Arch of the Foot

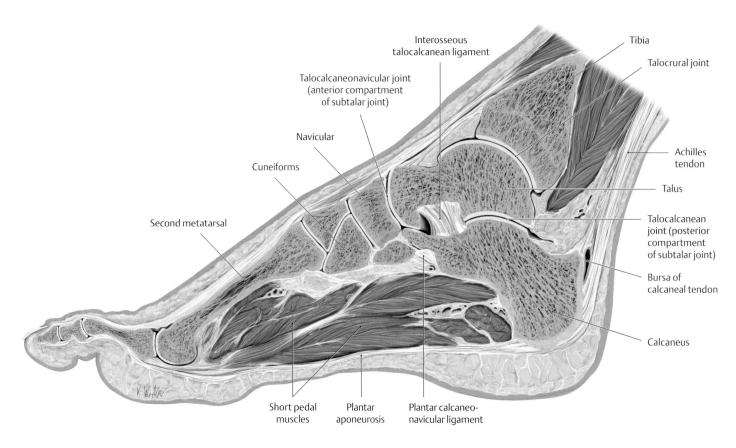

Interosseous
talocalcanean ligament

Talocalcaneonavicular joint
(anterior compartment
of subtalar joint)

Navicular

Cuneiforms

Second metatarsal

Tibia

Talocrural joint

Achilles
tendon

Talus

Talocalcanean
joint (posterior
compartment
of subtalar joint)

Bursa of
calcaneal tendon

Calcaneus

Short pedal
muscles

Plantar
aponeurosis

Plantar calcaneo-
navicular ligament

A Active stabilizers of the longitudinal arch

Sagittal section at the level of the second ray of a right foot, medial view. The second ray (consisting of the second toe, second metatarsal, intermediate cuneiform, navicular, and calcaneus) forms the highest arch within the overall longitudinal plantar arch, its height diminishing laterally. The main active stabilizers of the longitudinal arch are the *short muscles of the foot*: abductor hallucis, flexor hallucis brevis, flexor digitorum brevis, quadratus plantae, and abductor digiti minimi (drawn from a specimen in the Anatomical Collection of Kiel University).

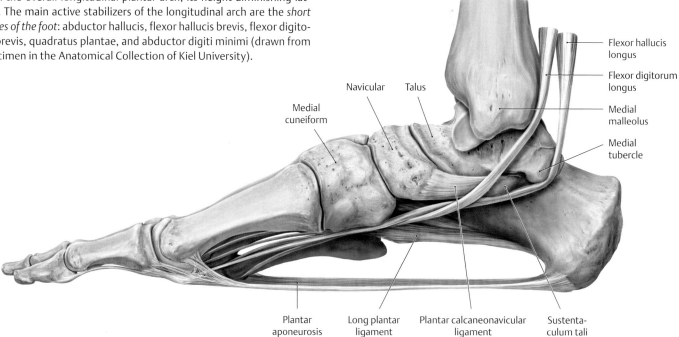

Navicular   Talus

Medial
cuneiform

Flexor hallucis
longus

Flexor digitorum
longus

Medial
malleolus

Medial
tubercle

Plantar
aponeurosis

Long plantar
ligament

Plantar calcaneonavicular
ligament

Sustenta-
culum tali

B Passive stabilizers of the longitudinal arch

Right foot, medial view. The main passive stabilizers of the longitudinal arch are the plantar aponeurosis, the long plantar ligament, and the plantar calcaneonavicular (spring) ligament. The plantar aponeurosis is particularly important owing to its long lever arm, while the plantar calcaneonavicular ligament is the weakest component (shortest distance from the apex of the longitudinal arch). The *tendons of insertion of the long flexors* of the foot (flexor hallucis longus and flexor digitorum longus) also help to prevent sagging of the longitudinal arch. The flexor hallucis longus, which runs beneath the sustentaculum tali, is particularly effective in tightening the longitudinal arch like the chord of an arc.

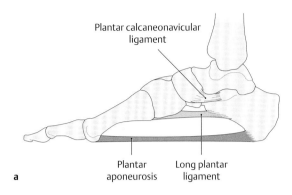

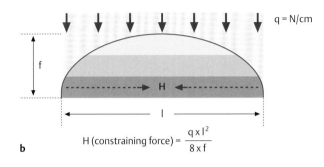

C Support of the longitudinal arch

a Ligamentous support of the longitudinal arch (right foot, medial view).

b Calculating the constraining force (H) needed to maintain the arch (after Rauber and Kopsch).

$$H \text{ (constraining force)} = \frac{q \times l^2}{8 \times f}$$

Comparing the longitudinal arch of the foot to a theoretical parabolic arch, we see that a constraining force (H) must be applied to maintain the arch curvature. The magnitude of this force depends on the load (q), the chord length of the arch (l), and the height of the arch (f). As a result, the structures that are most effective in maintaining the pedal arch are those closest to the ground, since the long lever arm of those structures requires the least expenditure of force. The formula also dictates that the constraining force must increase as the distance l between the points of support increases, or as the arch becomes flatter (smaller f).

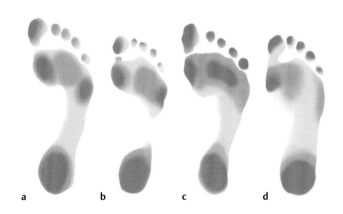

D Footprints (podograms) of right feet (after Rauber and Kopsch)

a Normal plantar arches (pes rectus).

b Increased height of the longitudinal arch (pes cavus).

c Loss of the transverse arch (splayfoot = pes transversoplanus).

d Loss of the longitudinal arch (flat foot = pes planus).

Foot deformities—deviations from a normal, healthy foot shape—may be congenital, or acquired through paralysis or trauma. Structural abnormalities caused by chronic loads imposed on the foot by the body weight are referred to specifically as *static deformities*.

E Location of pain associated with splayfoot and flat foot (after Loeweneck)

a Right splayfoot viewed from the plantar aspect. The collapse of the transverse arch results in a broadened forefoot (arrows) with greater pressure acting on the heads of the second through fourth metatarsals and the associated metatarsophalangeal joints. Typically, very painful calluses will form between the balls of the large and little toes in this situation.

b Right flat foot viewed from the medial aspect. With collapse of the longitudinal arch, marked by downward displacement of the talus and navicular (arrow), weight bearing often incites a diffuse foot pain that is most intense in the area of the stretched calcaneonavicular (spring) ligament. Calf pain may also develop as a result of sustained, increased tension on the calf muscles (and the pedal muscles as well, which must compensate for the deficient passive stabilizers).

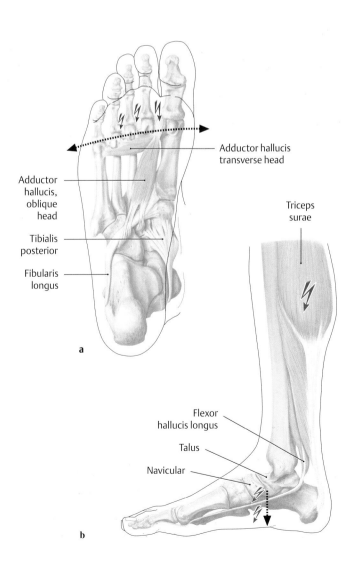

415

1.29 The Sesamoid Bones and Deformities of the Toes

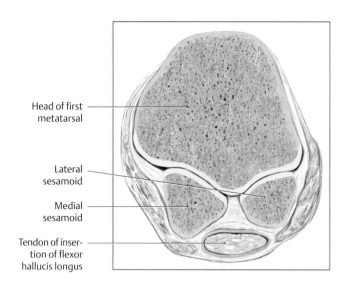

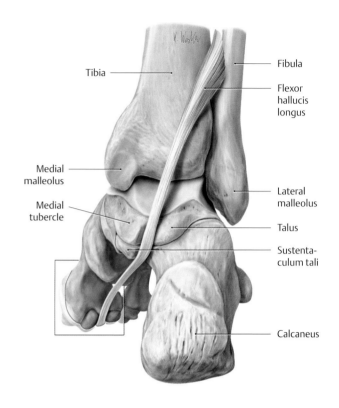

A Cross section through the head of the first metatarsal at the level of the sesamoids

Big toe of right foot, proximal view. The plane of section is indicated in **B**. The lateral and medial sesamoids are hemispherical bones, each presenting a slightly convex dorsal articular surface that articulates with the grooved plantar articular surfaces on the head of the first metatarsal. Sesamoids protect the tendons from excessive friction. They are important functionally for their ability to lengthen the effective lever arm of the muscle, so that muscular forces can be applied more efficiently. The development of sesamoids can be interpreted as a functional adaptation to the presence of pressure tendons.

B The sesamoids of the big toe

Right foot, posteromedial view. The tendon of flexor hallucis longus runs between the two sesamoids. The box around the sesamoids indicates the plane of section shown in **A**.

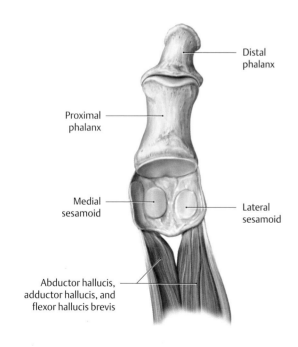

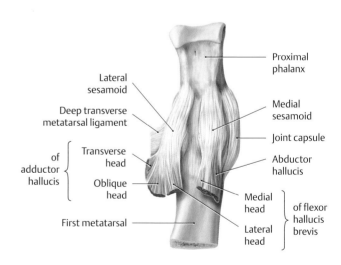

C The articular surfaces of the sesamoids

Dorsal view with the first metatarsal removed.

D The capsule and ligaments of the sesamoids and muscular attachments

First metatarsophalangeal joint of the right foot, plantar view. Both sesamoids are attached to the joint capsule and to the collateral ligaments of the metatarsophalangeal joint. They are embedded in the tendons of insertion of the following muscles:

- Medial sesamoid
  - Abductor hallucis
  - Medial head of flexor hallucis brevis

- Lateral sesamoid
  - Lateral head of flexor hallucis brevis
  - Transverse head of adductor hallucis
  - Oblique head of adductor hallucis

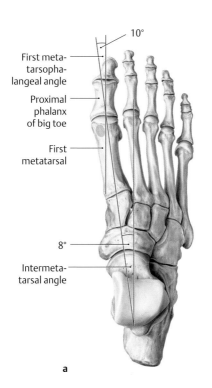

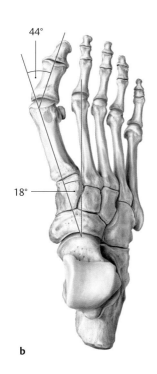

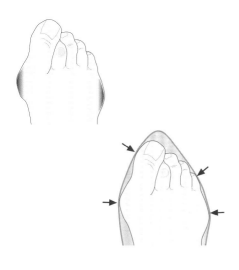

a

b

E Change in the first intermetatarsal angle and first metatarsophalangeal angle in hallux valgus

Right foot, superior view.

a Skeleton of a normal right foot.
b Lateral deviation of the first ray with subluxation of the metatarsophalangeal joint in hallux valgus.

In a normal foot, the *first intermetatarsal angle* (angle between the longitudinal axes of the first and second metatarsals) should not exceed 8°. The *first metatarsophalangeal angle* (angle between the longitudinal axes of the proximal phalanx of the big toe and the first metatarsal) should be less than 20°. In hallux valgus and also in splayfoot, which generally precedes it, both the intermetatarsal angle and metatarsophalangeal angle are significantly increased.

G Etiology of hallux valgus

Hallux valgus usually develops secondary to splayfoot. When a broadened forefoot is forced into a narrow, pointed shoe, the outer toes are crowded against the middle toes. This results in the pressure points and pain that are typical of hallux valgus and predominantly affect the medial side of the head of the first metatarsal, with chronic irritation of the first metatarsophalangeal joint and the overlying bursa (bursitis) in addition to reactive bone changes (exostosis). The middle toes are squeezed together anteriorly and become clawed (hammer toes, claw toes) (after Debrunner).

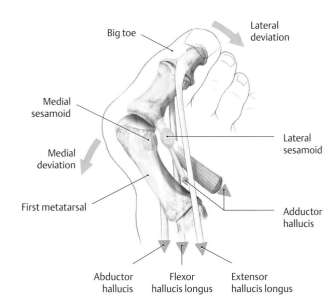

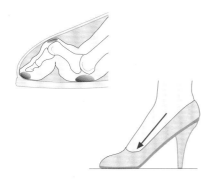

F Pathogenic mechanism of hallux valgus

Right forefoot, superior view. As the first metatarsal deviates medially and the big toe deviates laterally, a muscular imbalance develops marked by a change in the direction of tendon pull, which perpetuates and exacerbates the deformity. Most notably, the abductor hallucis moves laterally with the medial sesamoid, causing it to become an *adductor*. Meanwhile the long flexor and extensor tendons move laterally, reinforcing the lateral angulation at the first metatarsophalangeal joint.

H Claw toes and hammer toes

Toe deformities are a very common associated feature of hallux valgus and splayfoot. When the foot is placed into a tight shoe with a high heel, it tends to slide forward and downward, and the resulting pressure leads to a typical cramped deformity with degenerative changes in the toe joints and painful callus formation. The claw toe deformity is characterized by marked hyperextensibility of the metatarsophalangeal joint with flexion of the proximal and distal interphalangeal joints. With hammer toes, there is less pronounced dorsiflexion of the metatarsophalangeal joint.

417

1.30 Human Gait

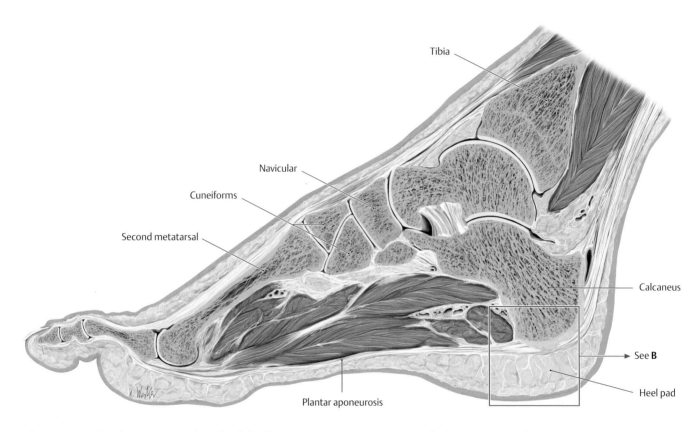

Tibia

Navicular

Cuneiforms

Second metatarsal

Calcaneus

See **B**

Heel pad

Plantar aponeurosis

A The pressure chamber system in the sole of the foot
Sagittal section through the right foot at the level of the second ray, medial view (see detail in **B**).
During walking and particularly in stance, large compressive forces are exerted on the heel pad and on the balls of the big and little toes. To distribute these concentrated stresses more evenly over a larger area, the sole of the foot is covered by a layer of subcutaneous connective tissue up to 2 cm thick. As a functional adaptation to these demands, the tissue has a "pressure chamber" construction which acts as a shock absorber while also enhancing the mechanical stability of the sole. Without this pressure chamber system, the loads on the foot would generate very high, localized stresses that would result in pressure necrosis (drawn from a specimen in the Anatomical Collection of Kiel University).

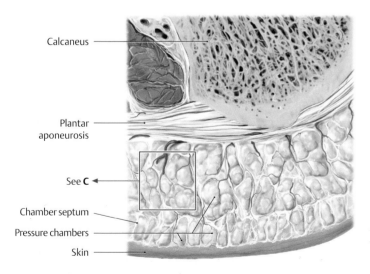

Calcaneus

Plantar aponeurosis

See **C**

Chamber septum

Pressure chambers

Skin

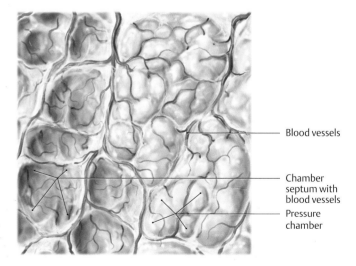

Blood vessels

Chamber septum with blood vessels

Pressure chamber

B The plantar pressure chambers
Detail from **A**.
Each of the pressure chambers contains an internal fibrofatty tissue covered externally by tough connective tissue made up of collagen fibers. These fibrous septa are firmly attached between the plantar aponeurosis and plantar corium and are supplied by an extensive network of blood vessels that further stabilize the walls of the pressure chambers (see close-up in **C**).

C Structure of the pressure chambers
Detail from **B**.
The fatty tissue has been removed from the chambers on the left side of the drawing to demonstrate the blood vessels that permeate the septa. (The sole of the foot is one of the most highly vascularized regions of the body surface.)

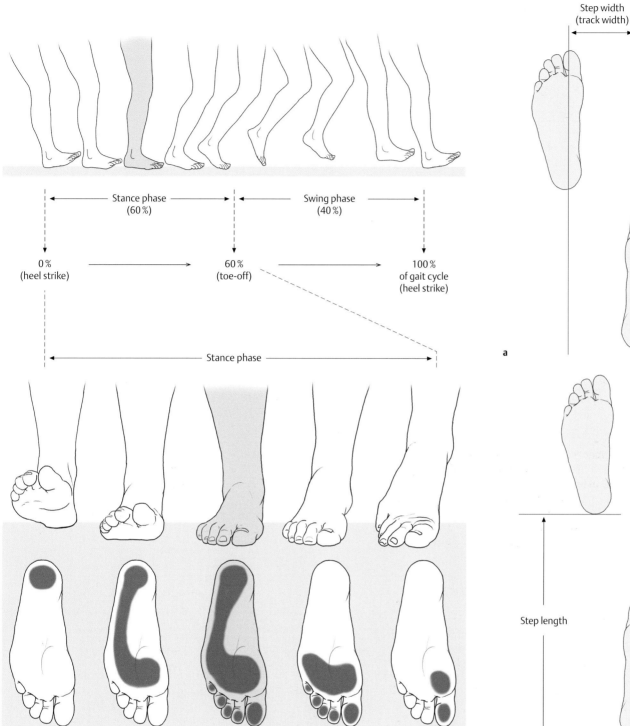

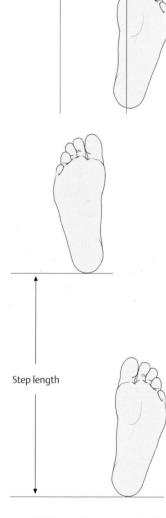

a

b

D Movements of the leg during one gait cycle

During normal walking, each leg functions alternately as the stance leg and swing leg. The stance phase begins when the heel contacts the ground (heel strike) and ends when the toes push off from the ground (toe-off). This phase makes up 60% of the gait cycle. The swing phase begins with the toe-off and ends with the heel strike. It makes up 40% of the gait cycle. (100% of gait cycle = the period between two heel strikes of the same foot.)

E Step width (a) and step length (b)

The step width (track width) is evaluated from behind. Generally it is narrower than the distance between the two hip joints. The step length (evaluated from the side) equals approximately 2 to 3 foot lengths.

The track width and step length define the area of support and thus play a critical role in stability. This is particularly important in hemiplegic patients, for example, in whom impaired proprioception can lead to instabilities of gait and stance.

2.1 The Muscles of the Lower Limb: Classification

In most mammals, the upper and lower limbs share many functions and have analogous functional groups of muscles. In humans, however, the specializations of the upper limb for manipulation and the lower limb for ambulation have imposed radically different requirements upon their respective muscle groups. For instance, the shoulder girdle has considerable freedom of motion on the trunk and is acted upon by an array of muscles, but the pelvic ring is firmly fixed to the vertebral column and changes position very little relative to the trunk, and has no comparable muscles to move it. In contrast, the hip and gluteal muscles have evolved into massive and powerful movers and stabilizers of the femur, counteracting the loads imposed by support of the whole body weight on two limbs and maintaining balance and stability during bipedal locomotion; these muscles are, in aggregate, larger than their counterparts that act upon the humerus, with a significantly different arrangement and orientation.

As with the upper limb (see p. 256), the muscles of the lower limb can be classified on the basis of origin, topography, function, and innervation. Each such classification system has advantages and disadvantages, and so several schemes are presented here. Segregation of muscles that act at the hip into specific functional groups is valid only for a particular joint position, because the axis of motion changes relative to the muscles as the joint is dynamically reoriented, causing abductors to become adductors, for example. Muscles surrounding the hip can be categorized topographically into an inner and outer group, relative to the pelvic girdle (see **A**). Muscles acting on the knee and foot can be grouped logically in an arrangement that uses both functional and topographical criteria, because these muscles tend to be clustered by functional groups into discrete compartments and act in a consistent way on joints with restricted ranges of motion. As with the upper limb, it is also instructive to categorize the lower limb's muscles by the pattern of their innervation (see **E**), a pattern that reveals the underlying logic of different clinical syndromes involving nerve damage.

A The hip and gluteal muscles

Inner hip muscles
- Psoas major
- Psoas minor   } Act in unison as the "iliopsoas"
- Iliacus

Outer hip muscles
- Gluteus maximus
- Gluteus medius
- Gluteus minimus
- Tensor fasciae latae
- Piriformis
- Obturator internus
- Gemelli
- Quadratus femoris

Muscles of the adductor group*
- Obturator externus
- Pectineus
- Adductor longus
- Adductor brevis
- Adductor magnus
- Adductor minimus
- Gracilis

* For functional reasons the muscles of the adductor group, all of which are located on the medial side of the thigh, are classified as hip muscles because they act mainly on the hip joint.

B The thigh muscles

Anterior thigh muscles
- Sartorius
- Quadriceps femoris
  - Rectus femoris
  - Vastus medialis
  - Vastus lateralis
  - Vastus intermedius
  - (Articularis genus, the "fifth head" of quadriceps femoris, see p. 428)

Posterior thigh muscles
- Biceps femoris
- Semimembranosus   } The hamstrings
- Semitendinosus

C The leg muscles

Anterior compartment
- Tibialis anterior
- Extensor digitorum longus
- Extensor hallucis longus
- Fibularis tertius

Lateral compartment
- Fibularis longus
- Fibularis brevis

Posterior compartment
Superficial part
- Triceps surae
  - Soleus
  - Gastrocnemius (medial and lateral heads)
- Plantaris

Deep part
- Tibialis posterior
- Flexor digitorum longus
- Flexor hallucis longus
- Popliteus

D The intrinsic muscles of the foot

Dorsal muscles
- Extensor digitorum brevis
- Extensor hallucis brevis

Plantar muscles
Medial compartment
- Abductor hallucis
- Flexor hallucis brevis (medial and lateral heads)

Lateral compartment
- Abductor digiti minimi
- Flexor digiti minimi brevis
- Opponens digiti minimi

Central compartment
- Flexor digitorum brevis
- Adductor hallucis (transverse and oblique heads)
- Quadratus plantae
- First through fourth lumbricals
- First through third plantar interossei
- First through fourth dorsal interossei

E Classification of muscles based on their motor innervation

All the muscles of the lower limb are supplied by branches of the lumbar plexus (T 12–L 4) and the sacral plexus (L 5–S 3). They may be supplied by short, direct branches or by long nerves emanating from the corresponding plexus (see p. 470).

Nerve or plexus	Muscles supplied
Lumbar plexus	
Direct branches (muscular branches)	Psoas major and minor
Nerves arising from the lumbar plexus	
Femoral nerve	Iliacus, pectineus; sartorius, quadriceps femoris
Obturator nerve	Obturator externus, pectineus, adductor longus, adductor brevis, adductor magnus (deep part), adductor minimus, gracilis
Sacral plexus	
Direct branches (muscular branches)	Piriformis, obturator internus, gemelli, quadratus femoris
Nerves arising from the sacral plexus	
Superior gluteal nerve	Tensor fasciae latae, gluteus medius and minimus
Inferior gluteal nerve	Gluteus maximus
Sciatic nerve (see also **F**)	Adductor magnus (superficial part, tibial part); Biceps femoris (long head, tibial part); Biceps femoris (short head, fibular part) Semimembranosus, semitendinosus (tibial part)
• Common fibular* nerve – Deep fibular nerve	Tibialis anterior, extensor digitorum longus and brevis, fibularis tertius, extensor hallucis longus and brevis
– Superficial fibular nerve	Fibularis longus and brevis
• Tibial nerve	Popliteus, triceps surae, plantaris, tibialis posterior, flexor digitorum longus, flexor hallucis longus
– Medial plantar nerve	Abductor hallucis, flexor hallucis brevis (medial head), flexor digitorum brevis, first and second lumbricals
– Lateral plantar nerve	Flexor hallucis brevis (lateral head), adductor hallucis, abductor digiti minimi, flexor digiti minimi brevis, opponens digiti minimi, quadratus plantae, third and fourth lumbricals, first through third plantar interossei, first through fourth dorsal interossei

* The common fibular nerve and its divisions are also referred to as "peroneal nerves."

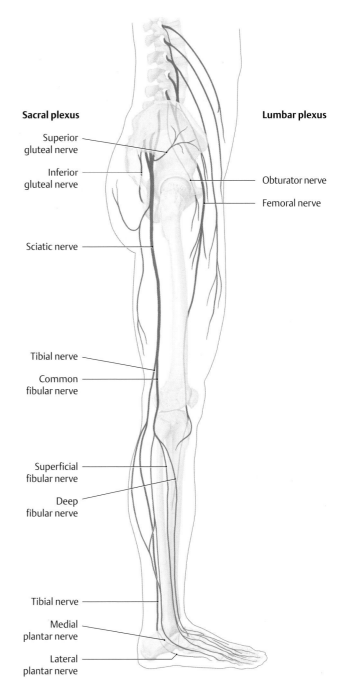

Sacral plexus
- Superior gluteal nerve
- Inferior gluteal nerve
- Sciatic nerve
- Tibial nerve
- Common fibular nerve
- Superficial fibular nerve
- Deep fibular nerve
- Tibial nerve
- Medial plantar nerve
- Lateral plantar nerve

Lumbar plexus
- Obturator nerve
- Femoral nerve

F The branches of the lumbosacral plexus that innervate the muscles of the lower limb

Right leg, lateral view. The ventral rami of the lumbar and sacral nerves, with contributions from the subcostal nerve and coccygeal nerve (not shown here), combine to form the lumbosacral plexus. While the branches arising from the lumbar plexus run *anterior to* the hip joint and mainly supply the muscles on the anterior and medial views of the thigh, the branches from the sacral plexus run *behind* the hip joint to supply the posterior thigh muscles and all the muscles of the leg and foot. The grossly visible division of the sciatic nerve into its two terminal branches (the tibial nerve and common fibular nerve) is generally located just above the knee joint, as pictured here (*low division*). But the nerve fibers that make up the two terminal branches become organized into bundles at a much more proximal level, where they already appear as separate nerve branches within their common fibrous sheath. In the *high division* pattern, the nerve divides into its terminal branches while still in the lesser pelvis (see p. 493).

421

2.2   The Hip and Gluteal Muscles: The Inner Hip Muscles

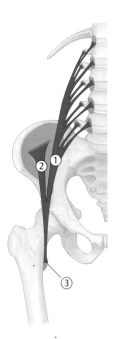

Origin:	• ① Psoas major (superficial layer): lateral surfaces of the T12 vertebral body, the L1–L4 vertebral bodies, and the associated intervertebral disks • ① Psoas minor (deep layer): costal processes of the L1–L5 vertebrae • ② Iliacus: the iliac fossa
Insertion:	Common insertion on the lesser trochanter of the femur as the iliopsoas ③ (psoas minor inserts into the iliopectineal arch (not depicted; see **B**)
Action:	• Hip joint: flexion and external rotation • Lumbar spine: unilateral contraction (with the femur fixed) bends the trunk laterally to the same side, bilateral contraction raises the trunk from the supine position
Innervation:	Femoral nerve (iliacus) and direct branches from the lumbar plexus (psoas) (L1–L3)

A Schematic of the inner hip muscles

Properties and clinical aspects of the iliopsoas muscle

The iliopsoas is classified as a hip flexor along with the rectus femoris, sartorius, and tensor fasciae latae. It is the most powerful flexor, its long vertical travel making it an important muscle for standing, walking, and running. As a typical postural muscle with a preponderance of slow-twitch red (type I) fibers, however, the iliopsoas is inherently susceptible to pathological shortening (particularly in older patients with a sedentary lifestyle or chronic immobilization conditions), and requires regular stretching to maintain normal tone (see p. 40).

Shortening (contracture) of the hip flexors leads to:

• increased anterior pelvic tilt,
• increased lumbar lordosis, and
• limitation of hip extension.

Unilateral shortening of the iliopsoas, in which the ilium on the affected side is tilted forward, can be diagnosed with the Thomas maneuver (see p. 386). This condition leads to pelvic torsion, in which the pelvis becomes twisted upon itself. This mainly alters the function of the sacroiliac joints but also compromises the intervertebral joints and the lumbosacral junction (increased lordosis of the lumbar spine with degenerative changes in the vertebral bodies, see p. 104). Patients with *bilateral* iliopsoas weakness or paralysis are unable to raise the trunk from the supine position, despite intact abdominal muscles, without using their arms and are greatly limited in their ability to walk and climb stairs without assistance.

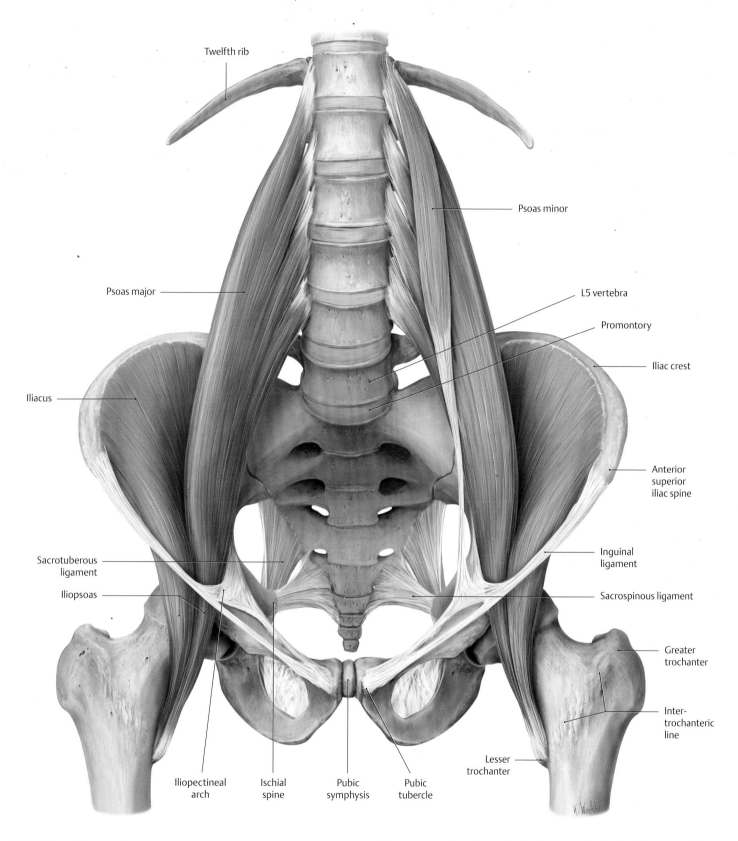

Twelfth rib

Psoas minor

Psoas major

L5 vertebra

Promontory

Iliac crest

Iliacus

Anterior
superior
iliac spine

Sacrotuberous
ligament

Inguinal
ligament

Iliopsoas

Sacrospinous ligament

Greater
trochanter

Inter-
trochanteric
line

Lesser
trochanter

Iliopectineal
arch

Ischial
spine

Pubic
symphysis

Pubic
tubercle

B The inner hip muscles
Anterior view.

The psoas major unites with the iliacus at the level of the inguinal liga-ment to form a conjoined muscle, the iliopsoas. Approximately 50% of the population also have a psoas minor muscle (as shown here), which arises from the T 12 and L 1 vertebrae and inserts into the iliopectineal arch (iliac fascia).

2.3 The Hip and Gluteal Muscles: The Outer Hip Muscles

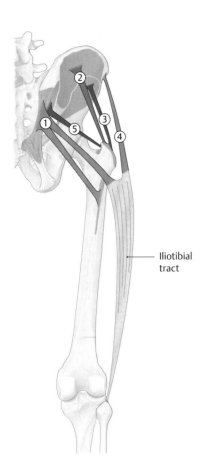

— Iliotibial tract

A Schematic of the vertically-oriented outer hip muscles

① **Gluteus maximus**

Origin:	Lateral part of the dorsal surface of the sacrum, posterior part of the gluteal surface of the ilium (behind the posterior gluteal line), also from the thoracolumbar fascia and sacrotuberous ligament
Insertion:	• Upper fibers: iliotibial tract • Lower fibers: gluteal tuberosity
Action:	• Entire muscle: extends and externally rotates the hip, stabilizes the hip in both the sagittal and coronal planes • Upper fibers: abduction • Lower fibers: adduction
Innervation:	Inferior gluteal nerve (L 5–S 2)

② **Gluteus medius**

Origin:	Gluteal surface of the ilium (below the iliac crest between the anterior and posterior gluteal line)
Insertion:	Lateral surface of the greater trochanter of the femur
Action:	• Entire muscle: abducts the hip, stabilizes the pelvis in the coronal plane • Anterior part: flexion and internal rotation • Posterior part: extension and external rotation
Innervation:	Superior gluteal nerve (L 4–S 1)

③ **Gluteus minimus**

Origin:	Gluteal surface of the ilium (below the origin of gluteus medius)
Insertion:	Anterolateral surface of the greater trochanter of the femur
Action:	• Entire muscle: abducts the hip, stabilizes the pelvis in the coronal plane • Anterior part: flexion and internal rotation • Posterior part: extension and external rotation
Innervation:	Superior gluteal nerve (L 4–S 1)

④ **Tensor fasciae latae**

Origin:	Anterior superior iliac spine
Insertion:	Iliotibial tract
Action:	• Tenses the fascia lata • Hip joint: abduction, flexion, and internal rotation
Innervation:	Superior gluteal nerve (L 4–S 1)

⑤ **Piriformis**

Origin:	Pelvic surface of the sacrum
Insertion:	Apex of the greater trochanter of the femur
Action:	• External rotation, abduction, and extension of the hip joint • Stabilizes the hip joint
Innervation:	Direct branches from the sacral plexus (L 5–S 2)

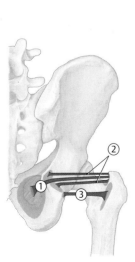

B Schematic of the horizontally-oriented outer hip muscles

① **Obturator internus**

Origin:	Inner surface of the obturator membrane and its bony boundaries
Insertion:	Medial surface of the greater trochanter
Action:	External rotation, adduction, and extension of the hip joint (also active in abduction, depending on the position of the joint)
Innervation:	Direct branches from the sacral plexus (L 5, S 1)

② **Gemelli**

Origin:	• Gemellus superior: ischial spine • Gemellus inferior: ischial tuberosity
Insertion:	Jointly with obturator internus tendon (medial surface, greater trochanter)
Action:	External rotation, adduction, and extension of the hip joint (also active in abduction, depending on the position of the joint)
Innervation:	Direct branches from the sacral plexus (L 5, S 1)

③ **Quadratus femoris**

Origin:	Lateral border of the ischial tuberosity
Insertion:	Intertrochanteric crest of the femur
Action:	External rotation and adduction of the hip joint
Innervation:	Direct branches from the sacral plexus (L 5, S 1)

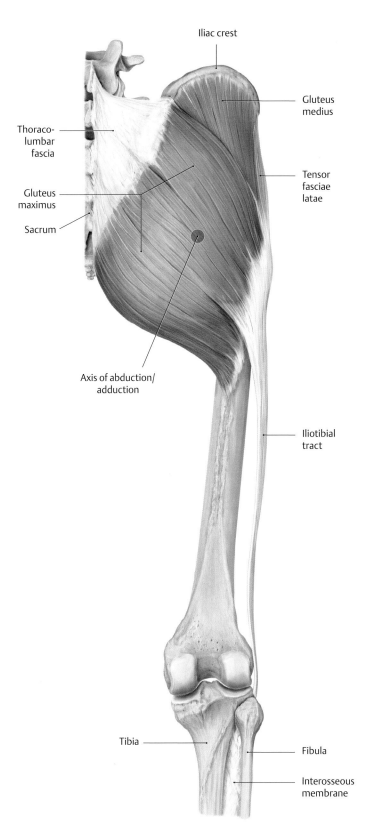

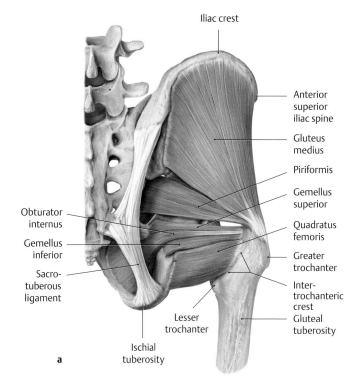

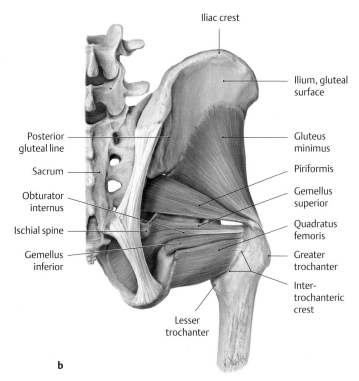

C The outer hip muscles: superficial layer

Right side, posterior view.

Note the position of the gluteus maximus muscle in relation to the axis of hip abduction and adduction. While the fibers of gluteus maximus that run *above* the axis and insert on the tibia via the iliotibial tract are active in abducting the hip joint, the muscle fibers that run *below* the axis are active in adduction.

D The outer hip muscles: deep layer

Right side, posterior view.

a With the gluteus maximus removed.
b With the gluteus medius removed.

If there is weakness or paralysis of the small gluteal muscles (gluteus medius and minimus), the pelvis can no longer be stabilized in the coronal plane and will tilt toward the unaffected side (positive Trendelenburg sign, see also p. 476).

2.4 The Hip and Gluteal Muscles: The Adductor Group

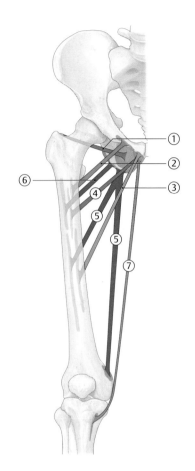

A Schematic of the adductors

① **Obturator externus**

Origin:	Outer surface of the obturator membrane and its bony boundaries
Insertion:	Trochanteric fossa of the femur
Action:	• Adduction and external rotation of the hip joint
	• Stabilizes the pelvis in the sagittal plane
Innervation:	Obturator nerve (L 3, L 4)

② **Pectineus**

Origin:	Pecten pubis
Insertion:	Pectineal line and the proximal linea aspera of the femur
Action:	• Adduction, external rotation, and slight flexion of the hip joint
	• Stabilizes the pelvis in the coronal and sagittal planes
Innervation:	Femoral nerve, obturator nerve (L 2, L 3)

③ **Adductor longus**

Origin:	Superior pubic ramus and anterior side of the symphysis
Insertion:	Linea aspera: medial lip in the middle third of the femur
Action:	• Adduction and flexion (up to 70°) of the hip joint (extends the hip past 80° of flexion)
	• Stabilizes the pelvis in the coronal and sagittal planes
Innervation:	Obturator nerve (L 2–L 4)

④ **Adductor brevis**

Origin:	Inferior pubic ramus
Insertion:	Linea aspera: medial lip in the upper third of the femur
Action:	• Adduction and flexion (up to 70°) of the hip joint (extends the hip past 80° of flexion)
	• Stabilizes the pelvis in the coronal and sagittal planes
Innervation	Obturator nerve (L 2, L 3)

⑤ **Adductor magnus**

Origin:	Inferior pubic ramus, ischial ramus, and ischial tuberosity
Insertion:	• Deep part ("fleshy insertion"): medial lip of linea aspera
	• Superficial part ("tendinous insertion"): medial epicondyle of the femur
Actions	• Adduction, external rotation, and extension of the hip joint (the tendinous insertion is also active in internal rotation)
	• Stabilizes the pelvis in the coronal and sagittal planes
Innervation:	• Deep part: obturator nerve (L 2–L 4)
	• Superficial part: tibial nerve (L 4)

⑥ **Adductor minimus (upper division of adductor magnus)**

Origin:	Inferior pubic ramus
Insertion:	Medial lip of the linea aspera
Action:	Adduction, external rotation and slight flexion of the hip joint
Innervation:	Obturator nerve (L 2–L 4)

⑦ **Gracilis**

Origin:	Inferior pubic ramus below the symphysis
Insertion:	Medial border of the tuberosity of the tibia (along with the tendons of sartorius and semitendinosus)
Action:	• Hip joint: adduction and flexion
	• Knee joint: flexion and internal rotation
Innervation:	Obturator nerve (L 2, L 3)

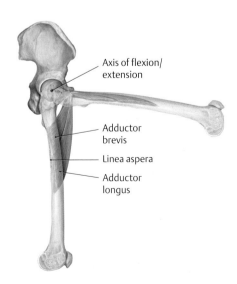

Axis of flexion/ extension

Adductor brevis

Linea aspera

Adductor longus

B Reversal of muscle actions, illustrated for the adductor brevis and longus

Right hip joint, lateral view. The femur in 80° of flexion is shown in lighter shading. In addition to their primary action as adductors, both muscles may also be active in flexion and extension, depending on the joint position.

• They assist in flexion from the neutral (zero-degree) position to approximately 70°.

• Their actions reverse past approximately 80° of flexion, and they become active in extension.

The flexor components of both muscles are transformed into extensor components as soon as their insertion (the linea aspera) moves higher than their origin (the inferior or superior pubic ramus).

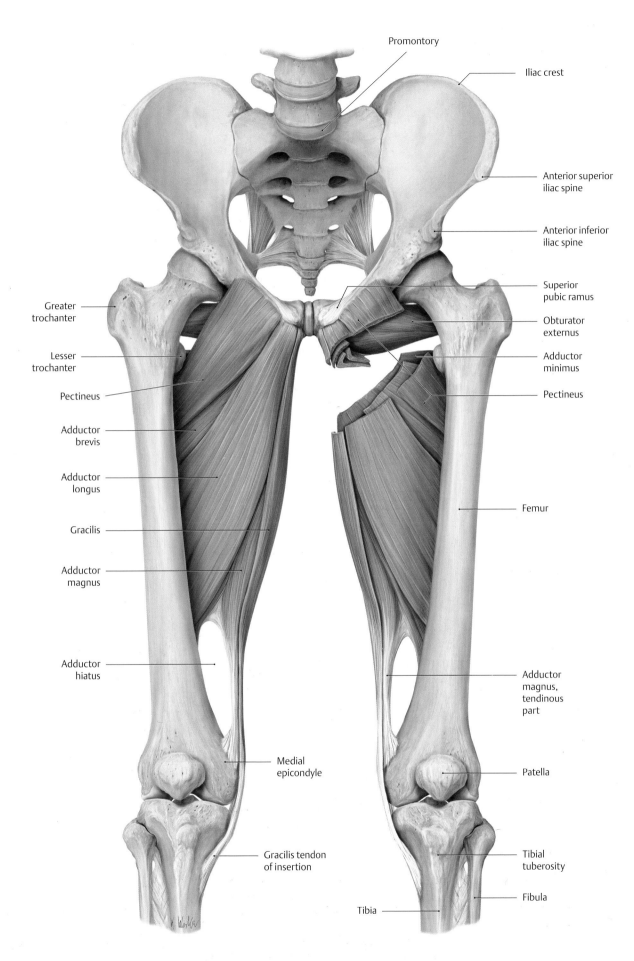

Promontory

Iliac crest

Anterior superior
iliac spine

Anterior inferior
iliac spine

Superior
pubic ramus

Obturator
externus

Adductor
minimus

Pectineus

Femur

Adductor
magnus,
tendinous
part

Patella

Tibial
tuberosity

Fibula

Tibia

Greater
trochanter

Lesser
trochanter

Pectineus

Adductor
brevis

Adductor
longus

Gracilis

Adductor
magnus

Adductor
hiatus

Medial
epicondyle

Gracilis tendon
of insertion

C The adductors (obturator externus; pectineus; adductores longus, brevis, magnus, and minimus; and gracilis)
Anterior view. A portion of the adductors, pectineus, and gracilis muscles on the left side have been removed just past their origins to demonstrate the course of obturator externus more clearly.

Note: Unilateral shortening of the adductors leads to functional leg shortening on the affected side.

427

2.5 The Anterior Thigh Muscles: The Extensor Group

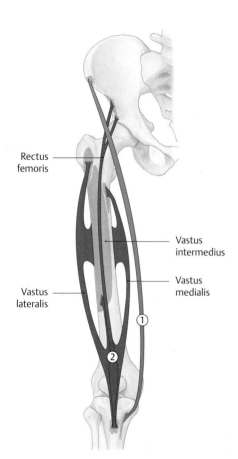

① Sartorius

Origin: Anterior superior iliac spine
Insertion: Medial to the tibial tuberosity (together with gracilis and semitendinosus)
Action:
- Hip joint: flexion, abduction, and external rotation
- Knee joint: flexion and internal rotation

Innervation: Femoral nerve (L 2, L 3)

② Quadriceps femoris

Origin:
- Rectus femoris: anterior inferior iliac spine, acetabular roof of the hip joint
- Vastus medialis: medial lip of the linea aspera, distal part of the intertrochanteric line
- Vastus lateralis: lateral lip of the linea aspera, lateral surface of the greater trochanter
- Vastus intermedius: anterior side of the femoral shaft
- Articularis genus (distal fibers of the vastus intermedius): anterior side of the femoral shaft at the level of the suprapatellar recess

Insertion:
- On the tibial tuberosity via the patellar ligament (entire muscle)
- Both sides of the tuberosity on the medial and lateral condyles via the medial and longitudinal patellar retinacula (vastus medialis and lateralis)
- The suprapatellar recess of the knee joint capsule (articularis genus)

Action:
- Hip joint: flexion (rectus femoris)
- Knee joint: extension (all parts), prevents entrapment of the capsule (articularis genus)

Innervation: Femoral nerve (L 2–L 4)

A Schematic of the extensors

B Deficient stabilization of the knee joint due to weakness or paralysis of quadriceps femoris
Right lower limb, lateral view.

a When the quadriceps femoris is intact and the knee is in slight flexion, the line of gravity (see p. 363) falls *behind* the transverse axis of knee motion. As the only extensor muscle of the knee joint, the quadriceps femoris keeps the body from tipping backward and ensures stability.

b With weakness or paralysis of the quadriceps femoris, the knee joint can no longer be actively extended. In order to stand upright, the patient must hyperextend the knee so that the line of gravity, and thus the whole-body center of gravity, is shifted forward, in front of the knee, to utilize gravity as the extending force. The joint is stabilized in this situation by the posterior capsule and ligaments of the knee.

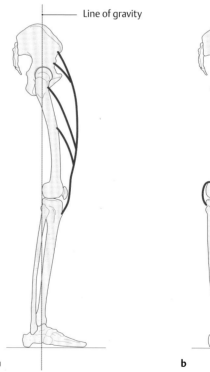

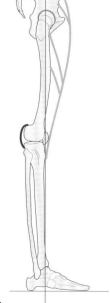

Line of gravity

a   b

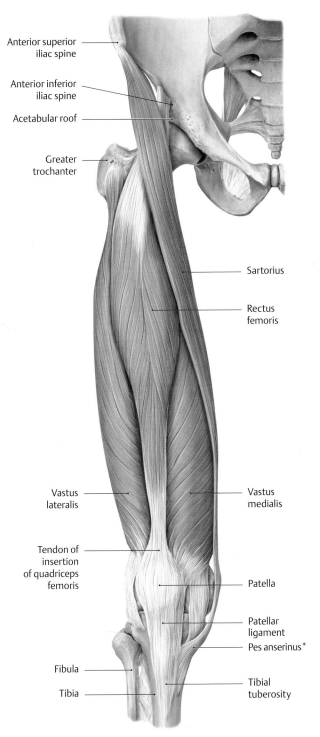

Anterior superior
iliac spine

Anterior inferior
iliac spine

Acetabular roof

Greater
trochanter

Sartorius

Rectus
femoris

Vastus
lateralis

Vastus
medialis

Tendon of
insertion
of quadriceps
femoris

Patella

Patellar
ligament

Pes anserinus*

Fibula

Tibia

Tibial
tuberosity

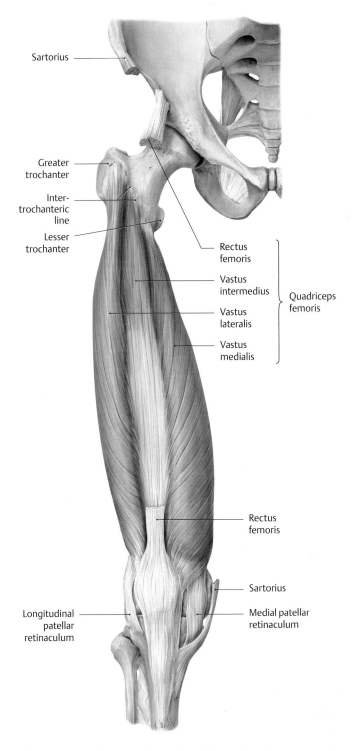

Sartorius

Greater
trochanter

Inter-
trochanteric
line

Lesser
trochanter

Rectus
femoris

Vastus
intermedius

Vastus
lateralis

Vastus
medialis

Quadriceps
femoris

Rectus
femoris

Sartorius

Longitudinal
patellar
retinaculum

Medial patellar
retinaculum

C The extensors (quadriceps femoris and sartorius)

Right side, anterior view. As its name implies, the quadriceps femoris is basically a four-headed muscle consisting of the rectus femoris and the vastus medialis, lateralis, and intermedius (the vastus intermedius, covered here by the rectus femoris, is visible in **D**). It may also be considered as having a fifth head, the articularis genus. The latter is composed of distal fibers of the vastus intermedius and so does not constitute a separate muscle. But because its fibers insert in the suprapatellar recess (not shown), unlike the other four parts which all attach to the patellar ligament, the articularis genus is often regarded as the fifth head of quadriceps femoris.

Note: The only biarticular part of quadriceps femoris is the rectus femoris, which acts on both the hip and knee joints.

* The pes anserinus is the common tendinous expansion for the gracilis, sartorius, and semitendinosus.

D The extensors (deep portion of quadriceps femoris)

Right side, anterior view. The sartorius and rectus femoris have been removed to their origins and insertions.

The area of origin of the rectus femoris is intimately related to the anterior aspect of the capsule of the hip joint, a relation with functional and clinical consequences. Pathological swelling of the joint capsule can cause pain that induces reflex reactions when the rectus is used for knee flexion; such reflex reactions are the basis of a useful test. With the patient lying prone, the examiner flexes the patient's knee. This causes passive stretching of the rectus femoris and adds significant pressure to a hip joint capsule already distended by effusion. The patient reflexively "escapes" the painful stimulus by raising the buttock, a positive "rectus sign."

2.6 The Posterior Thigh Muscles: The Flexor Group

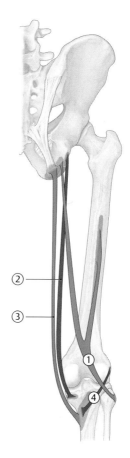

A Schematic of the flexors

① **Biceps femoris**

Origin:	• Long head: ischial tuberosity, sacrotuberous ligament (common head with semitendinosus) • Short head: lateral lip of the linea aspera in the middle third of the femur
Insertion:	Head of fibula
Action:	• Hip joint (long head): extends the hip, stabilizes the pelvis in the sagittal plane • Knee joint (entire muscle): flexion and external rotation
Innervation:	• Tibial nerve, L 5–S 2 (long head) • Common fibular nerve, L 5–S 2 (short head)

② **Semimembranosus**

Origin:	Ischial tuberosity
Insertion:	Medial tibial condyle, oblique popliteal ligament, popliteus fascia
Action:	• Hip joint: extends the hip, stabilizes the pelvis in the sagittal plane • Knee joint: flexion and internal rotation
Innervation:	Tibial nerve (L 5–S 2)

③ **Semitendinosus**

Origin:	Ischial tuberosity and sacrotuberous ligament (common head with long head of biceps femoris)
Insertion:	Medial to the tibial tuberosity in the pes anserinus (along with the tendons of gracilis and sartorius)
Action:	• Hip joint: extends the hip, stabilizes the pelvis in the sagittal plane • Knee joint: flexion and internal rotation
Innervation:	Tibial nerve (L 5–S 2)

④ **Popliteus**

Origin:	Lateral femoral condyle, posterior horn of the lateral meniscus
Insertion:	Posterior tibial surface (above the origin of soleus)
Action:	Flexion and internal rotation of the knee joint (stabilizes the knee)
Innervation:	Tibial nerve (L 4–S 1)

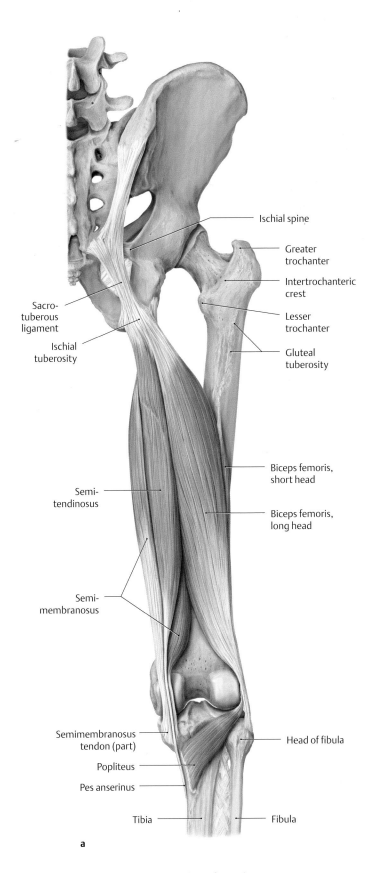

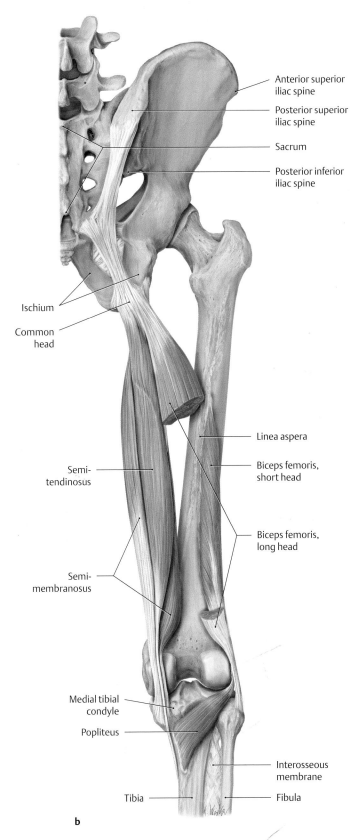

a

b

B The flexors (the hamstrings and popliteus)

Right side, posterior view.

a The *hamstrings* are the posterior thigh muscles that arise from the ischium and insert on the leg: biceps femoris, semimembrano-

sus, and semitendinosus. All but the short head of biceps femoris are "biarticular," spanning both the hip and knee joints.

b A portion of the long head of biceps femoris has been removed to display the short head and its origin from the lateral lip of the linea aspera.

431

2.7 The Leg Muscles: The Anterior and Lateral Compartments (Extensor and Fibularis Group)

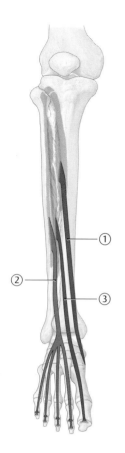

① Tibialis anterior

Origin: Upper two thirds of the lateral surface of the tibia, the crural interosseous membrane, and the highest part of the superficial crural fascia

Insertion: Medial and plantar surface of the medial cuneiform, the medial base of the first metatarsal

Action:
- Talocrural joint: dorsiflexion
- Subtalar joint: inversion (supination)

Innervation: Deep fibular nerve (L 4, L 5)

② Extensor digitorum longus

Origin: Lateral tibial condyle, head of the fibula, anterior border of the fibula, and the crural interosseous membrane

Insertion: By four slips to the dorsal aponeuroses of the second through fifth toes and the bases of the distal phalanges of the second through fifth toes

Action:
- Talocrural joint: dorsiflexion
- Subtalar joint: eversion (pronation)
- Extends the metatarsophalangeal and interphalangeal joints of the second through fifth toes

Innervation: Deep fibular nerve (L 5, S 1)

③ Extensor hallucis longus

Origin: Middle third of the medial surface of the fibula, the crural interosseous membrane

Insertion: Dorsal aponeurosis of the big toe and the base of its distal phalanx

Action:
- Talocrural joint: dorsiflexion
- Subtalar joint: active in both eversion and inversion (pronation/supination), depending on the initial position of the foot
- Extends the metatarsophalangeal and interphalangeal joints of the big toe

Innervation: Deep fibular nerve (L 5)

A Schematic of the anterior compartment

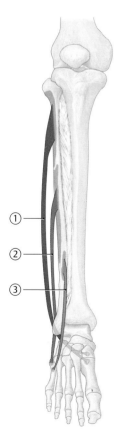

① Fibularis longus

Origin: Head of the fibula, proximal two-thirds of the lateral surface of the fibula (arising partly from the intermuscular septa)

Insertion: Plantar side of the medial cuneiform, base of the first metatarsal

Action:
- Talocrural joint: plantar flexion
- Subtalar joint: eversion (pronation)
- Supports the transverse arch of the foot

Innervation: Superficial fibular nerve (L 5, S 1)

② Fibularis brevis

Origin: Distal half of the lateral surface of the fibula, intermuscular septa

Insertion: Tuberosity at the base of the fifth metatarsal (with an occasional division to the dorsal aponeurosis of the fifth toe)

Action:
- Talocrural joint: plantar flexion
- Subtalar joint: eversion (pronation)

Innervation: Superficial fibular nerve (L 5, S 1)

③ Fibularis tertius (part of extensor digitorum longus)

Origin: Anterior border of the distal fibula

Insertion: Base of the fifth metatarsal

Action:
- Talocrural joint: dorsiflexion
- Subtalar joint: eversion (pronation)

Innervation: Deep fibular nerve (L 5, S 1)

B Schematic of the lateral compartment

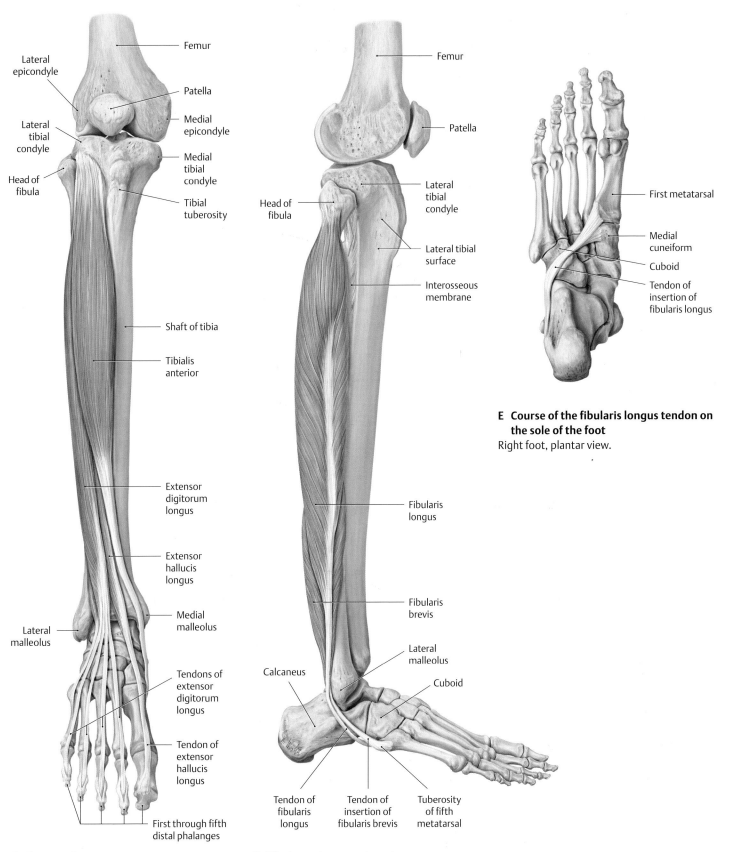

Lateral epicondyle

Lateral tibial condyle

Head of fibula

Femur

Patella

Medial epicondyle

Medial tibial condyle

Tibial tuberosity

Shaft of tibia

Tibialis anterior

Extensor digitorum longus

Extensor hallucis longus

Medial malleolus

Lateral malleolus

Tendons of extensor digitorum longus

Tendon of extensor hallucis longus

First through fifth distal phalanges

Femur

Patella

Head of fibula

Lateral tibial condyle

Lateral tibial surface

Interosseous membrane

Fibularis longus

Fibularis brevis

Lateral malleolus

Calcaneus

Cuboid

Tendon of fibularis longus

Tendon of insertion of fibularis brevis

Tuberosity of fifth metatarsal

First metatarsal

Medial cuneiform

Cuboid

Tendon of insertion of fibularis longus

E Course of the fibularis longus tendon on the sole of the foot
Right foot, plantar view.

**C The anterior compartment
(tibialis anterior, extensor digitorum longus, and extensor hallucis longus)**
Right leg, anterior view.

**D The lateral compartment
(fibularis longus and brevis)**
Right leg, lateral view.

433

2.8 The Leg Muscles: The Posterior Compartment (Superficial Flexor Group)

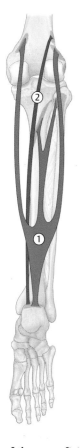

A Schematic of the superficial flexors

① **Triceps surae**

Origin:	• Soleus: posterior surface of the head and neck of the fibula; attached to the soleal line of the tibia via a tendinous arch
	• Gastrocnemius: Medial head—medial epicondyle of the femur
	Lateral head—lateral epicondyle of the femur
Insertion:	The calcaneal tuberosity via the Achilles tendon
Action:	• Talocrural joint: plantar flexion
	• Subtalar joint: inversion (supination)
	• Knee joint: flexion (gastrocnemius)
Innervation:	Tibial nerve (S 1, S 2)

② **Plantaris**

Origin:	Proximal to the lateral head of gastrocnemius
Insertion:	The calcaneal tuberosity via the Achilles tendon
Action:	Negligible due to its small cross section; may act to prevent compression of the posterior leg musculature during knee flexion
Innervation:	Tibial nerve (S 1, S 2)

B Rupture of the Achilles tendon

Right leg, posterior view. The Achilles tendon (calcanean tendon) is the common tendon of insertion of the muscles that comprise the triceps surae (the soleus and both heads of gastrocnemius). The tendon has an average length of 20–25 cm, a mean cross-sectional area of approximately 70–80 mm², and a breaking strength of 60–100 newtons/mm². A healthy tendon can thus bear a load of nearly one ton. It is very unlikely, then, that the Achilles tendon will rupture unless it has been subjected to chronic excessive loads (in high jumpers, for example). Repetitive microtrauma can compromise the blood supply to the tendon, causing it to degenerate and gradually lose its strength. This is particularly damaging in the area where the tendon already has the least blood flow: approximately 2–6 cm proximal to its insertion on the calcaneal tuberosity. This is the most common site of a degenerative Achilles tendon rupture, which is eventually precipitated by a trivial injury. The rupture is accompanied by a whip-like snapping sound. Afterward the patient loses active plantar flexion and has only residual flexion from the deep flexor muscles.

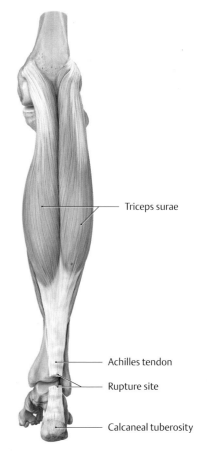

Triceps surae

Achilles tendon

Rupture site

Calcaneal tuberosity

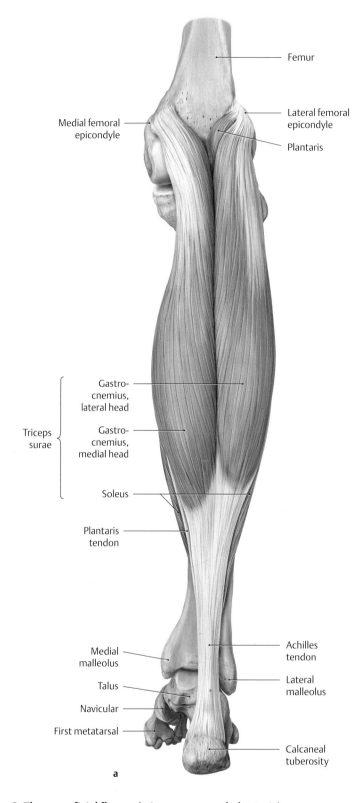

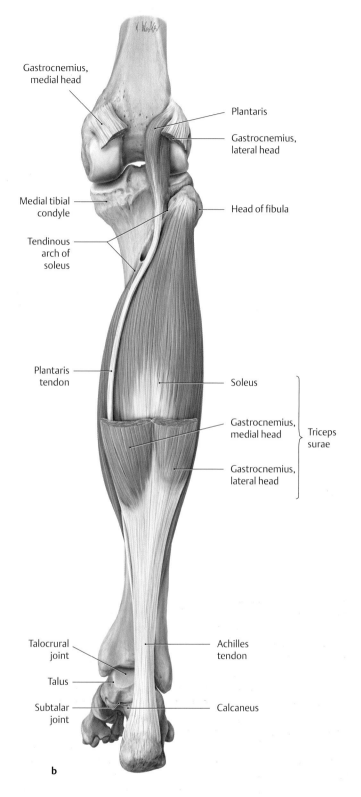

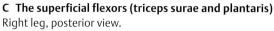

a

b

C The superficial flexors (triceps surae and plantaris)
Right leg, posterior view.

a The three heads of triceps surae are clearly distinguishable: the medial and lateral heads of gastrocnemius and the soleus. The plantaris, which arises proximal to the lateral head of gastrocnemius, is often viewed as the fourth head of triceps surae.

b Portions of the lateral and medial heads of gastrocnemius have been removed to expose the soleus and the plantaris with its long, narrow tendon of insertion.

2.9 The Leg Muscles: The Posterior Compartment (Deep Flexor Group)

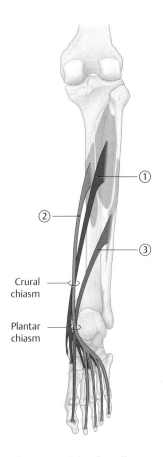

① **Tibialis posterior**

Origin: Crural interosseous membrane and the adjacent borders of the tibia and fibula
Insertion: Tuberosity of the navicular; medial, intermediate, and lateral cuneiforms; bases of the second through fourth metatarsals
Action: • Talocrural joint: plantar flexion
• Subtalar joint: inversion (supination)
• Supports the longitudinal and transverse arches of the foot
Innervation: Tibial nerve (L 4, L 5)

② **Flexor digitorum longus**

Origin: Middle third of the posterior surface of the tibia
Insertion: Bases of the second through fifth distal phalanges
Action: • Talocrural joint: plantar flexion
• Subtalar joint: inversion (supination)
• Metatarsophalangeal and interphalangeal joints of the second through fifth toes: plantar flexion
Innervation: Tibial nerve (L 5–S 2)

③ **Flexor hallucis longus**

Origin: Distal two-thirds of the posterior surface of the fibula, adjacent crural interosseous membrane
Insertion: Base of the distal phalanx of the big toe
Action: • Talocrural joint: plantar flexion
• Subtalar joint: inversion (supination)
• Metatarsophalangeal and interphalangeal joints of the big toe: plantar flexion
• Supports the medial longitudinal arch of the foot
Innervation: Tibial nerve (L 5–S 2)

A Schematic of the deep flexors

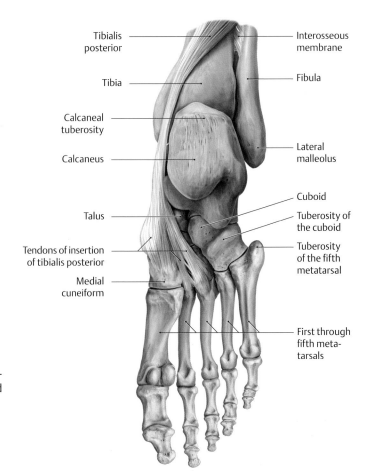

B Insertion of the tibialis posterior
Right foot in plantar flexion, plantar view. With its fan-shaped insertion, the tibialis posterior assists in stabilizing both the longitudinal and transverse arches of the foot.

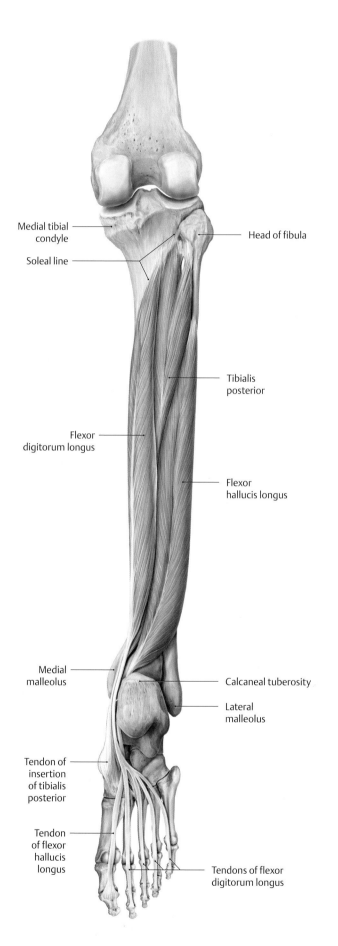

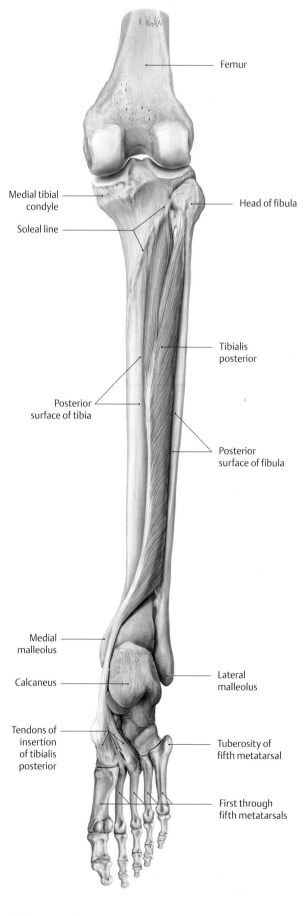

C The deep flexors (tibialis posterior, flexor digitorum longus, and flexor hallucis longus)
Right leg with the foot in plantar flexion, posterior view.

D The tibialis posterior
Right leg with the flexor digitorum longus and flexor hallucis longus removed. Foot in plantar flexion, posterior view.

437

2.10 The Intrinsic Muscles of the Foot: The Dorsum and Sole of the Foot (Lateral and Medial Compartments)

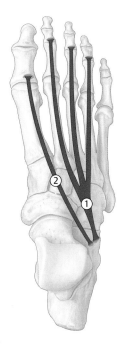

A Dorsal view of the short muscles

① **Extensor digitorum brevis**

Origin: Dorsal surface of the calcaneus
Insertion: Dorsal aponeurosis of the second through fourth toes, bases of the middle phalanges of these toes
Action: Extension of the metatarsophalangeal and proximal interphalangeal joints of the second through fourth toes
Innervation: Deep fibular nerve (L5, S1)

② **Extensor hallucis brevis**

Origin: Dorsal surface of the calcaneus
Insertion: Dorsal aponeurosis of the big toe, base of the proximal phalanx of the big toe
Action: Extension of the metatarsophalangeal joint of the big toe
Innervation: Deep fibular nerve (L5, S1)

① **Abductor hallucis**

Origin: Medial process of the calcaneal tuberosity, plantar aponeurosis
Insertion: Base of the proximal phalanx of the big toe via the medial sesamoid
Action: First metatarsophalangeal joint: flexion and medial abduction of the first toe; supports the longitudinal arch
Innervation: Medial plantar nerve (S1, S2)

② **Flexor hallucis brevis**

Medial cuneiform, intermediate cuneiform, plantar calcaneocuboid ligament
• Medial head: base of the proximal phalanx of the big toe via the medial sesamoid
• Lateral head: base of the proximal phalanx of the big toe via the lateral sesamoid
Flexes the first metatarsophalangeal joint, supports the longitudinal arch
• Medial head: medial plantar nerve (S1, S2)
• Lateral head: lateral plantar nerve (S1, S2)

③ **Adductor hallucis** (for clarity, the adductor hallucis is depicted here, although it is located in the central compartment)

Origin: • Oblique head: bases of the second through fourth metatarsals, cuboid, lateral cuneiform
• Transverse head: metatarsophalangeal joints of the third through fifth toes, deep transverse metatarsal ligament
Insertion: Base of the first proximal phalanx by a common tendon via the lateral sesamoid
Action: Flexes the first metatarsophalangeal joint, adducts the big toe; transverse head supports the transverse arch, oblique head supports the longitudinal arch
Innervation: Lateral plantar nerve (S2, S3)

④ **Abductor digiti minimi**

Origin: Lateral process and inferior surface of the calcaneal tuberosity, plantar aponeurosis
Insertion: Base of the proximal phalanx of the little toe, tuberosity of the fifth metatarsal
Action: Flexes the metatarsophalangeal joint of the little toe, abducts the little toe, supports the longitudinal arch
Innervation: Lateral plantar nerve (S1–S3)

⑤ **Flexor digiti minimi brevis**

Origin: Base of the fifth metatarsal, long plantar ligament
Insertion: Base of the proximal phalanx of the little toe
Action: Flexes the metatarsophalangeal joint of the little toe
Innervation: Lateral plantar nerve (S1, S2)

⑥ **Opponens digiti minimi** (often included with flexor digiti minimi brevis)

Origin: Long plantar ligament, plantar tendon sheath of the fibularis longus
Insertion: Fifth metatarsal
Action: Pulls the fifth metatarsal slightly in the plantar and medial direction
Innervation: Lateral plantar nerve (S1, S2)

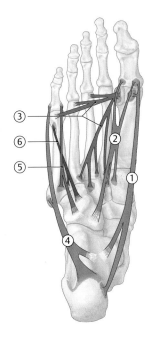

B Plantar view of the short muscles

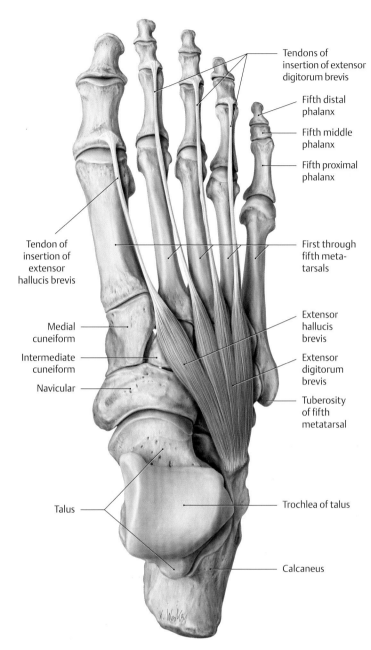

Tendons of insertion of extensor digitorum brevis

Fifth distal phalanx

Fifth middle phalanx

Fifth proximal phalanx

Tendon of insertion of extensor hallucis brevis

First through fifth meta-tarsals

Medial cuneiform

Extensor hallucis brevis

Intermediate cuneiform

Extensor digitorum brevis

Navicular

Tuberosity of fifth metatarsal

Talus

Trochlea of talus

Calcaneus

C The dorsal muscles of the foot (extensor digitorum brevis and extensor hallucis brevis)
Right foot, dorsal view.

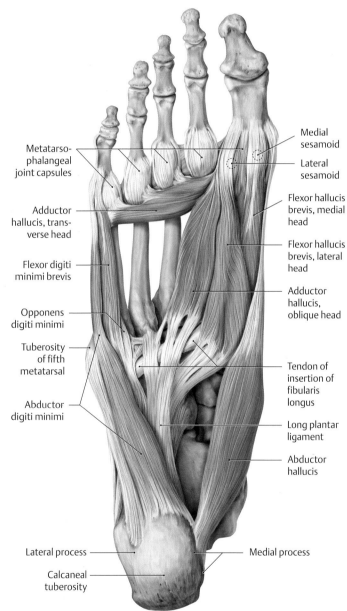

Metatarso-phalangeal joint capsules

Medial sesamoid

Lateral sesamoid

Adductor hallucis, trans-verse head

Flexor hallucis brevis, medial head

Flexor digiti minimi brevis

Flexor hallucis brevis, lateral head

Opponens digiti minimi

Adductor hallucis, oblique head

Tuberosity of fifth metatarsal

Tendon of insertion of fibularis longus

Abductor digiti minimi

Long plantar ligament

Abductor hallucis

Lateral process

Medial process

Calcaneal tuberosity

D The plantar muscles of the medial and lateral compartments (abductor hallucis, adductor hallucis*, flexor hallucis brevis, abductor digiti minimi, flexor digiti minimi, and opponens digiti minimi)
Right foot, plantar view.

* The adductor hallucis is considered part of the central compartment.

2.11 The Short Muscles of the Foot: The Sole of the Foot (Central Compartment*)

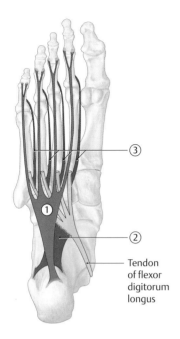

A Schematic of the flexor digitorum brevis, quadratus plantae, and the first through fourth lumbricals

① **Flexor digitorum brevis**

Origin:	Medial tubercle of the calcaneal tuberosity, plantar aponeurosis
Insertion:	The sides of the middle phalanges of the second through fifth toes
Action:	• Flexes the metatarsophalangeal and proximal interphalangeal joints of the second through fifth toes
	• Supports the longitudinal arch of the foot
Innervation:	Medial plantar nerve (S 1, S 2)

② **Quadratus plantae**

Origin:	Medial and plantar borders on the plantar side of the calcaneal tuberosity
Insertion:	Lateral border of the flexor digitorum longus tendon
Action:	Redirects and augments the pull of flexor digitorum longus
Innervation:	Lateral plantar nerve (S 1–S 3)

③ **First through fourth lumbricals**

Origin:	Medial borders of the flexor digitorum longus tendons
Insertion:	Dorsal aponeuroses of the second through fifth toes
Action:	• Flexes the metatarsophalangeal joints of the second through fifth toes
	• Extension of the interphalangeal joints of the second through fifth toes
	• Moves the toes closer together (adducts the second through fifth toes toward the big toe)
Innervation:	• First and second lumbricals: medial plantar nerve (S 2, S 3)
	• Second through fourth lumbricals: lateral plantar nerve (S 2, S 3)

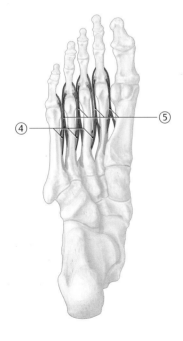

B Schematic of the first through third plantar interossei and the first through fourth dorsal interossei

④ **First through third plantar interossei**

Origin:	Medial border of the third through fifth metatarsals
Insertion:	Medial base of the proximal phalanx of the third through fifth toes
Action:	• Flexes the metatarsophalangeal joints of the third through fifth toes
	• Extension of the interphalangeal joints of the third through fifth toes
	• Moves the toes closer together (adducts the third through fifth toes toward the second toe)
Innervation:	Lateral plantar nerve (S 2, S 3)

⑤ **First through fourth dorsal interossei**

Origin:	By two heads from opposing sides of the first through fifth metatarsals
Insertion:	• First interosseus: medial base of the second proximal phalanx, dorsal aponeurosis of the second toe
	• Second through fourth interossei: lateral base of the second through fourth proximal phalanges, dorsal aponeurosis of the second through fourth toes
Action:	• Flexes the metatarsophalangeal joints of the second through fourth toes
	• Extension of the interphalangeal joints of the second through fourth toes
	• Spreads the toes apart (abducts the third and fourth toes from the second toe)
Innervation:	Lateral plantar nerve (S 2, S 3)

* The adductor hallucis, though part of the central compartment, is not pictured here (see p. 439).

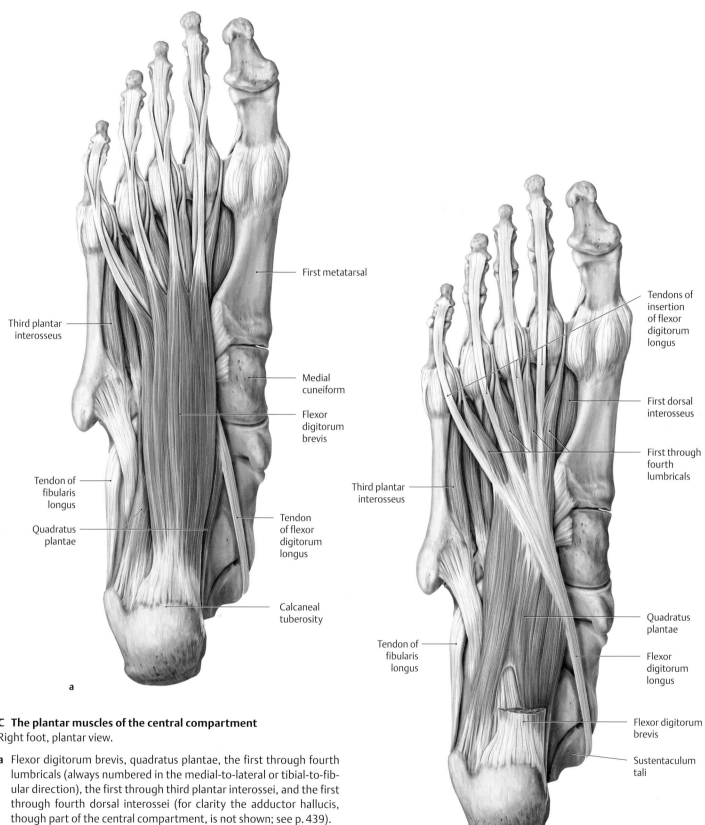

Third plantar interosseus

First metatarsal

Medial cuneiform

Flexor digitorum brevis

Tendon of fibularis longus

Quadratus plantae

Tendon of flexor digitorum longus

Calcaneal tuberosity

a

Tendons of insertion of flexor digitorum longus

First dorsal interosseus

First through fourth lumbricals

Third plantar interosseus

Quadratus plantae

Flexor digitorum longus

Tendon of fibularis longus

Flexor digitorum brevis

Sustentaculum tali

b

C The plantar muscles of the central compartment
Right foot, plantar view.

a Flexor digitorum brevis, quadratus plantae, the first through fourth lumbricals (always numbered in the medial-to-lateral or tibial-to-fibular direction), the first through third plantar interossei, and the first through fourth dorsal interossei (for clarity the adductor hallucis, though part of the central compartment, is not shown; see p. 439).
b Flexor digitorum brevis has been removed to its origin to display more clearly the insertion of quadratus plantae on the lateral margin of the flexor digitorum longus tendon.

Note the "movable origins" of the first through fourth lumbricals from the medial borders of the flexor digitorum longus tendons. When the flexor digitorum longus contracts and therefore shortens, the origins of the lumbricals move proximad. This "prestretching" of the lumbricals improves their ability to contract, enabling them to develop greater force.

441

3.1 The Muscles of the Thigh, Hip and Gluteal Region from the Medial and Anterior Views

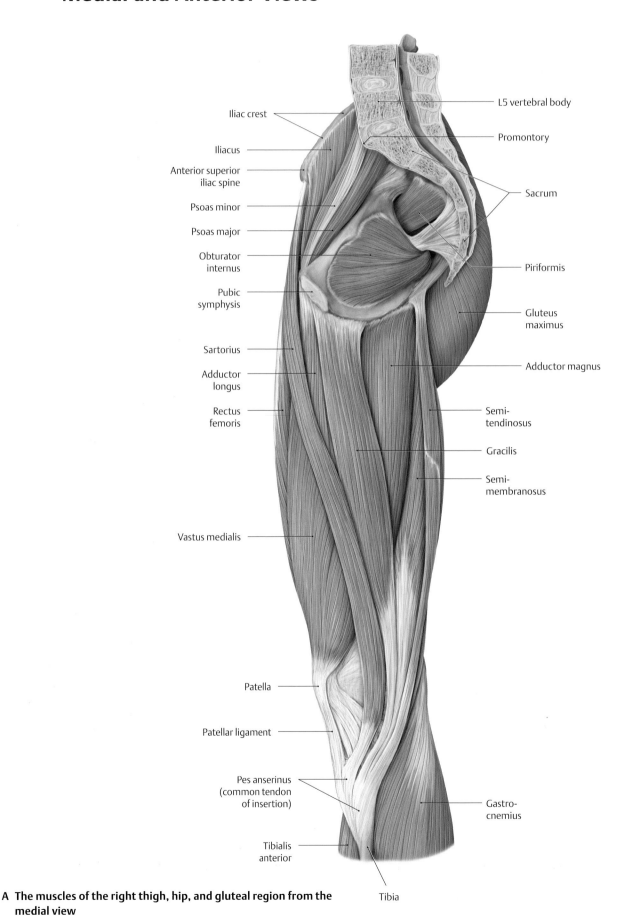

A The muscles of the right thigh, hip, and gluteal region from the medial view

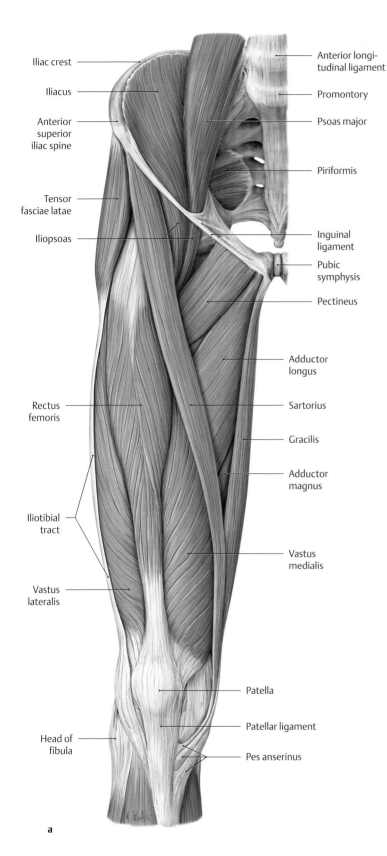

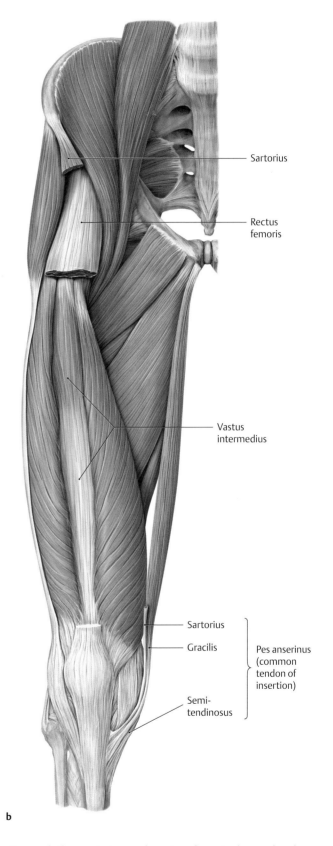

Iliac crest

Iliacus

Anterior superior iliac spine

Tensor fasciae latae

Iliopsoas

Rectus femoris

Iliotibial tract

Vastus lateralis

Head of fibula

Anterior longitudinal ligament

Promontory

Psoas major

Piriformis

Inguinal ligament

Pubic symphysis

Pectineus

Adductor longus

Sartorius

Gracilis

Adductor magnus

Vastus medialis

Patella

Patellar ligament

Pes anserinus

a

Sartorius

Rectus femoris

Vastus intermedius

Sartorius

Gracilis

Pes anserinus (common tendon of insertion)

Semi-tendinosus

b

B The muscles of the right thigh, hip, and gluteal region from the anterior view

a The fascia lata of the thigh (see p. 485) has been removed as far as the lateral iliotibial tract.

b Portions of the sartorius and rectus femoris have also been removed.

443

3.2 The Muscles of the Thigh, Hip, and Gluteal Region from the Anterior View; Origins and Insertions

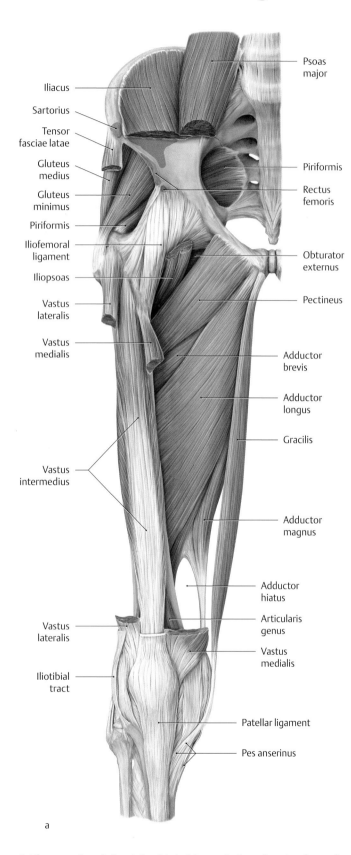

Iliacus

Sartorius

Tensor fasciae latae

Gluteus medius

Gluteus minimus

Piriformis

Iliofemoral ligament

Iliopsoas

Vastus lateralis

Vastus medialis

Vastus intermedius

Vastus lateralis

Iliotibial tract

Psoas major

Piriformis

Rectus femoris

Obturator externus

Pectineus

Adductor brevis

Adductor longus

Gracilis

Adductor magnus

Adductor hiatus

Articularis genus

Vastus medialis

Patellar ligament

Pes anserinus

a

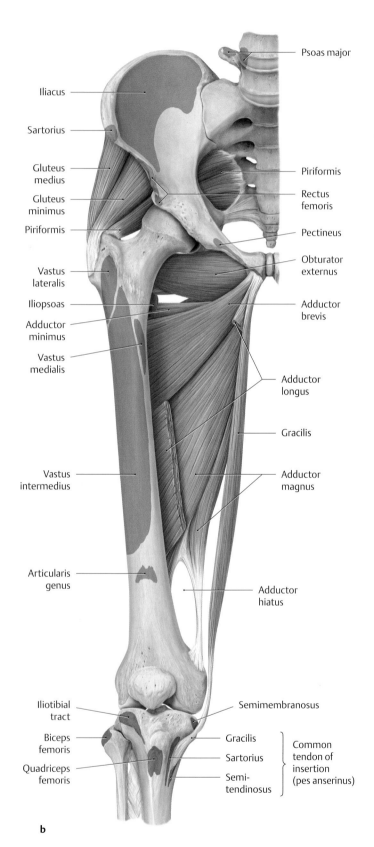

Iliacus

Sartorius

Gluteus medius

Gluteus minimus

Piriformis

Vastus lateralis

Iliopsoas

Adductor minimus

Vastus medialis

Vastus intermedius

Articularis genus

Iliotibial tract

Biceps femoris

Quadriceps femoris

Psoas major

Piriformis

Rectus femoris

Pectineus

Obturator externus

Adductor brevis

Adductor longus

Gracilis

Adductor magnus

Adductor hiatus

Semimembranosus

Gracilis

Sartorius

Semi-tendinosus

Common tendon of insertion (pes anserinus)

b

A The muscles of the right thigh, hip, and gluteal region from the anterior view
The origins and insertions of the muscles are indicated by color shading (red = origin, blue = insertion).

a The iliopsoas and tensor fasciae latae have been partially removed. The sartorius, rectus femoris, vastus lateralis, and vastus lateralis have been completely removed.

b The quadriceps femoris, iliopsoas, tensor fasciae latae, and pectineus have been completely removed. The midportion of adductor longus has been removed.

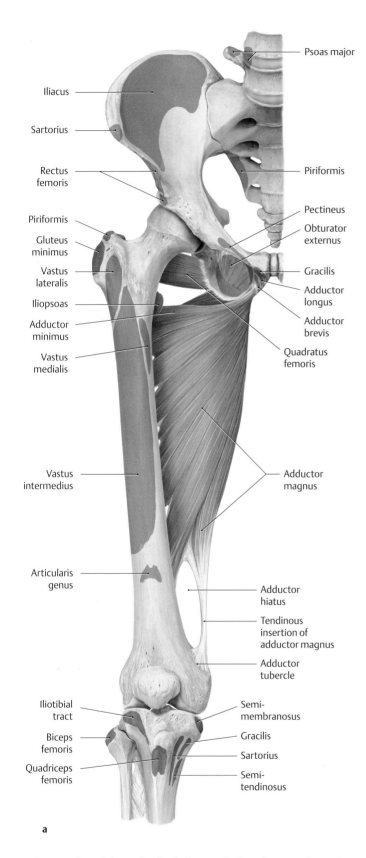

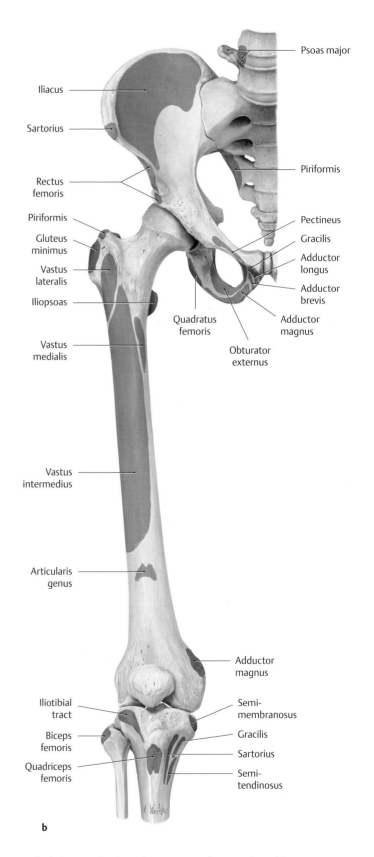

a

b

B The muscles of the right thigh, hip, and gluteal region from the anterior view

The origins and insertions of the muscles are indicated by color shading (red = origin, blue = insertion).

a All of the muscles have been removed except for adductor magnus and quadratus femoris.

b All of the muscles have been removed.

Note the adductor hiatus, through which the femoral artery and vein enter the popliteal fossa of the leg.

445

3.3 The Muscles of the Thigh, Hip, and Gluteal Region from the Lateral and Posterior Views

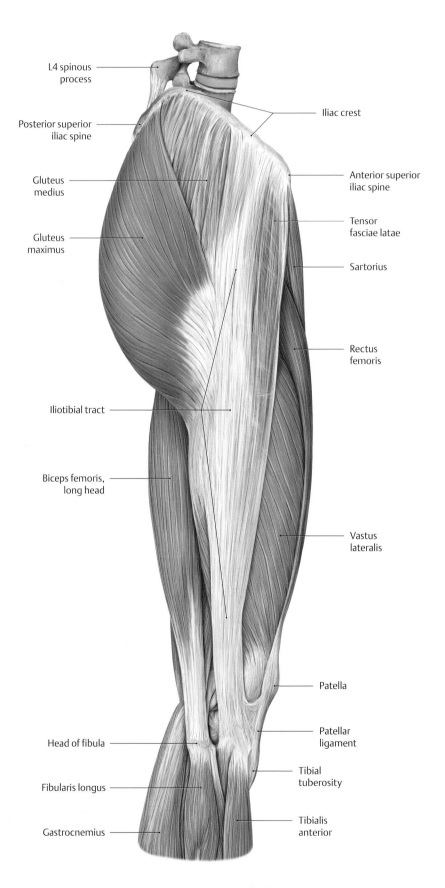

L4 spinous process

Iliac crest

Posterior superior iliac spine

Anterior superior iliac spine

Gluteus medius

Tensor fasciae latae

Gluteus maximus

Sartorius

Rectus femoris

Iliotibial tract

Biceps femoris, long head

Vastus lateralis

Patella

Head of fibula

Patellar ligament

Fibularis longus

Tibial tuberosity

Gastrocnemius

Tibialis anterior

A The muscles of the right thigh, hip, and gluteal region from the lateral view

Note the tensor fasciae latae and gluteus maximus muscles, whose tendons of insertion strengthen and thicken the lateral part of the fascia lata. This thickened band, called *the iliotibial tract* because it runs between the *iliac* crest and the lateral side of the upper *tibia*, functions mechanically as a tension band to reduce the bending loads on the proximal femur (after Pauwels, see also p. 367).

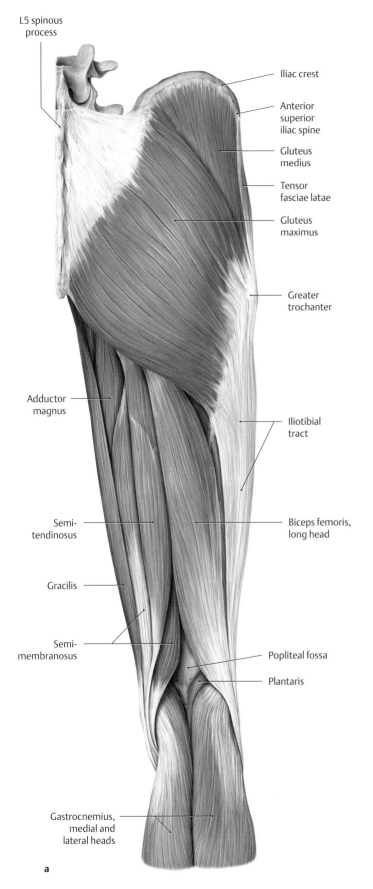

L5 spinous process

Iliac crest

Anterior superior iliac spine

Gluteus medius

Tensor fasciae latae

Gluteus maximus

Greater trochanter

Adductor magnus

Iliotibial tract

Semi-tendinosus

Biceps femoris, long head

Gracilis

Semi-membranosus

Popliteal fossa

Plantaris

Gastrocnemius, medial and lateral heads

a

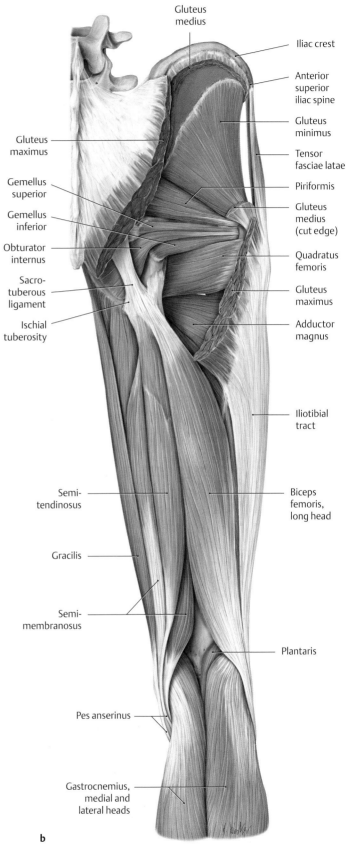

Gluteus medius

Gluteus maximus

Iliac crest

Anterior superior iliac spine

Gluteus minimus

Tensor fasciae latae

Gemellus superior

Piriformis

Gemellus inferior

Gluteus medius (cut edge)

Obturator internus

Quadratus femoris

Sacro-tuberous ligament

Gluteus maximus

Ischial tuberosity

Adductor magnus

Iliotibial tract

Semi-tendinosus

Biceps femoris, long head

Gracilis

Semi-membranosus

Plantaris

Pes anserinus

Gastrocnemius, medial and lateral heads

b

B The muscles of the right thigh, hip, and gluteal region from the posterior view

a The fascia lata has been removed as far as the iliotibial tract (the portion over the buttock is called the gluteal fascia).

b The gluteus maximus and gluteus medius have been partially removed.

447

3.4 The Muscles of the Thigh, Hip, and Gluteal Region from the Posterior View; Origins and Insertions

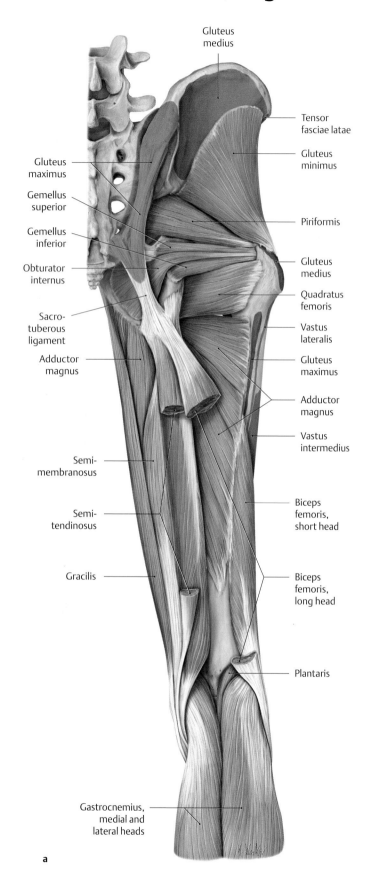

a

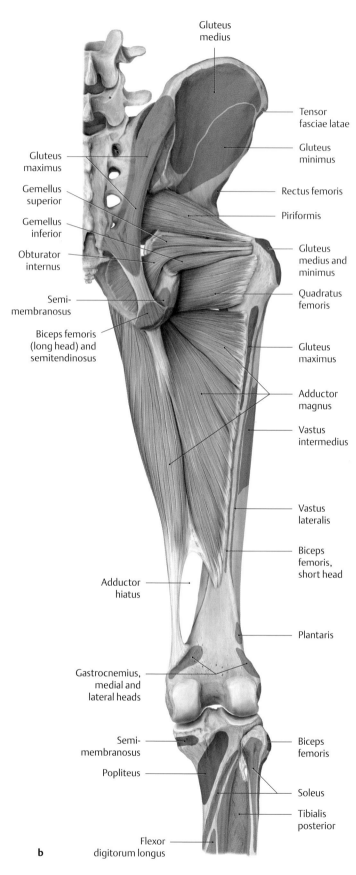

b

A The muscles of the right thigh, hip, and gluteal region from the posterior view

The origins and insertions of the muscles are indicated by color shading (red = origin, blue = insertion).

a The semitendinosus and biceps femoris have been partially removed. The gluteus maximus and medius have been completely removed.

b The hamstrings (semitendinosus, semimembranosus, and biceps femoris) and gluteus minimus have been completely removed.

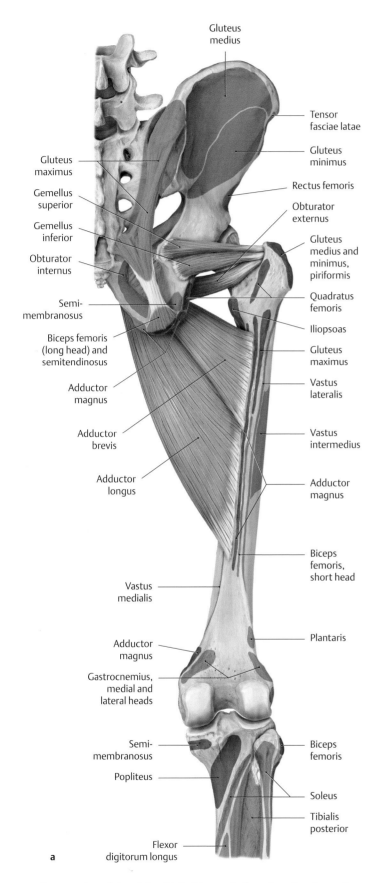

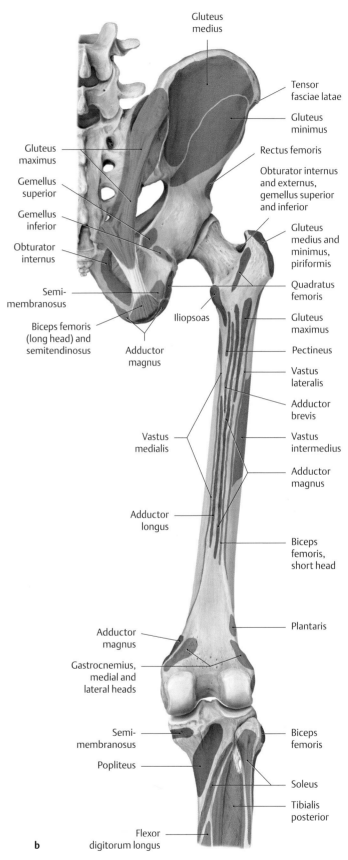

Gluteus medius

Gluteus maximus

Gemellus superior

Gemellus inferior

Obturator internus

Semi-membranosus

Biceps femoris (long head) and semitendinosus

Adductor magnus

Adductor brevis

Adductor longus

Vastus medialis

Adductor magnus

Gastrocnemius, medial and lateral heads

Semi-membranosus

Popliteus

Flexor digitorum longus

a

Tensor fasciae latae

Gluteus minimus

Rectus femoris

Obturator externus

Gluteus medius and minimus, piriformis

Quadratus femoris

Iliopsoas

Gluteus maximus

Vastus lateralis

Vastus intermedius

Adductor magnus

Biceps femoris, short head

Plantaris

Biceps femoris

Soleus

Tibialis posterior

Gluteus medius

Gluteus maximus

Gemellus superior

Gemellus inferior

Obturator internus

Semi-membranosus

Biceps femoris (long head) and semitendinosus

Adductor magnus

Iliopsoas

Vastus medialis

Adductor longus

Adductor magnus

Gastrocnemius, medial and lateral heads

Semi-membranosus

Popliteus

Flexor digitorum longus

b

Tensor fasciae latae

Gluteus minimus

Rectus femoris

Obturator internus and externus, gemellus superior and inferior

Gluteus medius and minimus, piriformis

Quadratus femoris

Gluteus maximus

Pectineus

Vastus lateralis

Adductor brevis

Vastus intermedius

Adductor magnus

Biceps femoris, short head

Plantaris

Biceps femoris

Soleus

Tibialis posterior

B The muscles of the right thigh, hip, and gluteal region from the posterior view
The origins and insertions of the muscles are indicated by color shading (red = origin, blue = insertion).

a All muscles have been removed except for the adductor brevis, adductor longus, gemellus superior and inferior, and obturator externus.
b All of the muscles have been removed.

449

3.5 The Muscles of the Leg from the Lateral and Anterior View; Origins and Insertions

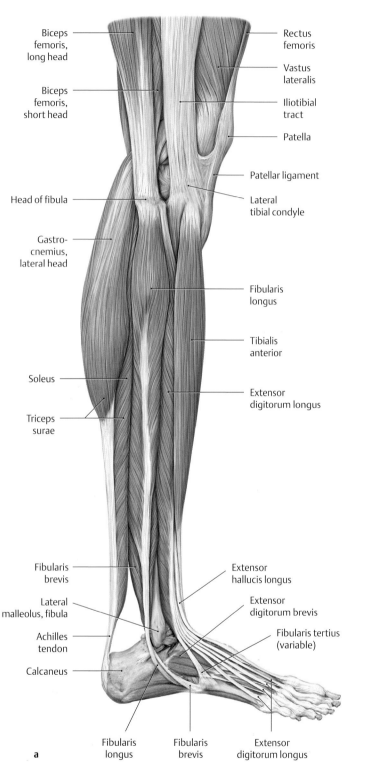

Biceps femoris, long head
Biceps femoris, short head
Head of fibula
Gastro-cnemius, lateral head
Soleus
Triceps surae
Fibularis brevis
Lateral malleolus, fibula
Achilles tendon
Calcaneus

Rectus femoris
Vastus lateralis
Iliotibial tract
Patella
Patellar ligament
Lateral tibial condyle
Fibularis longus
Tibialis anterior
Extensor digitorum longus
Extensor hallucis longus
Extensor digitorum brevis
Fibularis tertius (variable)

a

Fibularis longus
Fibularis brevis
Extensor digitorum longus

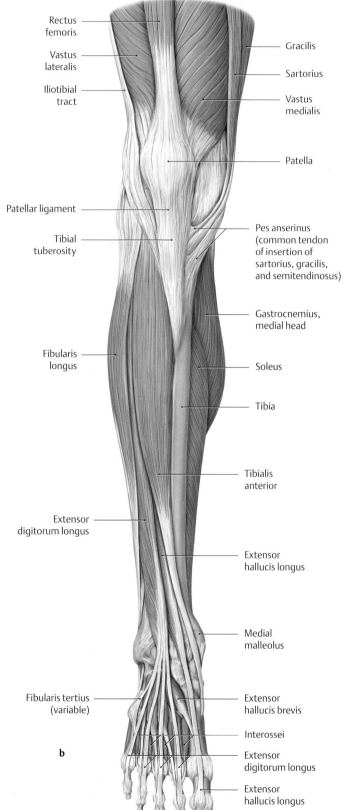

Rectus femoris
Vastus lateralis
Iliotibial tract
Patellar ligament
Tibial tuberosity
Fibularis longus
Extensor digitorum longus

Gracilis
Sartorius
Vastus medialis
Patella
Pes anserinus (common tendon of insertion of sartorius, gracilis, and semitendinosus)
Gastrocnemius, medial head
Soleus
Tibia
Tibialis anterior
Extensor hallucis longus
Medial malleolus
Extensor hallucis brevis
Interossei
Extensor digitorum longus
Extensor hallucis longus

Fibularis tertius (variable)

b

A The muscles of the right leg
a Lateral view, **b** anterior view.

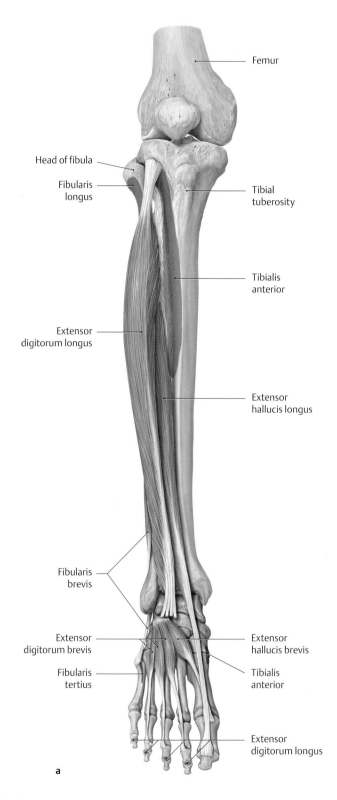

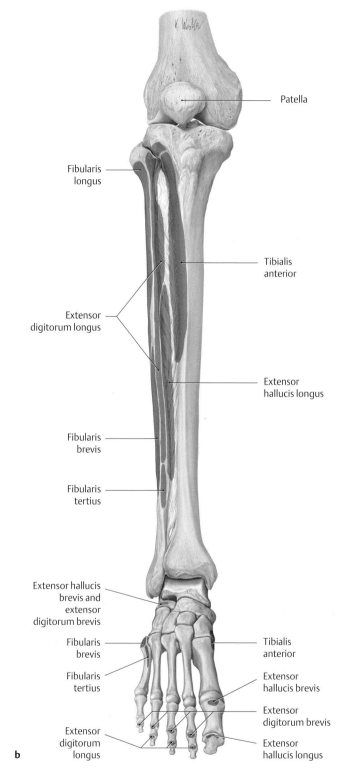

B The muscles of the right leg from the anterior view
The origins and insertions of the muscles are indicated by color shading
(red = origin, blue = insertion).

a The tibialis anterior and fibularis longus have been completely
removed, as have the distal portions of the extensor digitorum longus tendons. The fibularis tertius is a division of the extensor digitorum longus.

b All of the muscles have been removed.

3.6 The Muscles of the Leg from the Posterior View; Origins and Insertions

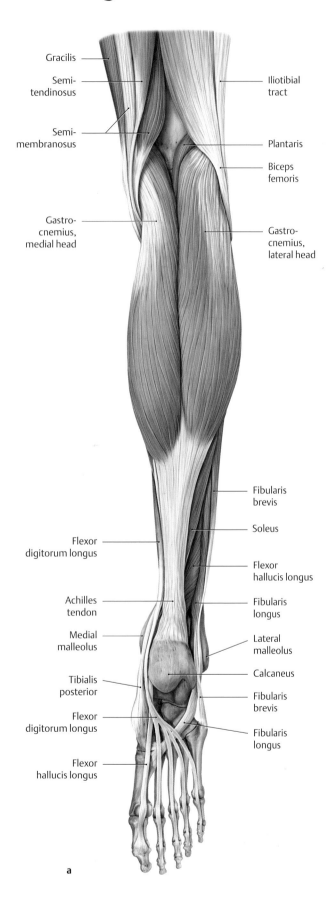

Gracilis

Semi-tendinosus

Semi-membranosus

Gastro-cnemius, medial head

Iliotibial tract

Plantaris

Biceps femoris

Gastro-cnemius, lateral head

Fibularis brevis

Soleus

Flexor digitorum longus

Flexor hallucis longus

Achilles tendon

Fibularis longus

Medial malleolus

Lateral malleolus

Tibialis posterior

Calcaneus

Flexor digitorum longus

Fibularis brevis

Fibularis longus

Flexor hallucis longus

a

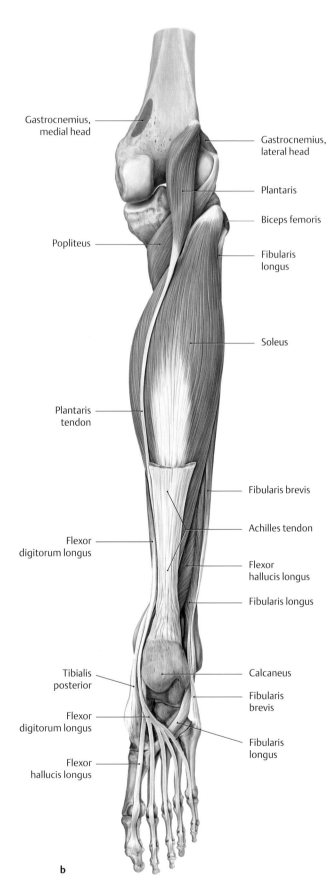

Gastrocnemius, medial head

Gastrocnemius, lateral head

Plantaris

Biceps femoris

Popliteus

Fibularis longus

Soleus

Plantaris tendon

Fibularis brevis

Achilles tendon

Flexor digitorum longus

Flexor hallucis longus

Fibularis longus

Tibialis posterior

Calcaneus

Fibularis brevis

Flexor digitorum longus

Fibularis longus

Flexor hallucis longus

b

A The muscles of the right leg from the posterior view
The origins and insertions of the muscles are indicated by color shading (red = origin, blue = insertion). The foot is shown in a plantar-flexed position to better demonstrate the plantar tendons.

a The bulge of the calf is produced mainly by the triceps surae muscle (= soleus plus the two heads of gastrocnemius).
b Both heads of gastrocnemius have been removed.

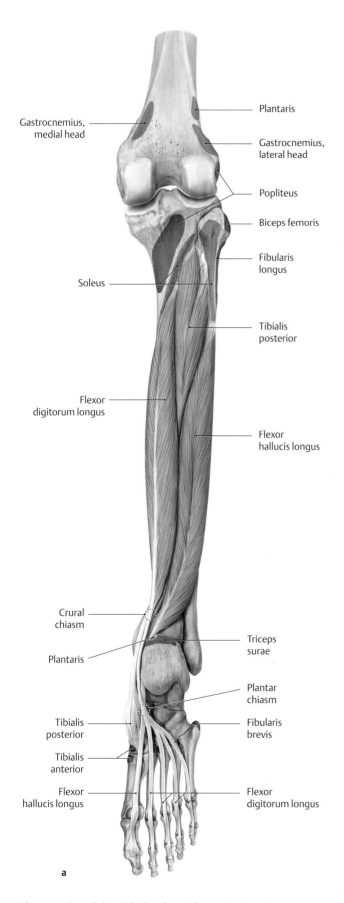

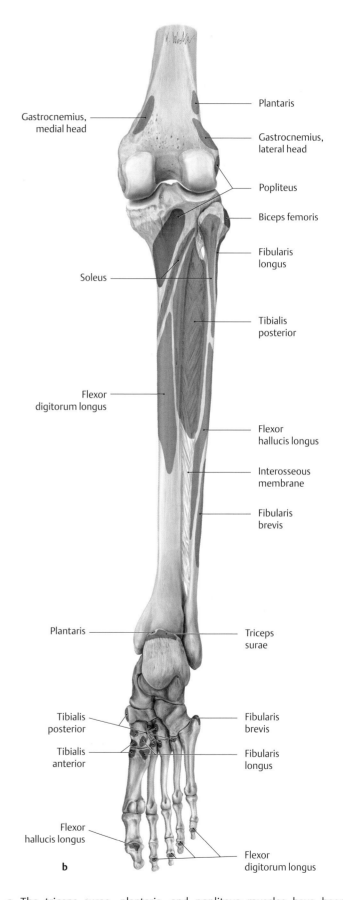

B The muscles of the right leg from the posterior view
The origins and insertions of the muscles are indicated by color shading (red = origin, blue = insertion). The foot is shown in a plantar-flexed position to better demonstrate the plantar tendons.

a The triceps surae, plantaris, and popliteus muscles have been removed.
b All of the muscles have been removed.

453

3.7 The Tendon Sheaths and Retinacula of the Foot

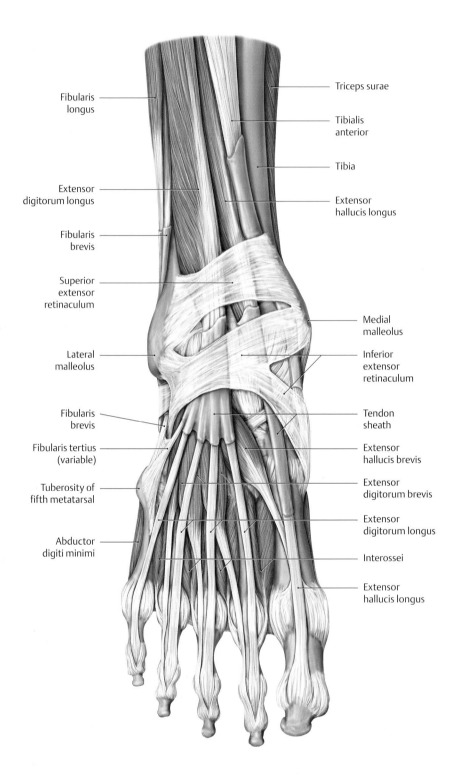

Fibularis longus

Triceps surae

Tibialis anterior

Tibia

Extensor digitorum longus

Extensor hallucis longus

Fibularis brevis

Superior extensor retinaculum

Medial malleolus

Lateral malleolus

Inferior extensor retinaculum

Fibularis brevis

Tendon sheath

Fibularis tertius (variable)

Extensor hallucis brevis

Tuberosity of fifth metatarsal

Extensor digitorum brevis

Extensor digitorum longus

Abductor digiti minimi

Interossei

Extensor hallucis longus

A The tendon sheaths and retinacula of the right foot from the anterior view

The foot is plantar-flexed, with superficial fascia removed, to display the deep fascial bands—*retinacula*—that hold in place the tendon sheaths of the long foot extensors and flexors. The superior and inferior extensor retinacula retain the long extensor tendons, allowing efficient redirection of the forces generated by their muscles (tibialis anterior, extensor digitorum longus, extensor hallucis longus, and fibularis tertius) while

preventing the tendons from rising away from the bones of the ankle when the foot is dorsiflexed. Similarly, the fibular retinacula, laterally, hold the fibular muscle tendons in place posterior to the lateral malleolus (see **B**, part **a**), and the flexor retinaculum retains the long flexor tendons behind the medial malleolus (see **B**, part **b**), preventing displacement of these tendons while enabling them to operate smoothly regardless of the orientation of the ankle joint.

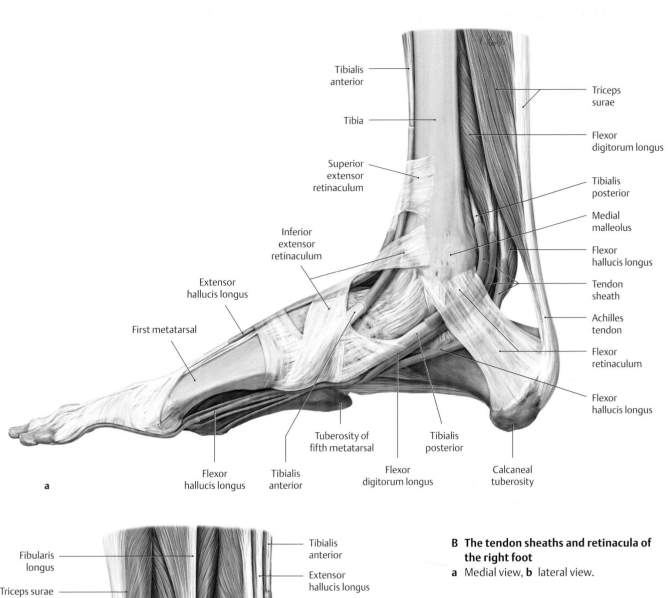

Tibialis anterior

Tibia

Superior extensor retinaculum

Inferior extensor retinaculum

Extensor hallucis longus

First metatarsal

Triceps surae

Flexor digitorum longus

Tibialis posterior

Medial malleolus

Flexor hallucis longus

Tendon sheath

Achilles tendon

Flexor retinaculum

Flexor hallucis longus

Tuberosity of fifth metatarsal

Tibialis posterior

Flexor hallucis longus

Tibialis anterior

Flexor digitorum longus

Calcaneal tuberosity

a

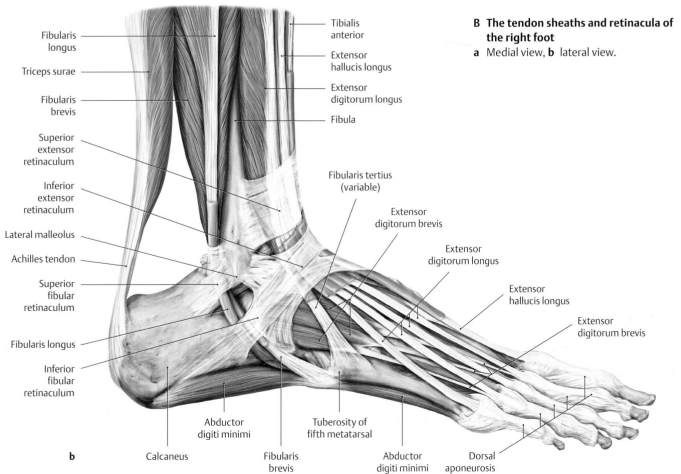

Fibularis longus

Triceps surae

Fibularis brevis

Superior extensor retinaculum

Inferior extensor retinaculum

Lateral malleolus

Achilles tendon

Superior fibular retinaculum

Fibularis longus

Inferior fibular retinaculum

Tibialis anterior

Extensor hallucis longus

Extensor digitorum longus

Fibula

Fibularis tertius (variable)

Extensor digitorum brevis

Extensor digitorum longus

Extensor hallucis longus

Extensor digitorum brevis

Abductor digiti minimi

Calcaneus

Fibularis brevis

Tuberosity of fifth metatarsal

Abductor digiti minimi

Dorsal aponeurosis

b

B The tendon sheaths and retinacula of the right foot

a Medial view, **b** lateral view.

3.8 The Intrinsic Foot Muscles from the Plantar View; the Plantar Aponeurosis

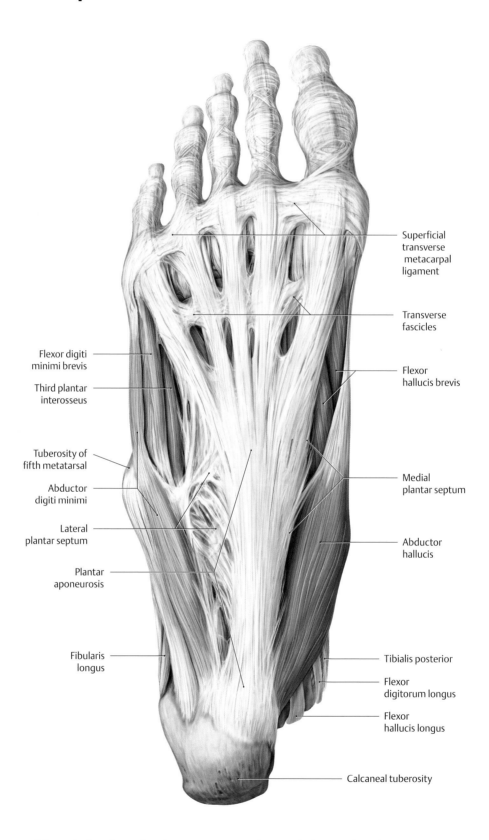

Superficial
transverse
metacarpal
ligament

Transverse
fascicles

Flexor digiti
minimi brevis

Third plantar
interosseus

Flexor
hallucis brevis

Tuberosity of
fifth metatarsal

Abductor
digiti minimi

Lateral
plantar septum

Medial
plantar septum

Plantar
aponeurosis

Abductor
hallucis

Fibularis
longus

Tibialis posterior

Flexor
digitorum longus

Flexor
hallucis longus

Calcaneal tuberosity

A The plantar aponeurosis of the right foot from the plantar view
The *plantar aponeu*rosis is a tough aponeurotic sheet that is thicker centrally than medially and laterally and blends with the dorsal fascia (not shown here) at the borders of the foot. Two sagittal expansions of the thick *central* aponeurosis (the medial and lateral plantar septa) extend deep to the bones of the foot, defining the boundaries of three muscle compartments in the plantar region: the medial compartment, lateral compartment, and central compartment (not labeled here, see p. 440). The main function of the plantar aponeurosis is to give *passive* support to the longitudinal arch (see also p. 415).

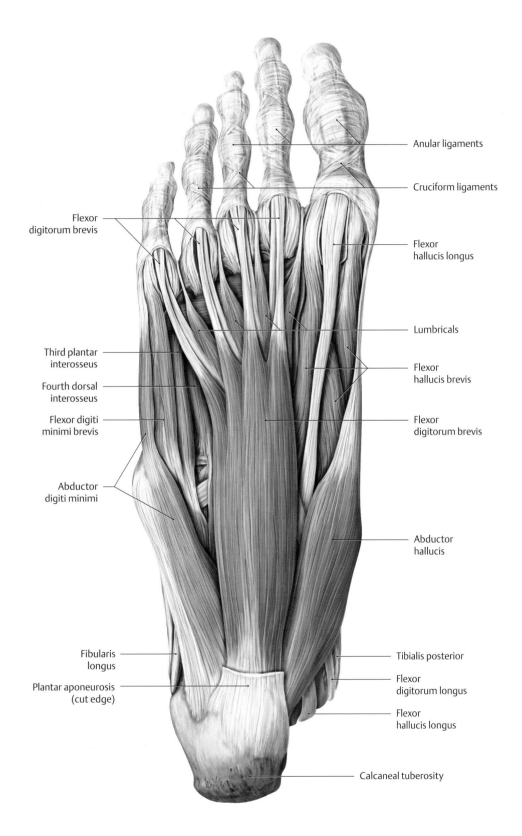

Anular ligaments

Cruciform ligaments

Flexor digitorum brevis

Flexor hallucis longus

Lumbricals

Third plantar interosseus

Flexor hallucis brevis

Fourth dorsal interosseus

Flexor digiti minimi brevis

Flexor digitorum brevis

Abductor digiti minimi

Abductor hallucis

Fibularis longus

Tibialis posterior

Plantar aponeurosis (cut edge)

Flexor digitorum longus

Flexor hallucis longus

Calcaneal tuberosity

B The intrinsic muscles of the right foot from the plantar view
The entire plantar aponeurosis, including the superficial transverse metacarpal ligament, has been removed.

Note the anular ligaments on the plantar side of the toes. Together with the oblique cruciform ligaments, they strengthen the tendon sheaths and help to hold the tendons in position.

3.9   The Intrinsic Foot Muscles from the Plantar View

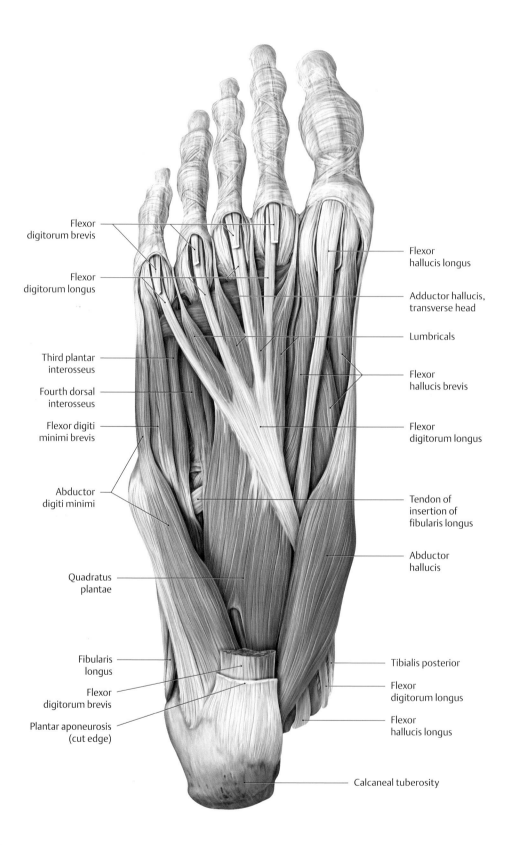

Flexor digitorum brevis

Flexor digitorum longus

Third plantar interosseus

Fourth dorsal interosseus

Flexor digiti minimi brevis

Abductor digiti minimi

Quadratus plantae

Fibularis longus

Flexor digitorum brevis

Plantar aponeurosis (cut edge)

Flexor hallucis longus

Adductor hallucis, transverse head

Lumbricals

Flexor hallucis brevis

Flexor digitorum longus

Tendon of insertion of fibularis longus

Abductor hallucis

Tibialis posterior

Flexor digitorum longus

Flexor hallucis longus

Calcaneal tuberosity

A The intrinsic muscles of the right foot from the plantar view
The plantar aponeurosis and flexor digitorum brevis have been removed.

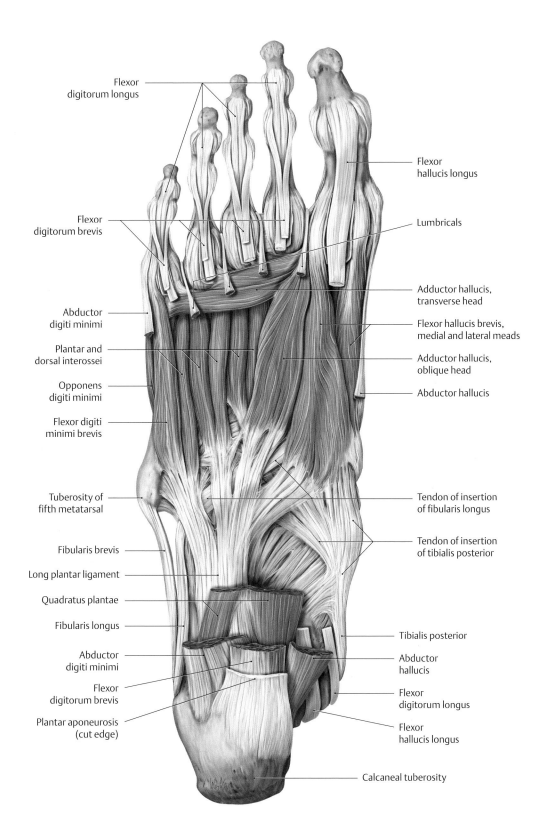

Flexor
digitorum longus

Flexor
digitorum brevis

Abductor
digiti minimi

Plantar and
dorsal interossei

Opponens
digiti minimi

Flexor digiti
minimi brevis

Tuberosity of
fifth metatarsal

Fibularis brevis

Long plantar ligament

Quadratus plantae

Fibularis longus

Abductor
digiti minimi

Flexor
digitorum brevis

Plantar aponeurosis
(cut edge)

Flexor
hallucis longus

Lumbricals

Adductor hallucis,
transverse head

Flexor hallucis brevis,
medial and lateral meads

Adductor hallucis,
oblique head

Abductor hallucis

Tendon of insertion
of fibularis longus

Tendon of insertion
of tibialis posterior

Tibialis posterior

Abductor
hallucis

Flexor
digitorum longus

Flexor
hallucis longus

Calcaneal tuberosity

B The intrinsic muscles of the right foot from the plantar view
The plantar aponeurosis has been removed in addition to the following muscles: flexor digitorum brevis, abductor digiti minimi, abductor hallucis, quadratus plantae, the lumbricals, and the tendons of insertion of flexor digitorum longus and flexor hallucis longus.

Note that each of the four tendons of insertion of flexor digitorum brevis divides into two slips, and that the tendons of flexor digitorum longus pass between these slips to insert on the distal phalanges.

459

3.10 The Intrinsic Foot Muscles from the Plantar View; Origins and Insertions

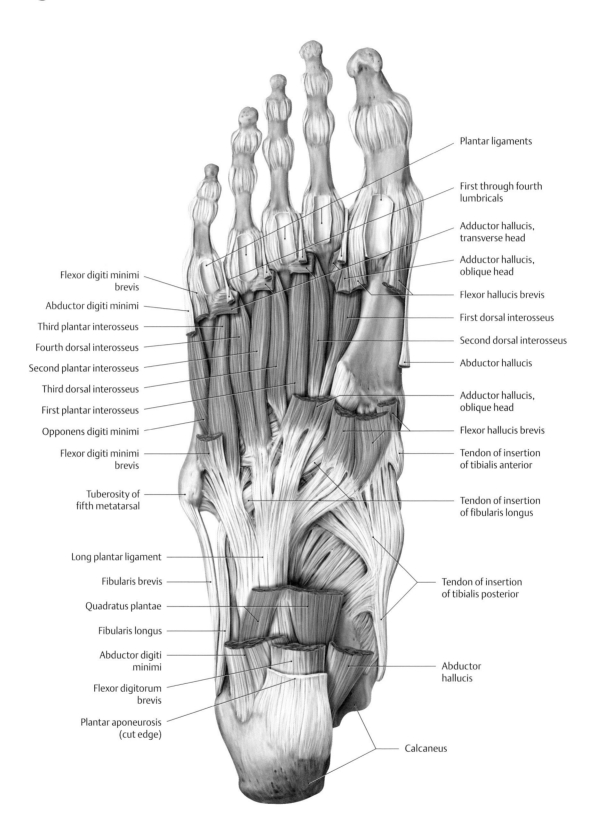

Flexor digiti minimi brevis

Abductor digiti minimi

Third plantar interosseus

Fourth dorsal interosseus

Second plantar interosseus

Third dorsal interosseus

First plantar interosseus

Opponens digiti minimi

Flexor digiti minimi brevis

Tuberosity of fifth metatarsal

Long plantar ligament

Fibularis brevis

Quadratus plantae

Fibularis longus

Abductor digiti minimi

Flexor digitorum brevis

Plantar aponeurosis (cut edge)

Plantar ligaments

First through fourth lumbricals

Adductor hallucis, transverse head

Adductor hallucis, oblique head

Flexor hallucis brevis

First dorsal interosseus

Second dorsal interosseus

Abductor hallucis

Adductor hallucis, oblique head

Flexor hallucis brevis

Tendon of insertion of tibialis anterior

Tendon of insertion of fibularis longus

Tendon of insertion of tibialis posterior

Abductor hallucis

Calcaneus

A The intrinsic muscles of the right foot from the plantar view
All of the short foot muscles except for the dorsal and plantar interossei have been removed, leaving behind their origins and insertions.

Note the course of the tibialis posterior and fibularis longus tendons of insertion, both of which help to support the transverse arch of the foot.

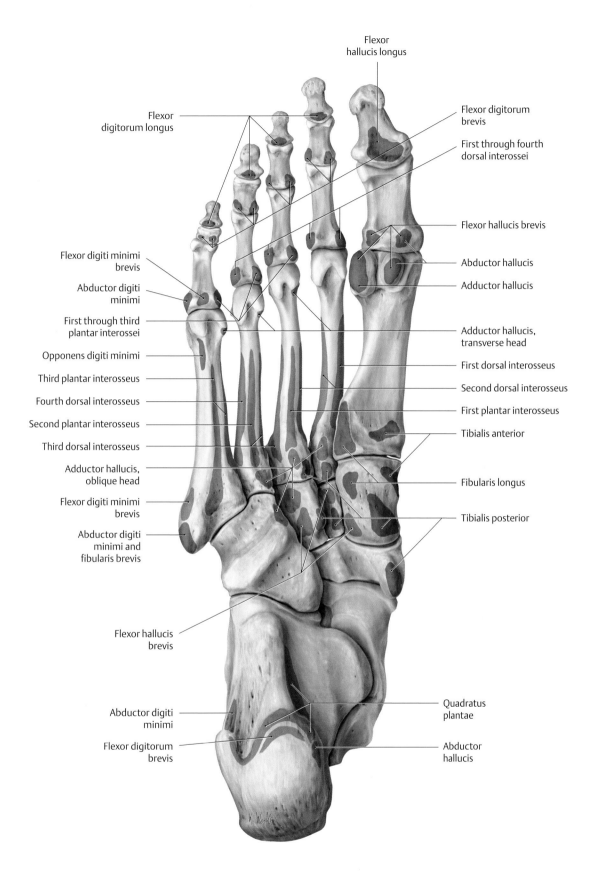

Flexor hallucis longus

Flexor digitorum longus

Flexor digiti minimi brevis

Abductor digiti minimi

First through third plantar interossei

Opponens digiti minimi

Third plantar interosseus

Fourth dorsal interosseus

Second plantar interosseus

Third dorsal interosseus

Adductor hallucis, oblique head

Flexor digiti minimi brevis

Abductor digiti minimi and fibularis brevis

Flexor hallucis brevis

Abductor digiti minimi

Flexor digitorum brevis

Flexor digitorum brevis

First through fourth dorsal interossei

Flexor hallucis brevis

Abductor hallucis

Adductor hallucis

Adductor hallucis, transverse head

First dorsal interosseus

Second dorsal interosseus

First plantar interosseus

Tibialis anterior

Fibularis longus

Tibialis posterior

Quadratus plantae

Abductor hallucis

B   Muscle origins and insertions on the plantar view of the right foot

The origins and insertions of the muscles are indicated by color shading (red = origin, blue = insertion).

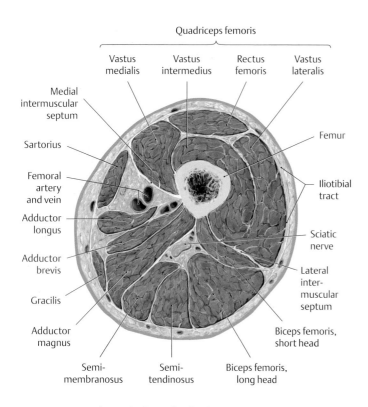

A Cross-section through the right thigh
Proximal view. The level of the section is shown in **C**.

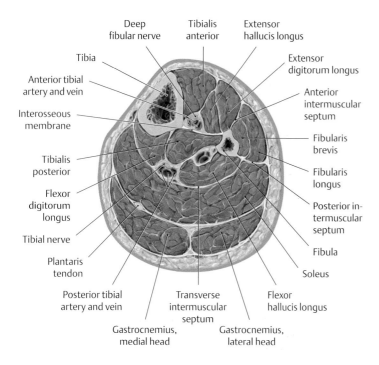

B Cross-section through the right leg
Proximal view. The level of the section is shown in **C**.

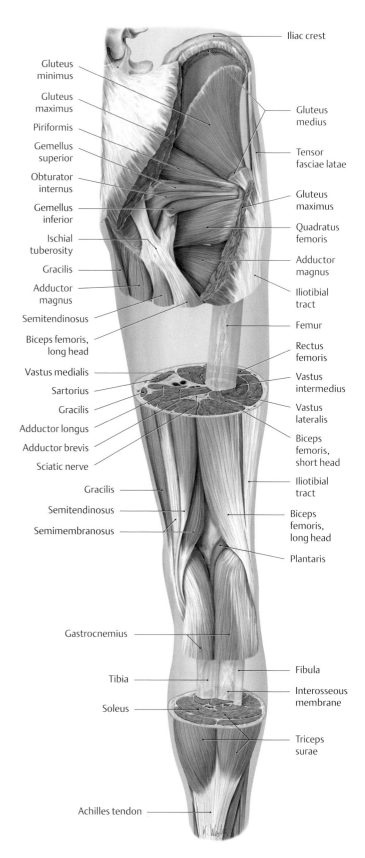

C "Windowed" dissection of the right lower limb
Posterior view. Portions of the gluteus maximus and medius have been removed (the removed cross-sections are shown in **A** and **B**). The lower limb is one of the body regions most frequently examined by tomographic methods, and a knowledge of its cross-sectional anatomy is critically important in the identification of landmarks in both radiological and magnetic-resonance (MR)-based images.

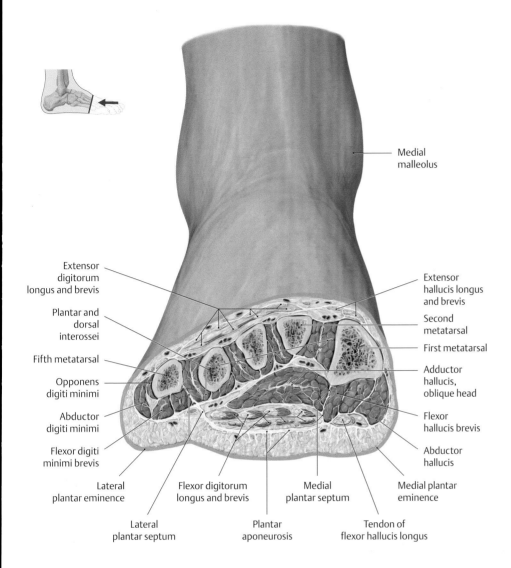

Extensor digitorum longus and brevis

Plantar and dorsal interossei

Fifth metatarsal

Opponens digiti minimi

Abductor digiti minimi

Flexor digiti minimi brevis

Medial malleolus

Extensor hallucis longus and brevis

Second metatarsal

First metatarsal

Adductor hallucis, oblique head

Flexor hallucis brevis

Abductor hallucis

Lateral plantar eminence

Flexor digitorum longus and brevis

Medial plantar septum

Medial plantar eminence

Lateral plantar septum

Plantar aponeurosis

Tendon of flexor hallucis longus

D Cross-section through the right foot at the level of the metatarsals

View of the distal cut surface. The muscle compartments of the foot are formed mainly by the plantar aponeurosis, the medial and lateral plantar septa, and the deep plantar fascia (see also **E**). Foot injuries, such as fracture-dislocations of the tarsus and metatarsus, may lead to *compartment syndromes of the foot*. They are caused by increased tissue pressure in the affected compartment due to the local extravasation of blood. The raised pressure in the compartment leads to impaired venous drainage and diminished capillary perfusion, manifested clinically by swelling and pain. This leads in turn to neuromuscular dysfunction with circulatory compromise that may culminate in muscle necrosis (drawn from a specimen in the Anatomical Collection of Kiel University).

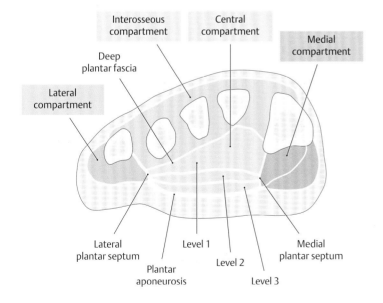

Interosseous compartment

Central compartment

Medial compartment

Deep plantar fascia

Lateral compartment

Lateral plantar septum

Level 1

Medial plantar septum

Plantar aponeurosis

Level 2

Level 3

E Location of the compartments of the foot
Schematic cross section through a right foot, distal view. The different muscle compartments are indicated by color shading.

F The four compartments of the foot and their muscular contents
(see also **E**)

Interosseous compartment
• Dorsal and plantar interossei

Medial compartment
• Abductor hallucis
• Flexor hallucis brevis
• Tendon of insertion of flexor hallucis longus

Lateral compartment
• Abductor digiti minimi
• Flexor digiti minimi
• Opponens digiti minimi

Central compartment, consisting of three levels
• Level 1: Adductor hallucis
• Level 2: Quadratus plantae, lumbricals, and flexor digitorum longus tendons
• Level 3: Flexor digitorum brevis

(after Mubarak and Hargens)

4.1 The Arteries

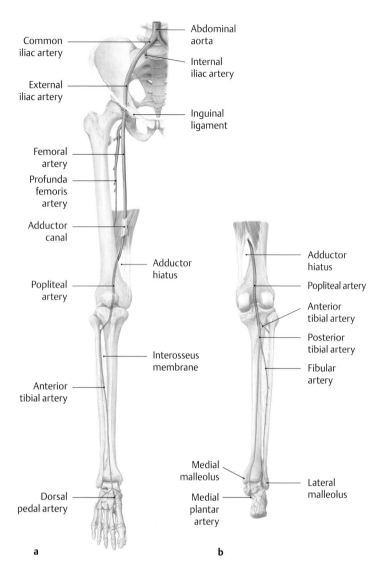

a   **b**

A Different segments of the arteries of the lower limb
a Right leg, anterior view; **b** right leg, posterior view. The different arterial segments are shown in different colors.

External iliac artery: arises with the internal iliac artery from the common iliac artery and descends along the medial border of psoas major through the lacuna vasorum (see p. 489). It becomes the femoral artery at the level of the inguinal ligament.

Femoral artery: the continuation of the external iliac artery, runs down the medial side of the thigh to the adductor canal, through which it passes from the anterior to the posterior side of the limb. On leaving the adductor hiatus, it becomes the popliteal artery.

Popliteal artery: runs from the adductor hiatus through the popliteal fossa to the popliteus, dividing at the inferior border of that muscle into its terminal branches, the anterior and posterior tibial arteries.

Anterior tibial artery: enters the extensor compartment of the leg at the upper border of the interosseous membrane and descends between the tibialis anterior and extensor hallucis longus. Distal to the extensor retinaculum, it continues onto the dorsum of the foot as the *dorsal pedal artery*.

Posterior tibial artery: the direct continuation of the popliteal artery, enters the flexor compartment of the leg and passes behind the medial malleolus. At that level it divides into its two terminal branches, the *medial* and *lateral plantar arteries* (the latter is shown in **D**), which continue onto the plantar side of the foot. The posterior tibial artery also gives rise to the fibular artery.

B Overview of the principal arteries of the lower limb
The arteries of the lower limb vary considerably in their origins and branching patterns (the main variants are reviewed in Chapter 5, Neurovascular Systems: Topographical Anatomy. The branches are listed in the order in which they arise from the parent vessels.

Branches of the external iliac artery
- Inferior epigastric artery
  - Cremasteric artery
  - Artery of the round ligament of the uterus
  - Pubic branch
- Deep circumflex iliac artery

Branches of the femoral* artery
- Superficial epigastric artery
- Superficial circumflex iliac artery
- Superficial external pudendal artery
- Deep external pudendal artery
- Profunda femoris artery
  - Medial circumflex femoral artery
  - Lateral circumflex femoral artery
  - Perforating branches
- Descending genicular artery

Branches of the popliteal artery
- Medial and lateral superior genicular arteries
- Sural arteries
- Middle genicular artery
- Medial and lateral inferior genicular arteries
  Note that the paired superior and inferior genicular arteries form the *arterial anastomotic network* around the knee.

Branches of the anterior tibial artery
- Anterior tibial recurrent artery
- Anterior lateral malleolar artery
- Anterior medial malleolar artery
- Dorsal pedal artery
  - Lateral tarsal artery
  - Medial tarsal artery
  - Arcuate artery with the dorsal metatarsal arteries
    (→ dorsal digital arteries)

Branches of the posterior tibial artery
- Posterior tibial recurrent artery (arterial network of the knee)
- Fibular artery
  - Perforating branch
  - Communicating branch
  - Lateral malleolar branches
  - Calcaneal branches
- Medial malleolar branch
- Calcaneal branches
- Medial plantar artery
  - Superficial branch
  - Deep branch (→ deep plantar arch)
- Lateral plantar artery (→ deep plantar arch)
- Plantar metatarsal arteries
- Common plantar digital arteries

* Often referred to clinically as the superficial femoral artery.
→ = is continuous with

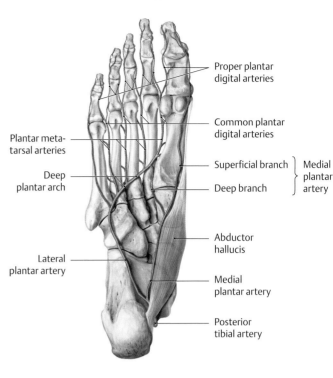

Abdominal aorta

Common iliac artery

Internal iliac artery

Superior and inferior gluteal arteries

External iliac artery

Inferior epigastric artery

External pudendal arteries

Medial circumflex femoral artery

Proper plantar digital arteries

Common plantar digital arteries

Superficial branch | Medial plantar artery

Deep branch

Plantar metatarsal arteries

Deep plantar arch

Lateral plantar artery

Abductor hallucis

Medial plantar artery

Posterior tibial artery

D The arteries of the sole of the foot
Right foot, plantar view.

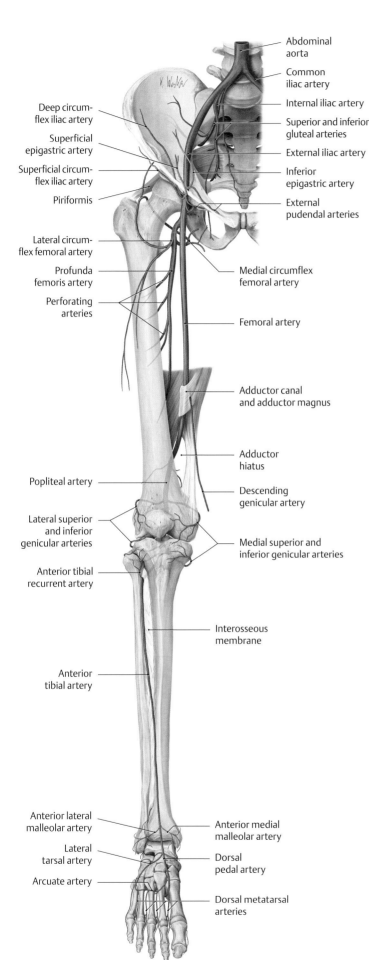

Deep circumflex iliac artery

Superficial epigastric artery

Superficial circumflex iliac artery

Piriformis

Lateral circumflex femoral artery

Profunda femoris artery

Perforating arteries

Femoral artery

Adductor canal and adductor magnus

Adductor hiatus

Descending genicular artery

Popliteal artery

Medial superior and inferior genicular arteries

Lateral superior and inferior genicular arteries

Anterior tibial recurrent artery

Interosseous membrane

Anterior tibial artery

Anterior lateral malleolar artery

Lateral tarsal artery

Arcuate artery

Anterior medial malleolar artery

Dorsal pedal artery

Dorsal metatarsal arteries

C The arteries of the lower limb
Right leg, anterior view with the foot in plantar flexion.

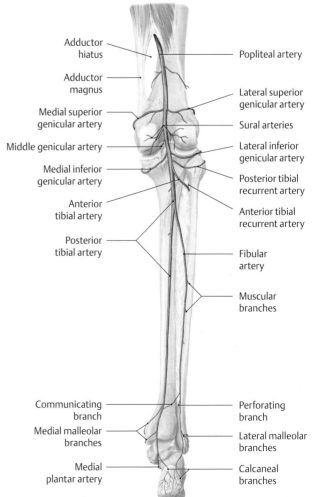

Adductor hiatus

Adductor magnus

Medial superior genicular artery

Middle genicular artery

Medial inferior genicular artery

Anterior tibial artery

Posterior tibial artery

Popliteal artery

Lateral superior genicular artery

Sural arteries

Lateral inferior genicular artery

Posterior tibial recurrent artery

Anterior tibial recurrent artery

Fibular artery

Muscular branches

Communicating branch

Medial malleolar branches

Medial plantar artery

Perforating branch

Lateral malleolar branches

Calcaneal branches

E The arteries of the popliteal fossa and leg
Right leg, posterior view.

465

4.2 The Veins

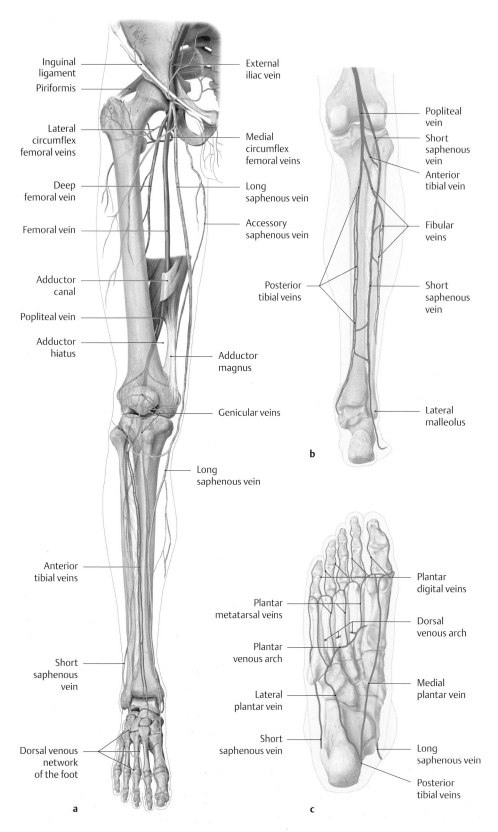

Inguinal ligament
Piriformis
Lateral circumflex femoral veins
Deep femoral vein
Femoral vein
Adductor canal
Popliteal vein
Adductor hiatus
Anterior tibial veins
Short saphenous vein
Dorsal venous network of the foot

External iliac vein
Medial circumflex femoral veins
Long saphenous vein
Accessory saphenous vein
Adductor magnus
Genicular veins
Long saphenous vein

a

Popliteal vein
Short saphenous vein
Anterior tibial vein
Fibular veins
Short saphenous vein
Posterior tibial veins
Lateral malleolus

b

Plantar metatarsal veins
Plantar venous arch
Lateral plantar vein
Short saphenous vein

Plantar digital veins
Dorsal venous arch
Medial plantar vein
Long saphenous vein
Posterior tibial veins

c

A The deep and superficial veins of the right lower limb

a Thigh, leg, and dorsum of the foot, anterior view.

b Leg, posterior view.

c Sole of the foot, plantar view.

For clarity, only the most important veins are demonstrated here.

B Overview of the principal veins of the lower limb

The veins of the lower limb are subdivided into three systems: a superficial (epifascial) system, a deep (intermuscular) system, and a *perforating* system that interconnects the superficial and deep veins. The upright human body posture places an exceptional load on the veins of the lower limb, which must act against the force of gravity in returning the blood to the heart (the deep venous system handles approximately 85 % of the venous return, the superficial veins approximately 15 %). A series of venous valves help to maintain the normal superficial-to-deep direction of blood flow (see also p. 467). Note that, for the sake of clarity, not all of the veins in the table below have been depicted in these illustrations.

Deep veins of the lower limb
- Femoral vein
- Deep femoral vein
- Medial and lateral circumflex femoral veins
- Popliteal vein
- Sural veins
- Genicular veins
- Anterior and posterior tibial veins
- Fibular veins
- Dorsal and plantar metatarsal veins (see **Ac**)
- Plantar digital veins (see **Ac**)

Superficial lower limb veins
- Long saphenous vein
- External pudendal veins
- Superficial circumflex iliac vein
- Superficial epigastric vein
- Accessory saphenous vein
- Posterior arch vein
- Short saphenous vein (see **Cb**)
- Femoropopliteal vein (see **Cb**)
- Dorsal venous network (see **Ca**)
- Dorsal venous arch
- Plantar venous network
- Plantar venous arch

Perforating veins
Of the many perforating veins in the leg, three groups have the greatest clinical importance (see **E**):
- The Dodd group (medial side of the thigh, middle third)
- The Boyd group (medial side of the leg below the knee)
- The Cockett group (medial side of the distal leg)

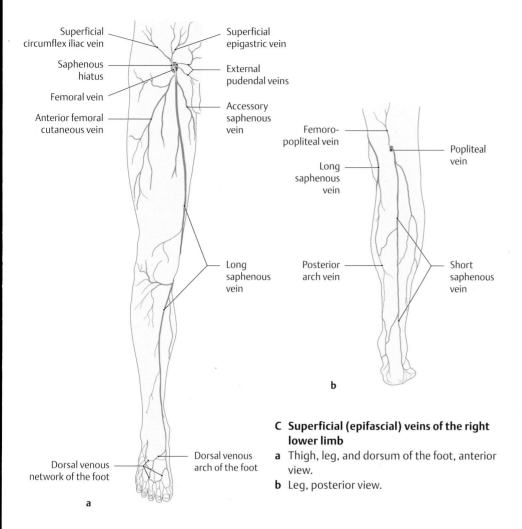

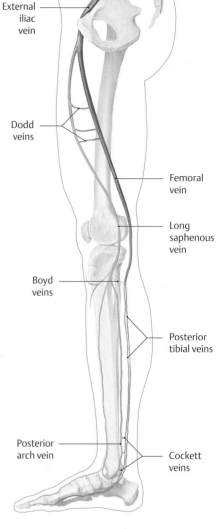

Superficial circumflex iliac vein

Saphenous hiatus

Femoral vein

Anterior femoral cutaneous vein

Superficial epigastric vein

External pudendal veins

Accessory saphenous vein

Long saphenous vein

Dorsal venous network of the foot

Dorsal venous arch of the foot

a

Femoro-popliteal vein

Long saphenous vein

Posterior arch vein

Popliteal vein

Short saphenous vein

b

C Superficial (epifascial) veins of the right lower limb
a Thigh, leg, and dorsum of the foot, anterior view.
b Leg, posterior view.

External iliac vein

Dodd veins

Boyd veins

Posterior arch vein

Femoral vein

Long saphenous vein

Posterior tibial veins

Cockett veins

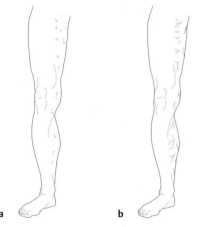

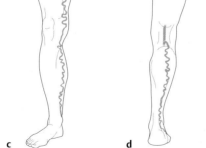

a **b** **c** **d**

E Clinically important perforating veins
Right leg, medial view. Numerous perforating veins interconnect the deep and superficial venous systems of the leg. Their venous valves normally prevent blood flow from the deep veins to the superficial cutaneous veins. The clinically important members of this system are located between the deep veins and the tributary region of the long saphenous vein:

- **Dodd veins:** located between the long saphenous vein and femoral vein at the level of the adductor canal.
- **Boyd veins:** located between the long saphenous vein and posterior tibial veins on the medial side of the proximal leg.
- **Cockett veins (I–III):** located between a curved branch of the long saphenous vein behind the medial malleolus (the posterior arch vein) and the posterior tibial veins. The Cockett veins on the medial side of the distal leg are of special clinical importance because of this region's susceptibility to ulceration.

D Varices of the superficial leg veins
a Spider veins (tiny intradermal varices).
b Reticular varices (weblike dilatations of small subcutaneous veins).
c Long saphenous varicosity.
d Short saphenous varicosity.

Varicose disease of the *superficial* leg veins is the most common *chronic* venous disease, affecting 15 % of the adult population. Varicose veins can be classified as primary idiopathic varices (75 %) or as secondary symptomatic varices. **Primary varices** generally result from degeneration of the vein wall leading to incompetence of the venous valves. **Secondary** varices result from chronic occlusion of the *deep* venous system with incompetence of the perforator veins and a reversal in the direction of venous flow. Besides chronic conditions, there are also important *acute* diseases that may affect the superficial venous system (e.g., thrombophlebitis) and deep venous system (e.g., venous thrombosis).

A The superficial lymphatic system of the right lower limb

a Anterior view, **b** posterior view. (The arrows indicate the main directions of lymphatic drainage.)

The lymph in the lower limb is drained by a superficial (epifascial) system and a deep (subfascial) system, similar to the arrangement in the arm. The largest lymph vessels, called collectors, basically follow the course of the superficial veins (long and short saphenous veins) and deep veins (popliteal vein, femoral vein) and are interconnected by anastomoses located mostly in the popliteal and inguinal regions. While the superficial lymph vessels primarily drain the skin and subcutaneous tissue, the deep system drains lymph from the muscles, joints, and nerves. The superficial lymphatics consist of an anteromedial bundle and a posterolateral bundle. The **anteromedial bundle** runs along the long saphenous vein to the superficial *inguinal* lymph nodes. It drains all of the skin and subcutaneous tissue of the lower limb except for the lateral border of the foot and a narrow strip on the calf. Those areas are drained by the **posterolateral bundle** (see **b**), which thus receives drainage from a considerably smaller region. The lymph in the posterolateral bundle first passes along the short saphenous vein to the superficial *popliteal* lymph nodes and then drains through the deep popliteal lymph nodes to the deep inguinal lymph nodes.

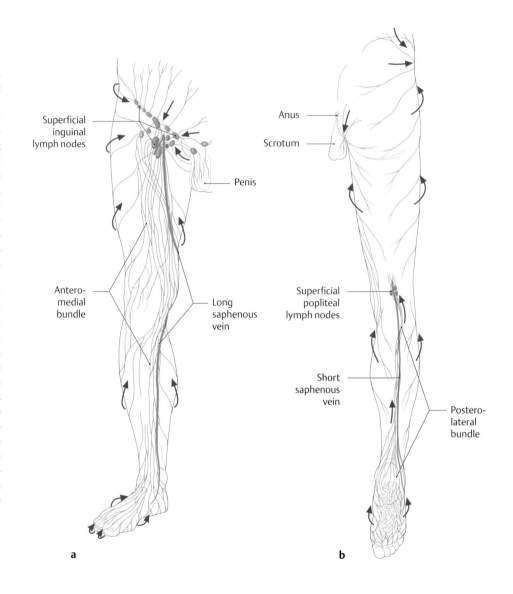

a

b

B The deep lymph nodes of the inguinal region

Right inguinal region after removal of the cribriform fascia about the saphenous hiatus, anterior view. The veins and lymphatic system above the inguinal ligament are shown in light shading. The deep inguinal lymph nodes are located near the termination of the long saphenous vein, medial to the femoral vein. They are important because *all the lymph from the limb* filters through them before reaching the iliac lymph nodes. The largest lymph node of this group (the *Rosenmüller lymph node*) is also the highest, placed at the level of the femoral canal. The group of pelvic lymph nodes, which includes the external iliac nodes, begins just above the inguinal ligament.

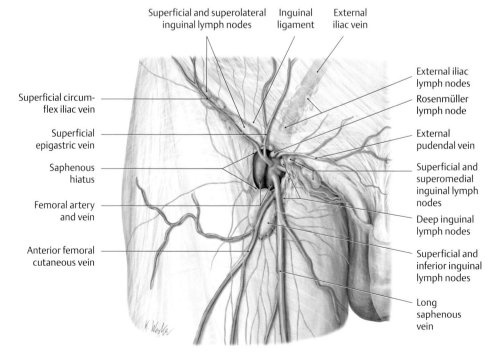

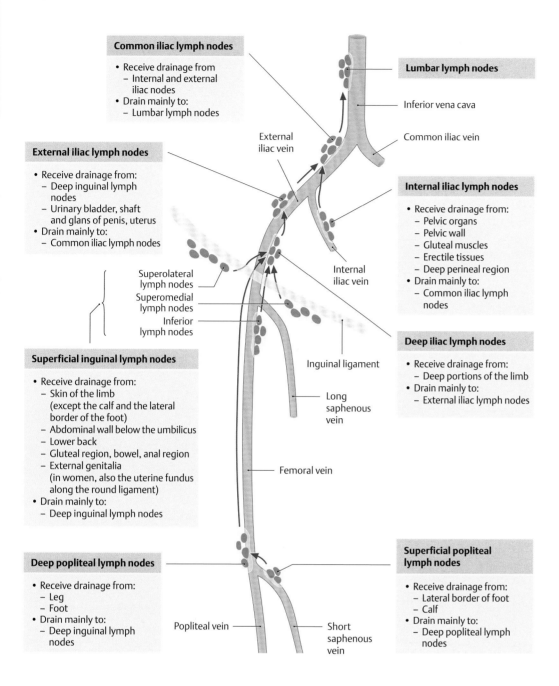

Common iliac lymph nodes

- Receive drainage from
  - Internal and external iliac nodes
- Drain mainly to:
  - Lumbar lymph nodes

External iliac lymph nodes

- Receive drainage from:
  - Deep inguinal lymph nodes
  - Urinary bladder, shaft and glans of penis, uterus
- Drain mainly to:
  - Common iliac lymph nodes

Superolateral lymph nodes
Superomedial lymph nodes
Inferior lymph nodes

Superficial inguinal lymph nodes

- Receive drainage from:
  - Skin of the limb (except the calf and the lateral border of the foot)
  - Abdominal wall below the umbilicus
  - Lower back
  - Gluteal region, bowel, anal region
  - External genitalia (in women, also the uterine fundus along the round ligament)
- Drain mainly to:
  - Deep inguinal lymph nodes

Deep popliteal lymph nodes

- Receive drainage from:
  - Leg
  - Foot
- Drain mainly to:
  - Deep inguinal lymph nodes

Lumbar lymph nodes

Inferior vena cava

Common iliac vein

External iliac vein

Internal iliac lymph nodes

- Receive drainage from:
  - Pelvic organs
  - Pelvic wall
  - Gluteal muscles
  - Erectile tissues
  - Deep perineal region
- Drain mainly to:
  - Common iliac lymph nodes

Internal iliac vein

Deep iliac lymph nodes

- Receive drainage from:
  - Deep portions of the limb
- Drain mainly to:
  - External iliac lymph nodes

Inguinal ligament

Long saphenous vein

Femoral vein

Popliteal vein

Short saphenous vein

Superficial popliteal lymph nodes

- Receive drainage from:
  - Lateral border of foot
  - Calf
- Drain mainly to:
  - Deep popliteal lymph nodes

C The lymph node stations and drainage pathways in the lower limb

Right limb, anterior view. The arrows indicate the main directions of lymph flow in the superficial and deep lymphatic systems.

Note: Lymph from the skin and subcutaneous tissues of the calf and the lateral border of the foot passes through the superficial and deep popliteal lymph nodes along the deep system of lymphatics *directly* to the deep inguinal lymph nodes. By contrast, lymph from the rest of the skin of the lower limb first drains through the anteromedial bundle along the long saphenous vein to the superficial inguinal lymph nodes (see also **A**).

The *superficial inguinal lymph nodes*, located on the fascia lata, consist of the following:

- Lymph nodes arranged parallel to the inguinal ligament (the superomedial and superolateral inguinal lymph nodes)
- Lymph nodes distributed vertically along the terminal segment of the long saphenous vein (the inferior inguinal lymph nodes)

These nodes first drain into the deep inguinal lymph nodes (see **B**) and then along the external iliac vein to the external and common iliac lymph nodes, finally reaching the lumbar lymph nodes.

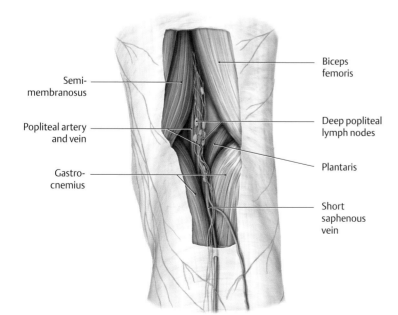

Semi-membranosus

Popliteal artery and vein

Gastro-cnemius

Biceps femoris

Deep popliteal lymph nodes

Plantaris

Short saphenous vein

D The deep lymph nodes of the popliteal region

The popliteal fossa of the right leg, posterior view. Lymph from the deep lymphatics of the leg drains (through the deep popliteal nodes between the posterior knee joint capsule and popliteal vessels) along the femoral vein and then anteriorly through the adductor hiatus to the deep inguinal lymph nodes.

4.4 The Structure of the Lumbosacral Plexus

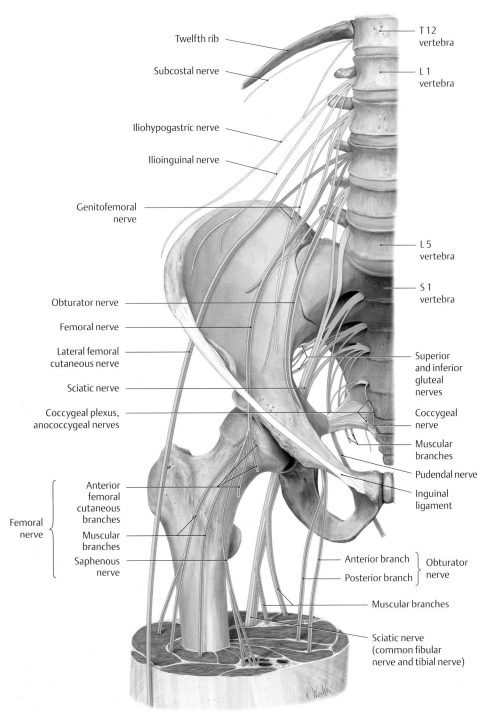

Twelfth rib

Subcostal nerve

Iliohypogastric nerve

Ilioinguinal nerve

Genitofemoral nerve

Obturator nerve

Femoral nerve

Lateral femoral cutaneous nerve

Sciatic nerve

Coccygeal plexus, anococcygeal nerves

Femoral nerve
- Anterior femoral cutaneous branches
- Muscular branches
- Saphenous nerve

T 12 vertebra

L 1 vertebra

L 5 vertebra

S 1 vertebra

Superior and inferior gluteal nerves

Coccygeal nerve

Muscular branches

Pudendal nerve

Inguinal ligament

Anterior branch ⎱ Obturator
Posterior branch ⎰ nerve

Muscular branches

Sciatic nerve (common fibular nerve and tibial nerve)

A The lumbosacral plexus and its branches

Right side, anterior view. For clarity, the muscles of the pelvis and lumbar spine have been removed. Lateral to the intervertebral foramina of the lumbar spine, the *ventral rami* of the first four *lumbar* spinal nerves (L1–L4) form the lumbar plexus and pass through the psoas major muscle. The smaller, muscular branches are distributed directly to the psoas major. The larger branches emerge from the muscle at various sites and pass sharply downward to reach the abdominal wall and thigh, except for the obturator nerve, which runs down the lateral wall of the lesser pelvis to the thigh. The ventral rami of the first four *sacral* spinal nerves (S1–S4) emerge from the anterior foramina of the sacrum and unite on the anterior surface of the piriformis to form the sacral plexus. The nerves from the sacral plexus are distributed to the back of the thigh, the leg, and the foot (after Mumenthaler).

B Spinal cord segments and nerves of the lumbosacral plexus

The lumbosacral plexus supplies sensory and motor innervation to the lower limb. It is formed by the ventral rami of the lumbar and sacral spinal nerves, with contributions from the subcostal nerve (T12) and coccygeal nerve (Co1) (see **D**). The lumbosacral plexus is subdivided into the lumbar plexus and sacral plexus based on its distribution and topography.

Lumbar plexus (T12–L4)
- Iliohypogastric nerve (T12–L1)
- Ilioinguinal nerve (L1)
- Genitofemoral nerve (L1, L2)
- Lateral femoral cutaneous nerve (L2, L3)
- Obturator nerve (L2–L4)
- Femoral nerve (L2–L4)
- Short, direct muscular branches to specific hip muscles

Sacral plexus (L5–S4)*
- Superior gluteal nerve (L4–S1)
- Inferior gluteal nerve (L5–S2)
- Posterior femoral cutaneous nerve (S1–S3)
- Sciatic nerve (L4–S3) with its two large branches:
  - Tibial nerve (L4–S3)
  - Common fibular nerve (L4–S2)
- Pudendal nerve (S2–S4)
- Short, direct muscular branches to specific hip muscles

* Often the sacral plexus is further subdivided into a sciatic plexus and a pudendal plexus. The main branch of the pudendal plexus, the pudendal nerve, supplies the skin and muscles of the pelvic floor, perineum, and external genitalia.

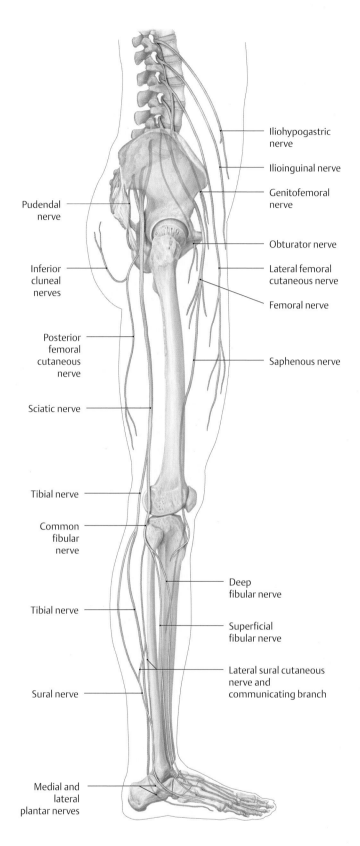

Pudendal nerve

Inferior cluneal nerves

Posterior femoral cutaneous nerve

Sciatic nerve

Tibial nerve

Common fibular nerve

Tibial nerve

Sural nerve

Medial and lateral plantar nerves

Iliohypogastric nerve

Ilioinguinal nerve

Genitofemoral nerve

Obturator nerve

Lateral femoral cutaneous nerve

Femoral nerve

Saphenous nerve

Deep fibular nerve

Superficial fibular nerve

Lateral sural cutaneous nerve and communicating branch

C Topography of the lumbosacral plexus
Right lower limb, lateral view. The nerves of the lumbar plexus reach the lower limb *in front of* the hip joint and mainly supply the *anterior side of the thigh*, while the nerves of the sacral plexus descend *behind* the hip joint and innervate the *posterior side of the thigh*, most of the *leg*, and the entire *foot*.

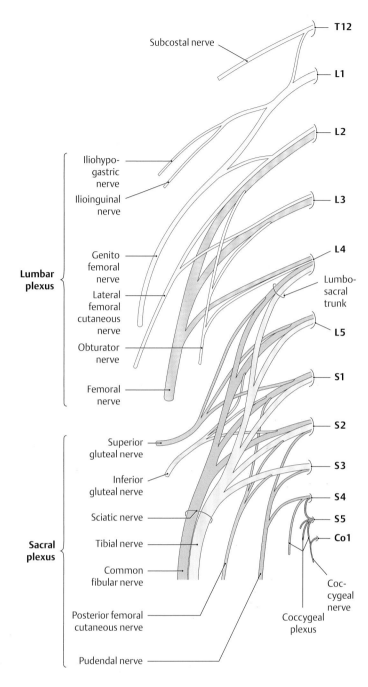

Subcostal nerve

T12
L1
L2
L3
L4
Lumbosacral trunk
L5
S1
S2
S3
S4
S5
Co1

Lumbar plexus

Iliohypogastric nerve

Ilioinguinal nerve

Genitofemoral nerve

Lateral femoral cutaneous nerve

Obturator nerve

Femoral nerve

Sacral plexus

Superior gluteal nerve

Inferior gluteal nerve

Sciatic nerve

Tibial nerve

Common fibular nerve

Posterior femoral cutaneous nerve

Pudendal nerve

Coccygeal nerve

Coccygeal plexus

D Structure of the lumbosacral plexus
The communicating branch passing between the lumbar plexus and sacral plexus contains fibers from the ventral ramus of L4 and is called the lumbosacral trunk. The last spinal nerve, the coccygeal nerve, emerges from the sacral hiatus. It unites with the ventral rami of the fourth and fifth sacral nerves to form the coccygeal plexus (see p. 482) (after Mumenthaler).

471

4.5 The Nerves of the Lumbar Plexus: The Iliohypogastric, Ilioinguinal, Genitofemoral, and Lateral Femoral Cutaneous Nerves

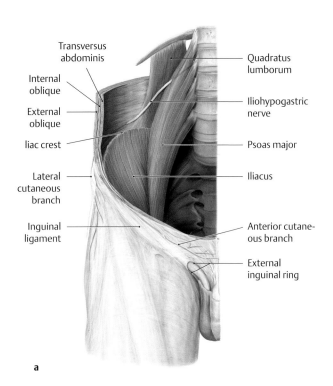

a

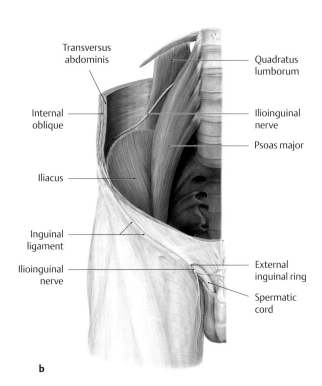

b

A Course of the iliohypogastric, ilioinguinal, genitofemoral, and lateral femoral cutaneous nerves after emerging from the lumbar plexus (after Mumenthaler).
Right lateral and posterior abdominal wall region, anterior view.

a The **iliohypogastric nerve** generally emerges with the ilioinguinal nerve (see **b**) at the lateral border of the psoas major and runs laterally and obliquely on the anterior surface of the quadratus lumborum. Approximately 3–4 cm past the lateral border of that muscle, it pierces the transversus abdominis and runs anteriorly above the iliac crest, passing between the transversus abdominis and internal oblique. After giving off several muscular branches to both of these muscles and a sensory lateral cutaneous branch to

the skin of the lateral hip region, the terminal branch of the iliohypogastric nerve courses medially, running parallel to the inguinal ligament. Above the external inguinal ring it pierces the aponeurosis of the external oblique muscle and supplies a sensory anterior cutaneous branch to the skin above the inguinal ligament.

b The **ilioinguinal nerve** generally courses with the iliohypogastric nerve (see **a**) on the quadratus lumborum but soon separates from it and runs at the level of the iliac crest to the lateral abdominal wall, which it pierces at a variable location. It runs medially at the level of the inguinal ligament between the transversus abdominis and internal oblique, supplying twigs to both muscles, and it distributes sensory fibers through the external inguinal ring to the skin over the symphysis and to the lateral portion of the labia majora or scrotum.

B Overview of the nerves of the lumbar plexus

Nerve	Segment	Innervated muscles	Cutaneous branches (to the region receiving sensory innervation, see **C** and pp. 474 and 475)
• Iliohypogastric nerve	T 12–L 1	• Transversus abdominis, internal oblique (the inferior portions of each)	• Anterior cutaneous branch • Lateral cutaneous branch
• Ilioinguinal nerve	L 1	• Transversus abdominis, internal oblique (the inferior portions of each)	• Anterior scrotal nerves in males, anterior labial nerves in females
• Genitofemoral nerve	L 1, L 2	• Cremaster in males (genital branch)	• Genital branch, femoral branch
• Lateral femoral cutaneous nerve	L 2, L 3		• Lateral femoral cutaneous nerve

• Obturator nerve (see p. 474)
  – Anterior branch
 	
  – Posterior branch
	L 2–L 4	• Obturator externus
		• Adductor longus, adductor brevis, gracilis, pectineus
		• Adductor magnus
			• Cutaneous branch

• Femoral nerve (see p. 474)	L 2–L 4	• Iliopsoas, pectineus, sartorius, quadriceps femoris	• Anterior cutaneous branches, saphenous nerve
• Short, direct muscular branches (see p. 474)	T 12–L 4	• Psoas major, quadratus lumborum, iliacus, intertransversarii lumborum	

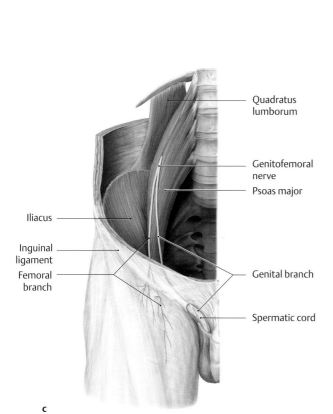

c

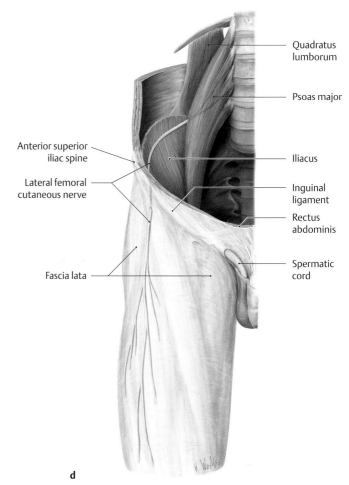

d

c The **genitofemoral nerve** pierces the psoas major and descends upon its anterior surface, dividing into its two terminal branches: the genital branch and femoral branch:

- The *purely sensory femoral branch* pierces the lacuna vasorum in the area of the saphenous hiatus (see p. 489) and becomes superficial, supplying the skin below the inguinal ligament in both sexes.
- The *mixed genital branch* runs in the spermatic cord in males. In females it initially passes through the inguinal canal accompanied by the round ligament of the uterus. In its further course it distributes sensory fibers to the scrotal skin in males and to the skin of the labia majora in females. It also supplies motor fibers to the cremaster muscle in males (see p. 148).

d The **lateral femoral cutaneous nerve** emerges from the lateral border of the psoas major and runs obliquely downward and laterally

beneath the iliacus fascia toward the anterior superior iliac spine. Medial to the iliac spine, the nerve leaves the pelvis through the lateral lacuna musculorum (see p. 489) and first runs beneath the fascia lata and then upon it to the skin of the anterior thigh, piercing the fascia approximately 2–3 cm below the anterior superior iliac spine. The nerve is susceptible to occasional mechanical injury at its site of emergence from the pelvis below the inguinal ligament, as it makes an approximately 80° angle at that site and is susceptible to stretching, especially on extension of the hip. The nerve also has only scant coverage by fatty tissue at that location. Stretch injuries are manifested by sensory disturbances (paresthesias) or pain in the *lateral* part of the thigh.

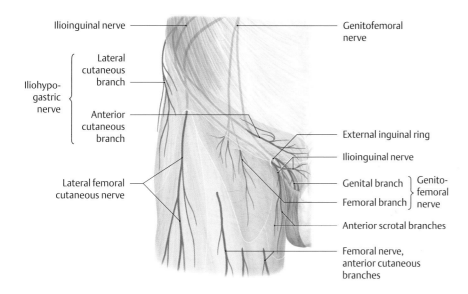

C Sensory innervation of the inguinal region and thigh

Right inguinal region of a male, anterior view. The territories of the various sensory nerves are indicated by different colors.

Note: Both the ilioinguinal nerve and the genital branch of the genitofemoral nerve pass through the external inguinal ring. The two nerves are frequently confused. The genital branch in males is located by first opening the spermatic cord. In females, the genital branch accompanies the uterine round ligament to supply the skin of the labia majora (see also **Ac**).

4.6 The Nerves of the Lumbar Plexus: The Obturator and Femoral Nerves

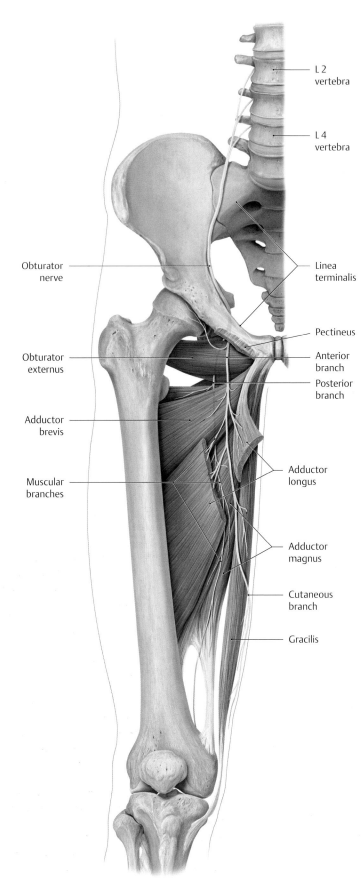

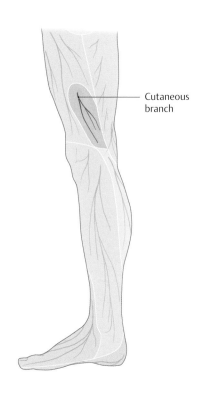

B Sensory distribution of the obturator nerve
Right leg, medial view.

A Course of the obturator nerve

The right inguinal region and thigh, anterior view. The obturator nerve receives fibers from the L 2–L 4 spinal segments. After leaving the lumbar plexus, it descends behind and medial to the psoas major (not shown here) toward the lesser pelvis and enters the obturator canal (not shown here, see p. 498) below the linea terminalis, accompanied by the obturator vessels. Farther distally it distributes muscular branches to the obturator externus and subsequently divides into an anterior branch and a posterior branch. These branches continue distally, passing respectively anterior and posterior to the adductor brevis, and supply motor innervation to the rest of the adductor muscles (pectineus, adductor longus, adductor brevis, adductor magnus, adductor minimus, and gracilis). The anterior branch gives off a terminal, sensory cutaneous branch at the anterior border of the gracilis, which pierces the fascia lata to supply a palm-sized area of skin on the medial view of the distal thigh. In evaluating motor deficits that are associated with obturator nerve injuries (e.g., intrapartum or due to pelvic fractures), it is important to know that the femoral nerve contributes to the supply of the pectineus muscle while the sciatic nerve helps to supply the adductor magnus.

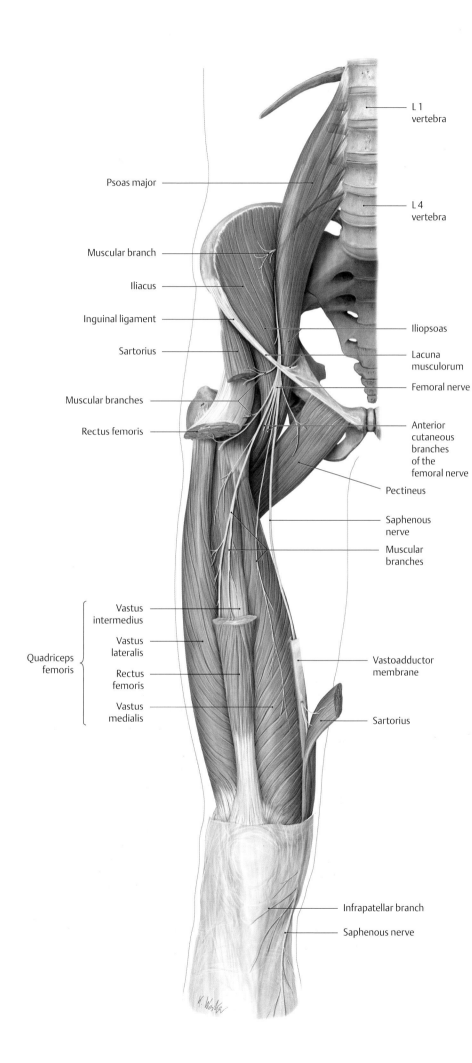

Psoas major

Muscular branch

Iliacus

Inguinal ligament

Sartorius

Muscular branches

Rectus femoris

Quadriceps femoris
- Vastus intermedius
- Vastus lateralis
- Rectus femoris
- Vastus medialis

L 1 vertebra

L 4 vertebra

Iliopsoas

Lacuna musculorum

Femoral nerve

Anterior cutaneous branches of the femoral nerve

Pectineus

Saphenous nerve

Muscular branches

Vastoadductor membrane

Sartorius

Infrapatellar branch

Saphenous nerve

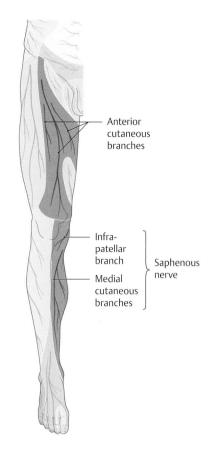

Anterior cutaneous branches

Infra- patellar branch

Medial cutaneous branches

Saphenous nerve

D Sensory distribution of the femoral nerve
Right leg, anterior view.

C Course of the femoral nerve
The right inguinal region and thigh, anterior view. As the largest and longest nerve of the lumbar plexus, the femoral nerve receives fibers from the second through fourth lumbar segments of the spinal cord. It supplies *motor* innervation to the iliopsoas, pectineus, sartorius, and quadriceps femoris muscles and *sensory* innervation to the skin of the anterior thigh, medial leg, and hindfoot (see **D**). The nerve, under cover of the psoas fascia, runs in a groove between psoas major and iliacus to the medial lacuna musculorum while giving off branches to both muscles. Approximately 8 cm below the inguinal ligament, the femoral nerve divides into numerous cutaneous branches (anterior cutaneous branches) and muscular branches as well as a long, terminal sensory branch that continues to the foot, the saphenous nerve. Initially the saphenous nerve enters the adductor canal with the femoral vessels (below the vastoadductor membrane) but then leaves the canal through the vastoadductor membrane and passes with the sartorius toward the medial side of the knee. After giving off a sensory infrapatellar branch to the skin of the medial knee, it follows the long saphenous vein to the skin of the medial leg and foot.

475

4.7 The Nerves of the Sacral Plexus: The Superior Gluteal, Inferior Gluteal, and Posterior Femoral Cutaneous Nerves

A Nerves of the sacral plexus (part I)

(The motor and sensory nerves of the sacral plexus are reviewed in parts II and III, see pp. 478 and 482.)

Nerve	Segment	Innervated muscles	Cutaneous branches
• Superior gluteal nerve	L4–S1	• Gluteus medius • Gluteus minimus • Tensor fasciae latae	
• Inferior gluteal nerve	L5–S2	• Gluteus maximus	
• Posterior femoral cutaneous nerve	S1–S3		• Posterior femoral cutaneous nerve – Inferior cluneal nerves – Perineal branches (see **F** for sensory distribution)
• *Direct branches from the plexus:* – Nerve of piriformis – Nerve of obturator internus – Nerve of quadratus femoris	 L5, S2 L5, S1 L5, S1	 • Piriformis • Obturator internus • Gemelli • Quadratus femoris	

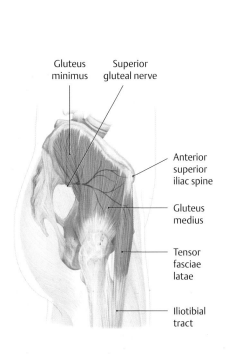

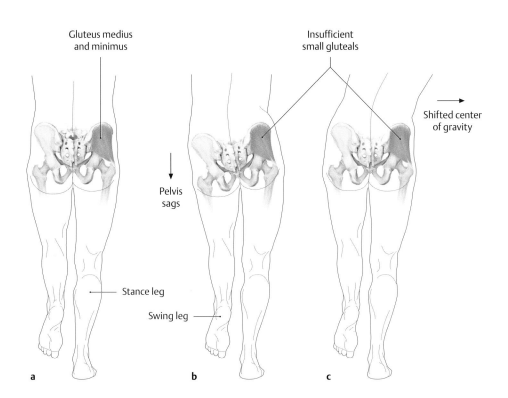

B Motor distribution of the superior gluteal nerve

Right hip region, lateral view. Accompanied by blood vessels with the same name, the superior gluteal nerve leaves the lesser pelvis through the greater sciatic foramen superior to the piriformis (see p. 494), runs in the intergluteal space, and supplies motor fibers to the small gluteal muscles (gluteus medius and minimus) and tensor fasciae latae.

C Clinical indicators of small gluteal muscle weakness: the Trendelenburg sign and the Duchenne limp

Lower half of body, posterior view.

a In normal one-legged stance, the small gluteal muscles on the stance side can stabilize the pelvis in the coronal plane.

b Weakness or paralysis of the small gluteal muscles (e.g., due to a faulty intramuscular injection causing damage to the superior gluteal nerve) is manifested by weak abduc-tion of the affected hip joint and an inability to stabilize the pelvis in the coronal plane. In a positive Trendelenburg test, the pelvis sags toward the *normal* unsupported side.

c Tilting the upper body toward the affected side shifts the center of gravity onto the stance side, thereby elevating the pelvis on the swing side (*Duchenne limp*). With bilateral loss of the small gluteals, the patient exhibits a typical waddling gait.

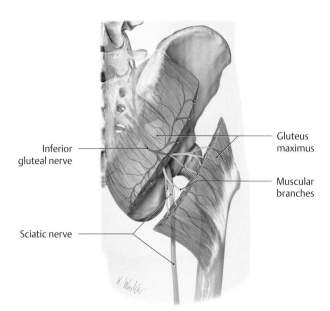

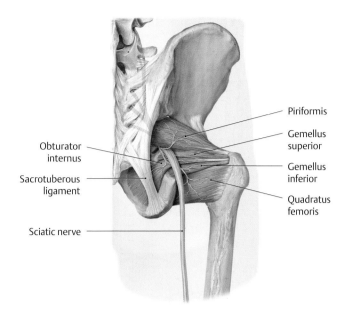

D Motor distribution of the inferior gluteal nerve

Right half of the pelvis, posterior view. The inferior gluteal nerve leaves the lesser pelvis with the sciatic nerve through the greater sciatic foramen inferior to the piriformis (see p. 494) and supplies numerous muscular branches to the gluteus maximus. Paralysis of the gluteus maximus causes little impairment of normal gait on even ground because the deficit is well compensated by the hamstrings (see p. 430). The affected patient is unable to run, jump, or climb stairs, however.

E Muscles that are supplied by direct branches from the sacral plexus

Right half of the pelvis, posterior view. The direct branches of the sacral plexus are listed in **A**.

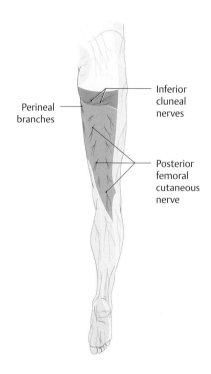

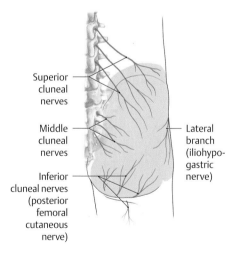

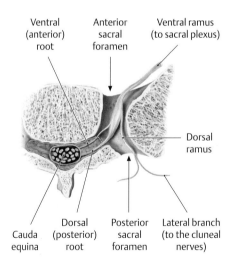

F Sensory distribution of the posterior femoral cutaneous nerve

Right lower limb, posterior view. Besides the skin of the posterior thigh, the posterior femoral cutaneous nerve distributes several branches to the skin of the gluteal sulcus (inferior cluneal nerves), and its perineal branches supply the skin of the perineal region (darker shading indicates the exclusive area).

G Sensory innervation of the gluteal region

Right buttock, posterior view.
The gluteal region receives sensory innervation from portions of the sacral plexus and lumbar plexus (ventral rami of the spinal nerves) and also from dorsal rami:

- From the sacral plexus: inferior cluneal nerves (from the posterior femoral cutaneous nerve).
- From the lumbar plexus: the lateral branch of the iliohypogastric nerve.
- From dorsal rami of the spinal nerves: the superior cluneal nerves (dorsal rami of L 1–L 3) and middle cluneal nerves (dorsal rami of S 1–S 3).

H An emerging sacral nerve

Horizontal section through the right half of the sacrum at the level of the sacral foramina. While the ventral ramus of a sacral nerve emerges from the sacrum through an *anterior* sacral foramen, the corresponding dorsal ramus passes through the *posterior* sacral foramen to supply the skin of the buttock.

4.8 The Nerves of the Sacral Plexus: The Sciatic Nerve (Overview and Sensory Distribution)

A The motor and sensory nerves of the sacral plexus (part II)

The largest and longest of the peripheral nerves, the sciatic nerve, leaves the lesser pelvis through the greater sciatic foramen inferior to the piriformis and passes below the gluteus maximus to the back of the thigh. It divides into its two main branches, the tibial and common fibular nerves, at a variable level but generally before entering the popliteal fossa. The *muscular branches* of the sciatic nerve, however, can already be identified as consisting of a *fibular part* (Fib) and a *tibial part* (Tib) while still proximal to the bifurcation (see also p. 480). Injuries of the sciatic nerve may be caused by compression of the nerve at its emergence inferior to the piriformis (usually by extrinsic pressure, such as sitting). Other potential causes are misdirected intramuscular injections (in which the nerve is accidentally pricked), pelvic fractures, and surgical procedures (e.g., hip replacement).

Nerve	Segment	Innervated muscles	Cutaneous branches

Sciatic nerve	L 4–S 3	• Semitendinosus (Tib)
		• Semimembranosus (Tib)
		• Biceps femoris
		  – Long head (Tib)
		  – Short head (Fib)
		• Adductor magnus (Tib), medial part	

• Common fibular nerve	L 4–S 2		• Lateral sural cutaneous nerve • Fibular communicating branch
– Superficial fibular nerve		• Fibularis longus • Fibularis brevis	• Medial dorsal cutaneous nerve • Intermediate dorsal cutaneous nerve
– Deep fibular nerve		• Tibialis anterior • Extensor digitorum longus • Extensor digitorum brevis • Extensor hallucis longus • Extensor hallucis brevis • Fibularis tertius	• Lateral cutaneous nerve of the big toe • Medial cutaneous nerve of the second toe
• Tibial nerve	L 4–S 3	• Triceps surae • Plantaris • Popliteus • Tibialis posterior • Flexor digitorum longus • Flexor hallucis longus	• Medial sural cutaneous nerve (⟶ sural nerve) • Lateral calcaneal branches • Medial calcaneal branches • Lateral dorsal cutaneous nerve
– Medial plantar nerve		• Abductor hallucis • Flexor digitorum brevis • Flexor hallucis brevis, medial head • First and second lumbricals	• Proper plantar digital nerves
– Lateral plantar nerve		• Flexor hallucis brevis, lateral head • Quadratus plantae • Abductor digiti minimi • Flexor digiti minimi brevis • Opponens digiti minimi • Third and fourth lumbricals • First through third plantar interossei • First through fourth dorsal interossei • Adductor hallucis	• Proper plantar digital nerves

⟶ = is continuous with

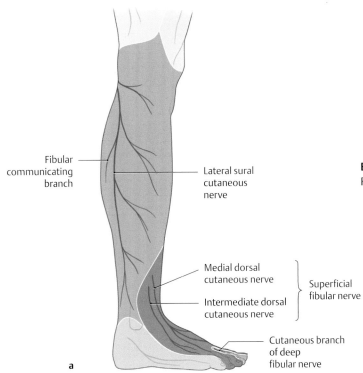

Fibular communicating branch

Lateral sural cutaneous nerve

Medial dorsal cutaneous nerve

Intermediate dorsal cutaneous nerve

Superficial fibular nerve

Cutaneous branch of deep fibular nerve

a

B Sensory distribution of the sciatic nerve
Right leg. **a** Lateral view, **b** anterior view, **c** posterior view.

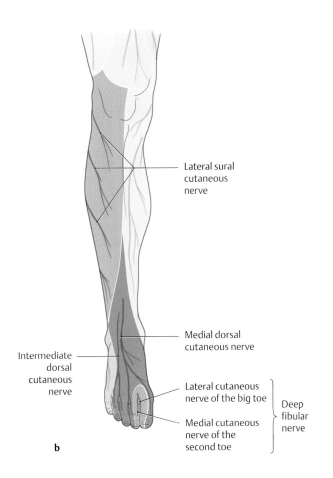

Lateral sural cutaneous nerve

Intermediate dorsal cutaneous nerve

Medial dorsal cutaneous nerve

Lateral cutaneous nerve of the big toe

Medial cutaneous nerve of the second toe

Deep fibular nerve

b

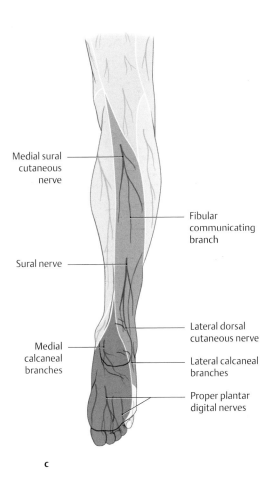

Medial sural cutaneous nerve

Fibular communicating branch

Sural nerve

Medial calcaneal branches

Lateral dorsal cutaneous nerve

Lateral calcaneal branches

Proper plantar digital nerves

c

4.9 The Nerves of the Sacral Plexus: The Sciatic Nerve (Course and Motor Distribution)

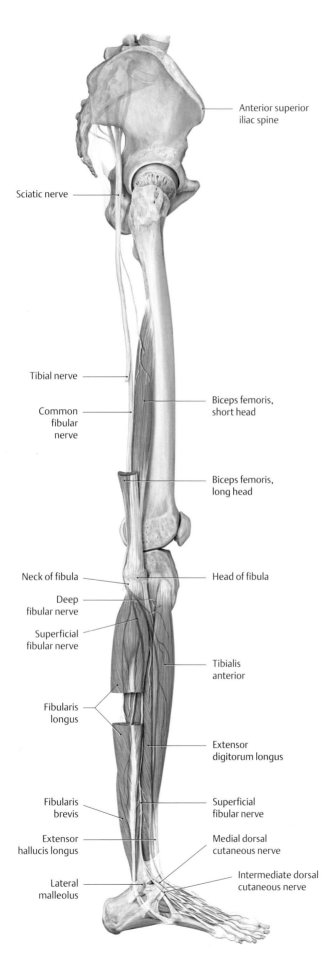

Sciatic nerve

Anterior superior iliac spine

Tibial nerve

Common fibular nerve

Biceps femoris, short head

Biceps femoris, long head

Neck of fibula

Head of fibula

Deep fibular nerve

Superficial fibular nerve

Tibialis anterior

Fibularis longus

Extensor digitorum longus

Fibularis brevis

Superficial fibular nerve

Extensor hallucis longus

Medial dorsal cutaneous nerve

Lateral malleolus

Intermediate dorsal cutaneous nerve

A Course and motor distribution of the sciatic nerve: the fibular part (common fibular nerve)

Right lower limb, lateral view. After giving off several muscular branches from its fibular part (to the short head of biceps femoris), the sciatic nerve consistently divides in the lower third of the thigh into the tibial nerve and common fibular nerve. The common fibular nerve then follows the medial border of biceps femoris to the head of the fibula and winds around the neck of the fibula to the front of the leg. Immediately after entering the fibularis longus, it divides into its two terminal branches, the *deep* fibular nerve and *superficial* fibular nerve. The superficial fibular nerve supplies the fibularis muscles and runs between the fibularis longus and fibula to the dorsum of the foot. The deep fibular nerve runs through the interosseus membrane to enter the extensor compartment. After supplying the tibialis anterior, extensor digitorum longus, and extensor hallucis longus, it runs in a groove between tibialis anterior and extensor hallucis longus on the crural interosseous membrane, accompanied by the anterior tibial vessels, to the dorsum of the foot.

- If the nerve is damaged at the level of the fibular neck (a very exposed location!) before dividing into its two terminal branches, the result is weakness or paralysis of the anterior and lateral compartment muscles, resulting in foot drop with some inversion.
- If the nerve is damaged after dividing into its terminal branches, the result may be an isolated weakness or paralysis of the anterior compartment or the lateral muscles, depending on whether the deep fibular or the superficial fibular nerve is affected. Accordingly, the result may be weak dorsiflexion or weakness of eversion. An isolated lesion of the superficial fibular nerve generally affects only the sensory terminal branch, with pain involving the distal leg and dorsum of the foot. Gait disturbance will occur only with an isolated lesion of the deep fibular nerve (as in compartment syndrome caused by anterior compartment hemorrhage, see p. 507), resulting in foot drop and a "steppage gait". Increased flexion of the hip and knee joints is necessary to keep the toe from dragging the ground during the swing phase of gait.

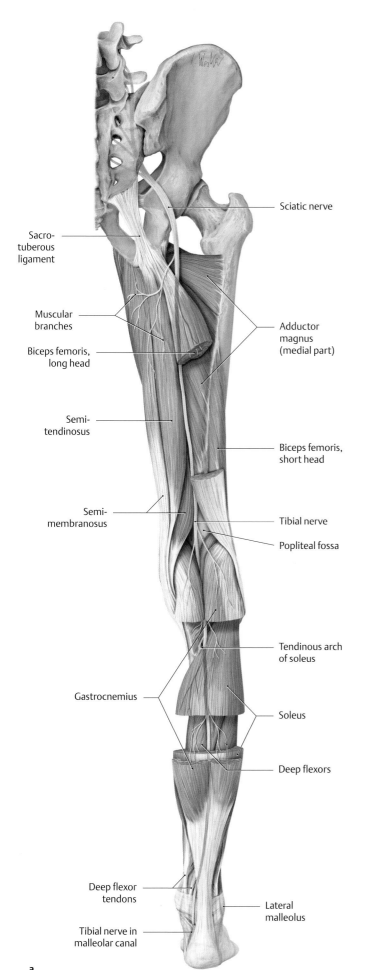

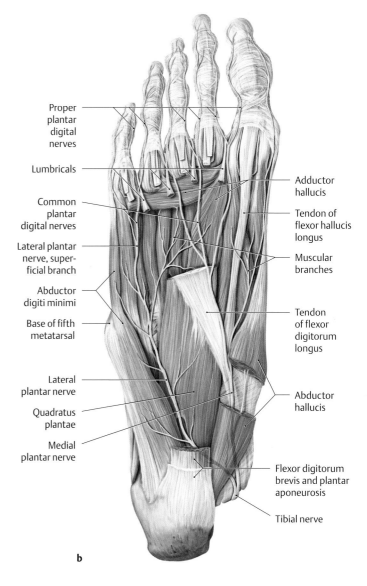

b

B Course and motor distribution of the sciatic nerve: the tibial part (tibial nerve)

a Right lower limb, posterior view; **b** right foot, plantar view. While still in the thigh, the tibial part of the sciatic nerve distributes several muscular branches to the semitendinosus, semimembranosus, biceps femoris (long head), and adductor magnus (medial part). After division of the sciatic nerve, the tibial nerve continues straight down through the center of the popliteal fossa and runs below the tendinous arch of the soleus muscle to the superficial and deep plantar flexors, which it supplies. In the deep posterior compartment, the tibial nerve continues distally in a neurovascular bundle with the posterior tibial vessels (not shown here) and passes through the tarsal tunnel, accompanied by the deep flexor tendons, to the plantar side of the foot (**b**). In passing through the tarsal tunnel, the tibial nerve divides into its two terminal branches (the lateral and medial plantar nerves), which supply all the muscles on the plantar side of the foot. Compression of the tibial nerve or its terminal branches at this site leads to an entrapment syndrome (= tarsal tunnel syndrome). This can result in pain and sensory disturbances affecting the sole of the foot or even palsies of the intrinsic foot muscles, particularly following severe nerve trauma in connection with a fracture of the tibial shaft or medial malleolus.

.

4.10 The Nerves of the Sacral Plexus: The Pudendal and Coccygeal Nerves

A The nerves of the sacral plexus (part III)

The pudendal nerve, the lowest branch of sacral plexus, arises from a separate small plexus formed by the ventral rami of S 1–S 4; hence it is occasionally referred to as the *pudendal plexus*.

Nerve	Segment	Innervated muscles	Cutaneous branches

• Pudendal nerve (*pudendal plexus*)	S2–S4	• Pelvic floor muscles
		  – Levator ani
		  – Superficial transverse perineal
		  – Deep transverse perineal
		  – Bulbospongiosus
		  – External anal sphincter
		  – Urethral sphincter
			• Inferior rectal nerves
			• Perineal nerves
			  – Posterior labial nerves in females
			  – Posterior scrotal nerves in males
			  – Dorsal clitoral nerve in females

• Coccygeal nerve (*coccygeal plexus*)	S5–Co2	• Coccygeus	• Anococcygeal nerve (ventral rami) • Dorsal rami

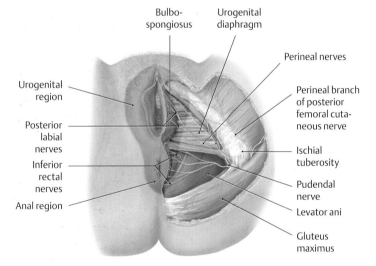

Bulbo-spongiosus — Urogenital diaphragm
Urogenital region
Posterior labial nerves
Inferior rectal nerves
Anal region
Perineal nerves
Perineal branch of posterior femoral cutaneous nerve
Ischial tuberosity
Pudendal nerve
Levator ani
Gluteus maximus

B The cutaneous branches of the pudendal nerve and its sensory distribution in the female

Lithotomy position, inferior view. The skin layers have been removed on the left side to demonstrate the terminal branches of the pudendal nerve in the ischioanal fossa (see p. 496). The area of cutaneous sensory innervation is color-shaded. Large portions of the urogenital region and anal region receive their sensory supply from the pudendal nerve. The skin area supplied by the pudendal nerve can be anesthetized during childbirth by infiltration anesthesia or a nerve block, enabling the obstetrician to perform and repair an episiotomy without pain (see p. 202). This can be done either by infiltrating the perineum between the anus and posterior fornix with a local anesthetic or by temporarily blocking the pudendal nerve with local anesthetic injected near the ischial spine (before the nerve has branched; see diagram in **C**).

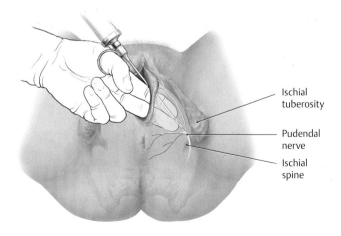

Ischial tuberosity
Pudendal nerve
Ischial spine

C Technique of a left-sided pudendal nerve block

Lithotomy position, inferior view. The most common type of conduction anesthesia used in vaginal deliveries is the pudendal nerve block, which renders the perineum, vulva, and lower third of the vagina insensitive to pain. In the *transvaginal approach*, a special guide cannula is introduced into the vagina, and 10 mL of a local anesthetic solution is injected approximately 1 cm above and 1 cm lateral to the palpable ischial spine on each side. An injection at this site will block the pudendal nerve *before* it has entered the pudendal canal (Alcock's canal) and *before* it has divided into its terminal branches. Often the nerve block is administered at the end of the expulsion stage to relieve stretch pain in the perineal region (see p. 202).

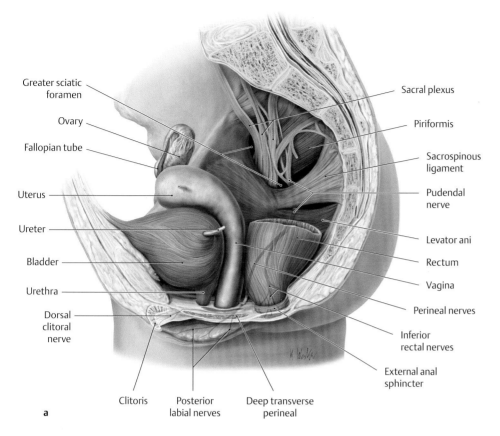

Greater sciatic foramen
Ovary
Fallopian tube
Uterus
Ureter
Bladder
Urethra
Dorsal clitoral nerve
Clitoris
Posterior labial nerves
Deep transverse perineal

a

Sacral plexus
Piriformis
Sacrospinous ligament
Pudendal nerve
Levator ani
Rectum
Vagina
Perineal nerves
Inferior rectal nerves
External anal sphincter

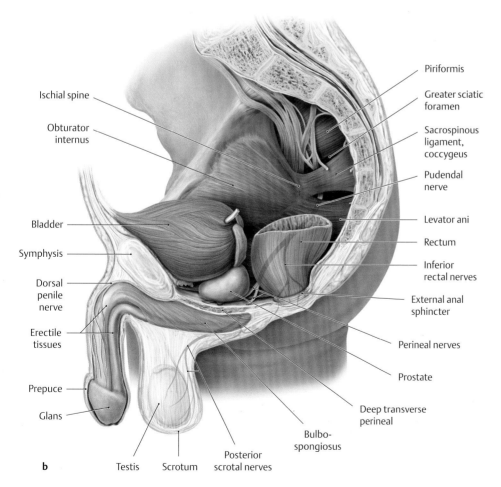

Ischial spine
Obturator internus
Bladder
Symphysis
Dorsal penile nerve
Erectile tissues
Prepuce
Glans

b

Testis
Scrotum
Posterior scrotal nerves
Bulbo-spongiosus
Deep transverse perineal
Prostate
Perineal nerves
External anal sphincter
Inferior rectal nerves
Rectum
Levator ani
Pudendal nerve
Sacrospinous ligament, coccygeus
Greater sciatic foramen
Piriformis

D Course of the pudendal nerve and coccygeal nerve in the female and male

a Sagittal section through the female pelvis, left lateral view.

b Sagittal section through the male pelvis, left lateral view.

The **pudendal nerve** emerges from the lesser pelvis through the *greater* sciatic foramen. It then courses around the ischial spine and sacrospinous ligament and passes through the *lesser* sciatic foramen into the ischioanal (ischiorectal) fossa (see p. 496). It runs forward in the lateral wall of the fossa, embedded in a duplication of the obturator internus fascia (pudendal canal = Alcock's canal) and accompanied by the internal pudendal vessels (see p. 495). Below the symphysis it passes to the dorsum of the penis or the clitoris. The pudendal nerve gives off numerous *branches* from within the perineum:

- The *inferior rectal nerves* supply motor innervation to the external anal sphincter and sensory innervation to the skin around the anus.
- The *perineal nerves* distribute motor branches to the muscles of the perineum (see p. 136) and sensory branches to the skin of the posterior scrotum or labia majora and minora, to the skin of the penis or clitoris, and to the glans, prepuce, and erectile tissues.

Damage to the pudendal nerve (e.g., resulting from perineal injuries during childbirth) leads to loss of function of the muscles of the perineum, especially the sphincter muscles of the bladder and bowel, causing urinary and fecal incontinence. Pudendal nerve lesions can also lead to sexual dysfunction (e.g., male impotence).

The ventral rami of the fifth sacral nerve and the first or second coccygeal nerve form the **coccygeal nerve** (synonym: *coccygeal plexus*). This nerve and its terminal sensory branches, the anococcygeal nerves, pass along the anococcygeal ligament to supply the skin between the coccyx and anus.

483

5.1 Surface Anatomy and Superficial Nerves and Vessels: Anterior View

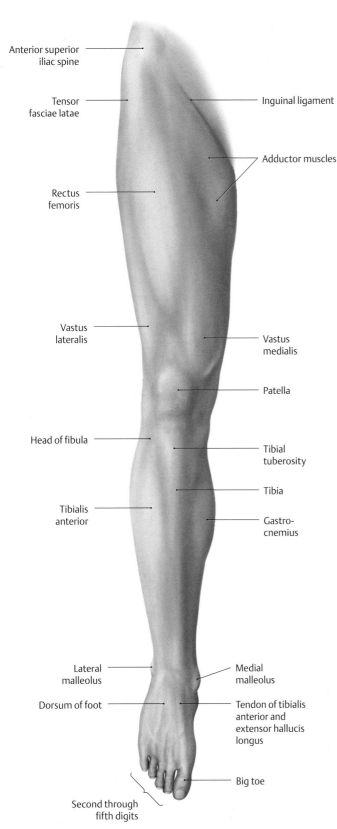

Anterior superior iliac spine

Tensor fasciae latae

Inguinal ligament

Adductor muscles

Rectus femoris

Vastus lateralis

Vastus medialis

Patella

Head of fibula

Tibial tuberosity

Tibia

Tibialis anterior

Gastro-cnemius

Lateral malleolus

Medial malleolus

Dorsum of foot

Tendon of tibialis anterior and extensor hallucis longus

Big toe

Second through fifth digits

A Surface anatomy of the right lower limb
Palpable *bony prominences* on the lower limb are reviewed on p. 361.

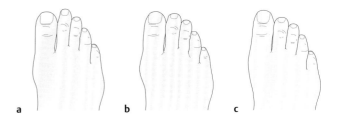

a   b   c

B The most common variants of the forefoot and toes (after Debrunner and Lelievre)

Three types of foot shape are distinguished based on the relative lengths of the first and second toes:

a The "Greek" type, in which the second toe is longer than the first.
b The square type, in which the first and second toes are of equal length.
c The "Egyptian" type, in which the first toe is longer than the second.

In the "Greek" type, the second metatarsal is generally longer than the metatarsal of the big toe. As a result, the head of the second metatarsal is often subject to painful overloading, especially when high heels are worn.

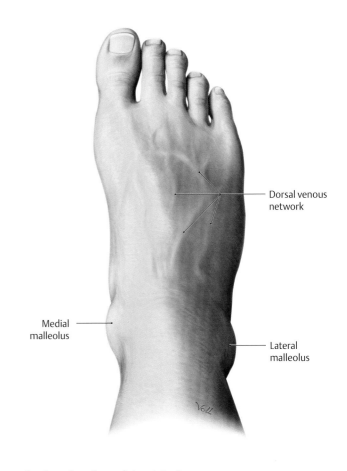

Dorsal venous network

Medial malleolus

Lateral malleolus

C The dorsal surface of the right foot
The superficial venous network is visible on the dorsum of the foot (compare with **D**).

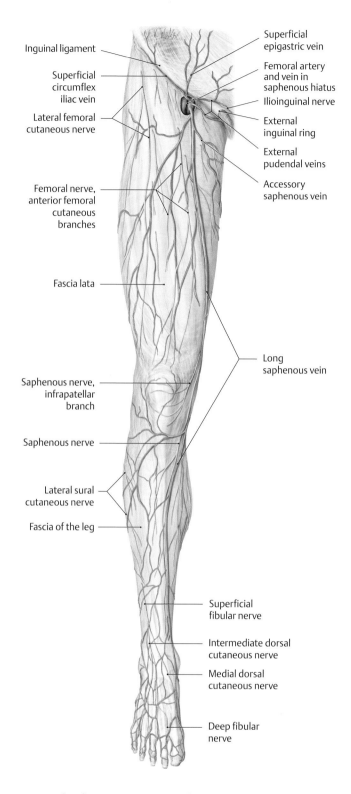

Labels (left figure, D):
- Inguinal ligament
- Superficial circumflex iliac vein
- Lateral femoral cutaneous nerve
- Femoral nerve, anterior femoral cutaneous branches
- Fascia lata
- Saphenous nerve, infrapatellar branch
- Saphenous nerve
- Lateral sural cutaneous nerve
- Fascia of the leg
- Superficial epigastric vein
- Femoral artery and vein in saphenous hiatus
- Ilioinguinal nerve
- External inguinal ring
- External pudendal veins
- Accessory saphenous vein
- Long saphenous vein
- Superficial fibular nerve
- Intermediate dorsal cutaneous nerve
- Medial dorsal cutaneous nerve
- Deep fibular nerve

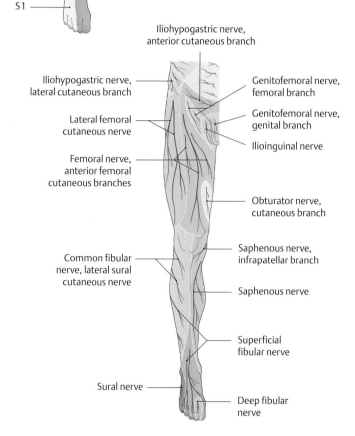

Labels (right figures, E and F):
- T11, T12, L1, S2, L2, L3, L4, L5, S1
- Iliohypogastric nerve, anterior cutaneous branch
- Iliohypogastric nerve, lateral cutaneous branch
- Lateral femoral cutaneous nerve
- Femoral nerve, anterior femoral cutaneous branches
- Common fibular nerve, lateral sural cutaneous nerve
- Sural nerve
- Genitofemoral nerve, femoral branch
- Genitofemoral nerve, genital branch
- Ilioinguinal nerve
- Obturator nerve, cutaneous branch
- Saphenous nerve, infrapatellar branch
- Saphenous nerve
- Superficial fibular nerve
- Deep fibular nerve

E Segmental or radicular cutaneous innervation pattern (dermatomes) in the right lower limb

As in the arm, the outgrowth of the lower limb during development causes the sensory cutaneous segments to become elongated and drawn out into narrow bands. The L 4, L 5, and S 1 segments in particular move so far peripherally that they no longer have any connection with the corresponding segments of the trunk.

Note that the dermatomes of the lumbar trunk segments lie mostly on the front of the leg while those of the sacral segments are mostly on the back of the leg (see p. 65). This can be of diagnostic importance in patients with a herniated disk, for example, in order to determine the level of the herniation (after Mumenthaler).

D Superficial cutaneous veins and nerves of the right lower limb

Anterior view. The dorsal venous network of the foot is drained by two large venous trunks (the long and short saphenous veins), which receive a variable pattern of cutaneous veins. While the short saphenous vein (see p. 487) enters the popliteal vein at the level of the popliteal fossa, the long saphenous vein extends up the medial side of the leg to a point just below the inguinal ligament, where it passes through the saphenous hiatus of the fascia lata to enter the femoral vein. The superficial veins of the lower limb are commonly affected by varicosity, causing them to become thickened, tortuous, and distinctly visible and palpable (see also p. 467).

F Pattern of peripheral sensory innervation in the right lower limb

As in the arm, the sensory distribution in the lower limb corresponds to the branching patterns of the peripheral cutaneous nerves in the subcutaneous connective tissue. The territories of the individual peripheral nerves overlap, especially at their margins. Hence the clinically determined *exclusive area* of a particular cutaneous nerve (the area supplied by that nerve alone) tends to be considerably smaller than the *maximum area* that can be demonstrated anatomically. For this reason, the traumatic disruption of a nerve causes a complete loss of sensation (anesthesia) in the exclusive area but often will cause only diminished sensation (hypoesthesia) at the perimeter of that area.

Note that the sensory loss resulting from a peripheral nerve injury presents a completely different pattern from that caused by injury to a nerve root (see p. 64) (after Mumenthaler).

485

5.2 Surface Anatomy and Superficial Nerves and Vessels: Posterior View

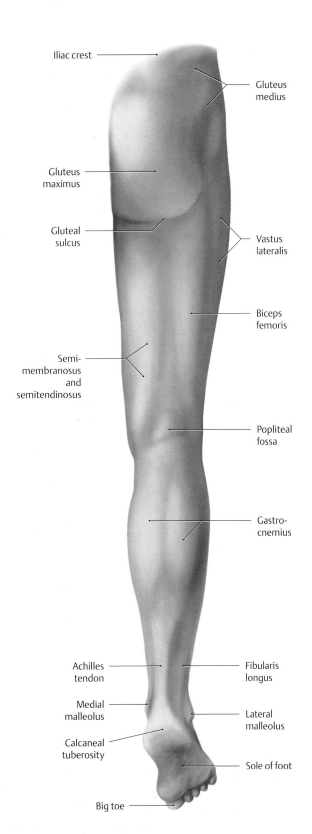

A Surface anatomy of the right lower limb
The foot is in plantar flexion. (Palpable *bony prominences* on the lower limb are reviewed on p. 361.)

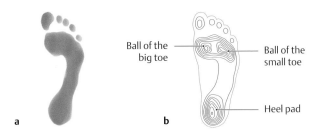

B Footprints (podograms) of the normal right foot in an adult
A podogram provides a graphic representation of the loads borne by the foot. Besides visual inspection of the sole of the foot, analysis of the podogram supplies the most useful information on the weight-bearing dynamics of the foot.

a Footprint created with an ink pad.
b Pressure podogram showing a normal weight-bearing pattern on the foot. The concentric lines indicate that the pressure is evenly distributed over all the major points of support. These three areas are clearly defined, while the intervening plantar arches bear essentially no weight (see p. 412).

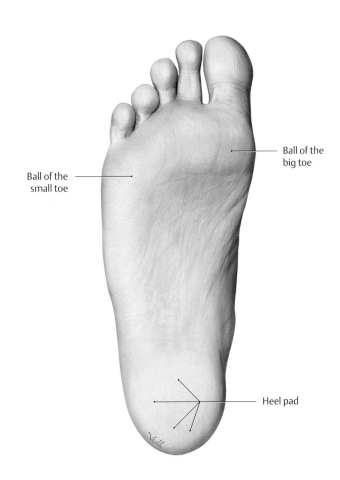

C The plantar surface of the right foot
The skin on the plantar surface of the foot serves as a sensory organ for contact with the ground, perceiving its consistency during stance and locomotion by means of receptors in the sole of the foot. Stresses acting on the heel pad and the balls of the big and little toes generate high local compressive forces at those sites, to which the subcutaneous connective tissue has adapted functionally by developing a system of *pressure chambers* (see p. 418).

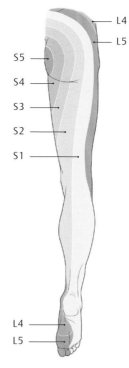

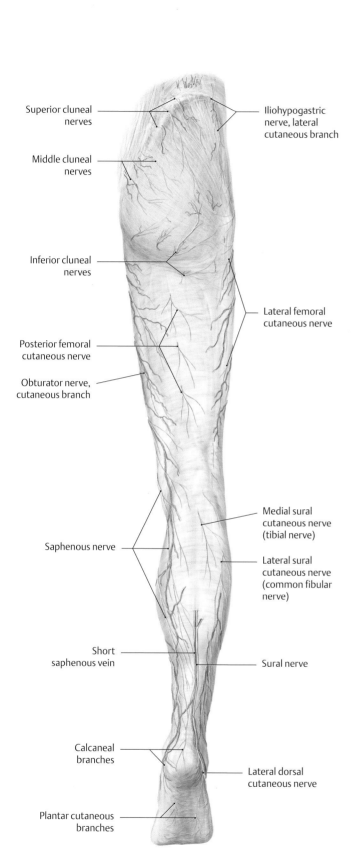

E Segmental or radicular cutaneous innervation pattern (dermatomes) of the right lower limb

As in the arm, the outgrowth of the lower limb during development causes the sensory cutaneous segments to become elongated into narrow bands. The L4, L5, and S1 segments in particular move so far peripherally that they no longer have any connection with the corresponding segments of the trunk.

Note that the dermatomes of the lumbar trunk segments lie mostly on the front of the leg while those of the sacral segments are mostly on the back of the leg (see p. 65). This can be of diagnostic importance in patients with a herniated disk, for example, in order to determine the level of the herniation (after Mumenthaler).

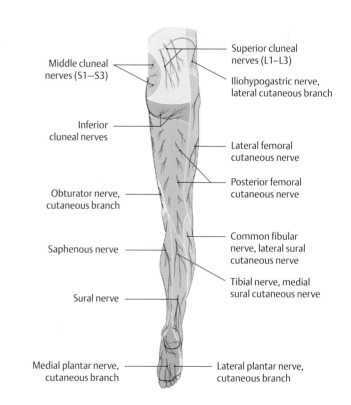

F Pattern of peripheral sensory innervation in the right lower limb

As in the arm, the sensory distribution in the lower limb corresponds to the branching patterns of the peripheral cutaneous nerves in the subcutaneous connective tissue. The territories of the individual peripheral nerves overlap, especially at their margins. Hence the clinically determined *exclusive area* of a particular cutaneous nerve (the area supplied by that nerve alone) tends to be considerably smaller than the *maximum area* that can be demonstrated anatomically. For this reason, the traumatic disruption of a nerve causes a complete loss of sensation (anesthesia) in the exclusive area but often will cause only diminished sensation (hypoesthesia) at the perimeter of that area.

Note that the sensory loss resulting from a peripheral nerve injury presents a completely different pattern from that caused by injury to a nerve root (see p. 64) (after Mumenthaler).

D The epifascial cutaneous veins and nerves of the right lower limb
Posterior view.

5.3 The Anterior Femoral Region Including the Femoral Triangle

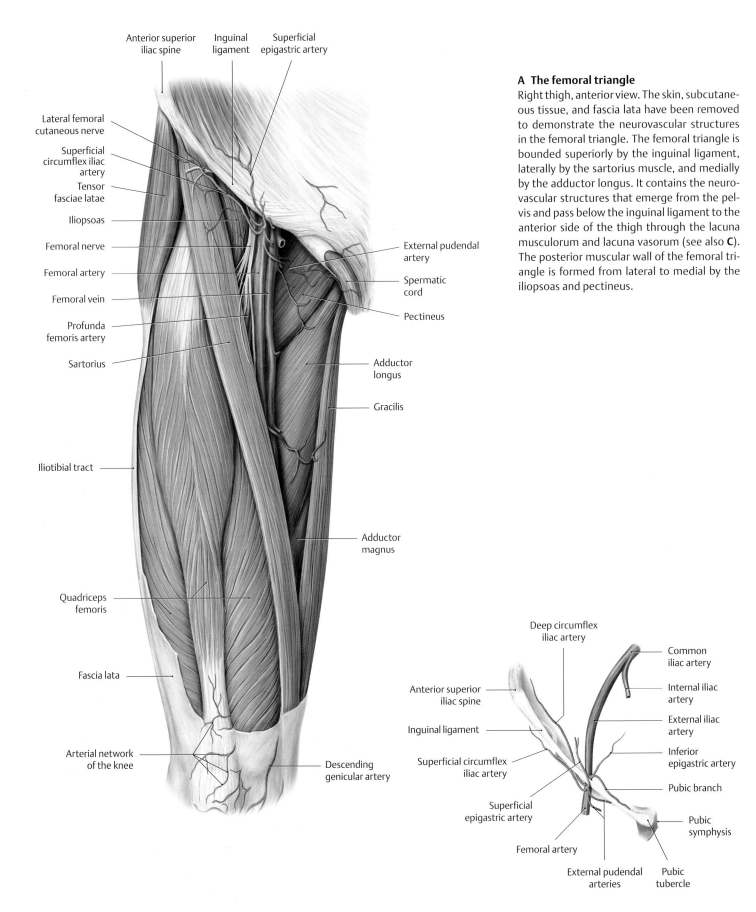

Anterior superior iliac spine

Inguinal ligament

Superficial epigastric artery

Lateral femoral cutaneous nerve

Superficial circumflex iliac artery

Tensor fasciae latae

Iliopsoas

Femoral nerve

Femoral artery

Femoral vein

Profunda femoris artery

Sartorius

Iliotibial tract

Quadriceps femoris

Fascia lata

Arterial network of the knee

External pudendal artery

Spermatic cord

Pectineus

Adductor longus

Gracilis

Adductor magnus

Descending genicular artery

A The femoral triangle

Right thigh, anterior view. The skin, subcutaneous tissue, and fascia lata have been removed to demonstrate the neurovascular structures in the femoral triangle. The femoral triangle is bounded superiorly by the inguinal ligament, laterally by the sartorius muscle, and medially by the adductor longus. It contains the neurovascular structures that emerge from the pelvis and pass below the inguinal ligament to the anterior side of the thigh through the lacuna musculorum and lacuna vasorum (see also **C**). The posterior muscular wall of the femoral triangle is formed from lateral to medial by the iliopsoas and pectineus.

Deep circumflex iliac artery

Common iliac artery

Anterior superior iliac spine

Internal iliac artery

Inguinal ligament

External iliac artery

Superficial circumflex iliac artery

Inferior epigastric artery

Pubic branch

Superficial epigastric artery

Pubic symphysis

Femoral artery

External pudendal arteries

Pubic tubercle

B The branches of the external iliac artery at its junction with the femoral artery in the region of the inguinal ligament

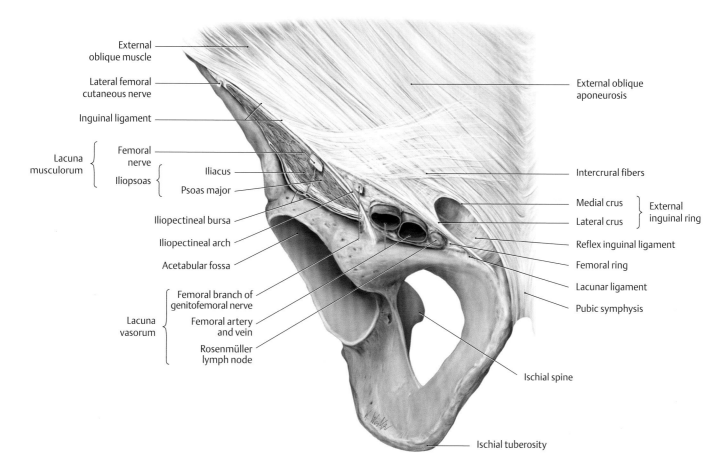

External oblique muscle
Lateral femoral cutaneous nerve
Inguinal ligament
Lacuna musculorum
Femoral nerve
Iliopsoas
Iliacus
Psoas major
Iliopectineal bursa
Iliopectineal arch
Acetabular fossa
Lacuna vasorum
Femoral branch of genitofemoral nerve
Femoral artery and vein
Rosenmüller lymph node

External oblique aponeurosis
Intercrural fibers
Medial crus
Lateral crus
External inguinal ring
Reflex inguinal ligament
Femoral ring
Lacunar ligament
Pubic symphysis
Ischial spine
Ischial tuberosity

C Inguinal region and the contents of the lacuna musculorum and lacuna vasorum

Anterior view. The drawing shows a portion of the right hip bone and the adjacent anterior inferior abdominal wall with the external inguinal ring and the contents of the lacuna musculorum and lacuna vasorum below the inguinal ligament. The site of emergence of the muscles and vessels, bounded by the inguinal ligament and the superior pelvic rim, is subdivided by the fibrous iliopectineal arch into a lateral muscular port (lacuna musculorum) and a medial vascular port (lacuna vasorum).

The **lacuna vasorum** is located medial to the iliopectineal arch. This "vascular portal" is traversed from lateral to medial by the femoral branch of the genitofemoral nerve, the femoral artery and vein, and the deep inguinal lymphatic vessels (only one lymph node is shown here). The part of the lacuna vasorum that lies medial to the femoral vein is

called the *femoral ring*. The lymph vessels from the thigh pass through that ring to enter the pelvis. The femoral ring is covered by a thin sheet of connective tissue called the femoral septum (not shown here), which usually contains a lymph node (the Rosenmüller node) belonging to the group of deep inguinal lymph nodes (see also p. 468).

The **lacuna musculorum** is lateral to the iliopectineal arch. This "muscular portal" is traversed by the iliopsoas muscle, femoral nerve, and lateral femoral cutaneous nerve.

Note the iliopectineal bursa located below the iliopsoas. It is the largest bursa of the hip region and communicates in 15 % of cases with the joint cavity of the hip. For this reason, an inflammatory disease of the hip joint may incite inflammation of this bursa (bursitis). When inflamed, the iliopectineal bursa is frequently painful and swollen and may occasionally be mistaken for a neoplasm on MR images.

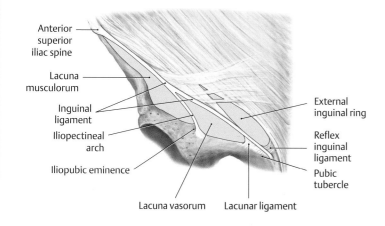

Anterior superior iliac spine
Lacuna musculorum
Inguinal ligament
Iliopectineal arch
Iliopubic eminence
Lacuna vasorum
Lacunar ligament
External inguinal ring
Reflex inguinal ligament
Pubic tubercle

D The connective-tissue and bony boundaries of the lacuna musculorum and lacuna vasorum

Diagram of the right inguinal region, anterior view. The connective-tissue boundary between the lacuna musculorum and lacuna vasorum is formed by the iliopectineal arch, a thickened band in the medial portion of the iliacus fascia. It extends between the inguinal ligament and the iliopubic eminence. The fibrous band that curves downward from the medial attachment of the inguinal ligament is called the lacunar ligament. This sharp-edged ligament defines the medial boundary of the lacuna *vasorum* (femoral ring) and may entrap the hernial sac in patients with a femoral hernia (see p. 186). Above the inguinal ligament is the external (superficial) inguinal ring, which is the external opening of the inguinal canal (see p. 182). The lacuna *musculorum* is bounded laterally by the anterior superior iliac spine.

5.4 Arterial Supply to the Thigh

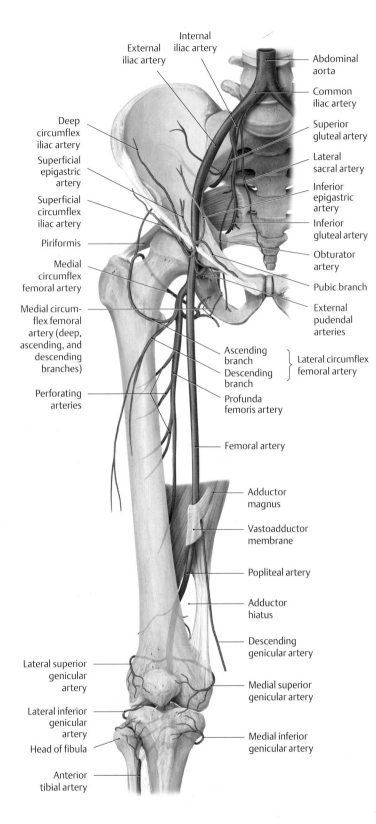

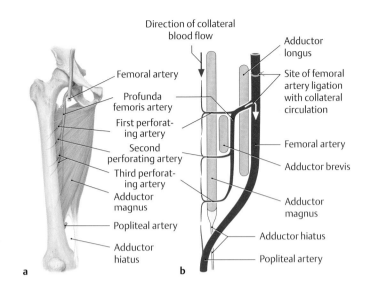

B Course of the profunda femoris artery and sites where the perforating arteries pierce the adductor muscles
a Right thigh, anterior view; **b** schematic longitudinal section through the adductor muscles at the level of the perforating arteries. The profunda femoris artery has approximately 3–5 terminal branches that pass from the front to the back of the thigh through the femoral insertions of the adductor muscles (= first through third perforating arteries) to supply the hamstring muscles (biceps femoris, semitendinosus, and semimembranosus). Generally the arteries pierce the adductor muscles above and below the adductor brevis and just above the adductor hiatus. Ligation of the femoral artery proximal to the origin of the profunda femoris artery is relatively well tolerated owing to a good collateral supply from branches of the internal iliac artery (superior gluteal artery and obturator artery).

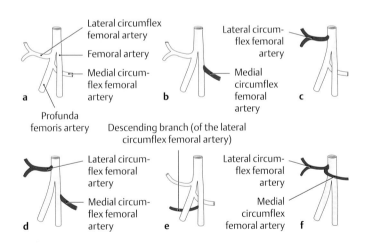

C Variants in the femoral artery branching pattern (after Lippert and Pabst)
a Usually the profunda femoris artery and medial and lateral circumflex femoral arteries arise from the femoral artery by a common trunk (58 % of cases, also shown in the other figures on this page).
b The medial circumflex femoral artery arises directly from the femoral artery (18 % of cases).
c The lateral circumflex femoral artery arises directly from the femoral artery (15 % of cases).
d The circumflex arteries arise separately from the femoral artery (4 % of cases).
e The descending branch of the lateral circumflex femoral artery springs directly from the femoral artery (3 % of cases).
f The circumflex arteries arise by a common trunk (1 % of cases).

A Course and branches of the femoral artery
The femoral artery, the distal continuation of the external iliac artery, runs along the medial side of the thigh to the adductor canal, through which it passes to the back of the leg. After emerging from the adductor hiatus, it becomes the popliteal artery. In clinical parlance the femoral artery is often called the *superficial* femoral artery because of its superficial course down the front of the thigh, distinguishing it from the more deeply placed *profunda femoris* artery that arises from it (see **D**).

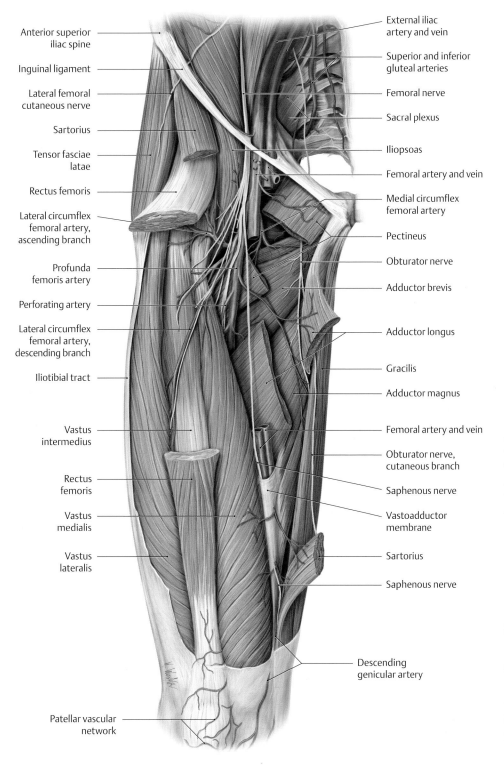

Anterior superior iliac spine

Inguinal ligament

Lateral femoral cutaneous nerve

Sartorius

Tensor fasciae latae

Rectus femoris

Lateral circumflex femoral artery, ascending branch

Profunda femoris artery

Perforating artery

Lateral circumflex femoral artery, descending branch

Iliotibial tract

Vastus intermedius

Rectus femoris

Vastus medialis

Vastus lateralis

Patellar vascular network

External iliac artery and vein

Superior and inferior gluteal arteries

Femoral nerve

Sacral plexus

Iliopsoas

Femoral artery and vein

Medial circumflex femoral artery

Pectineus

Obturator nerve

Adductor brevis

Adductor longus

Gracilis

Adductor magnus

Femoral artery and vein

Obturator nerve, cutaneous branch

Saphenous nerve

Vastoadductor membrane

Sartorius

Saphenous nerve

Descending genicular artery

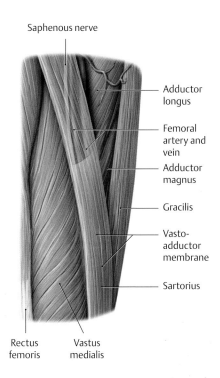

Saphenous nerve

Adductor longus

Femoral artery and vein

Adductor magnus

Gracilis

Vasto-adductor membrane

Sartorius

Rectus femoris

Vastus medialis

E The location of the adductor canal

Right thigh, anterior view. The saphenous nerve passes down the adductor canal on the anterior side of the thigh, accompanied by the femoral artery and vein. While both vessels continue toward the popliteal fossa through the adductor hiatus, the saphenous nerve pierces the vastoadductor membrane along with the descending genicular artery and passes to the medial side of the knee joint (see also **F**).

F The boundaries and contents of the adductor canal

Boundaries
- Adductor longus and magnus (posterior)
- Sartorius (medial)
- Vastoadductor membrane (anterior)
- Vastus medialis (lateral and anterior)

Contents
- Femoral artery
- Femoral vein
- Saphenous nerve ⎱ pierce the
- Descending ⎰ vastoadductor
  genicular artery ⎱ membrane

D The blood supply to the thigh from the profunda femoris artery

Right thigh, anterior view. The sartorius, rectus femoris, adductor longus, and pectineus muscles have been partially removed along with the central portion of the femoral artery to demonstrate the course of the profunda femoris artery in the thigh. For clarity, the veins have also been removed to the level of the external iliac vein. This dissection does not show the anterior abdominal wall or the pelvic and abdominal organs above the level of the inguinal ligament. While the branches of the medial and lateral circumflex arteries mainly supply blood to the hip joint and extensors and adductors of the thigh, the terminal branches of the profunda femoris artery (the first through third perforating arteries, see **B**) on the medial side of the femur pass to the back of the thigh through gaps in the insertions of the adductor muscles and supply the hamstrings (biceps femoris, semitendinosus, and semimembranosus).

Note: The vastoadductor membrane is pierced by the descending genicular artery and saphenous nerve (see **E** and **F**).

491

5.5 The Gluteal Region: Overview of its Vessels and Nerves

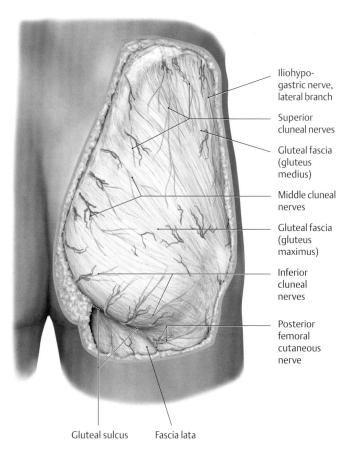

Iliohypo-
gastric nerve,
lateral branch

Superior
cluneal nerves

Gluteal fascia
(gluteus
medius)

Middle cluneal
nerves

Gluteal fascia
(gluteus
maximus)

Inferior
cluneal
nerves

Posterior
femoral
cutaneous
nerve

Gluteal sulcus   Fascia lata

A The fasciae and cutaneous nerves of the superficial gluteal region

Right gluteal region, posterior view. The gluteal region is covered by the gluteal fascia, which is part of the fascia lata (although the term "fascia lata" strictly refers only to the part below the gluteus medius and maximus). The fascia covering the gluteus maximus forms septa-like invaginations between the muscle bundles. At the junction of the gluteal region with the back of the upper thigh is the gently curved gluteal sulcus, in which thickened fiber tracts of the fascia lata run transversely across the thigh at the level of the ischial tuberosity.

Note on surface anatomy: The oblique inferior border of the gluteus maximus (see **B**) *crosses* the gluteal sulcus. Its course, then, is not identical to that of the gluteal sulcus.

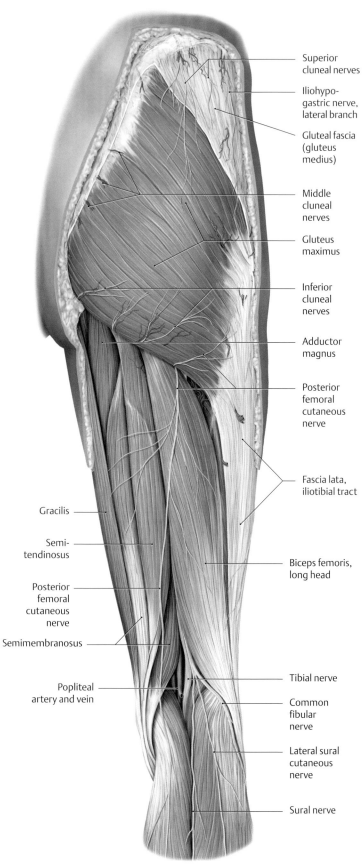

Superior
cluneal nerves

Iliohypo-
gastric nerve,
lateral branch

Gluteal fascia
(gluteus
medius)

Middle
cluneal
nerves

Gluteus
maximus

Inferior
cluneal
nerves

Adductor
magnus

Posterior
femoral
cutaneous
nerve

Fascia lata,
iliotibial tract

Gracilis

Semi-
tendinosus

Posterior
femoral
cutaneous
nerve

Semimembranosus

Popliteal
artery and vein

Biceps femoris,
long head

Tibial nerve

Common
fibular
nerve

Lateral sural
cutaneous
nerve

Sural nerve

B The gluteal region and thigh with the fasciae removed
Right side, posterior view. With the fascia lata removed, the main trunk of the posterior femoral cutaneous nerve, which is subfascial over much of its course, can be traced into the popliteal fossa.

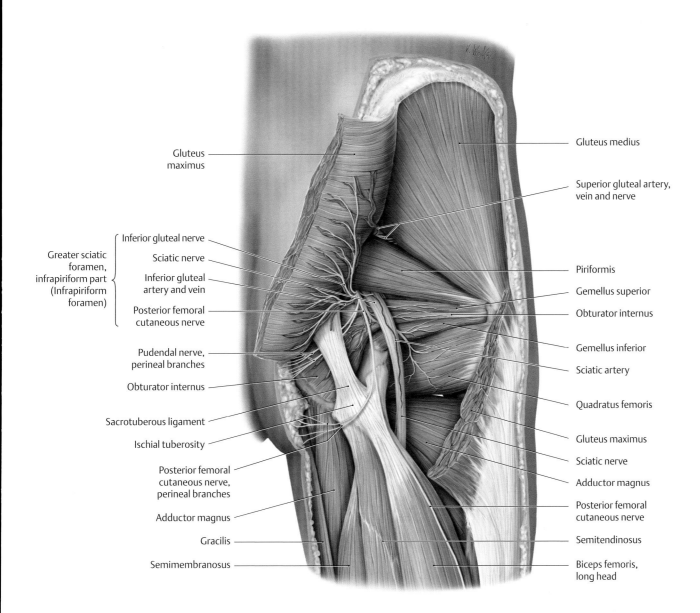

Gluteus maximus

Greater sciatic foramen, infrapiriform part (Infrapiriform foramen) {
Inferior gluteal nerve
Sciatic nerve
Inferior gluteal artery and vein
Posterior femoral cutaneous nerve
}

Pudendal nerve, perineal branches

Obturator internus

Sacrotuberous ligament

Ischial tuberosity

Posterior femoral cutaneous nerve, perineal branches

Adductor magnus

Gracilis

Semimembranosus

Gluteus medius

Superior gluteal artery, vein and nerve

Piriformis

Gemellus superior

Obturator internus

Gemellus inferior

Sciatic artery

Quadratus femoris

Gluteus maximus

Sciatic nerve

Adductor magnus

Posterior femoral cutaneous nerve

Semitendinosus

Biceps femoris, long head

C The vessels and nerves of the deep gluteal region
Right side, posterior view, with the gluteus maximus partially removed. The neurovascular structures of the deep gluteal region traverse an extensive fatty and connective-tissue space below the gluteus maximus. The floor of this space is formed by the piriformis, obturator internus, gemellus superior, and quadratus femoris muscles. It communicates through the sciatic foramina with the connective-tissue spaces of the lesser pelvis and ischioanal fossa (not shown here). A useful topographic landmark is the piriformis, which extends from the pelvic surface of the sacrum through the greater sciatic foramen to the tip of the greater trochanter (see **A**, p. 494).

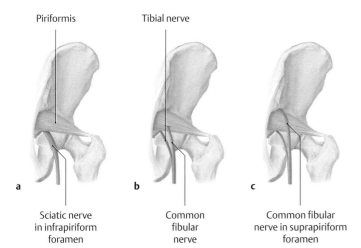

Piriformis

Tibial nerve

a

b

c

Sciatic nerve in infrapiriform foramen

Common fibular nerve

Common fibular nerve in suprapiriform foramen

D Variable course of the sciatic nerve in relation to the piriformis
(after Rauber/Kopsch)
a The sciatic nerve leaves the lesser pelvis inferior to the piriformis (almost 85 % of cases).
b This variant illustrates a *high division* of the sciatic nerve (approximately 15 % of cases). In this pattern the fibular division (common fibular nerve) and sometimes the posterior femoral cutaneous nerve pass through the piriformis muscle and may become compressed at that location, causing a "piriformis syndrome." Usually this term refers to the complaints that may develop following trauma to the gluteal region and are marked by severe gluteal pain. It is still uncertain whether these complaints are actually referable to the compression of sciatic nerve segments.
c In this variant the fibular part of the sciatic nerve leaves the lesser pelvis above the piriformis (rare, only about 0.5 % of cases).

493

5.6 The Gluteal Region: The Sciatic Foramen and Sciatic Nerve

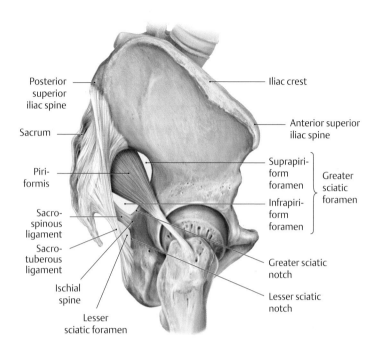

A Location of the greater and lesser sciatic foramina
Right hip bone, lateral view.

B The boundaries of the sciatic foramina and the structures that traverse them
The subgluteal connective-tissue space communicates through the sciatic foramina with the connective-tissue spaces of the lesser pelvis and the ischioanal fossa.

Foramen	Boundaries	Transmitted structures
• Greater sciatic foramen	• Greater sciatic notch • Sacrospinous ligament • Sacrum	• *Suprapiriform portion* – Superior gluteal artery and vein – Superior gluteal nerve • *Infrapiriform portion* – Inferior gluteal artery and vein – Inferior gluteal nerve – Internal pudendal artery and vein – Pudendal nerve – Sciatic nerve – Posterior femoral cutaneous nerve
• Lesser sciatic foramen	• Lesser sciatic notch • Sacrospinous ligament • Sacrotuberous ligament	– Internal pudendal artery and vein – Pudendal nerve – Obturator internus

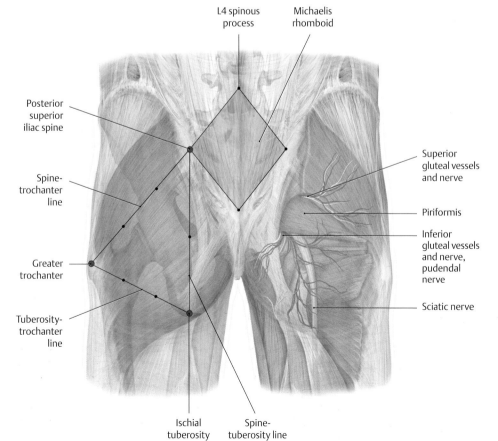

C Reference lines used for locating neurovascular structures in the gluteal region
Right and left gluteal regions, posterior view. The reference lines are drawn between the following points: the posterior superior iliac spine (lateral point of the Michaelis rhomboid), the ischial tuberosity, and the greater trochanter.

- **Spine-trochanter line:** The superior gluteal vessels emerge from the suprapiriform foramen between the middle and upper thirds of this line.
- **Tuberosity-trochanter line:** The sciatic nerve runs downward between the middle and medial thirds of this line.
- **Spine-tuberosity line:** The sciatic nerve, inferior gluteal nerve, and the pudendal and inferior gluteal vessels emerge from the infrapiriform foramen at the midpoint of this line.

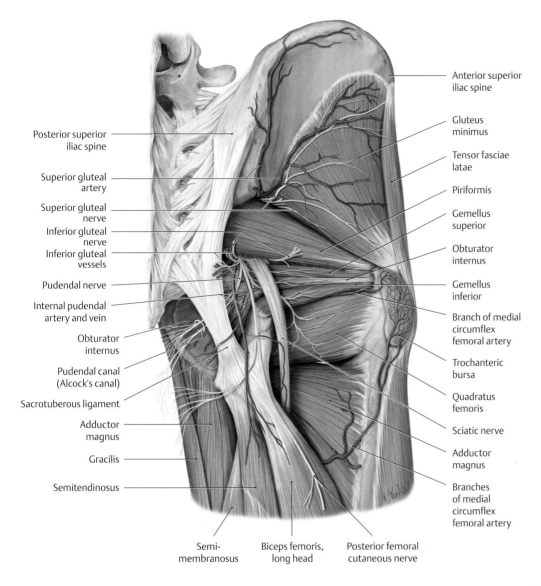

Posterior superior iliac spine

Superior gluteal artery

Superior gluteal nerve

Inferior gluteal nerve

Inferior gluteal vessels

Pudendal nerve

Internal pudendal artery and vein

Obturator internus

Pudendal canal (Alcock's canal)

Sacrotuberous ligament

Adductor magnus

Gracilis

Semitendinosus

Anterior superior iliac spine

Gluteus minimus

Tensor fasciae latae

Piriformis

Gemellus superior

Obturator internus

Gemellus inferior

Branch of medial circumflex femoral artery

Trochanteric bursa

Quadratus femoris

Sciatic nerve

Adductor magnus

Branches of medial circumflex femoral artery

Semi-membranosus

Biceps femoris, long head

Posterior femoral cutaneous nerve

D The vessels and nerves of the gluteal region and ischioanal fossa

Right gluteal region, posterior view, with the gluteus maximus and medius removed.

Note the course of the pudendal vessels and pudendal nerve in the lateral wall of the ischioanal fossa. They run in the pudendal canal (Alcock's canal), which is formed by the obturator internus fascia (see p. 424).

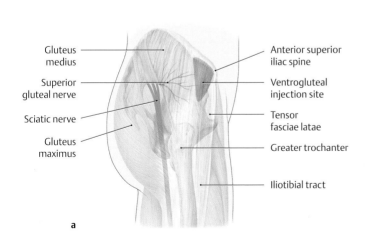

Gluteus medius

Superior gluteal nerve

Sciatic nerve

Gluteus maximus

Anterior superior iliac spine

Ventrogluteal injection site

Tensor fasciae latae

Greater trochanter

Iliotibial tract

a

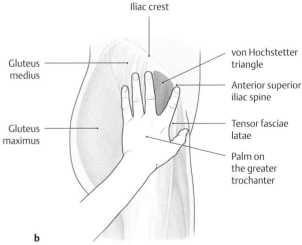

Iliac crest

Gluteus medius

Gluteus maximus

von Hochstetter triangle

Anterior superior iliac spine

Tensor fasciae latae

Palm on the greater trochanter

b

E Location of the sciatic nerve and superior gluteal nerves and their protection during intragluteal injections

Right gluteal region, lateral view.

a Two very important nerves are found in the gluteal region: the sciatic nerve and the superior gluteal nerve. To avoid jeopardizing these nerves during intramuscular injections, the needle should be inserted with the greatest possible safety margin with respect to these structures. Making the injection within the "von Hochstetter triangle" ensures that this safety margin is maintained.

b Locating the von Hochstetter triangle: The target site is located in the anterolateral gluteal region (accounting for the term "ventrogluteal injection"). To give an intramuscular injection on the right side, for example, place the palm of the left hand on the greater trochanter and the tip of the index finger on the anterior superior iliac spine. Keeping the hand in place, abduct the middle finger away from the index finger and introduce the needle perpendicular to the skin surface within the triangular zone between the two fingers and the iliac crest.

5.7 The Ischioanal Fossa

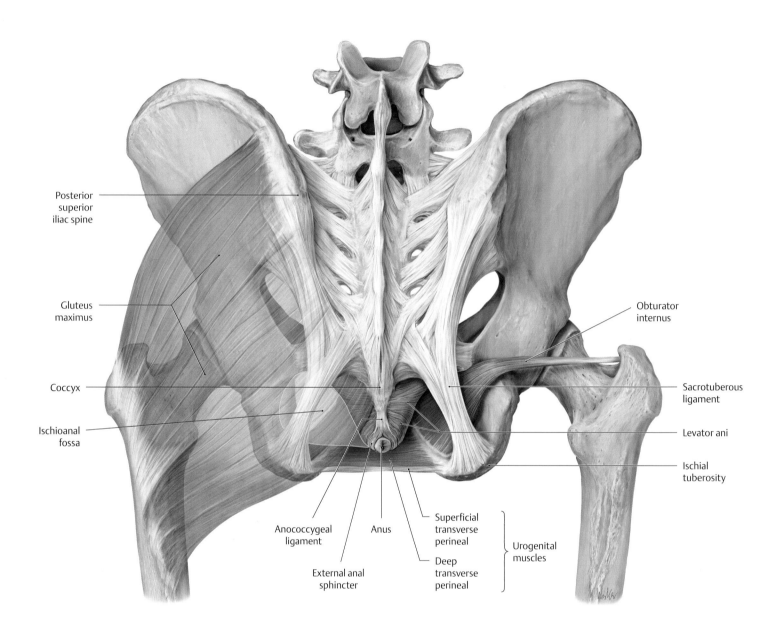

Posterior superior iliac spine

Gluteus maximus

Coccyx

Ischioanal fossa

Obturator internus

Sacrotuberous ligament

Levator ani

Ischial tuberosity

Anococcygeal ligament

Anus

Superficial transverse perineal

Deep transverse perineal

Urogenital muscles

External anal sphincter

A The muscular boundaries of the ischioanal fossa
Left and right gluteal region, posterior view. The ischioanal fossa is a pyramid-shaped space located lateral to the levator ani muscle on each side. The tip of the three-sided pyramid points toward the symphysis, and the base of the pyramid faces posteriorly. The ischioanal fossa is bounded by the following muscles:

- Superamedially by the levator ani
- Laterally by the obturator internus
- Inferiorly by the deep transverse perineal
- The entrance to the ischioanal fossa is bounded posteriorly by the gluteus maximus and sacrotuberous ligament.

The fatty tissue that occupies most of the ischioanal fossa (the fat pad of the ischioanal fossa) functions as a mobile pad that can slide downward and backward, for example, during bowel evacuation or during labor. It is traversed by the branches of the internal pudendal vessels and pudendal nerve (see **B**), whose trunks run in the pudendal canal or Alcock's canal; see **A**, p. 498.

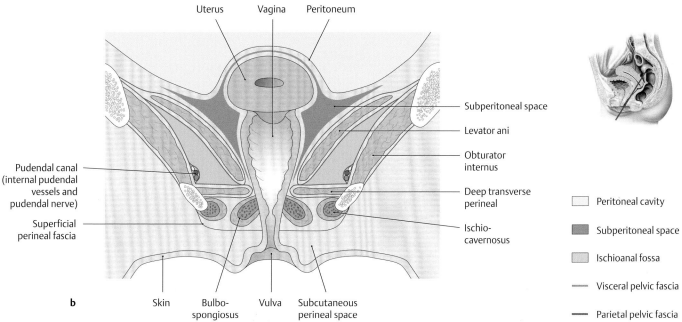

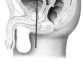

Prostate Bladder Peritoneum

Obturator foramen

Pudendal canal (Alcock's canal) with the internal pudendal vessels and pudendal nerve

Subperitoneal space

Levator ani

Obturator internus

Deep transverse perineal

Ischio-cavernosus

a Superficial perineal fascia Bulb of penis with bulbospongiosus Skin Subcutaneous perineal space

Uterus Vagina Peritoneum

Pudendal canal (internal pudendal vessels and pudendal nerve)

Superficial perineal fascia

Subperitoneal space

Levator ani

Obturator internus

Deep transverse perineal

Ischio-cavernosus

b Skin Bulbo-spongiosus Vulva Subcutaneous perineal space

☐ Peritoneal cavity

▨ Subperitoneal space

▨ Ischioanal fossa

— Visceral pelvic fascia

— Parietal pelvic fascia

B The ischioanal fossa
a Coronal section through the male pelvis at the level of the prostate.
b Oblique coronal section through the female pelvis at the level of the vagina.

The pelvic organs make varying contributions to the shape of the peritoneal cavity and subperitoneal space, but they are not represented in the ischioanal fossa. While the peritoneal cavity is lined by the parietal peritoneum and the visceral peritoneum (on intraperitoneal organs such as the ovary), the subperitoneal space is lined by the pelvic fasciae (composed of parietal and visceral layers, see p. 155).

5.8 The Pudendal Canal and Perineal Region (Urogenital and Anal Region)

A Location of the pudendal canal (Alcock's canal) and the neurovascular structures it contains

Right half of the pelvis, medial view. All of the muscles have been removed except for the psoas major, piriformis, and obturator internus. For clarity, the individual veins are not shown. The pudendal canal is formed by the obturator internus fascia. It begins just below the ischial spine and courses in the lateral wall of the ischioanal fossa below the tendinous arch of levator ani, passing toward the pubic symphysis and the posterior border of the urogenital muscles (see p. 136). The neurovascular structures that are transmitted by the canal (the internal pudendal vessels, of which only the artery is shown, and the pudendal nerve, see **B**) exit the lesser pelvis through the greater sciatic foramen and enter the pudendal canal through the lesser sciatic foramen. They pass through the canal toward the pubic symphysis and the posterior border of the urogenital muscles.

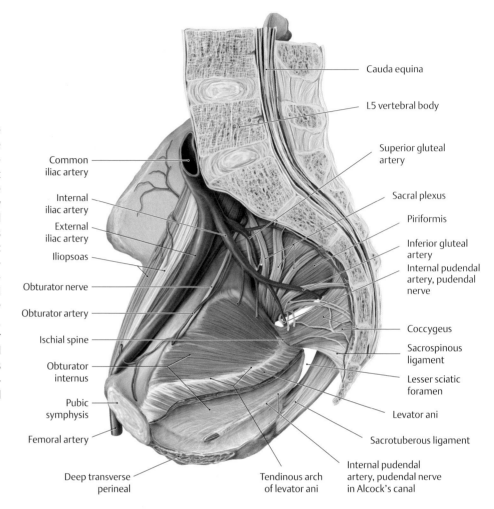

Common iliac artery
Internal iliac artery
External iliac artery
Iliopsoas
Obturator nerve
Obturator artery
Ischial spine
Obturator internus
Pubic symphysis
Femoral artery
Deep transverse perineal

Cauda equina
L5 vertebral body
Superior gluteal artery
Sacral plexus
Piriformis
Inferior gluteal artery
Internal pudendal artery, pudendal nerve
Coccygeus
Sacrospinous ligament
Lesser sciatic foramen
Levator ani
Sacrotuberous ligament
Internal pudendal artery, pudendal nerve in Alcock's canal
Tendinous arch of levator ani

B Distribution of the pudendal nerve and internal pudendal vessels to the anus, perineum, and external genitalia

Gluteal region and ischioanal fossa on the right side, posterior view. The gluteus maximus and sacrotuberous ligament have been partially removed and all fatty tissue has been removed from the ischioanal fossa to demonstrate the course of the pudendal nerve and the internal pudendal vessels. On their way through the pudendal canal (not shown here in order to display the course of the nerve and vessels below the sacrotuberous ligament), the various neural and vascular branches are successively distributed in a fan-shaped pattern to the anus, perineum, and external genitalia. It is very common in obstetrics to perform a pudendal nerve block by anesthetizing the pudendal nerve at the level of the ischial spine (i. e., before it branches into the inferior rectal, perineal, dorsal clitoral, and posterior labial nerves; see p. 482).

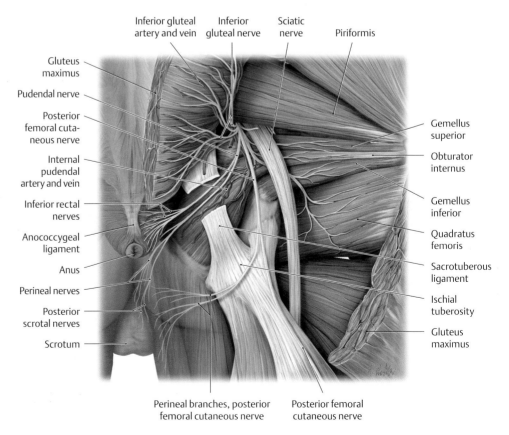

Inferior gluteal artery and vein
Inferior gluteal nerve
Sciatic nerve
Piriformis
Gluteus maximus
Pudendal nerve
Posterior femoral cutaneous nerve
Internal pudendal artery and vein
Inferior rectal nerves
Anococcygeal ligament
Anus
Perineal nerves
Posterior scrotal nerves
Scrotum

Gemellus superior
Obturator internus
Gemellus inferior
Quadratus femoris
Sacrotuberous ligament
Ischial tuberosity
Gluteus maximus

Perineal branches, posterior femoral cutaneous nerve
Posterior femoral cutaneous nerve

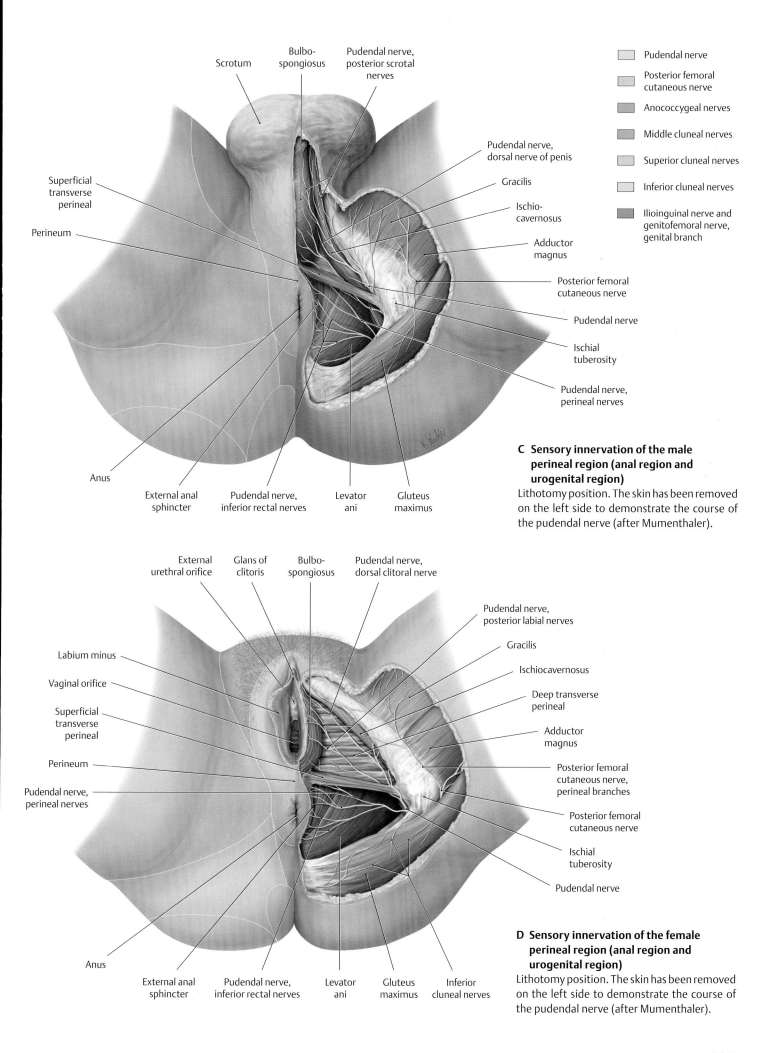

Scrotum

Bulbo-spongiosus

Pudendal nerve, posterior scrotal nerves

Pudendal nerve, dorsal nerve of penis

Gracilis

Ischio-cavernosus

Adductor magnus

Posterior femoral cutaneous nerve

Pudendal nerve

Ischial tuberosity

Pudendal nerve, perineal nerves

Superficial transverse perineal

Perineum

Anus

External anal sphincter

Pudendal nerve, inferior rectal nerves

Levator ani

Gluteus maximus

Pudendal nerve

Posterior femoral cutaneous nerve

Anococcygeal nerves

Middle cluneal nerves

Superior cluneal nerves

Inferior cluneal nerves

Ilioinguinal nerve and genitofemoral nerve, genital branch

C Sensory innervation of the male perineal region (anal region and urogenital region)
Lithotomy position. The skin has been removed on the left side to demonstrate the course of the pudendal nerve (after Mumenthaler).

External urethral orifice

Glans of clitoris

Bulbo-spongiosus

Pudendal nerve, dorsal clitoral nerve

Pudendal nerve, posterior labial nerves

Gracilis

Ischiocavernosus

Deep transverse perineal

Adductor magnus

Posterior femoral cutaneous nerve, perineal branches

Posterior femoral cutaneous nerve

Ischial tuberosity

Pudendal nerve

Labium minus

Vaginal orifice

Superficial transverse perineal

Perineum

Pudendal nerve, perineal nerves

Anus

External anal sphincter

Pudendal nerve, inferior rectal nerves

Levator ani

Gluteus maximus

Inferior cluneal nerves

D Sensory innervation of the female perineal region (anal region and urogenital region)
Lithotomy position. The skin has been removed on the left side to demonstrate the course of the pudendal nerve (after Mumenthaler).

499

5.9 The Posterior Thigh Region and Popliteal Region

A The vessels and nerves of the posterior thigh

Right thigh, posterior view. To demonstrate the vessels and nerves in their course from the gluteal region down the back of the thigh to the popliteal fossa (see **C**), the skin and muscle fasciae have been removed and the following muscles have been partially removed: gluteus maximus, gluteus medius, and biceps femoris. The semimembranosus has been retracted slightly medially to display the adductor hiatus (transmits the femoral artery and vein) (deeper neurovascular structures in the popliteal fossa are shown in **F**). The posterior femoral region receives most of its blood supply from branches of the profunda femoris artery (the first through third perforating arteries) and the deep branch (not shown) of the medial circumflex femoral artery. The proximal part of the sciatic nerve is supplied by the sciatic artery, which is a branch of the inferior gluteal artery, and its distal part is supplied by branches of the first through third perforating arteries.

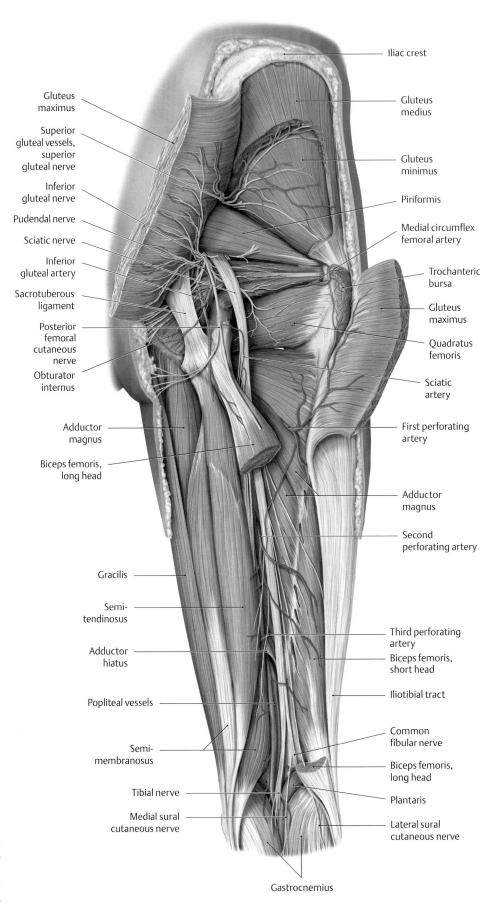

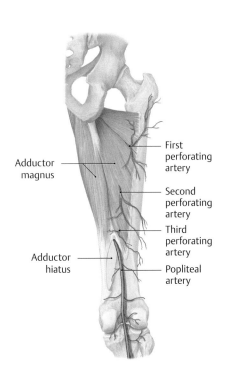

B Sites of emergence of the perforating arteries on the back of the thigh

Right thigh, posterior view. All of the muscles have been removed except for the adductor magnus.

Note: The femoral artery enters the popliteal fossa through the adductor hiatus, thereafter becoming the popliteal artery.

500

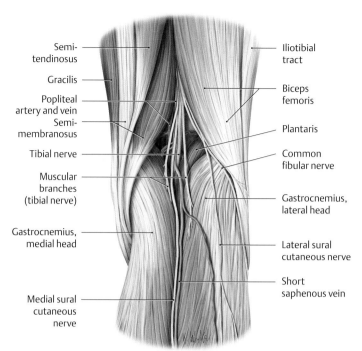

C The muscular boundaries of the popliteal fossa

Right popliteal fossa, posterior view. For clarity the skin, fasciae, and fat pads have been removed.

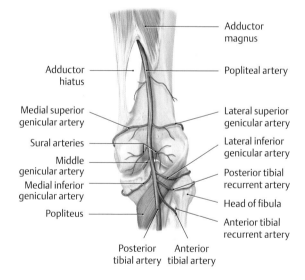

D Branches of the popliteal artery that course in the popliteal fossa

Right knee joint, posterior view. The popliteal artery begins at the outlet of the adductor canal and ends at the level of the popliteus muscle, where it divides into the anterior tibial artery and posterior tibial artery.

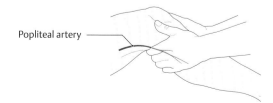

E Palpation of the popliteal artery in the popliteal fossa

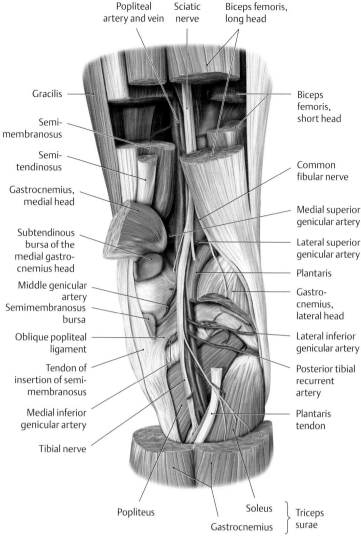

F Deep neurovascular structures in the popliteal fossa

Right knee joint, posterior view. Portions of both heads of the gastrocnemius and portions of the hamstrings have been removed to demonstrate the course of the deep neurovascular structures in the popliteal fossa. Five vessels, some paired, branch from the middle portion of the popliteal artery to supply the knee joint (see **D**):

- Lateral and medial superior genicular arteries
- Middle genicular artery
- Lateral and medial inferior genicular arteries

One of these vessels, the middle genicular artery, pierces the joint capsule of the knee in the area of the oblique popliteal ligament and supplies the cruciform ligaments. The other vessels run forward on the medial and lateral sides to form the arterial network (articular rete) of the knee. The posterior and anterior tibial recurrent arteries contribute to the articular rete. The paired sural arteries supply the two heads of the gastrocnemius (see **D**, removed in **F**).

Note on the medial side the subtendinous bursa of the gastrocnemius, which consistently communicates with the joint cavity of the knee, and the bursa of the semimembranosus, which occasionally communicates with the bursa of the gastrocnemius head (this forms an extensive recess in the joint cavity of the knee, which may become abnormally enlarged to form a Baker cyst; see p. 392).

5.10 The Posterior Leg Region and the Tarsal Tunnel

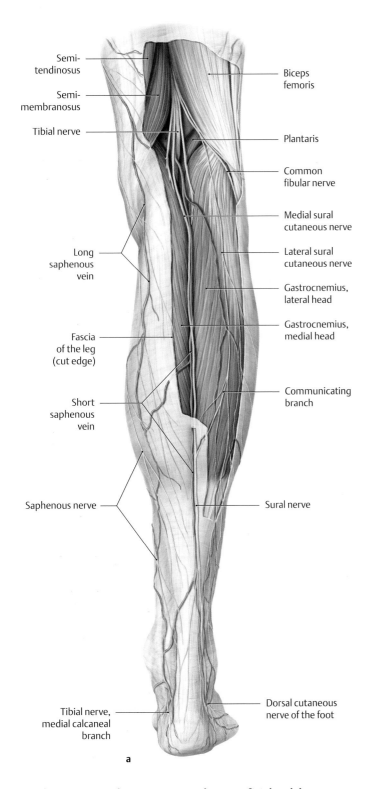

Semi-tendinosus

Semi-membranosus

Tibial nerve

Long saphenous vein

Fascia of the leg (cut edge)

Short saphenous vein

Saphenous nerve

Tibial nerve, medial calcaneal branch

Biceps femoris

Plantaris

Common fibular nerve

Medial sural cutaneous nerve

Lateral sural cutaneous nerve

Gastrocnemius, lateral head

Gastrocnemius, medial head

Communicating branch

Sural nerve

Dorsal cutaneous nerve of the foot

a

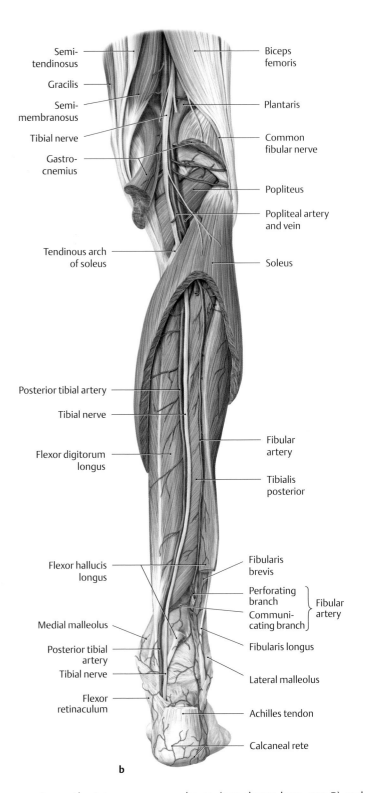

Semi-tendinosus

Gracilis

Semi-membranosus

Tibial nerve

Gastro-cnemius

Tendinous arch of soleus

Posterior tibial artery

Tibial nerve

Flexor digitorum longus

Flexor hallucis longus

Medial malleolus

Posterior tibial artery

Tibial nerve

Flexor retinaculum

Biceps femoris

Plantaris

Common fibular nerve

Popliteus

Popliteal artery and vein

Soleus

Fibular artery

Tibialis posterior

Fibularis brevis

Perforating branch

Communi-cating branch

Fibularis longus

Lateral malleolus

Achilles tendon

Calcaneal rete

Fibular artery

b

A The neurovascular structures in the superficial and deep posterior compartments

Right leg, posterior view.

a Neurovascular structures in the *superficial posterior compartment:* The superficial layer of the fascia of the leg ensheaths the triceps surae and has been partially removed proximally.

b Neurovascular structures in the *deep posterior compartment* after partial removal of the triceps surae and the deep layer of the fascia of the leg. The popliteal artery divides into the anterior and posterior tibial arteries at the distal border of the popliteus. The anterior tibial artery

pierces the interosseous membrane (not shown here, see **B**) and passes to the anterior side of the leg, entering the anterior compartment. The posterior tibial artery, accompanied by the tibial nerve, passes below the tendinous arch of the soleus into the deep posterior compartment, almost immediately gives off the fibular artery, and then continues distally behind the medial malleolus to the plantar side of the foot. The deep posterior compartment is one of four poorly distensible muscle compartments in the leg ("fibro-osseous canals"), which are potential sites for the development of a compartment syndrome following a vascular injury (see p. 507).

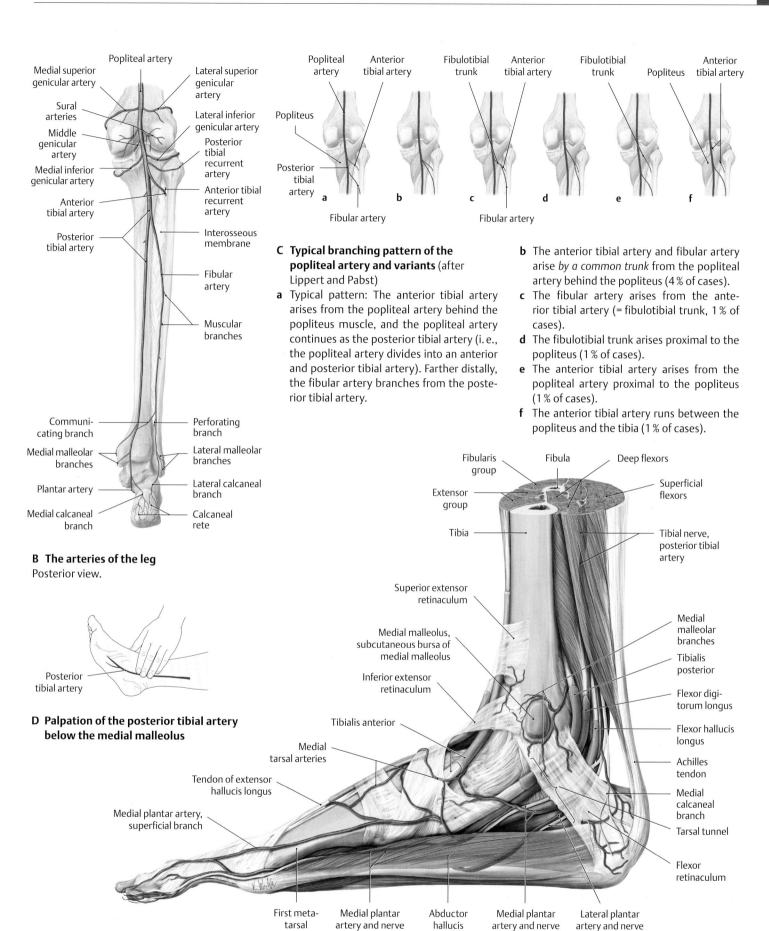

B The arteries of the leg
Posterior view.

D Palpation of the posterior tibial artery below the medial malleolus

C Typical branching pattern of the popliteal artery and variants (after Lippert and Pabst)

a Typical pattern: The anterior tibial artery arises from the popliteal artery behind the popliteus muscle, and the popliteal artery continues as the posterior tibial artery (i.e., the popliteal artery divides into an anterior and posterior tibial artery). Farther distally, the fibular artery branches from the posterior tibial artery.

b The anterior tibial artery and fibular artery arise *by a common trunk* from the popliteal artery behind the popliteus (4% of cases).

c The fibular artery arises from the anterior tibial artery (= fibulotibial trunk, 1% of cases).

d The fibulotibial trunk arises proximal to the popliteus (1% of cases).

e The anterior tibial artery arises from the popliteal artery proximal to the popliteus (1% of cases).

f The anterior tibial artery runs between the popliteus and the tibia (1% of cases).

E The neurovascular structures of the medial malleolar region
Right foot, medial view. The neurovascular structures pass from the deep flexor compartment to the plantar side of the foot through the tarsal tunnel, between the flexor retinaculum and medial malleolus. They are accompanied by the tendons of insertion of the long flexors (tibialis posterior, flexor digitorum longus, flexor hallucis longus) in their synovial sheaths.

Note the division of the posterior tibial nerve into the medial and lateral plantar nerves and the division of the posterior tibial artery into the medial and lateral plantar arteries within the malleolar canal. Compression of the nerves at this site can cause a medial or posterior tarsal tunnel syndrome (see p. 481).

5.11   The Sole of the Foot

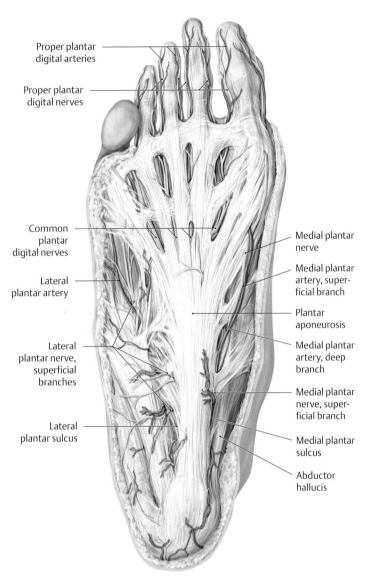

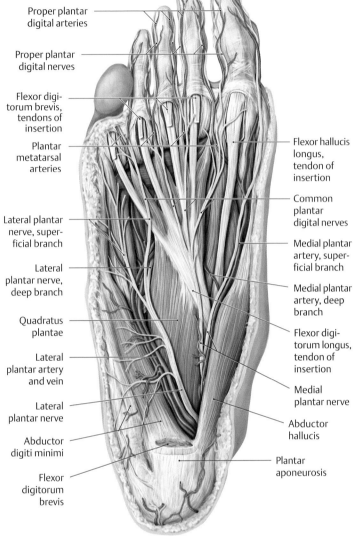

A The plantar arteries and nerves of the foot (superficial layer)
Right foot, plantar view. The skin and subcutaneous tissue have been removed to demonstrate the plantar aponeurosis and superficial neurovascular structures.

B The plantar arteries and nerves of the foot (middle layer)
Right foot, plantar view, with the plantar aponeurosis and flexor digitorum brevis removed.

C The plantar arteries of the foot: possible variants
Right foot, plantar view. Any of four basic anatomical variants may be seen (after Lippert and Pabst):

a The deep plantar arch and the plantar metatarsal arteries arising from it are supplied entirely by the deep plantar branch of the dorsal pedal artery (53 % of cases).

b The first through third plantar metatarsal arteries are supplied by the deep plantar branch of the dorsal pedal artery, the fourth plantar metatarsal artery by the deep branch of the lateral plantar artery (19 % of cases).

c The first and second plantar metatarsal arteries are supplied by the deep plantar branch of the dorsal pedal artery, the third and fourth metatarsal arteries by the deep branch of the lateral plantar artery (13 % of cases).

d The deep plantar arch and the first through fourth plantar metatarsal arteries are supplied entirely by the deep branch of the lateral plantar artery (7 % of cases).

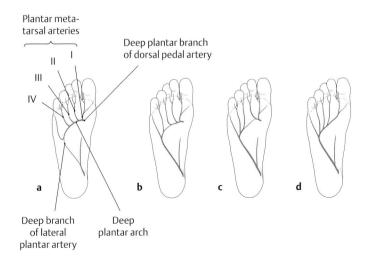

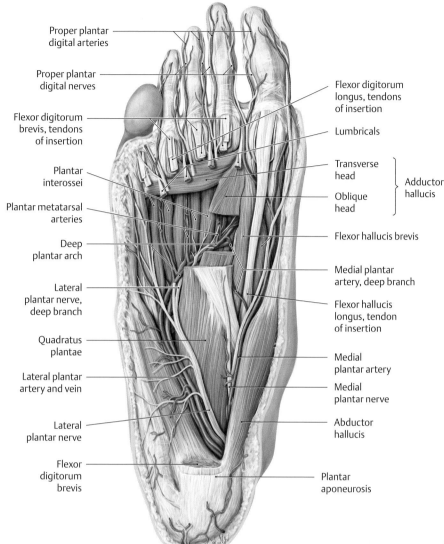

Proper plantar digital arteries

Proper plantar digital nerves

Flexor digitorum brevis, tendons of insertion

Plantar interossei

Plantar metatarsal arteries

Deep plantar arch

Lateral plantar nerve, deep branch

Quadratus plantae

Lateral plantar artery and vein

Lateral plantar nerve

Flexor digitorum brevis

Flexor digitorum longus, tendons of insertion

Lumbricals

Transverse head

Oblique head

⎫ Adductor hallucis ⎬

Flexor hallucis brevis

Medial plantar artery, deep branch

Flexor hallucis longus, tendon of insertion

Medial plantar artery

Medial plantar nerve

Abductor hallucis

Plantar aponeurosis

D The plantar arteries and nerves of the foot (deep layer)

Right foot, plantar view. The plantar aponeurosis, flexor digitorum brevis, the tendons of flexor digitorum longus, and the oblique head of adductor hallucis have been removed to demonstrate the deep plantar arch and the deep branch of the lateral plantar nerve.

Note: The superficial branch of the lateral plantar nerve and the lateral plantar artery course in the *lateral plantar sulcus* while the superficial branches of the medial plantar nerve and medial plantar artery course in the *medial plantar sulcus* (see **A**). The superficial branches of the medial and lateral plantar arteries help to supply the critically important pressure-chamber system in the sole of the foot (see p. 418).

E Overview of the plantar arteries of the foot

Right foot, plantar view.

The *deep plantar arch* is an arterial arcade in the sole of the foot that is formed by the deep plantar branch of the *dorsal pedal artery* and also by the deep branch of the *lateral plantar artery*. Often these two arteries that supply the deep plantar arch differ in size and thus make different contributions to the first through fourth plantar metatarsal arteries that consistently branch from the deep plantar arch (see **C**).

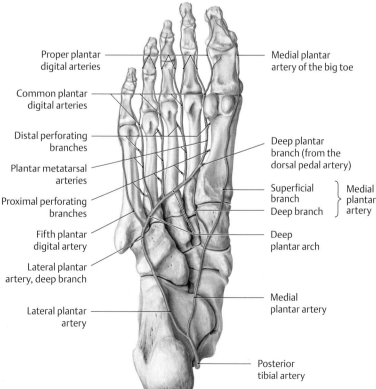

Proper plantar digital arteries

Common plantar digital arteries

Distal perforating branches

Plantar metatarsal arteries

Proximal perforating branches

Fifth plantar digital artery

Lateral plantar artery, deep branch

Lateral plantar artery

Medial plantar artery of the big toe

Deep plantar branch (from the dorsal pedal artery)

Superficial branch

Deep branch

⎫ Medial plantar artery ⎬

Deep plantar arch

Medial plantar artery

Posterior tibial artery

505

5.12 The Anterior Leg Region and Dorsum of the Foot: Cutaneous Innervation

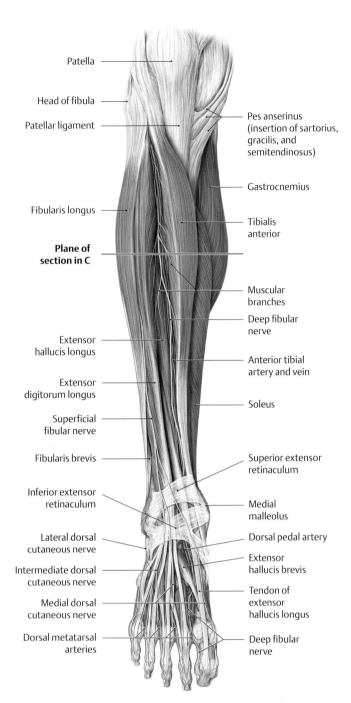

A The neurovascular structures of the anterior compartment and dorsum of the foot

Right leg with the foot in plantar flexion, anterior view. The skin, subcutaneous tissue, and fasciae have been removed and the tibialis anterior and extensor hallucis longus muscles have been retracted to demonstrate the anterior tibial vessels (= anterior tibial artery and vein). The *anterior tibial artery* crosses beneath the tendon of extensor hallucis longus at the junction of the leg with the dorsum of the foot. Below the extensor retinaculum it becomes the *dorsal pedal artery*, which runs lateral to the hallucis longus tendon on the dorsum of the foot, accompanied by the terminal branch of the *deep fibular nerve* (the site for taking the pedal pulse is shown in **E**). The *deep fibular nerve* may be compressed in its passage beneath the inferior extensor retinaculum (with sensory disturbances affecting the first and second toes).

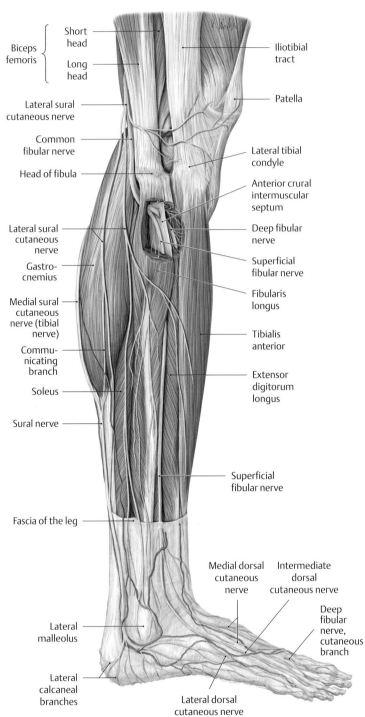

B Division of the common fibular nerve into the deep and superficial fibular nerves

Right leg, lateral view. The origins of the fibularis longus and extensor digitorum longus have been excised below the head of the fibula and the lateral tibial condyle. After the *common fibular nerve* bifurcates in the proximal part of the lateral compartment, the *superficial fibular nerve* remains in the lateral compartment. The *deep fibular nerve* pierces the anterior intermuscular septum and descends with the anterior tibial vessels in the extensor compartment (**C** gives a sectional view of the compartments in the leg).

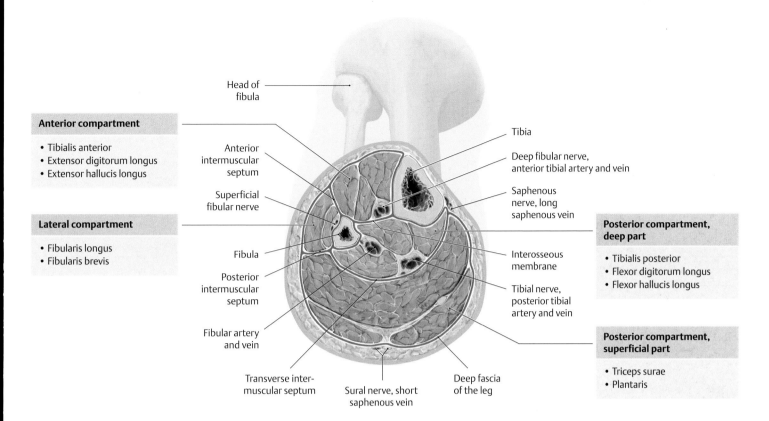

Anterior compartment

- Tibialis anterior
- Extensor digitorum longus
- Extensor hallucis longus

Lateral compartment

- Fibularis longus
- Fibularis brevis

Posterior compartment, deep part

- Tibialis posterior
- Flexor digitorum longus
- Flexor hallucis longus

Posterior compartment, superficial part

- Triceps surae
- Plantaris

Head of fibula

Anterior intermuscular septum

Superficial fibular nerve

Fibula

Posterior intermuscular septum

Fibular artery and vein

Transverse inter- muscular septum

Sural nerve, short saphenous vein

Tibia

Deep fibular nerve, anterior tibial artery and vein

Saphenous nerve, long saphenous vein

Interosseous membrane

Tibial nerve, posterior tibial artery and vein

Deep fascia of the leg

C The compartments and neurovascular structures in the leg
Cross section through a right leg one handwidth below the neck of the fibula, distal view (the level of the section is shown in **A**). The intermuscular septa and interosseous membrane, together with the superficial and deep layers of the fascia of the leg, define the boundaries of four distinct, poorly distensible fibro-osseous compartments in which the neurovascular structures descend through the leg. A rise in tissue pressure, which may result from conditions such as muscular edema or a fracture hematoma, can lead to neurovascular compression, inducing a local ischemia that can cause irreversible neuromuscular damage within a few hours (compartment syndromes such as the tibialis anterior syn-

drome). At greatest risk are the neurovascular structures of the deep posterior compartment (the posterior tibial artery and veins and the tibial nerve) and the anterior compartment (the anterior tibial artery and veins and the deep fibular nerve). Tibialis anterior syndrome is characterized in its acute stage by severe pain and an inability to dorsiflex the toes due to the unopposed action of the plantar flexors. This causes the toes to "claw up." Generally the only effective treatment option at this stage is emergency incision of the fascia of the leg. This immediately decompresses the compartment and relieves the pressure on the vessels that supply the muscles.

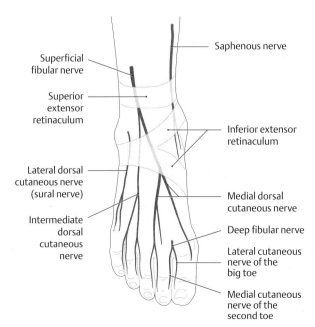

Saphenous nerve

Superficial fibular nerve

Superior extensor retinaculum

Inferior extensor retinaculum

Lateral dorsal cutaneous nerve (sural nerve)

Intermediate dorsal cutaneous nerve

Medial dorsal cutaneous nerve

Deep fibular nerve

Lateral cutaneous nerve of the big toe

Medial cutaneous nerve of the second toe

D The cutaneous nerves on the dorsum of the foot
Right foot, dorsal view.

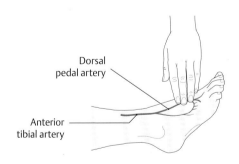

Dorsal pedal artery

Anterior tibial artery

E Palpation of the pedal pulse
The dorsal pedal artery is palpable on the dorsum of the foot, just lateral to the extensor hallucis longus tendon. In addition to determining regional skin temperature, checking the pedal pulse is an important step in the examination of patients with suspected lower limb arterial disease (one foot is markedly colder or paler than the other due to diminished blood flow). It is generally best to begin by palpating the femoral artery at the groin crease, then proceed distally to the popliteal fossa (popliteal artery), the medial malleolus (posterior tibial artery), and finally to the dorsum of the foot (dorsal pedal artery, which is the terminal branch of the anterior tibial artery). The palpable pulses should always be compared between the right and left sides. It should be noted that the pedal pulses may be difficult or impossible to palpate when peripheral edema is present, and so it is best to examine the supine patient.

5.13 The Arteries of the Dorsum of the Foot

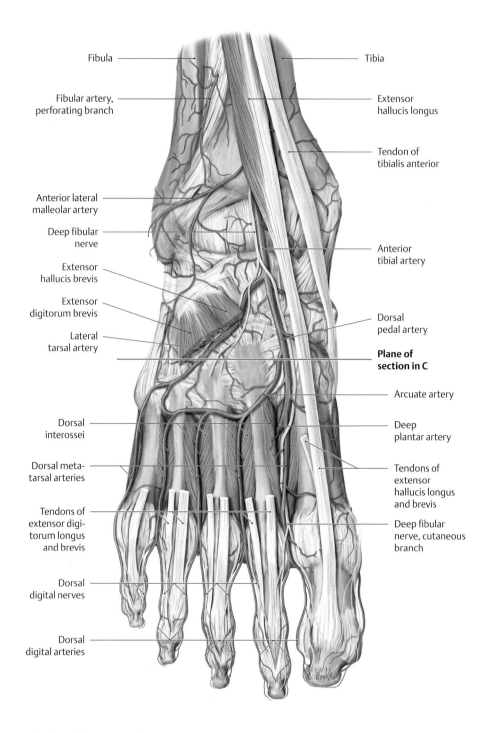

Fibula

Fibular artery, perforating branch

Anterior lateral malleolar artery

Deep fibular nerve

Extensor hallucis brevis

Extensor digitorum brevis

Lateral tarsal artery

Dorsal interossei

Dorsal meta-tarsal arteries

Tendons of extensor digitorum longus and brevis

Dorsal digital nerves

Dorsal digital arteries

Tibia

Extensor hallucis longus

Tendon of tibialis anterior

Anterior tibial artery

Dorsal pedal artery

Plane of section in C

Arcuate artery

Deep plantar artery

Tendons of extensor hallucis longus and brevis

Deep fibular nerve, cutaneous branch

A The dorsal arteries and nerves of the foot

Right foot in plantar flexion, dorsal view. The skin, subcutaneous tissue, and superficial and deep layers of the dorsal pedal fascia have been removed for clarity, along with the extensor digitorum longus tendons and the extensor digitorum brevis and extensor hallucis brevis muscles. Possible variants of the arteries are shown in **D**.

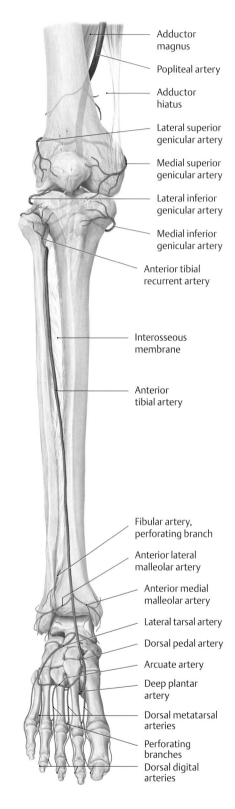

Adductor magnus

Popliteal artery

Adductor hiatus

Lateral superior genicular artery

Medial superior genicular artery

Lateral inferior genicular artery

Medial inferior genicular artery

Anterior tibial recurrent artery

Interosseous membrane

Anterior tibial artery

Fibular artery, perforating branch

Anterior lateral malleolar artery

Anterior medial malleolar artery

Lateral tarsal artery

Dorsal pedal artery

Arcuate artery

Deep plantar artery

Dorsal metatarsal arteries

Perforating branches

Dorsal digital arteries

B The arteries of the leg and foot

Right lower limb, anterior view.

Note: The dorsum of the foot is supplied mainly by branches of the anterior tibial artery.

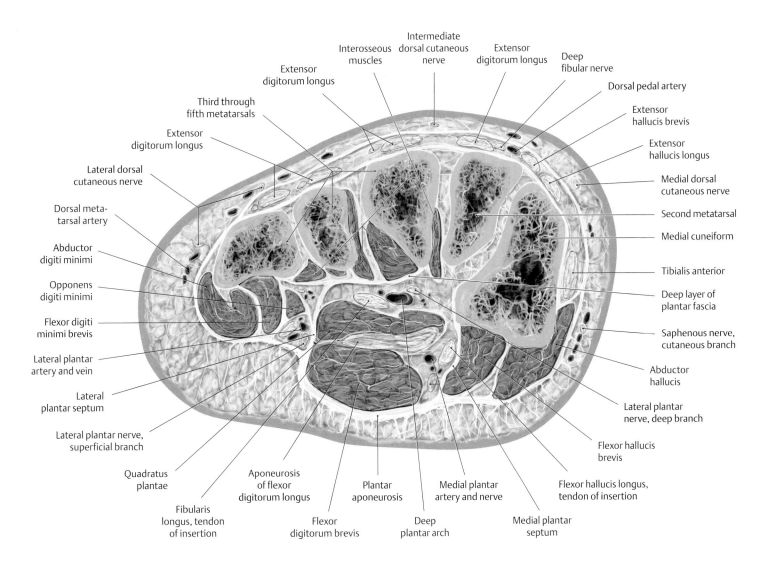

Intermediate
Interosseous — dorsal cutaneous — Extensor
muscles — nerve — digitorum longus — Deep
Extensor — fibular nerve
digitorum longus — Dorsal pedal artery
Third through — Extensor
fifth metatarsals — hallucis brevis
Extensor — Extensor
digitorum longus — hallucis longus
Lateral dorsal — Medial dorsal
cutaneous nerve — cutaneous nerve
Dorsal meta- — Second metatarsal
tarsal artery — Medial cuneiform
Abductor — Tibialis anterior
digiti minimi
Opponens — Deep layer of
digiti minimi — plantar fascia
Flexor digiti — Saphenous nerve,
minimi brevis — cutaneous branch
Lateral plantar — Abductor
artery and vein — hallucis
Lateral — Lateral plantar
plantar septum — nerve, deep branch
Lateral plantar nerve, — Flexor hallucis
superficial branch — brevis
Quadratus — Aponeurosis — Medial plantar — Flexor hallucis longus,
plantae — of flexor — Plantar — artery and nerve — tendon of insertion
digitorum longus — aponeurosis
Fibularis — Flexor — Deep — Medial plantar
longus, tendon — digitorum brevis — plantar arch — septum
of insertion

C The neurovascular structures in the sole of the foot
Cross section through the right foot at the level of the medial cuneiform bone (the location of the section is shown in **A**), distal view (after Rauber and Kopsch).

Note the deep layer of the plantar fascia, in which the deep neurovascular structures of the sole (the deep plantar arch and deep branch of the lateral plantar nerve) are embedded in connective tissue which cushions and protects them (for the arrangement of the pedal compartments, see p. 463).

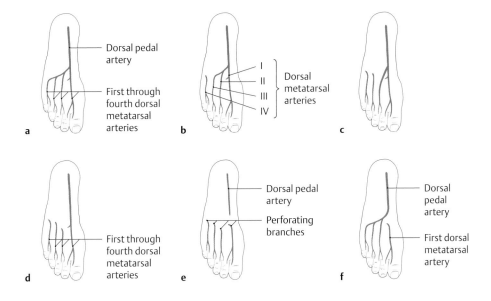

a — Dorsal pedal artery / First through fourth dorsal metatarsal arteries

b — I, II, III, IV Dorsal metatarsal arteries

c

d — First through fourth dorsal metatarsal arteries

e — Dorsal pedal artery / Perforating branches

f — Dorsal pedal artery / First dorsal metatarsal artery

D Variants in the dorsal arterial supply of the foot (after Lippert and Pabst)
a All of the dorsal metatarsal arteries arise from the dorsal pedal artery (20 % of cases).
b The fourth dorsal metatarsal artery is supplied by a perforating branch from the plantar side of the foot (6 % of cases).
c The third and fourth dorsal metatarsal arteries are supplied by perforating branches from the plantar metatarsal arteries (5 % of cases).
d The first dorsal metatarsal artery is the only branch of the dorsal pedal artery (40 % of cases).
e All of the dorsal metatarsal arteries are supplied by perforating branches from the plantar metatarsal arteries (10 %).
f Only the first dorsal metatarsal artery is supplied by a perforating branch (5 %).

Appendix

References

Bähr, M., M. Frotscher: Duus' Neurologisch-topische Diagnostik, 8th ed. Thieme, Stuttgart 2003

Baumgartl, F.: Das Kniegelenk. Springer, Berlin 1969

Chassard, J., C. Lapiné: Étude radiologique de l'arcade pubienne chez la femme enceinte. J Radiol Electrol 7 (1923), 113

Christ, B., F. Wachtler: Medizinische Embryologie. Ullstein Medical, Wiesbaden 1998

Debrunner, A. M.: Orthopädie. Die Störungen des Bewegungsapparates in Klinik und Praxis, 2nd ed. Hans Huber, Stuttgart 1985

Debrunner, H. U.: Gelenkmessung (Neutral-O-Methode), Längenmessung, Umfangmessung. AO-Bulletin, Bern 1971

Drews, U.: Color Atlas of Embryology. Thieme, Stuttgart 1996

Faller, A.: Anatomie in Stichworten. Enke, Stuttgart 1980

Feneis, H., W. Dauber: Anatomisches Bildwörterbuch, 8th ed. Thieme, Stuttgart 1999

Ficat, P.: Pathologie Fémoro-Patellaire. Masson, Paris 1970

Földi, M., S. Kubik: Lehrbuch der Lymphologie. G. Fischer, Stuttgart 1993

Frick, H., H. Leonhardt, D. Starck: Allgemeine und spezielle Anatomie. Taschenlehrbuch der gesamten Anatomie, Vols 1 and 2, 4th ed. Thieme, Stuttgart 1992

Fritsch, H., W. Kühnel: Taschenatlas der Anatomie, Vol 2, Thieme, Stuttgart 2001

Goerke, K.: Taschenatlas der Geburtshilfe. Thieme, Stuttgart 2002

Grants Anatomie: Lehrbuch und Atlas (A. M. R. Agur), Enke, Stuttgart 1999

Hansen, K., K. Schliack: Segmentale Innervation, 2nd ed. Thieme, Stuttgart 1962

Hees, H.: Grundriss und Atlas der Mikroskopischen Anatomie des Menschen, Vol 1: Zytologie und Allgemeine Histologie, 12th ed. Gustav Fischer, Stuttgart 1996

Henne-Bruns, D., M. Dürig, B. Kremer: Chirurgie, 2nd ed. Thieme, Stuttgart 2003

Hepp, W. R.: Radiologie des Femoro-Patellargelenkes. Bücherei des Orthopäden, Vol 37, Enke, Stuttgart 1983

Hilgenreiner, H.: Zur Frühdiagnose der angeborenen Hüftgelenksverrenkung. Med Klein. 21, 1925, Hippokrates, Stuttgart 1981

Hochschild, J.: Strukturen und Funktionen begreifen, Vols 1 and 2, Thieme, Stuttgart 1998 und 2002

Hüter-Becker, A., H. Schewe, W. Heipertz: Physiotherapie Vol 1: Biomechanik, Arbeitsmedizin, Ergonomie. Thieme, Stuttgart 1999

Junghanns, H.: Die funktionelle Pathologie der Zwischenwirbelscheibe als Grundlage für klinische Betrachtungen. Langenbecks Arch. Klin. Chir. 267 (1951), 393–417

Kahle, W., M. Frotscher: Color Atlas and Textbook of Human Anatomy, Vol 3, Thieme, Stuttgart 2003

Kapandji, I. A.: Funktionelle Anatomie der Gelenke, Vols 1–3, 2nd ed. Enke, Stuttgart 1992

Kaufmann, P.: Reife Plazenta. In: Becker, V., T. H. Schiebler, F. Kubli (eds.): Die Plazenta des Menschen. Thieme, Stuttgart 1981

Klinke, R., S. Silbernagl: Lehrbuch der Physiologie, 3rd ed. Thieme, Stuttgart 2001

Koebke, J.: Anatomie des Handgelenkes und der Handwurzel, Unfallchirurgie 14 (1988), 74–79

Kristic, R. V.: General Histology of the Mammals. Springer, Berlin 1985

Kubik, S.: Lymphsystem der oberen Extremität. In: Lehrbuch der Lymphologie für Mediziner und Physiotherapeuten (eds: M. Földi and S. Kubik), G. Fischer, Stuttgart 1989

Kummer, B.: Biomechanik der Wirbelgelenke. In: Meinicke, F.-W.: Die Wibelbogengelenke. Hippokrates, Stuttgart 1983

Lehnert, G.: Dopplersonographische Diagnostik der erektilen Dysfunktion unter Anwendung des Papaverintests, Dissertation, University of Kiel (Medical Faculty) 1995

Lelièvre, J.: Pathologie du Pied, 2nd ed. Masson, Paris 1961

Lippert, H., R. Pabst: Arterial Variations in Man. Bergmann, Munich 1985

Loeweneck, H.: Diagnostische Anatomie. Springer, Berlin 1981

Lüllmann-Rauch, R.: Histologie. Thieme, Stuttgart 2003

Lundborg, G., R. Myrhage, B. Rydevik: The vascularization of human flexor tendons within the digital synovial sheath region – structural and functional aspects. J. Hand Surg. 2 (1977), 417–427

Luschka, H.: Die Halbgelenke des menschlichen Körpers. Reiner, Berlin 1858

Masuhr, K. F., M. Neumann: Neurologie (Duale Reihe), 4th ed. Hippokrates, Stuttgart 1998

Möller, T. B., E. Reif: Taschenatlas der Röntgenanatomie, 2nd ed. Thieme, Stuttgart 1998

Mubarak, S. J., A. R. Hargens: Compartment Syndromes and Volkamn's Contracture, W. B. Sanders, Philadelphia 1981

Mumenthaler, M., M. Stöhr, H. Müller-Vahl: Läsion peripherer Nerven und radikuläre Syndrome, 8th ed. Thieme, Stuttgart 2003

Netter, F. H.: Farbatlanten der Medizin. Thieme, Stuttgart

Niethard, F. U., J. Pfeil: Orthopädie (Duale Reihe), 3rd ed. Hippokrates, Stuttgart 1997

Niethard, F. U.: Kinderorthopädie. Thieme, Stuttgart 1997

O'Rahilly, R., F. Müller: Developmental Stages in Human Embryos. Carnegie Institution of Washington, Publication 637 (1987)

Pauwels, F.: Eine neue Theorie über den Einfluss mechanischer Reize auf die Differenzierung der Stützgewebe (X). Beitrag zur funktionellen Anatomie und kausalen Morphologie des Stützapparates. Z. Anat. Entwickl.-Gesch. 121 (1968), 478–515

Petersen, W., B. Tillmann: Z. Orthop. 137 (1999), 31–37

Pette, D., R. S. Staron: Transitions of muscle fiber phenotypic profiles. Histochem Cell Biol 115 (5) (2001), 359–379

Platzer, W.: Color Atlas and Textbook of Human Anatomy, Vol 1, Thieme, Stuttgart 2004

Platzer, W.: Atlas der topographischen Anatomie. Thieme, Stuttgart 1982

Rauber/Kopsch: Anatomie des Menschen, Vols 1–4, Thieme, Stuttgart. Vol 1, 2nd ed.: 1997, Vols 2 and 3: 1987, Vol 4: 1988

Rohen, J. W.: Topographische Anatomie, 10th ed. Schattauer, Stuttgart 2000

Rohen, J. W., C. Yokochi, E. Lütjen-Drecoll: Anatomie des Menschen, 4th ed. Schattauer, Stuttgart 2000

Romer, A. S., T. S. Parson: Vergleichende Anatomie der Wirbeltiere, 5th ed. Paul Parey, Hamburg und Berlin 1983

513

Sadler, T. W.: Medizinische Embryologie, 10th ed. Thieme, Stuttgart 2003

Scheldrup, E. W.: Tendon sheath patterns in the hand. Surg. Gynec. Obestetr. 93 (1951), 16–22

Schmidt, H. M., U. Lanz: Chirurgische Anatomie der Hand, 2nd ed. Thieme, Stuttgart 2003

Schumpelick, V.: Hernien, 4th ed. Thieme, Stuttgart 2000

Schünke, M.: Funktionelle Anatomie – Topographie und Funktion des Bewegungssystems. Thieme, Stuttgart 2000

Silbernagl, S., A. Despopoulos, Taschenatlas der Physiologie, 6th ed. Thieme, Stuttgart 2003

Sökeland, J., H. Schulze, H. Rübben: Urologie, 12th ed. Thieme, Stuttgart 2002

Starck, D.: Embryologie, 3rd ed. Thieme, Stuttgart 1975

Streeter, G. L.: Developmental horizons in human embryos: age group XI, 13–20 somites and age group XII, 21–29 somites. Contrib Embryol 30 (1942), 211

Vahlensieck, M., M. Reiser (eds): MRT des Bewegungsapparates, 2nd revised and expanded ed. Thieme, Stuttgart 2001

von Hochstetter, A., H. K. von Rechenberg, R. Schmidt: Die intragluteale Injektion, Thieme, Stuttgart 1958

von Lanz, T., W. Wachsmuth: Praktische Anatomie, Vol 1/3, Arm, 2nd ed. Springer, Berlin 1959

von Lanz, T., W. Wachsmuth: Praktische Anatomie, Vol 1/4, Bein und Statik, Springer, Berlin 1972

Weber, U.: Orthopädische Mikrochirurgie (eds. Weber, Greulich, Sparmann), Thieme, Stuttgart 1993

Wiberg, G.: Roentgenographic and anatomic studies on the femoropatellar joint. With special reference to chondromalacia patellae. Acta Orthop Scand 12 (1941), 319–410

Wiberg, G.: Studies on dysplastic acetabulum and congenital subluxation of the hip joint with special reference of the complication of osteoarthritis. Acta Chir Scand. 83 (suppl), 1939, 58

Wolpert, L., R. Beddington, J. Brockes, T. Jessel, P. Lawrence, E. Meyerowitz: Entwicklungsbiologie. Spektrum Verlag, Weinheim 1999

Index